Emergency General Surgery

Carlos V. R. Brown • Kenji Inaba
Matthew J. Martin • Ali Salim
Editors

Emergency General Surgery

A Practical Approach

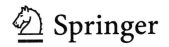
Springer

Editors
Carlos V. R. Brown
Dell Medical School
University of Texas at Austin
Austin, TX
USA

Matthew J. Martin
Madigan Army Medical Center
Tacoma, WA
USA

Kenji Inaba
Trauma and Surgical Critical Care
University of Southern California
Los Angeles, CA
USA

Ali Salim
Brigham and Womens's Hospital
Harvard Medical School
Boston, MA
USA

ISBN 978-3-319-96285-6   ISBN 978-3-319-96286-3   (eBook)
https://doi.org/10.1007/978-3-319-96286-3

Library of Congress Control Number: 2018957607

This Springer imprint is published by the registered company Springer Nature Switzerland AG
The registered company address is: Gewerbestrasse 11, 6330 Cham, Switzerland

Preface

The field of emergency general surgery encompasses a wide array of surgical diseases, ranging from the simple to the complex. Emergency general surgeons are tasked with caring for patients with emergent surgical diseases emanating from the emergency department or inpatient consultations. These diseases range from inflammatory, infectious, and hemorrhagic diseases spanning the entire gastrointestinal tract, complications of abdominal wall hernias, compartment syndromes, skin and soft tissue infections, and surgical diseases significantly complicated in special populations including elderly, obese, pregnant, immunocompromised, and cirrhotic patients.

The *Emergency General Surgery* textbook is a real-time and at-the-fingertip resource for surgeons and surgery residents, providing a practical and evidence-based approach to diagnosing and managing the wide array of surgical diseases encountered on emergency general surgery call. The chapters in this new and cutting-edge textbook are written by leading experts in the field and are filled with pearls of wisdom from surgeons with decades of experience taking emergency general surgery call. This compilation of thorough and cutting-edge content also serves as an excellent review for residency in-service exams, qualifying and certifying board exams, as well as up-to-date information for continuous certification in general surgery.

We wish to thank the professional editorial efforts of Springer and to acknowledge our peers, coworkers, friends, and family for their support throughout this project. Without the help of so many, this project could not have been brought to fruition.

Austin, TX, USA   Carlos V. R. Brown
Los Angeles, CA, USA   Kenji Inaba
Tacoma, WA, USA   Matthew J. Martin
Boston, MA, USA   Ali Salim

Contents

Contributors

Hasan B. Alam, MD Department of Surgery, University of Michigan Hospital, Ann Arbor, MI, USA

Essa M. Aleassa, MD, MSc, FRCSC Department of Surgery, Cleveland Clinic, Cleveland, OH, USA

Jared L. Antevil Cardiothoracic Surgery Service, Department of Surgery, Uniformed Services University of the Health Sciences and the Walter Reed National Military Medical Center, Bethesda, MD, USA

Reza Askari, MD Department of Surgery, Brigham and Women's Hospital, Harvard Medical School, Boston, MA, USA

Brittany Bankhead-Kendall, MD, MS Department of Surgery and Perioperative Care, University of Texas at Austin, Dell Medical School, Austin, Texas, USA

Andrew C. Bernard, MD Section of Trauma and Acute Care Surgery, Department of Surgery, University of Kentucky College of Medicine, UK Healthcare, Lexington, KY, USA

Anuradha R. Bhama, MD Department of Colorectal Surgery, Cleveland Clinic Foundation, Cleveland, OH, USA

Ben E. Biesterveld, MD Department of Surgery, Section of General Surgery, University of Michigan Hospital, Ann Arbor, MI, USA

Col (Ret) Mark W. Bowyer, MD, FACS, DMCC Uniformed Services University of the Health Sciences, Bethesda, MD, USA

Karen J. Brasel, MD, MPH Department of Surgery, Oregon Health and Science University, Portland, OR, USA

Stacy Brethauer, MD, FACS Department of Surgery, Cleveland Clinic, Cleveland, OH, USA

Alexandra Brito, MD Department of Surgery, UC San Diego Medical Center, San Diego, CA, USA

Carlos V. R. Brown, MD Department of Surgery and Perioperative Care, Dell Medical School at The University of Texas Austin, Dell Seton Medical Center at The University of Texas, Austin, TX, USA

Ronald Buczek, DO Department of Surgery, University of Utah, Salt Lake City, UT, USA

Milos Buhavac, MBBS, MA Department of Surgery, University of Utah School of Medicine, University of Utah, Salt Lake City, UT, USA

Marko Bukur, MD Department of Surgery, NYU Langone Medical Center, New York, NY, USA

Clay Cothren Burlew, MD FACS Department of Surgery, Denver Health Medical Center/University of Colorado, Denver, CO, USA

Andre R. Campbell, MD Department of Surgery, University of California San Francisco, San Francisco, CA, USA

Eric M. Campion, MD FACS Department of Surgery, Denver Health Medical Center/University of Colorado, Denver, CO, USA

Michael C. Chang, MD Department of Surgery, University of South Alabama School of Medicine, Mobile, AL, USA

C. Yvonne Chung, MD, MPH Department of Surgery and Perioperative Care, Dell Medical School at The University of Texas Austin Dell Seton Medical Center at The University of Texas, Austin, TX, USA

Jaclyn Clark, MD Department of Surgery, NYU Langone Medical Center, New York, NY, USA

K. Conley Coleman, DO Department of Surgery, West Virginia University, Morgantown, WV, USA

Marie L. Crandall, MD University of Florida, Jacksonville, FL, USA

Mitchell J. Daley, PharmD, FCCM, BCPS Department of Pharmacy, Dell Seton Medical Center at the University of Texas, Austin, TX, USA

Kimberly A. Davis, M.D., MBA, FACS, FCCM Department of Surgery, Yale School of Medicine, New Haven, CT, USA

Marc de Moya, MD FACS Division of Trauma/Acute Care Surgery, Medical College of Wisconsin-Froedtert Trauma Center, Milwaukee, WI, USA

Molly R. Deane, MD Department of Surgery, Harbor-UCLA Medical Center, Torrance, CA, USA

Paul J. Deramo, MD Methodist Dallas Medical Center, Dallas, TX, USA

Chris Dodgion, MD, MSPH, MBA, FACS Division of Trauma/Acute Care Surgery, Medical College of Wisconsin-Froedtert Trauma Center, Milwaukee, WI, USA

Joseph J. DuBose, MD Department of Surgery, University of Maryland School of Medicine, Baltimore, MD, USA

Paula Ferrada, MD FACS VCU Surgery Trauma, Critical Care and Emergency Surgery, Richmond, VA, USA

W. Drew Fielder, MD, FACS University of Texas at Austin, Dell Medical School, Austin, TX, USA

Elisa Furay, MD University of Texas at Austin, Dell Medical School, Austin, TX, USA

Stephen C. Gale, MD East Texas Medical Center, Tyler, TX, USA

Mathew Giangola, MD Trauma, Burn and Critical Care Surgery, Brigham and Women's Hospital, Boston, MA, USA

Daniel Grabo, MD, FACS Department of Surgery, West Virginia University, Morgantown, WV, USA

Mohammad Hamidi, MD Division of Trauma, Critical Care, Burns & Emergency Surgery, Department of Surgery, Banner – University Medical Center Tucson, Tucson, AZ, USA

Joaquim M. Havens, MD Department of Surgery, Brigham and Women's Hospital, Boston, MA, USA

Sameer A. Hirji, MD Department of Surgery, Brigham and Women's Hospital, Harvard Medical School, Boston, MA, USA

Emily K. Hodge, PharmD, BCCCP Department of Pharmacy, Dell Seton Medical Center at the University of Texas, Austin, TX, USA

Franchesca Hwang, MD Department of Surgery, Rutgers New Jersey Medical School, Newark, NJ, USA

Dirk C. Johnson, MD, FACS Department of General Surgery, Trauma and Acute Medical Care, Yale University, New Haven, CT, USA

Bellal Joseph, MD Division of Trauma, Critical Care, Burns & Emergency Surgery, Department of Surgery, Banner – University Medical Center Tucson, Tucson, AZ, USA

Lillian S. Kao, MD, MS Department of Surgery, McGovern Medical School at the University of Texas Health Science Center at Houston, Houston, TX, USA

Katherine A. Kelley, MD Department of Surgery, Oregon Health and Sciences University, Portland, OR, USA

Anthony W. Kim, MD Division of Thoracic Surgery, Keck University School of Medicine of the University of Southern California, Los Angeles, CA, USA

Dennis Y. Kim, MD Department of Surgery, Harbor-UCLA Medical Center, Torrance, CA, USA

Leslie Kobayashi, MD, FACS Department of Surgery, Division of Trauma, Surgical Critical Care, Acute Care Surgery and Burns, UC San Diego Medical Center, San Diego, CA, USA

Anastasia Kunac, MD FACS Department of Surgery, Rutgers New Jersey Medical School, Newark, NJ, USA

Sang W. Lee, MD, FACS, FASCRS Department of Colon & Rectal Surgery, University of Southern California, Keck School of Medicine, Los Angeles, CA, USA

Meghan Lewis, MD FACS Division of Trauma and Surgical Critical Care, LAC+USC Medical Center, University of Southern California, Los Angeles, CA, USA

Eric J. Ley, MD Department of Surgery, Cedars Sinai Medical Center, Los Angeles, CA, USA

Kazuhide Matsushima, MD Division of Trauma and Surgical Critical Care, LAC+USC Medical Center, Los Angeles, CA, USA

Emily Miraflor, MD Department of Surgery, UCSF-East Bay Surgery Program, Oakland, CA, USA

John D. Mitchell, MD Division of Cardiothoracic Surgery, University of Colorado School of Medicine, Aurora, CO, USA

Amirreza T. Motameni, MD The Hiram C. Polk Jr. Department of Surgery, University of Louisville School of Medicine, Louisville, KY, USA

Philip S. Mullenix Cardiothoracic Surgery Service, Department of Surgery, Uniformed Services University of the Health Sciences and the Walter Reed National Military Medical Center, Bethesda, MD, USA

Ram Nirula, MD Department of Surgery, University of Utah School of Medicine, University of Utah, Salt Lake City, UT, USA

Andrew M. Nunn, MD Department of Surgery, Wake Forest School of Medicine, Winston Salem, NC, USA

Rebecca E. Plevin, MD Department of Surgery, Zuckerberg San Francisco General Hospital, University of California San Francisco, San Francisco, CA, USA

Jessica K. Reynolds, MD Section of Trauma and Acute Care Surgery, Department of Surgery, University of Kentucky College of Medicine, UK Healthcare, Lexington, KY, USA

Erik Q. Roedel, MD, FACS Department of Surgery, Tripler Army Medical Center, Honolulu, HI, USA

Dusten T. Rose, PharmD, BCPS (AQ-ID), AAHIVP Department of Pharmacy, Dell Seton Medical Center at the University of Texas, Austin, TX, USA

Jack A. Sava, MD Department of General Surgery, Trauma Service, Washington Hospital Center, Washington, DC, USA

John Saydi, MD Michael E. DeBakey Department of Surgery, Baylor College of Medicine, Houston, TX, USA

Morgan Schellenberg, MD MPH Division of Trauma and Surgical Critical Care, LAC+USC Medical Center, Los Angeles, CA, USA

Andrew T. Schlussel, DO, FACS Department of Surgery, Madigan Army Medical Center, Tacoma, WA, USA

Martin A. Schreiber, MD Department of Surgery, Division of Trauma, Critical Care & Acute Care Surgery, Oregon Health & Science University, Portland, OR, USA

Kevin M. Schuster, MD Yale University, New Haven, CT, USA

Shahid Shafi, MD Baylor Scott and White Health System, Dallas, TX, USA

Meryl A. Simon, MD USAF, MC, David Grant USAF Medical Center; University of California Davis Medical Center, Division of Vascular and Endovascular Surgery, Sacramento, CA, USA

Jason W. Smith, MD PhD, FACS The Hiram C. Polk Jr. Department of Surgery, University of Louisville School of Medicine, Louisville, KY, USA

Sawyer Smith, MD Department of Surgery, Oregon Health and Sciences University, Portland, OR, USA

Steven C. Stain, MD, FACS Department of Surgery, Albany Medical College, Albany, NY, USA

Scott R. Steele, MD Department of Colorectal Surgery, Cleveland Clinic, Cleveland, OH, USA

Marcel Tafen, MD, FACS Department of Surgery, Albany Medical College, Albany, NY, USA

Sharven Taghavi, MD Department of Surgery, Brigham and Women's Hospital, Harvard Medical School, Boston, MA, USA

James M. Tatum, MD Department of Surgery, Cedars Sinai Medical Center, Los Angeles, CA, USA

Pedro G. R. Teixeira, MD, FACS Department of Surgery and Perioperative Care, University of Texas at Austin, Dell Medical School, Austin, TX, USA

Shawn Tejiram, MD General Surgery, Medstar Washington Hospital, Washington, DC, USA

S. Rob Todd, MD, FACS Michael E. DeBakey Department of Surgery, Baylor College of Medicine, Houston, TX, USA

Shirin Towfigh, MD FACS Beverly Hills Hernia Center, Beverly Hills, CA, USA

Michael S. Truitt, MD Department of Surgery, Methodist Dallas Medical Center, Dallas, TX, USA

Marc D. Trust, MD Department of Surgery and Perioperative Care, Dell Medical School at The University of Texas Austin, Dell Seton Medical Center at The University of Texas, Austin, TX, USA

Aela P. Vely, MD Division of Acute Care Surgical Services, Virginia Commonwealth University, Richmond, VA, USA

Neil Venardos, MD Division of Cardiothoracic Surgery, University of Colorado School of Medicine, Aurora, CO, USA

Gregory Victorino, MD UCSF Medical Center, San Francisco, CA, USA

Shuyan Wei, MD Department of Surgery, McGovern Medical School at the University of Texas Health Science Center at Houston, Houston, TX, USA

Jaye Alexander Weston, MD Division of Thoracic Surgery, Keck University School of Medicine of the University of Southern California, Los Angeles, CA, USA

Carey Wickham, MD Department of Colon & Rectal Surgery, University of Southern California, Keck School of Medicine, Los Angeles, CA, USA

Aaron M. Williams, MD Department of Surgery, Section of General Surgery, University of Michigan Hospital, Ann Arbor, MI, USA

Anna Yegiants Case Western Reserve University School of Medicine, Cleveland, OH, USA

Definition of Emergency General Surgery (EGS) and Its Burden on the Society

Stephen C. Gale, Kevin M. Schuster,
Marie L. Crandall, and Shahid Shafi

Defining Emergency General Surgery (EGS)

The American Association for the Surgery of Trauma (AAST) was the first to develop a formal definition of emergency general surgery (EGS) in 2013 [49]. The EGS patient was conceptually defined as "any patient (inpatient or emergency department) requiring an emergency surgical evaluation (operative or non-operative) for diseases within the realm of general surgery as defined by the American Board of Surgery" [49]. To define the actual scope of EGS practice, data were obtained from seven acute care surgeons in academic practice. Using a Delphi process, a consensus was generated over a list of International Classification of Diseases (ICD 9) diagnostic codes that encompassed EGS (Table 1.1). The list included several major disease categories including resuscitation, general abdominal conditions, upper gastrointestinal tract, hepatic-pancreatic-biliary, colorectal, hernias, soft tissue, vascular, cardiothoracic, and others. It should be noted that these surgeons practiced exclusively in relatively urban academic medical centers where the distribution of cases may be different than more rural or private practice settings. Despite this limitation, this ICD-9 code-based definition has spurred research in EGS, including early outcomes research measuring morbidity, mortality, and costs associated with EGS patients. All large-scale data analytics of EGS as a specialty must be interpreted within the context of how it is defined by ICD-9/10 codes.

At the present time, every acute care hospital with an emergency room and a general surgeon on staff cares for EGS patients. However, it is likely that the scope of EGS practice varies from center to center and from surgeon to surgeon within a center, depending upon local resources and expertise. Not all institutions will have adequate resources for addressing every EGS disease and severity. Hence, we believe that individual hospitals should define their scope of EGS practice, based upon local capabilities and ability to transfer patients to another center for a higher level of care.

S. C. Gale
East Texas Medical Center, Tyler, TX, USA

K. M. Schuster
Yale University, New Haven, CT, USA

M. L. Crandall
University of Florida, Jacksonville, FL, USA

S. Shafi (✉)
Baylor Scott and White Health, Dallas, TX, USA
e-mail: shahid.shafi@bswhealth.org

© Springer International Publishing AG, part of Springer Nature 2019
C. V. R. Brown et al. (eds.), *Emergency General Surgery*, https://doi.org/10.1007/978-3-319-96286-3_1

Table 1.1 Common emergency general surgery diseases

Surgical area	Clinical conditions
Resuscitation	Acute respiratory failure, shock
General abdominal conditions	Abdominal pain, abdominal mass, peritonitis, hemoperitoneum, retroperitoneal abscesses
Intestinal obstruction	Adhesions, incarcerated hernias, cancers, volvulus, intussusceptions
Upper gastrointestinal tract	Upper gastrointestinal bleed, peptic ulcer disease, fistulae, gastrostomy, small intestinal cancers, ileus, Meckel's diverticulum, bowel perforations, appendix
Hepatic-pancreatic-biliary	Gallstones and related diseases, pancreatitis, hepatic abscesses
Colorectal	Lower gastrointestinal bleed, diverticular disease, inflammatory bowel disease, colorectal cancers, colitis, colonic perforations, megacolon, regional enteritis, colostomy/ileostomy, hemorrhoids, perianal and perirectal fistulas and infections, anorectal stenosis, rectal prolapse
Hernias	Inguinal, femoral, umbilical, incisional, ventral, diaphragmatic
Soft tissue	Cellulitis, abscesses, fasciitis, wound care, pressure ulcers, compartment syndrome
Vascular	Ruptured aneurysms, acute intestinal ischemia, acute peripheral ischemia, phlebitis
Cardiothoracic	Cardiac tamponade, empyema, pneumothorax, esophageal perforation
Others	Tracheostomy, foreign bodies, bladder rupture

Source: Shafi et al. [49]

Defining the Anatomic Severity of EGS Disease

EGS patient outcomes are related to the severity of illness, based upon preexisting medical conditions, anatomic severity of disease, and physiologic derangements [39, 41]. However, until recently, there was no unified mechanism for measuring anatomic severity of EGS diseases. Hence, AAST developed a new grading system using a defined framework based upon a combination of clinical, radiographic, endoscopic, operative, and pathologic findings (Table 1.2) [11, 48, 58]. Sixteen disease

Table 1.2 American Association for the Surgery of Trauma anatomic grading system for measuring severity of emergency general surgery diseases

Grade	Description
Grade I	Local disease confined to the organ with minimal abnormality
Grade II	Local disease confined to the organ with severe abnormality
Grade III	Local extension beyond the organ
Grade IV	Regional extension beyond the organ
Grade V	Widespread extension beyond the organ

Source: Shafi et al. [48]

grading schemas were first produced for infectious or inflammatory EGS diseases, including acute appendicitis, breast infections, acute cholecystitis, acute diverticulitis, esophageal perforation, hernias, infectious colitis, small bowel obstruction due to adhesions, bowel ischemia due to arterial insufficiency, acute pancreatitis, pelvic inflammatory disease, perforated peptic ulcer, perineal abscess, pleural space infection, and surgical site infection. These grading scales were developed empirically by consensus experts but have subsequently been validated across several conditions including diverticulitis and appendicitis [20, 50]. Once validated, this anatomic grading system will be a powerful tool for research, quality improvement, and national tracking of emergency general surgical diseases. There are multiple physiologic scoring systems that have been applied to EGS patients [36]. Examples include the Sequential Organ Failure Assessment (SOFA) score, the Acute Physiology and Chronic Health Evaluation (APACHE) score, the American Society of Anesthesiologists Physical Status (ASA-PS), and various forms of the Physiological and Operative Severity Score for the enumeration of Mortality and Morbidity (POSSUM). Disease-specific scores include the Colonic Peritonitis Severity Score, Mannheim Peritonitis Index, and the Boey score for outcome prediction in perforated peptic ulcer disease [5, 7].

Burden of Disease for Emergency General Surgery

Perhaps the most remarkable aspect of EGS is the sheer volume of patients and the burden on the society that these patients represent in terms of level of acuity, manpower needs, and costs of care. Much like the societal burden of trauma care which went unrecognized until the 1980s [46], EGS is now being recognized as one of the major underappreciated public health crises of the twenty-first century [15, 38].

EGS Volume

Using definitions created by the AAST [49], researchers have estimated EGS hospitalizations and described patient demographics, operative needs, and major outcomes [9, 15, 32,

45]. Recent examinations of the Nationwide Inpatient Sample (NIS), the country's largest all-payer hospital database, demonstrate that EGS diseases account for nearly three million inpatient admissions annually (7% of all hospitalizations), at more than 4700 different hospitals in the United States in 2010 [34, 15]. These studies further show that EGS volumes are steadily increasing each year [15]. Nearly 30% of EGS patients required a major surgical procedure during their initial hospital stay (Fig. 1.1). Five EGS diagnostic groups accounted for more than 90% of admissions: hepatobiliary, colorectal including appendix, upper gastrointestinal, soft tissue, and intestinal

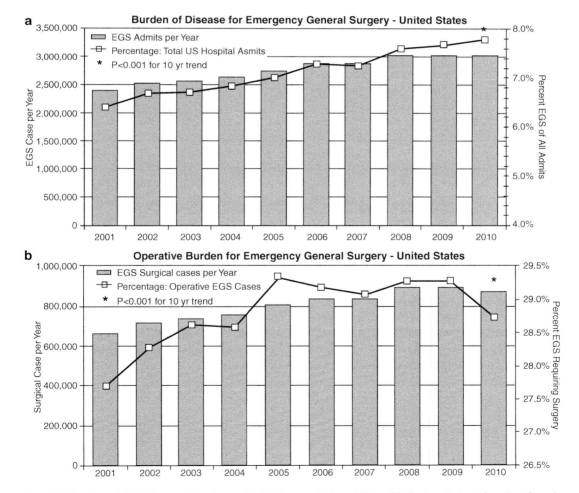

Fig. 1.1 Number of all EGS cases (**a**) and operative EGS cases (**b**) from 2001 to 2010 using National Inpatient Sample data (Source: Gale et al. [15])

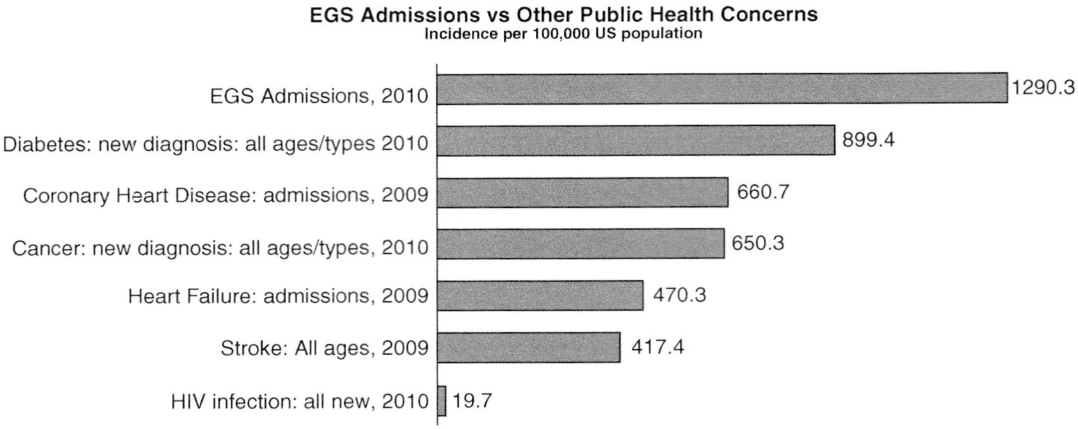

EGS Admissions vs Other Public Health Concerns
Incidence per 100,000 US population

EGS Admissions, 2010	1290.3
Diabetes: new diagnosis: all ages/types 2010	899.4
Coronary Heart Disease: admissions, 2009	660.7
Cancer: new diagnosis: all ages/types, 2010	650.3
Heart Failure: admissions, 2009	470.3
Stroke: All ages, 2009	417.4
HIV infection: all new, 2010	19.7

Fig. 1.2 Burden of EGS admissions compared to other common diseases (Source: Gale et al. [15])

obstruction. Cyclic seasonal variations exist in EGS hospitalizations, similar to trauma, and increase during the summer [60].

As a public health issue, the burden of EGS is very large, and population-based estimates reveal 1290 EGS admissions per 100,000 [15] – higher than many other common public health concerns including new-onset diabetes, heart disease admissions, and new cancer diagnoses, among others (Fig. 1.2).

These findings underestimate the total burden of EGS diseases, as these estimated do not include:

- Patients treated and released from the emergency room and urgent care centers (such as those with biliary colic and reducible hernias, minor soft tissue infections)
- Patients who require elective surgical procedures later in their course (such as colostomy reversal, hernia repair after reduction, delayed colectomy for diverticulitis)

- Patients who develop EGS diseases after being admitted for other conditions (such as intestinal ischemia after cardiovascular surgery, infected decubitus after prolonged mechanical ventilation, acalculous cholecystitis after prolonged parenteral nutrition)

Operative Burden

Operative rates for EGS conditions are consistent across studies at roughly one-third of admitted patients [15, 51, 52]. Further, Scott and colleagues [45] demonstrated that for patients requiring major surgery, more than 80% of procedures fall into only seven groupings: appendectomy, cholecystectomy, lysis of adhesions, colectomy, small bowel resection, hemorrhage control, and laparotomy (Fig. 1.3). These same procedures also account for more than 80% of EGS complications, deaths, and costs (Fig. 1.4) [15, 32, 35, 45].

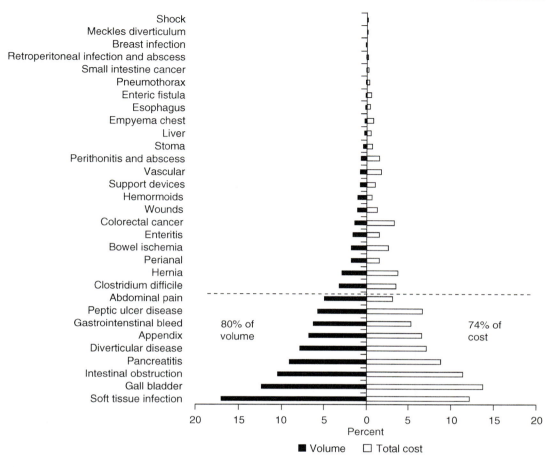

Fig. 1.3 Frequency of common EGS diseases with volume and costs (Source: Ogola and Shafi [35])

Fig. 1.4 Cumulative national burden of emergency general surgery procedures by rank. Each line represents the proportion of cumulative national burden of procedure volume, patient deaths, complications, and costs. The vertical dotted line delineates the top 7 ranked procedures, which accounted for approximately 80% of all cumulative burden. Data were obtained from the National Inpatient Sample for admissions between 2008 and 2011 (Source: Scott et al. [45])

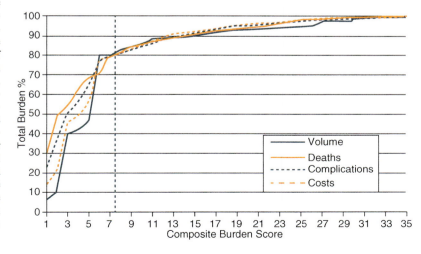

Demographics

Most studies demonstrate a mean age near 60 years for EGS patients [15, 18, 32, 51, 52] with 10% being octogenarians or older [45, 51, 55]. There is a slight female preponderance (53%) and approximately 25% are non-White [49]. Compared to elective general surgery patients, they have higher comorbidity rates [18], and most have at least one major preexisting medical condition [15, 18, 39]. Payer mix varies between studies, but uninsured rates are reported between 8% and 12%, commercial insurers provide roughly 33% of coverage, and government insurance (Medicare or Medicaid) covers the rest – more than 50% of all EGS patients [15, 32, 35, 45, 51].

Outcomes

Patient outcomes vary between EGS conditions and are dependent on multiple factors, such as anatomic severity of diseases, physiologic derangement at presentation [20, 30, 43, 50], age [40, 51, 52, 54, 55], need for and type of surgery [45], and patient comorbidities [51, 54].

Risk Assessment

Risk assessments and outcome predictions for EGS patients are aided by validated scoring systems including Charlson age-comorbidity index (CACI) [54], frailty scores [22, 27, 37], Emergency Surgery Score (ESS) [8, 39], and the Physiological and Operative Severity Score for the enumeration of Mortality and Morbidity (POSSUM) [21, 57]. In addition, the AAST has developed a grading system for reporting anatomic severity of multiple EGS conditions [14, 20, 43, 58, 59]. Further, the American College of Surgeons National Surgical Quality Improvement Program (NSQIP) universal Surgical Risk Calculator is available online and through smartphone apps [4]. However, NSQIP data are limited to operative cases, and some have questioned whether the same risk stratification tools should be used for both emergent and elective procedures [8, 39]. Other risk factors associated with poor outcomes of EGS patients include lack of insurance (associated with complex presentation [44] and mortality [51]) and treatment at rural [51] or low-volume hospitals [34] which carry higher mortality.

Morbidity and Mortality

Large cohort studies indicate that complication rates are approximately 15% for EGS patients requiring surgery [45]. Wound-related complications are most common, followed by pulmonary issues [26]. Postoperative stroke, major bleeding, and acute myocardial infarction present the highest risks for death [26]. Overall, mortality rates are relatively low, around 1.5% across multiple large studies [15, 45, 51], and have declined over time despite increasing volume [15]. Those requiring surgery have significantly higher mortality [26, 39].

Hospital length of stay has decreased over time [15] with median length of stay (LOS) of approximately four (4) days [15, 32, 51]. ICU admission rates are around 11% [32, 50, 54].

Other Outcomes: Readmissions, Reoperations, Loss of Independence, and Years of Life Lost

Havens [17] described a 5.9% readmission rate over 5 years for EGS patients – most commonly for surgical site infection – and found that Charlson Comorbidity Index score ≥ 2, patients leaving against medical advice, and public insurance were the greatest risk factors. Muthuvel [31] described a 15.2% postoperative readmission rate using ACS-NSQIP data and proposed using the surgical Apgar score (SAS) developed by Gawande [16] as a predictor. In that study, multivariable analysis demonstrated that SAS < 6 independently predicted 30-day readmission (odds ratio 3.3, 95% C.I. 1.1–10.1, $p < 0.04$). Hospital LOS > 12 days and ASA class ≥ 3 were also predictive. Shah and colleagues [53] analyzed more than 69,000 records from ACS-NSQIP and reported a 4.0% unplanned reoperation rate for EGS conditions. Appendiceal disorders were the most common underlying disease, and exploratory laparotomy was the most often required procedure. In that cohort, reoperation led to significant morbidity, increased mortality, and prolonged LOS.

EGS conditions pose a severe threat to independence, especially for older patients. In 2016 St. Louis and others [55] found that patients aged ≥80 were over four times more likely to require discharge to a facility other than home (odds ratio 4.72, 95% C.I. 1.27–17.54, $p < 0.02$). McIsaac and colleagues [27] reported on "frailty" in operative elderly EGS patients and identified 25.6% of 77,184 as frail. These patients had double the mortality rate and four times the institutional discharge rate (odds ratio 5.82, 95% C.I. 5.53–6.12; $p < 0.0001$). Berian [3] reported that of 570 elderly (aged ≥ 65) patients undergoing major EGS surgery in NSQIP database, 448 (78.6%) had some loss of independence. Many elderly and frail patients also have poor health-related quality of life (HRQOL) after EGS admission and may have indications for evaluation by palliative care clinicians [25]. The 2010 Global Burden of Disease Study [56] demonstrated a marked decline in death and disability related to EGS conditions from 1990 to 2010, and these data also indicate that 287 years

of life (YLL) and 358 disability-adjusted life years (DALY) are lost per 100,000 population indicating a massive *worldwide* burden – disproportionately borne by low- and middle-income countries with poor access to emergency surgical care.

Costs

Data on the financial burden of EGS has been limited to costs associated with inpatient admission [32, 35, 52]. Factors affecting costs of care include age [52], severity of disease [32], ICU admission [32], type of hospital [32], and need for surgery [45]. Admission costs vary by study and range from $8246 [32] to $13,241 per admissions [45]. In 2010 NIS data, average adjusted cost per admission for all EGS conditions was $10,744 (95% C.I. $10,615–$10,874) [33]. For 2,640,725 inpatient admissions in 2010, total cost to care for EGS patients was $28.37 billion (95% C.I. $28.03–$28.73 billion). Recently, Ogola used US Census Bureau's population projections to conclude that by 2060, costs for EGS hospitalizations would increase by 45% to over $41 billion annually – mostly related to the aging population [33] (Fig. 1.5). As mentioned before,

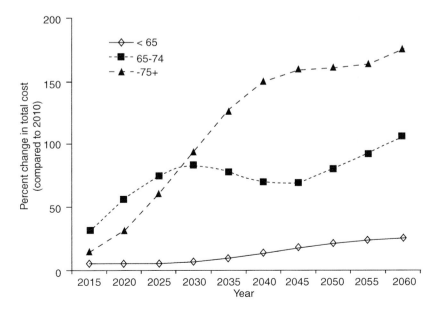

Fig. 1.5 Projected increase in cost of EGS care 2010–2060 (Source: [33])

these are underestimates due to lack of data on cost of services provided in emergency departments, urgent care centers, short-stay hospitals, post-acute care facilities (i.e., skilled nursing facilities or rehabilitation centers), physician offices, and patients' homes.

Policy and EGS Regionalization

In 2006, the Institute of Medicine described emergency care in the United States at a "breaking point" [23]; that same year the American College of Surgeons released "A Growing Crisis in Patient Access to Emergency Care" [13] outlining the issues surrounding the shortage of surgeons willing or able to provide EGS coverage. Reasons include declining reimbursement, uncompensated care, increased surgical specialization, aging of the surgeon workforce, and liability concerns. Further, as reimbursement models evolve from "fee for service" toward "value-based care," there exists a concern that the greater complexity [10] of EGS patients that results in higher complication rates, readmission rates [29], and costs [19] may place surgeons and hospitals at risk for financial penalties [61] and poor performance on published quality ratings [10]. These and other issues have led some to call for regionalization of EGS care – similar to the development of the national trauma system over the previous decades [2, 6, 12, 24, 34, 42]. Proponents argue that regionalization would capitalize on and further improve expertise, consolidate and make better use of limited resources, and ultimately lead to improved outcomes [6, 12, 24, 34]. Indeed Ogola postulated that 23.5% of EGS-related deaths in low-volume hospitals may be preventable by transfer to higher-volume hospitals [34]. Obviously costs are added with transporting patients between hospitals [28], delaying definitive care, and adding providers in tertiary centers, yet significant cost savings would occur with improved outcomes [34]. Detractors warn that, much like the evolution of trauma care, regionalization could lead to sanctioned repudiation of all EGS care – independent of severity or hospital capability –

resulting in a net transfer of complex, poorly compensated care to already overburdened tertiary care centers. In the NIS database in 2010, over 80% of hospitals caring for EGS patients were "non-teaching," and 40.8% were "rural" [34]; the logistics of large-scale EGS patient transfers need to be considered, as well. Hence, given the complex financial implications [28] and large, heterogeneous EGS patient volume, much remains unknown with regard to regionalization efforts.

Data Sources and Future Work

Data sources currently available to study EGS conditions and outcomes include local institutional registries, the NSQIP database, and various administrative discharge databases including State Inpatient Databases (SID) and the NIS. Each is limited by its scope, nonstandard format, and retrospective nature. In addition, most are not designed for collecting EGS-specific clinical data including physiologic, severity of disease, and operative details further limiting their clinical and research usefulness. To improve our understanding of EGS diseases and their treatment, allow outcomes benchmarking for hospitals and surgeons, facilitate research, and serve as a quality improvement tool, a dedicated national EGS registry, modeled on the NSQIP, is a critical next step and is currently being pursued [1, 47].

References

1. Becher RD, Meredith JW, Chang MC, Hoth JJ, Beard HR, Miller PR. Creation and implementation of an emergency general surgery registry modeled after the National Trauma Data Bank. J Am Coll Surg. 2012;214(2):156–63. https://doi.org/10.1016/j.jamcollsurg.2011.11.001.
2. Beecher S, O'Leary DP, McLaughlin R. Increased risk environment for emergency general surgery in the context of regionalization and specialization. Int J Surg. 2015;21:112–4. https://doi.org/10.1016/j.ijsu.2015.06.070.
3. Berian JR, Mohanty S, Ko CY, Rosenthal RA, Robinson TN. Association of loss of independence

with readmission and death after discharge in older patients after surgical procedures. JAMA Surg. 2016;151(9):e161689. https://doi.org/10.1001/jamasurg.2016.1689.

4. Bilimoria KY, Liu Y, Paruch JL, Zhou L, Kmiecik TE, Ko CY, Cohen ME. Development and evaluation of the universal ACS NSQIP surgical risk calculator: a decision aid and informed consent tool for patients and surgeons. J Am Coll Surg. 2013;217(5):833–842 e831. https://doi.org/10.1016/j.jamcollsurg.2013.07.385.

5. Biondo S, Ramos E, Fraccalvieri D, Kreisler E, Rague JM, Jaurrieta E. Comparative study of left colonic peritonitis severity score and Mannheim peritonitis index. Br J Surg. 2006;93(5):616–22. https://doi.org/10.1002/bjs.5326.

6. Block EF, Rudloff B, Noon C, Behn B. Regionalization of surgical services in Central Florida: the next step in acute care surgery. J Trauma Acute Care Surg. 2010;69(3):640–3.; discussion 643-644. https://doi.org/10.1097/TA.0b013e3181efbed9.

7. Boey J, Choi SK, Poon A, Alagaratnam TT. Risk stratification in perforated duodenal ulcers. A prospective validation of predictive factors. Ann Surg. 1987;205(1):22–6.

8. Bohnen JD, Ramly EP, Sangji NF, de Moya M, Yeh DD, Lee J, Velmahos GC, Chang DC, Kaafarani HM. Perioperative risk factors impact outcomes in emergency versus nonemergency surgery differently: time to separate our national risk-adjustment models? J Trauma Acute Care Surg. 2016;81(1):122–30. https://doi.org/10.1097/TA.0000000000001015.

9. Bruns BR, Tesoriero R, Narayan M, Klyushnenkova EN, Chen H, Scalea TM, Diaz JJ. Emergency general surgery: defining burden of disease in the state of Maryland. Am Surg. 2015;81(8):829–34.

10. Chen LM, Epstein AM, Orav EJ, Filice CE, Samson LW, Joynt Maddox KE. Association of practice-level social and medical risk with performance in the medicare physician value-based payment modifier program. JAMA. 2017;318(5):453–61. https://doi.org/10.1001/jama.2017.9643.

11. Crandall ML, Agarwal S, Muskat P, Ross S, Savage S, Schuster K, Tominaga GT, Shafi S, American Association for the Surgery of TraumaCommittee on Patient A, Outcomes. Application of a uniform anatomic grading system to measure disease severity in eight emergency general surgical illnesses. J Trauma Acute Care Surg. 2014;77(5):705–8. https://doi.org/10.1097/TA.0000000000000444.

12. Diaz JJ, Jr., Norris PR, Gunter OL, Collier BR, Riordan WP, Morris JA, Jr. (2011) Does regionalization of acute care surgery decrease mortality? J Trauma Acute Care Surg 71 (2):442–446. doi:https://doi.org/10.1097/TA.0b013e3182281fa2.

13. Division of Advocacy and Health Policy. A growing crisis in patient access to emergency surgical care. Bull Am Coll Surg. 2006;91(8):8–19.

14. Emergency General Surgery Anatomic Severity Scales. http://www.aast.org/emergency-general-surgery-anatomic-grading-scales. Accessed 22 Aug 2017.

15. Gale SC, Shafi S, Dombrovskiy VY, Arumugam D, Crystal JS. The public health burden of emergency general surgery in the United States: a 10-year analysis of the Nationwide inpatient sample--2001 to 2010. J Trauma Acute Care Surg. 2014;77(2):202–8. https://doi.org/10.1097/TA.0000000000000362.

16. Gawande AA, Kwaan MR, Regenbogen SE, Lipsitz SA, Zinner MJ. An Apgar score for surgery. J Am Coll Surg. 2007;204(2):201–8. https://doi.org/10.1016/j.jamcollsurg.2006.11.011.

17. Havens JM, Olufajo OA, Cooper ZR, Haider AH, Shah AA, Salim A. Defining rates and risk factors for readmissions following emergency general surgery. JAMA Surg. 2016;151(4):330–6. https://doi.org/10.1001/jamasurg.2015.4056.

18. Havens JM, Peetz AB, Do WS, Cooper Z, Kelly E, Askari R, Reznor G, Salim A. The excess morbidity and mortality of emergency general surgery. J Trauma Acute Care Surg. 2015;78(2):306–11. https://doi.org/10.1097/TA.0000000000000517.

19. Healy MA, Mullard AJ, Campbell DA Jr, Dimick JB. Hospital and payer costs associated with surgical complications. JAMA Surg. 2016;151(9):823–30. https://doi.org/10.1001/jamasurg.2016.0773.

20. Hernandez MC, Aho JM, Habermann EB, Choudhry AJ, Morris DS, Zielinski MD. Increased anatomic severity predicts outcomes: Validation of the American Association for the Surgery of Trauma's Emergency General Surgery score in appendicitis. J Trauma Acute Care Surg. 2017;82(1):73–9. https://doi.org/10.1097/TA.0000000000001274.

21. Horwood J, Ratnam S, Maw A. Decisions to operate: the ASA grade 5 dilemma. Ann R Coll Surg Engl. 2011;93(5):365–9. https://doi.org/10.1308/003588411X581367.

22. Joseph B, Zangbar B, Pandit V, Fain M, Mohler MJ, Kulvatunyou N, Jokar TO, O'Keeffe T, Friese RS, Rhee P. Emergency general surgery in the elderly: too old or too frail? J Am Coll Surg. 2016;222(5):805–13. https://doi.org/10.1016/j.jamcollsurg.2016.01.063.

23. Kellermann AL. Crisis in the emergency department. New Engl J Med. 2006;355(13):1300–3. https://doi.org/10.1056/NEJMp068194.

24. Kreindler SA, Zhang L, Metge CJ, Nason RW, Wright B, Rudnick W, Moffatt ME. Impact of a regional acute care surgery model on patient access and outcomes. Can J Surg. 2013;56(5):318–24.

25. Lilley EJ, Cooper Z. The high burden of palliative care needs among older emergency general surgery patients. J Palliat Med. 2016;19(4):352–3. https://doi.org/10.1089/jpm.2015.0502.

26. McCoy CC, Englum BR, Keenan JE, Vaslef SN, Shapiro ML, Scarborough JE. Impact of specific postoperative complications on the outcomes of emergency general surgery patients. J Trauma Acute Care Surg. 2015;78(5):912–8.; discussion 918-919. https://doi.org/10.1097/TA.0000000000000611.

27. McIsaac DI, Moloo H, Bryson GL, van Walraven C. The association of frailty with outcomes and resource use after emergency general surgery: a population-based cohort study. Anesth Analg. 2017;124(5):1653–61. https://doi.org/10.1213/ANE.0000000000001960.

28. Menke TJ, Wray NP. When does regionalization of expensive medical care save money? Health Serv Manag Res. 2001;14(2):116–24. https://doi.org/10.1258/0951484011912618.

29. Merkow RP, Ju MH, Chung JW, Hall BL, Cohen ME, Williams MV, Tsai TC, Ko CY, Bilimoria KY. Underlying reasons associated with hospital readmission following surgery in the United States. JAMA. 2015;313(5):483–95. https://doi.org/10.1001/jama.2014.18614.

30. Mullen MG, Michaels AD, Mehaffey JH, Guidry CA, Turrentine FE, Hedrick TL, Friel CM. Risk associated with complications and mortality after urgent surgery vs elective and emergency surgery: implications for defining "quality" and reporting outcomes for urgent surgery. JAMA Surg. 2017;152(8):768–74. https://doi.org/10.1001/jamasurg.2017.0918.

31. Muthuvel G, Tevis SE, Liepert AE, Agarwal SK, Kennedy GD. A composite index for predicting readmission following emergency general surgery. J Trauma Acute Care Surg. 2014;76(6):1467–72. https://doi.org/10.1097/TA.0000000000000223.

32. Narayan M, Tesoriero R, Bruns BR, Klyushnenkova EN, Chen H, Diaz JJ. Acute care surgery: defining the economic burden of emergency general surgery. J Am Coll Surg. 2016;222(4):691–9. https://doi.org/10.1016/j.jamcollsurg.2016.01.054.

33. Ogola GO, Gale SC, Haider A, Shafi S. The financial burden of emergency general surgery: national estimates 2010 to 2060. J Trauma Acute Care Surg. 2015;79(3):444–8. https://doi.org/10.1097/TA.0000000000000787.

34. Ogola GO, Haider A, Shafi S. Hospitals with higher volumes of emergency general surgery patients achieve lower mortality rates: a case for establishing designated centers for emergency general surgery. J Trauma Acute Care Surg. 2017;82(3):497–504. https://doi.org/10.1097/TA.0000000000001355.

35. Ogola GO, Shafi S. Cost of specific emergency general surgery diseases and factors associated with high-cost patients. J Trauma Acute Care Surg. 2016;80(2):265–71. https://doi.org/10.1097/TA.0000000000000911.

36. Oliver CM, Walker E, Giannaris S, Grocott MP, Mooneesinghe SR. Risk assessment tools validated for patients undergoing emergency laparotomy: a systematic review. Br J Anaesth. 2015;115(6):849–60. https://doi.org/10.1093/bja/aev350.

37. Orouji Jokar T, Ibraheem K, Rhee P, Kulavatunyou N, Haider A, Phelan HA, Fain M, Mohler MJ, Joseph B. Emergency general surgery specific frailty index: a validation study. J Trauma Acute Care Surg. 2016;81(2):254–60. https://doi.org/10.1097/TA.0000000000001120.

38. Paul MG. The public health crisis in emergency general surgery: who will pay the price and bear the burden? JAMA Surg. 2016;151(6):e160640. https://doi.org/10.1001/jamasurg.2016.0640.

39. Peponis T, Bohnen JD, Sangji NF, Nandan AR, Han K, Lee J, Yeh DD, de Moya MA, Velmahos GC, Chang DC, Kaafarani HMA. Does the emergency surgery score accurately predict outcomes in emergent laparotomies? Surgery. 2017;162(2):445–52. https://doi.org/10.1016/j.surg.2017.03.016.

40. Rubinfeld I, Thomas C, Berry S, Murthy R, Obeid N, Azuh O, Jordan J, Patton JH. Octogenarian abdominal surgical emergencies: not so grim a problem with the acute care surgery model? J Trauma Acute Care Surg. 2009;67(5):983–9. https://doi.org/10.1097/TA.0b013e3181ad6690.

41. Sangji NF, Bohnen JD, Ramly EP, Yeh DD, King DR, DeMoya M, Butler K, Fagenholz PJ, Velmahos GC, Chang DC, Kaafarani HM. Derivation and validation of a novel emergency surgery acuity score (ESAS). J Trauma Acute Care Surg. 2016;81(2):213–20. https://doi.org/10.1097/TA.0000000000001059.

42. Santry HP, Janjua S, Chang Y, Petrovick L, Velmahos GC. Interhospital transfers of acute care surgery patients: should care for nontraumatic surgical emergencies be regionalized? World J Surg. 2011;35(12):2660–7. https://doi.org/10.1007/s00268-011-1292-3.

43. Savage SA, Klekar CS, Priest EL, Crandall ML, Rodriguez BC, Shafi S, Committee APA. Validating a new grading scale for emergency general surgery diseases. J Surg Res. 2015;196(2):264–9. https://doi.org/10.1016/j.jss.2015.03.036.

44. Scott JW, Havens JM, Wolf LL, Zogg CK, Rose JA, Salim A, Haider AH. Insurance status is associated with complex presentation among emergency general surgery patients. Surgery. 2017;161(2):320–8. https://doi.org/10.1016/j.surg.2016.08.038.

45. Scott JW, Olufajo OA, Brat GA, Rose JA, Zogg CK, Haider AH, Salim A, Havens JM. Use of national burden to define operative emergency general surgery. JAMA Surg. 2016;151(6):e160480. https://doi.org/10.1001/jamasurg.2016.0480.

46. Segui-Gomez M, MacKenzie EJ. Measuring the public health impact of injuries. Epidemiol Rev. 2003;25:3–19.

47. Shafi S. Pursuing quality – emergency general surgery quality improvement program (EQIP). Am Coll Surg Surg News. 2015;11.

48. Shafi S, Aboutanos M, Brown CV, Ciesla D, Cohen MJ, Crandall ML, Inaba K, Miller PR, Mowery NT, American Association for the Surgery of Trauma Committee on Patient A, Outcomes. Measuring anatomic severity of disease in emergency general surgery. J Trauma Acute Care Surg. 2014;76(3):884–7. https://doi.org/10.1097/TA.0b013e3182aafdba.

49. Shafi S, Aboutanos MB, Agarwal S Jr, Brown CV, Crandall M, Feliciano DV, Guillamondegui O, Haider A, Inaba K, Osler TM, Ross S, Rozycki GS, Tominaga GT. Emergency general surgery: definition

and estimated burden of disease. J Trauma Acute Care Surg. 2013;74(4):1092–7. https://doi.org/10.1097/TA.0b013e31827e1bc7.

50. Shafi S, Priest EL, Crandall ML, Klekar CS, Nazim A, Aboutanos M, Agarwal S, Bhattacharya B, Byrge N, Dhillon TS, Eboli DJ, Fielder D, Guillamondegui O, Gunter O, Inaba K, Mowery NT, Nirula R, Ross SE, Savage SA, Schuster KM, Schmoker RK, Siboni S, Siparsky N, Trust MD, Utter GH, Whelan J, Feliciano DV, Rozycki G, American Association for the Surgery of Trauma Patient Assessment C. Multicenter validation of American Association for the Surgery of Trauma grading system for acute colonic diverticulitis and its use for emergency general surgery quality improvement program. J Trauma Acute Care Surg. 2016;80(3):405–10.; discussion 410-401. https://doi.org/10.1097/TA.0000000000000943.

51. Shah AA, Haider AH, Zogg CK, Schwartz DA, Haut ER, Zafar SN, Schneider EB, Velopulos CG, Shafi S, Zafar H, Efron DT. National estimates of predictors of outcomes for emergency general surgery. J Trauma Acute Care Surg. 2015;78(3):482–90; discussion 490-481. https://doi.org/10.1097/TA.0000000000000555.

52. Shah AA, Zafar SN, Kodadek LM, Zogg CK, Chapital AB, Iqbal A, Greene WR, Cornwell EE 3rd, Havens J, Nitzschke S, Cooper Z, Salim A, Haider AH. Never giving up: outcomes and presentation of emergency general surgery in geriatric octogenarian and nonagenarian patients. Am J Surg. 2016;212(2):211–20 e213. https://doi.org/10.1016/j.amjsurg.2016.01.021.

53. Shah AA, Zogg CK, Havens JM, Nitzschke SL, Cooper Z, Gates JD, Kelly EG, Askari R, Salim A. Unplanned reoperations in emergency general surgery: risk factors and burden. J Am Coll Surg. 2015;221(4):S44.

54. St-Louis E, Iqbal S, Feldman LS, Sudarshan M, Deckelbaum DL, Razek TS, Khwaja K. Using the age-adjusted Charlson comorbidity index to predict outcomes in emergency general surgery. J Trauma Acute Care Surg. 2015;78(2):318–23. https://doi.org/10.1097/TA.0000000000000457.

55. St-Louis E, Sudarshan M, Al-Habboubi M, El-Husseini Hassan M, Deckelbaum DL, Razek TS, Feldman LS, Khwaja K. The outcomes of the elderly

in acute care general surgery. Eur J Trauma Emerg Surg. 2016;42(1):107–13. https://doi.org/10.1007/s00068-015-0517-9.

56. Stewart B, Khanduri P, McCord C, Ohene-Yeboah M, Uranues S, Vega Rivera F, Mock C. Global disease burden of conditions requiring emergency surgery. Br J Surg. 2014;101(1):e9–22. https://doi.org/10.1002/bjs.9329.

57. Stonelake S, Thomson P, Suggett N. Identification of the high risk emergency surgical patient: which risk prediction model should be used? Ann Med Surg (Lond). 2015;4(3):240–7. https://doi.org/10.1016/j.amsu.2015.07.004.

58. Tominaga GT, Staudenmayer KL, Shafi S, Schuster KM, Savage SA, Ross S, Muskat P, Mowery NT, Miller P, Inaba K, Cohen MJ, Ciesla D, Brown CV, Agarwal S, Aboutanos MB, Utter GH, Crandall M, American Association for the Surgery of Trauma Committee on Patient A. The American Association for the Surgery of Trauma grading scale for 16 emergency general surgery conditions: disease-specific criteria characterizing anatomic severity grading. J Trauma Acute Care Surg. 2016;81(3):593–602. https://doi.org/10.1097/TA.0000000000001127.

59. Utter GH, Miller PR, Mowery NT, Tominaga GT, Gunter O, Osler TM, Ciesla DJ, Agarwal SK Jr, Inaba K, Aboutanos MB, Brown CV, Ross SE, Crandall ML, Shafi S. ICD-9-CM and ICD-10-CM mapping of the AAST emergency general surgery disease severity grading systems: conceptual approach, limitations, and recommendations for the future. J Trauma Acute Care Surg. 2015;78(5):1059–65. https://doi.org/10.1097/TA.0000000000000608.

60. Zangbar B, Rhee P, Pandit V, Hsu CH, Khalil M, Okeefe T, Neumayer L, Joseph B. Seasonal variation in emergency general surgery. Ann Surg. 2016;263(1):76–81. https://doi.org/10.1097/SLA.0000000000001238.

61. Zielinski MD, Thomsen KM, Polites SF, Khasawneh MA, Jenkins DH, Habermann EB. Is the Centers for Medicare and Medicaid Service's lack of reimbursement for postoperative urinary tract infections in elderly emergency surgery patients justified? Surgery. 2014;156(4):1009–15. https://doi.org/10.1016/j.surg.2014.06.073.

Evaluating the Acute Abdomen

2

Sawyer Smith and Martin A. Schreiber

Introduction

Acute abdominal pain is one of the most common complaints leading to patients seeking medical care, accounting for between 5% and 7% of all US emergency department visits [1, 2]. Due to the frequency of patients presenting with abdominal pain and the vast number of causes, a thorough and directed evaluation is necessary to rule out causes that require emergent intervention from those that may be managed conservatively. A surgeon must start making their differential diagnosis from the moment they meet the patient; keying in on pertinent positives and negatives in the patient's history of presenting illness, past medical and surgical history, and the physical exam will narrow the possible diagnoses. Determining the gravity of the patient's current physiologic state through vital signs, laboratory tests, and imaging will identify the criticalness of the patient's illness and the speed at which intervention is necessary. A thorough understanding about the potential disease processes is also necessary for a surgeon to have to make sure that all

possibilities for the patient's symptoms are accounted for so that the proper diagnosis leads to the most appropriate treatment for the patient in a timely manner.

History

Taking a thorough, concise history is essential to narrowing the differential diagnosis of the patient's abdominal pain. A surgeon must ask the pertinent questions to help guide the decision-making, imaging choice, and ultimate management of the patient, while eliminating many other causes of abdominal pain. One must take into account not only the most common causes for a patient's symptoms, but rule out less frequent life-threatening causes or other diagnoses that the patient may be predisposed to due to their previous medical history or demographics. When asking questions about a patient's pain, below is a list of categories that are essential to delineate (Table 2.1):

- *Onset:* The timing of the patient's symptoms is important as typical problems present similar time cadences. The pain can either be immediate (onset in minutes), progressive (1–4 h), or indolent (4–24 h).
- *Location*: The surgeon must differentiate between localized and generalized abdominal symptoms. If the patient's pain is located in a

S. Smith
Department of Surgery, Oregon Health & Sciences University, Portland, OR, USA

M. A. Schreiber (✉)
Department of Surgery, Division of Trauma, Critical Care & Acute Care Surgery, Oregon Health & Science University, Portland, OR, USA
e-mail: schreibm@ohsu.edu

© Springer International Publishing AG, part of Springer Nature 2019
C. V. R. Brown et al. (eds.), *Emergency General Surgery*, https://doi.org/10.1007/978-3-319-96286-3_2

specific area, this can help narrow the differential diagnosis. Localizing the symptoms to a specific quadrant will drive the next steps in evaluation and can lead to more specific lab and imaging tests. Generalized abdominal symptoms are worrisome for a more widespread process.

- *Quality/Character*: The type of pain (dull, sharp, electric, etc.) should also be elucidated. The physician should inquire about specific things that may improve or worsen the pain. Signs that point toward peritonitis include increased pain with movement, pain when hitting bumps while driving, or pain with coughing.
- *Radiation*: Certain pathology will classically have pain symptoms that radiate from one portion of the abdomen to other locations in the body. Pancreatitis typically radiates from the epigastrium to the spine. Urogenital pathology may radiate to the inguinal area or down into the scrotum of males.
- *Associated Symptoms*: Other symptoms in concert with severe abdominal pain such as nausea, emesis, diarrhea, constipation, hematemesis, or hematochezia are important to identify.

Table 2.1 Essential components of history taking

| History of present illness |
| Onset |
| Location |
| Quality/character |
| Radiation |
| Associated symptoms |
| Past medial history |
| Past surgical history |
| Family history |
| Medications |

Care should be taken to not just focus on the history of the present illness, but also on the patient's prior medical history. A careful medical history and review of systems will help identify any risk factors that the patient may have that either could be the cause of their presenting symptoms or contribute to their overall presentation. A cardiac history including any history of coronary artery disease or arrhythmias including atrial fibrillation would put the patient at risk for mesenteric ischemia from either thrombotic or embolic causes. Uncontrolled diabetes mellitus can blunt some abdominal pain symptoms due to neuropathy from chronic hyperglycemia. Prior history of malignancy or radiation would put the patient at risk for either recurrence of the primary tumor, metastatic disease, or radiation enteritis leading to their symptoms. A history of peptic ulcer disease would put the patient at risk for stomach or duodenal perforation or intraluminal hemorrhage. A thorough gynecologic history in female patients will help identify patients at risk for pelvic inflammatory disease, endometriosis, or ectopic pregnancy.

Nonsurgical causes of abdominal pain can be misleading. Etiologies include cardiopulmonary, metabolic, toxic ingestions, hematologic, immunologic, and infectious (Table 2.2).

A thorough surgical history should be obtained from every patient that is being worked up for surgical pathology but especially in the case of an acute abdomen. Knowledge of prior surgeries will give an understanding of any altered anatomy, identify any complications the patient may be at risk for, or eliminate certain pathology from consideration. Prior surgeries, such as bariatric procedures, can alter the patient's intestinal anatomy which can lead to many different

Table 2.2 Medical causes for acute abdominal pain

Cardiopulmonary	Metabolic	Toxic	Hematologic	Infectious
Myocardial infarction	Addison's crisis	Withdrawal syndromes	Sickle cell crisis	Gastroenteritis
Pericarditis	Diabetic ketoacidosis	Corrosive ingestion	Lymphadenopathy	Parasitic disease
Pneumonia	Hypercalcemia	Lead poisoning	Hemorrhage due to anticoagulants	Malaria
		Drug packing		Typhoid

pathological entities. An understanding of the patient's prior operations will also alert the surgeon to potential complications or pitfalls that will help with the planning and approach if the patient requires an operation. Lastly, prior surgeries can put patients at risk for hernias leading to incarcerated or strangulated bowel that should be added to the differential diagnosis.

Physical Exam

The physical exam of the patient presenting with acute abdominal findings begins as the surgeon walks into the room. Initial visual inspection of the patient's general appearance, position on the bed, and mannerisms will tell a great deal about their condition. Patients with peritonitis will often be ill appearing and moving minimally while patients with renal or biliary colic may be writhing in pain unable to get comfortable. Along with the initial inspection of the patient, vital signs (heart rate, blood pressure, respiratory rate, oxygen saturation, and temperature) should be noted. Severe intra-abdominal processes can push the patient into shock with inadequate tissue oxygen delivery. Patients in shock will be tachycardic and hypotensive and have decreased oxygen saturation. If shock is due to sepsis, hyperthermia or hypothermia may be present. These quick determinations of the patients overall appearance along with determining if the patient is in shock will help the surgeon determine if immediate action is needed to stabilize the patient or if there is time for further evaluation prior to determining the first treatment options.

A systematic physical exam should be performed with a focus on the heart, lungs, and abdomen. Cardiac and pulmonary exams are important not just to identify abnormalities that may lead to a nonsurgical diagnosis as the cause of the abdominal pain, but also to identify any comorbidities that may preclude or need further workup prior to the patient obtaining a general anesthetic if the patient requires surgery. Cardiac examination should identify any murmurs or arrhythmias, while the pulmonary exam should

focus on overall work of breathing, equal breath sounds, and auscultation of crackles consistent with pulmonary edema.

The abdominal exam should start with inspection looking for abdominal distention, previous incisions, asymmetry, or any obvious deformities consistent with a hernia. Auscultation of the abdomen, although classically taught in physical exam, is not as helpful with abdominal pathology as it is for aiding in the diagnosis in other regions of the body. There is low sensitivity and specificity along with auscultative findings being inconsistent from surgeon to surgeon [3, 4]. Percussion of the abdomen can help identify organ enlargement (hepatomegaly or splenomegaly) along with being able to help identify any free fluid such as ascites. Palpation of the abdomen will identify any signs of peritonitis with voluntary or involuntary guarding. Signs of peritonitis can be either localized to a certain area of the abdomen or diffuse throughout the abdomen. When palpating the abdomen, the surgeon should also be assessing for masses, fluid within the abdominal cavity, and any abdominal wall defects.

Examination of the inguinal canal should be completed in every patient with abdominal complaints looking for signs of incarcerated or strangulated hernias. Hernias that are extremely tender, unable to be reduced, or have overlying skin erythema are concerning for containing compromised intestine. Rectal examination and stool-occult blood testing can identify either gross or microscopic intestinal bleeding. All female patients with acute abdominal symptoms, particularly lower abdominal complaints, should have a pelvic exam including both bimanual examination and a speculum examination to identify gynecologic causes of acute abdominal pain such as ectopic pregnancy, ovarian torsion, or pelvic inflammatory disease.

Depending on a patient's presenting symptoms, further maneuvers may aid in determining the diagnosis. Rebound tenderness can be an indicator of peritonitis. This maneuver is positive when the patient has increased pain upon release of pressure on the abdomen as opposed to when the abdomen is palpated. Rovsing's sign is another maneuver that is positive when the patient has pain in the right lower quadrant of the abdomen at the time of palpation in the left lower quadrant. This sign is associated with acute appendicitis. Murphy's sign is a physical exam maneuver that classically is associated with cholecystitis. This maneuver is performed by having the patient exhale completely, palpating deeply in the right upper quadrant, and then having the patient take a deep breath in. If the patient has severe increased pain and arrests inspiration, this points toward cholecystitis.

Laboratory Studies

Although the mainstay of the diagnosis of the patient who presents with an acute abdomen is the history and physical exam, laboratory tests can aid in determining the cause of the patients' symptoms. While these tests can help, they should be used as an adjunct to the information gained from the history and physical exam, not as the mode of making the diagnosis. Along with aiding in diagnosis, laboratory tests will also show any metabolic or hematologic abnormalities that may need correction prior to the patient undergoing surgery (Table 2.3).

A complete metabolic panel will identify any electrolyte disturbances such as sodium, potassium, or chloride abnormalities. These changes in electrolytes could be associated with the primary process (emesis or diarrhea) or secondary to kidney injury due to hypovolemia or sepsis. Electrolyte disturbances can have implications with anesthetics and should be addressed prior to taking the patient to the operating room.

Table 2.3 Necessary laboratory tests for patients with acute abdominal pain

Laboratory tests
Complete metabolic panel
Complete blood count
Lipase
Amylase
PT/INR
PTT
Urinalysis
Pregnancy assessment (females of child-bearing age)
Stool studies

Creatinine and blood urea nitrogen (BUN) levels will give the clinician information about the patient's renal function. Metabolic panels will also provide liver enzymes, bilirubin, alkaline phosphatase, and albumin levels. Liver enzymes and bilirubin may be elevated from hepatobiliary processes or due to ischemia from hypotension due to other causes. Lipase and amylase are elevated with pancreatic inflammation with lipase being more specific for pancreatic inflammation. Pancreatitis is most commonly due to gallstone disease in the Western population but also may be due to alcohol abuse, hypercalcemia, hypertriglyceridemia, or autoimmune disease.

Complete blood counts and coagulation panels can also aid in the diagnosis but are essential for any patient prior to surgery. The white blood cell count can be elevated or depressed from normal values due to sepsis from an intra-abdominal infection. Hemoglobin and hematocrit levels can be depressed if hemorrhage is present but also in the setting of chronic illness. The platelet count, prothrombin time/international normalized ratio (PT/INR), and the partial thromboplastin time (PTT) are the classic indicators used to evaluate coagulopathy. Thrombelastography (TEG) is also used at some institutions giving the surgeon generalized functional coagulation information. These coagulation parameters are imperative for both the surgical and anesthesia team to evaluate prior to any operation to help minimize blood loss and correct any underlying abnormalities.

Urinalysis is another important lab to obtain for any patient with abdominal pain. Identification of a urinary tract infection that could account for the patient's symptoms should be done prior to more in-depth and expensive tests. Stool studies such as occult blood tests, fecal leukocytes, and ova and parasite examination can be helpful with patients who have symptoms of hematochezia, melena, or diarrhea and concern for gastrointestinal infection.

Imaging Studies

As medicine has evolved, there are multitudes of imaging studies that are available, many of which have various roles in evaluating patients with acute abdominal pain. Again, imaging studies should be used to assist in the diagnosis or for surgical planning. The specific imaging studies to obtain should be determined after a thorough history and physical exam have been done. After the history and physical exam, a physician should be able to narrow the differential diagnosis which can then direct the necessary imaging studies to be obtained. Reducing unnecessary tests will reduce radiation exposure, false-positive/false-negative studies, and overall cost to the patient and the healthcare system [5].

Standard X-rays, or plain films, of the abdomen provide limited anatomical information but can be very useful in the right situation. These images can readily identify obstructive or nonobstructive intestinal gas patterns. Patients with small intestinal obstruction will typically have multiple dilated loops of small bowel in the central abdomen with air/fluid levels. Plain films should be obtained with the patient in the upright or lateral decubitus position to utilize gravity to allow for visualization of air/fluid levels, which will be less apparent or not visualized on a supine radiograph. Upright and lateral decubitus images will also allow for identification of free intraperitoneal air which can be present if perforated viscous is the cause of the patient's presentation (Fig. 2.1).

Giving patients contrast, either by mouth or by rectum, can be used to identify specific problems within the gastrointestinal tract (GI tract). Upper gastrointestinal series (UGI) is used to image the esophagus, stomach, and small intestine. This can help identify perforations within these portions of the GI tract, hiatal hernias, or bowel obstructions. Barium or water-soluble contrast (i.e., gastrografin) are generally the intraluminal contrast that the patient will drink for the study. If the patient is at risk for aspiration, water-soluble contrast should not be used as it can cause intense pulmonary edema as the osmotic pressure draws fluid into the alveoli. If there is a risk for perforation, then barium should not be used as leakage into the peritoneal cavity can cause an inflammatory response and barium can persist in the peritoneal cavity making future studies more difficult to interpret.

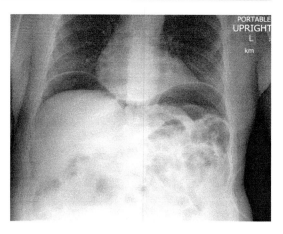

Fig. 2.1 Upright plain film of the abdomen with free intraperitoneal air that can be seen under the diaphragm

Ultrasound is another imaging modality that can be utilized to gain more information on a patient with an acute abdomen. Ultrasound is readily available, does not use radiation, and is inexpensive. The graded-compression technique is used when evaluating the abdomen with ultrasound, where the operator gradually increases the pressure to move the underlying fat and intestine out of the way. This technique can be used to identify free fluid, abscesses, or occasionally free intraperitoneal air which is represented by gas echoes that act as an obstacle to deeper imaging. Ultrasound is also the imaging modality of choice when patients present with acute right upper quadrant abdominal pain concerning for biliary pathology (Fig. 2.2). Although ultrasound has its benefits and is without radiation, it is operator dependent, and the reliability of the imaging is reliant upon the experience of the operator. Obese patients are also more difficult to image with ultrasound as the sound waves are less likely to penetrate the deeper, more dependent areas of the abdomen that are of interest.

Computed tomography (CT) is the mainstay for imaging of the acute abdomen as it shows the greatest anatomic and pathologic detail while being relatively quick to obtain. CT obtains axial slices of variable thickness, most commonly 5–7 mm, of the entire abdomen and pelvis. These images can be reconstructed to give the clinician multiplanar views of the abdomen, traditionally

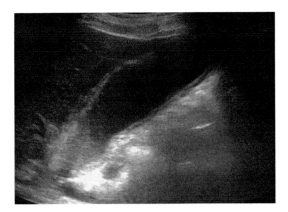

Fig. 2.2 Ultrasound of the gallbladder with a thickened perihepatic gallbladder wall, pericholecystic fluid, and sludge in the neck of the gallbladder in a patient with cholecystitis

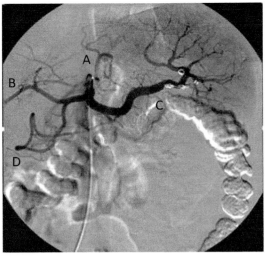

Fig. 2.3 Visceral angiogram showing the celiac truck with the left gastric (A), common hepatic (B), splenic (C), and gastroduodenal arteries (D)

coronal and sagittal images in addition to the originally obtained axial views. This allows for viewing of the abdomen from multiple view-points. These images can be enhanced with the use of intestinal (oral, rectal, or both) contrast with a water-soluble contrast agent or barium along with the use of iodinated contrast given intravenously (IV). Iodinated IV contrast should be used cautiously in patients with chronic or acute renal impairment; therefore laboratory examination of renal function with a current creatinine level should be obtained prior to administering the IV contrast. CT images can help identify perforations with either free intraperitoneal air or leakage of contrast material. Intestinal wall thickening indicates an inflammatory response which can be due to many different causes. Decreased IV contrast uptake of the intestine indicates ischemia in that area. Other pathology such as appendicitis, diverticulitis, neoplasm, obstruction, trauma, or foreign bodies can also be diagnosed using CT imaging.

Another method for evaluating the blood flow to the abdominal organs is visceral angiography (Fig. 2.3). This is generally performed through accessing either femoral artery and passing a catheter up through the abdominal aorta to visualize its branches. Contrast is deployed with subsequent visualization of the abdominal vascular supply. This method can be both diagnostic and therapeutic for ischemia. Stenosis, thrombosis, or

emboli can be identified. When the lesion is located, intra-arterial thrombolysis and percutaneous transluminal angioplasty with or without stent placement are possible therapeutic interventions. Lesions that are not amenable to percutaneous interventions will give the surgeon specific information for operative planning. Visceral angiography can also be used for acute gastrointestinal hemorrhage, again for both therapeutic and diagnostic purposes. For visceral angiography to be able to locate the site of bleeding, the hemorrhage must be at a rate > 0.5 ml/min. If located, embolization can stop the ongoing bleeding. Patient factors must be taken into account prior to using angiography. Patients with iodinated contrast allergy or acute/chronic kidney disease may require either premedication prior to angiography or, depending on the severity, have absolute contraindications for angiography.

Nuclear medicine imaging tests also can be helpful in certain patients with acute abdominal pain. In patients with suspected cholecystitis and equivocal imaging, cholescintigraphy (HIDA scan) is a reasonable option. HIDA scan uses technetium-99 m iminodiacetic acid (Tc99m IDA) analogue to image the biliary system. This tracer is taken up by hepatocytes and then excreted into the biliary system. When the gallbladder does not fill with this tracer, obstruction of the cystic duct confirms the diagnosis of cholecystitis. False-positive studies may occur in patients who have been NPO for prolonged periods or who have extremely slow radiotracer uptake and biliary excretion by the liver.

Technetium-99 m-labeled erythrocytes can be used for scintigraphy, also known as a tagged red blood cell scan. This imaging modality is another option for localization of an acute gastrointestinal hemorrhage. This imaging study can be performed relatively quickly and only requires a bleeding rate > 0.1 ml/min for reliable detection of hemorrhage. Knowledge of the location of hemorrhage can help with planning for either endoscopic, angiographic, or surgical intervention. The tagged red blood cell scan is diagnostic and does not allow for therapeutic intervention. False-positive rates may be as high as 25% [6]. The most common reason for false-positive tests is rapid transit of intraluminal blood causing the imaging to indicate that the hemorrhage is more distal in the gastrointestinal tract than it actually is. Localization of GI hemorrhage is less accurate utilizing the tagged red blood cell scan compared to arteriography.

Differential Diagnosis

When approaching any patient, the surgeon should start formulating their differential diagnosis as they walk into the room. This holds true when evaluating the patient with acute abdominal pain. Formulating the differential diagnosis while taking the patient's history, observing the patient, and performing the physical exam will drive the surgeon's decisions on laboratory tests, imaging examinations, and ultimately the management decisions that will need to be made. The differential for acute abdominal pain can be broad, but applying physiology, the patient's history, exam findings, and diagnostic tests will help the surgeon narrow it greatly.

Differential diagnosis can be approached in many ways, but the most common methods are either by location of pain or by anatomical systems. A common method is to break the abdomen

up into quadrants and narrow the diagnosis based on the location of the abdominal pain. The abdomen can be divided into the right upper, left upper, right lower, and left lower quadrants. While there are a number of pathologic findings that are not limited to one particular location in the abdomen, this approach can make certain diagnoses much less likely if the patient's symptoms are not in a typical location. If a patient's symptoms span multiple quadrants or are diffuse across the entire abdomen, this also narrows the options for a diagnosis as there are limited disease processes that will cause this type of diffuse pain.

Right upper quadrant abdominal pain is classically hepatobiliary in origin. Gallbladder pathology is the most common cause of right upper quadrant abdominal pain. Gallbladder causes generally are sequela of cholelithiasis, or gallstones, and can present along a spectrum of diseases. The most benign is symptomatic cholelithiasis, or biliary colic. This generally presents as pain after eating in the right upper quadrant but lacks any laboratory or imaging signs of inflammation of the gallbladder. If there is inflammation of the gallbladder, ultrasound imaging can show thickening of the gallbladder wall adjacent to the liver and pericholecystic fluid collections along with an elevated white blood count. Choledocholithiasis, or gallstones that are lodged in the common bile duct, can present with or without cholecystitis. Choledocholithiasis will also have ultrasound findings of a dilated common bile duct along with elevated bilirubin, aspartate aminotransferase (AST), alanine aminotransferase (ALT), and alkaline phosphatase from the obstruction of bile excretion from the liver. Gallstones can also lodge further down the biliary tree causing obstruction of the pancreatic duct leading to pancreatitis. Pancreatitis from gallstones can lead to intense pain and an inflammatory response and can present with or without signs of cholecystitis.

There are also non-biliary causes for right upper quadrant abdominal pain. Hepatic causes for right upper quadrant pain included acute alcohol intoxication, viral hepatitis, hepatic abscess (Fig. 2.4), and ruptured hepatic adenoma.

Processes involving the stomach or duodenum such as gastritis, gastroesophageal reflux disease, or peptic ulcer disease (Fig. 2.5) can also present with right upper quadrant pain. Pneumonia causing pleuritic pain may also cause pain in the right upper quadrant. Less commonly, but depending on the location of the appendix, appendicitis can rarely present with right upper quadrant pain instead of the more classic right lower quadrant pain. Right-sided colonic diverticulitis, although less common, can be a cause of right upper quadrant abdominal pain.

Left upper quadrant abdominal pain is less common and has fewer causes than other regions of the abdomen. Pancreatitis can present with isolated left upper quadrant pain or in conjunction with epigastric or right upper quadrant pain. Peptic ulcers are much rarer in the fundus and cardia, which are located in the left upper quadrant, but still can occur. Pathology involving the spleen such as abscess, infarct, or rupture can lead to severe left upper quadrant pain. Rupture of the spleen is most frequently due to trauma but can occur spontaneously from splenic enlargement seen with portal hypertension or lymphoma. Infarcts of the spleen can occur in patients with sickle-cell anemia, generally in their youth, or in patients with hypercoagulable disorders. Splenic aneurysms can rupture and lead to intraperitoneal hemorrhage, a disease entity more commonly problematic in pregnant patients. Splenic flexure colorectal adenocarcinoma can lead to acute abdominal pain, generally once the mass has grown to a critical size causing obstruction.

Right lower quadrant abdominal pain is a common presenting complaint for patients, most often due to appendicitis (Fig. 2.6). Appendicitis can initially present with periumbilical pain that

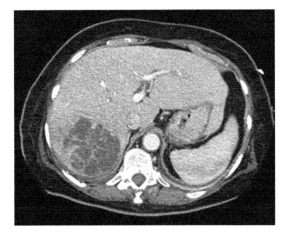

Fig. 2.4 CT axial image with a large hepatic abscess in the posterior aspect of the right lobe

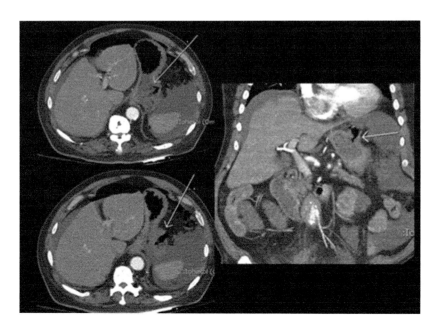

Fig. 2.5 Axial and sagittal CT images showing a perforated gastric ulcer (arrows) with extravasation of intraluminal fluid and air

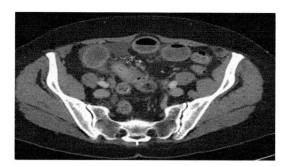

Fig. 2.6 Axial CT image showing acute appendicitis with thickened appendiceal wall (arrow) and surrounding fat stranding

migrates to the right lower quadrant, classically with pain over McBurney's point, or two-thirds of the way between the umbilicus and the anterior superior iliac spine. The pain can be associated with fevers along with nausea, vomiting, and anorexia that classically occur after the pain starts. Although appendicitis is a very common entity seen as the cause of acute abdominal pain in the right lower quadrant, there are a myriad of other causes that the surgeon must take into account and rule out prior to proceeding with operative management for appendicitis. Crohn's disease flares commonly occur in the distal ileum and can present with very similar symptoms and imaging showing inflammation similar to appendicitis. Meckel's diverticulum is a remnant of the omphalomesenteric duct and it occurs in about 2% of the population. This diverticulum is located in the distal ileum and can become inflamed leading to acute right lower quadrant pain. Sigmoid diverticulitis can also present with right lower quadrant pain in the patient with a redundant sigmoid. Urogenital disease processes such as pyelonephritis, perinephric abscess, urolithiasis, or urinary tract infections can all cause right lower quadrant pain. In female patients, gynecologic causes of right lower quadrant pain must also be excluded. For all female patients of childbearing age, pregnancy testing should always be part of the workup for any abdominal pain to rule out ectopic pregnancy, which can be a surgical emergency. This information is also critical as it could significantly alter the medical and/or surgical approach to the pathology responsible

for the abdominal pain. Other gynecologic causes include ruptured follicular or corpus luteum cyst, ovarian torsion, pelvic inflammatory disease, or salpingitis. Infectious causes such as viral gastroenteritis, Yersinia infections, and mesenteric adenitis can all mimic appendicitis with acute right lower quadrant abdominal pain. Abdominal wall defects, such as ventral and inguinal hernias, can also cause acute onset of abdominal pain in this region if intestinal contents become incarcerated or strangulated within the hernia.

Causes of left lower quadrant abdominal pain include many of the disease processes that cause pain in the right lower quadrant with some variability in the likelihood of certain diagnoses. Diverticulitis of the sigmoid colon more frequently causes left lower quadrant pain (Fig. 2.7). Out-pouches of the colon, or diverticulum, are common in the Western population and increase in frequency with age. These diverticula can become inflamed and lead to localized pain, perforation, abscess, and more rarely gross contamination of the abdominal cavity. Similar to right lower quadrant symptoms, urogenital and gynecologic causes of pain along with abdominal wall defects can also present with left lower quadrant pain if the process occurs on the left side.

Many of the disease entities that can present with localized pain can also lead to more diffuse abdominal pain depending on the timeline of symptoms. Any cause of perforated viscus, whether it is due to a peptic ulcer, small bowel obstruction, appendicitis, or colonic diverticulitis, can lead to diffuse abdominal pain throughout

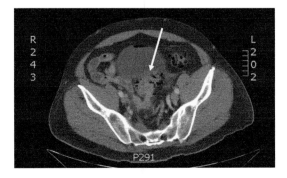

Fig. 2.7 Axial CT images of a patient with sigmoid diverticulitis and associated colovesicle fistula (arrow)

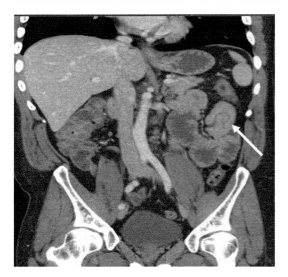

Fig. 2.8 Intussusception of the small intestine in the left upper quadrant (arrow) and proximally dilated bowel

any or all quadrants. The peritonitis that ensues when intestinal contents are spilled into the abdomen leads to a swift inflammatory response and the sensitive nature of the lining of the peritoneum can lead to excruciating pain. Inflammatory bowel disease, such as Crohn's disease or ulcerative colitis, can lead to diffuse abdominal pain. Intussusception is another entity, where a proximal piece of intestine telescopes into a more distal piece of intestine, which can cause obstruction and vascular compromise to the piece telescoping inside (Fig. 2.8). This can happen anywhere throughout the abdomen and therefore can cause pain in any location. Intestinal ischemia can also occur throughout the abdomen and lead to either localized or diffuse symptoms.

Management Considerations

After taking a history and performing a physical exam, reviewing the laboratory and radiographic results and narrowing the differential diagnosis, then the decision must be made on what to do for the patient. The ultimate decision will depend on many factors involving the patient's hemodynamic status, goals of care, and disease processes. While many causes of acute abdominal pain may

require urgent surgical intervention, others may require a period of observation or be able to be managed nonoperatively. The patient and the surgeon should have a discussion to consider the options for management, outline what those options entail, the risks involved with each option, and answer any questions that the patient has about the proposed procedure or disease process. It is important to not just consider the immediate short-term expectations and risks, but what the long-term sequela and recovery period will be like for the patient and tailor it to consider the patients' other comorbidities. If the patient is unable to participate either due to prior medical conditions or altered mental status, then these discussions should take place with the patient's legal representative. Each state has laws that govern the hierarchy for which of the patient's family members or representatives would be in charge of making decisions for them if they are unable to and do not have a medical power of attorney or physician's order for life-sustaining therapy (POLST) already established.

Endoscopic interventions can be used to address a multitude of issues leading to acute abdominal pain. Esophagogastroduodenoscopy can evaluate any lesions in the esophagus, stomach, and duodenum (Fig. 2.9). Peptic ulcers, although less common now with the widespread use of proton-pump inhibitors, can be intervened on with endoscopy if they have not led to a perforation. For complicated gallstone disease, endoscopic retrograde cholangiopancreatography (ERCP) can also be used. This is especially useful in the patient who presents with acute abdominal pain and is found to have gallstone pancreatitis as relieving the obstructing gallstone from the ampulla of Vater in a timely manner is essential to reducing the morbidity. Foreign body ingestion can also lead to acute abdominal pain, and upper endoscopy can be used to remove many objects as long as they have not traveled past the duodenum into the jejunum. Colonoscopy also has a role in patients with acute lower gastrointestinal hemorrhage and can be diagnostic and therapeutic by either clipping a bleeding vessel or using other methods to stop hemorrhage.

Fig. 2.9 Endoscopic images showing a duodenal ulcer with adherent clot

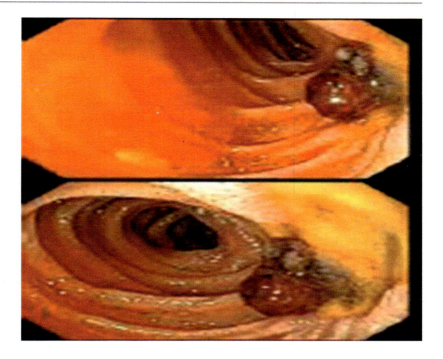

There are many disease processes that require surgical intervention to relieve the patient's symptoms. Appendicitis is one of the most common causes for acute abdominal pain and traditionally has been a disease process that has been managed surgically. There have been many studies and conflicting data, but some advocate for nonoperative treatment with antibiotics. Nonoperative treatment has higher failure rates but may avoid the risks of surgery in some patients [7, 8]. Acute cholecystitis is another very common cause of acute abdominal pain. For patients that do not have associated pancreatitis and are surgical candidates, operative cholecystectomy is the treatment of choice. In patients that are not good surgical candidates, due to other comorbidities or instability due to sepsis, cholecystostomy tube placement for decompression and source control is another option with the possibility of future cholecystectomy when the patient is more stable and optimized for the operating room.

Over the last few decades, a push toward more minimally invasive surgery with laparoscopy and now robotic-assisted laparoscopy has led to shorter hospitalizations and improved outcomes for many general surgery procedures. Although some patients presenting with acute abdominal pain are either not candidates or have contraindications for laparoscopy, minimally invasive techniques still have a large role in acute care surgery and patients with acute abdominal symptoms. Not only is laparoscopy generally used for common operations, such as appendectomy and cholecystectomy, it can also be used to explore the abdomen in a patient who still does not have a definitive diagnosis after their initial workup. Laparoscopy may be performed when certain pathology such as bowel obstruction, intussusception, or ischemic bowel is suspected but not confirmed with imaging. By starting with this technique, the surgeon can explore most parts of the abdomen quickly and, if no pathology is identified, only leave the patient with a few small incisions greatly reducing postoperative pain and morbidity. If concerning findings are identified on laparoscopic exploration, depending on the disease process, the patient's status, and the surgeons minimally invasive skills, the issue can often be addressed laparoscopically. If conversion to a laparotomy is necessary, this can be done easily and quickly. Patients who have had extensive prior abdominal operations are hemo-dynamically unstable, or if preoperative workup indicates the need for operative intervention that the surgeon does not feel can be completed laparoscopically, laparotomy is indicated.

Midline laparotomy is the approach for many patients who require surgical intervention after presenting with acute onset abdominal pain. Many disease processes will require an open approach, as opposed to the minimally invasive approach described earlier. But, it is not always the disease process that mandates a more invasive approach but rather the patient's condition. Patients with hemodynamic instability should not undergo laparoscopy. The insufflation of the abdomen with carbon dioxide reduces the venous return from the inferior vena cava and therefore decreases preload. This may worsen a patient's hemodynamics to a critical point and can lead to cardiovascular collapse. This increased intra-abdominal pressure with laparoscopy also may preclude laparoscopy in patients with underlying pulmonary disease causing hypercapnia as the increased pressure can make ventilation difficult. Patients who have had multiple prior abdominal surgeries also present an increased risk when performing laparoscopy and should be approached with an open operation due to likely dense scar tissue and risk of injuring the underlying bowel. Uncorrectable coagulopathy is also a contraindication to laparoscopic intervention due to the concern for not being able to control bleeding adequately that may occur. Although not an absolute contraindication, laparoscopy should be used with caution in patients with bowel obstruction and severely dilated small intestine due to the increased risk for iatrogenic injury.

The postoperative care of patients is a crucial part of their management. The care after the operation is as essential as any other step in the diagnosis or treatment. After undergoing abdominal operations, patients are at risk for many different complications, some inherent to the specific operation, but there are many that are ubiquitous to all operations.

Infection, mainly wound infections, is a common complication after abdominal surgery and is increased if there is leakage or resection of the intestine involved in the operation. Wounds should be examined daily for signs of infection such as erythema, increased pain, or drainage. Patients are also at risk for other infections such as pneumonia or urinary tract infections. Respiratory care with incentive spirometry, early mobilization, and adequate pain control to facilitate deep breathing and coughing are key to reducing the risk of pneumonia. Proper Foley catheter insertion and care help reduce the risk of urinary tract infections, and early removal of the Foley postoperatively is critical. Intra-abdominal infections can also be seen after abdominal operations, and again the risk is increased if there is gross contamination or resection of bowel is necessary. If a resection and anastomosis is performed, there is a risk that the new anastomosis may leak postoperatively.

Surgery and immobilization also puts patients at risk for deep vein thrombosis (DVT) and pulmonary embolism (PE). Hospitalized patients who have decreased mobility after surgery should be placed on prophylactic anticoagulation with either unfractionated heparin, low-molecular-weight heparin, or fondaparinux [9]. DVT can cause morbidity with leg swelling and pain due to venous congestion, but the concerning sequela of DVT is dislodgement of the thrombosis leading to pulmonary embolism. Other postoperative complications include myocardial infarction, intra-abdominal adhesions leading to bowel obstruction, hernia at the site of the incision, or injury to other intra-abdominal organs that were not involved in the original operation.

Special Populations

Certain populations of patients are at increased risk of developing particular disease processes or have distinct considerations that a surgeon must take into account when caring for them. These populations can also require variations in postoperative management that may influence their ultimate outcome.

Elderly patients are becoming an increasing demographic and require more medical care than their younger counterparts. Elderly patients are more likely to be frail and malnourished and have more comorbidities than younger patients which puts them at higher risk for postoperative complications. Frailty in elderly patients requiring an emergency surgical procedure is associated with increased mortality, ICU and total length of stay, institutional discharge, and cost of care [10]. One particular postoperative complication that occurs commonly in the elderly is delirium after general anesthesia which affects around 20% of patients >65 years in the general emergency surgery population [11]. Using minimally invasive techniques, nonnarcotic pain control, radiologic interventions, and early recognition of symptoms can lead to improved outcomes in the elderly experiencing delirium.

The pregnant patient also brings unique challenges to dealing with an acute abdomen. Pregnancy causes many different physiologic changes in the mother and adds the extra element of the care for the unborn fetus while approaching these patients. While there can be diagnostic challenges when working up a pregnant patient with acute abdominal pain, it is important to decrease any fetal risk when possible but never at the expense of the safety of the mother. When working up a pregnant patient with acute abdominal pain, the imaging test of choice is ultrasound whenever possible as this does not expose the fetus to radiation. While it is important to minimize the radiation to the fetus, critical imaging such as CT can be done with reasonable risks of future malignancies [12]. While there are risks of general anesthesia to the fetus, current recommendations support proceeding with an indicated operation regardless of term of pregnancy. Postponing necessary surgery until after the baby is delivered can lead to increased complication rates for both the mother and fetus.

When a pregnant patient requires an operation, there are a few very important things to consider. Patient positioning is very important, and pregnant patients in the supine position should have a bump placed under their right flank to reduce the pressure on the IVC from the gravid uterus when laying supine and facilitating venous return. Laparoscopy can safely be performed in the pregnant patient regardless of term of gesta-

tion. Entrance into the abdomen should be done using an open (Hasson) technique, and adjustment of port placement should take the fundal height into account. Insufflation pressures during laparoscopy should be maintained between 12 and 15 mmHg. Prior to taking a patient to the operating room, consultation with the obstetrics team and discussion of intraoperative fetal monitoring should also be considered. Current recommendations recommend against prophylactic tocolytic therapy, but these should be initiated if there are any signs of preterm labor preoperatively, during the operation, or postoperatively [13].

Another population that can present a unique set of challenges for a surgeon evaluating acute abdominal pain is the immunocompromised patient. Whether the immunodeficiency is congenital or acquired from malignancy, acquired immunodeficiency syndrome (AIDS), post-organ transplantation, or chronic steroid use, these patients can present with severe pathology but only minimal symptoms and therefore require a thorough workup. These minimal or atypical presentations are due to the depressed immune response that these patients will mount. Due to this, immunocompromised patients can decompensate quickly. Patients with intestinal lymphoma leading to perforation are not uncommon and this may be the presenting event. Other types of therapies the patient may need in the near future, such as chemotherapy for lymphoma, should be taken into consideration if resection of bowel is necessary as this may affect the decision to make an anastomosis or opt for an ostomy.

Conclusion

When evaluating a patient who presents with acute abdominal pain, the surgeon must be thorough and systematic in their approach. Outcomes for many patients presenting with acute abdominal pain rely on prompt and accurate diagnosis and proper management. Some of the most difficult decisions a surgeon will make are when to and when not to operate. The ability to take a focused history, perform a proper physical exam, and know what confirmatory laboratory and imaging studies is the key to elucidating the correct management. Early diagnosis and management is critical to reducing morbidity in patients presenting with acute abdominal pain.

References

1. Pitts SR, Niska RW, Xu J, Burt CW. National Hospital Ambulatory Medical Care Survey: 2006 emergency department summary. Natl Health Stat Report. 2008;(7):1–38.
2. Kamin RA, Nowicki TA, Courtney DS, Powers RD. Pearls and pitfalls in the emergency department evaluation of abdominal pain. Emerg Med Clin North Am. 2003;21(1):61–72. vi
3. Felder S, Margel D, Murrell Z, Fleshner P. Usefulness of bowel sound auscultation: a prospective evaluation. J Surg Educ. 2014;71(5):768–73.
4. Breum BM, Rud B, Kirkegaard T, Nordentoft T. Accuracy of abdominal auscultation for bowel obstruction. World J Gastroenterol. 2015;21(34):10018–24.
5. Stoker J, van Randen A, Lameris W, Boermeester MA. Imaging patients with acute abdominal pain. Radiology. 2009;253(1):31–46.
6. Ghassemi KA, Jensen DM. Lower GI bleeding: epidemiology and management. Curr Gastroenterol Rep. 2013;15(7):333.
7. Mason RJ, Moazzez A, Sohn H, Katkhouda N. Meta-analysis of randomized trials comparing antibiotic therapy with appendectomy for acute uncomplicated (no abscess or phlegmon) appendicitis. Surg Infect. 2012;13(2):74–84.
8. Di Saverio S, Sibilio A, Giorgini E, Biscardi A, Villani S, Coccolini F, et al. The NOTA study (non operative treatment for acute appendicitis): prospective study on the efficacy and safety of antibiotics (amoxicillin and clavulanic acid) for treating patients with right lower quadrant abdominal pain and long-term follow-up of conservatively treated suspected appendicitis. Ann Surg. 2014;260(1):109–17.
9. Douketis JD, Spyropoulos AC, Spencer FA, Mayr M, Jaffer AK, Eckman MH, et al. Perioperative management of antithrombotic therapy: antithrombotic therapy and prevention of thrombosis, 9th ed: American College of Chest Physicians Evidence-Based Clinical Practice Guidelines. Chest. 2012;141(2 Suppl):e326S–e50S.
10. McIsaac DI, Moloo H, Bryson GL, van Walraven C. The association of frailty with outcomes and resource use after emergency general surgery: a population-based cohort study. Anesth Analg. 2017;124(5):1653–61.
11. Moug SJ, Stechman M, McCarthy K, Pearce L, Myint PK, Hewitt J. Frailty and cognitive impairment: unique challenges in the older emergency surgical patient. Ann R Coll Surg Engl. 2016;98(3):165–9.
12. American College of O, Gynecologists' Committee on Obstetric P. Committee Opinion No. 656: Guidelines for diagnostic imaging during pregnancy and lactation. Obstet Gynecol. 2016;127(2):e75–80.
13. Pearl J, Price RR, Tonkin AE, Richardson WS, Stefanidis D. Society of american gastrointestinal and endoscopic surgeons. SAGES guidelines for the use of laparoscopy during pregnancy. 2017. SAGES: USA.

Imaging in Emergency General Surgery

Mathew Giangola and Joaquim M. Havens

The modalities of imaging patients with abdominal pain vary greatly. From plain film X-rays to nuclear imaging, all tests must be pertinent, sensitive, and specific in that they will change management depending on their results. The quickest exams such as a chest or abdominal X-ray may show signs of an emergent pathology which preclude further, more time-consuming, and expensive imaging. However, if initial tests are negative, more powerful tools such as ultrasound, multidetector computed tomography (CT), or magnetic resonance imaging (MRI) may be needed. Nuclear imaging has a role in further delineating the pathology if these subsequent studies require further characterization. Invasive radiologic procedures can be ordered as well, such as endoscopic ultrasound (EUS) and endoscopic retrograde cholangiography (ERCP) and angiography (Table 3.1).

Generalized Abdominal Pain

Abdominal pain in the acute setting can be a diagnostic challenge for which radiologic tests become increasingly useful. The most common causes of the acute abdomen are appendicitis, bowel obstruction, urinary tract disorders, and diverticulitis [1]; however when a physical exam fails to localize pain and laboratory tests cannot predict the most likely pathology, the recommended imaging is a CT scan with IV contrast. In a prospective study of 584 patients, CT improved diagnostic certainty to 92% from 70.5% and altered management in 42% of cases. In that study, 24.1% of patients who were planned to be admitted but subsequently underwent a CT scan were able to be discharged due to the findings on imaging [2]. Given the clinical suspicion, postsurgical/trauma state, chronicity, or underlying comorbidity, this can be altered to forgo or include oral contrast. A CT scan with IV and oral contrast may aid in visualizing mucosal pathology which can be common in the immunocompromised or HIV-/CMV-infected patients. Multiple studies have shown CT scans for acute abdominal pain do not require oral contrast, however, as most radiologists determine that no further information would have been provided by enteric contrast [3, 4]. Additionally, omitting oral contrast speeds throughput in the emergency room, and rarely do patients require additional imaging

M. Giangola
Trauma, Burn and Critical Care Surgery, Brigham and Women's Hospital, Boston, MA, USA

J. M. Havens (✉)
Department of Surgery, Brigham and Women's Hospital, Boston, MA, USA
e-mail: jhavens@bwh.harvard.edu

© Springer International Publishing AG, part of Springer Nature 2019
C. V. R. Brown et al. (eds.), *Emergency General Surgery*, https://doi.org/10.1007/978-3-319-96286-3_3

Table 3.1 Types of radiologic imaging

Modality	Common indications	Possible limitations
Chest X-ray	Perforated viscus Hiatal/paraesophageal hernia	Limited view of the abdomen, nonspecific
Abdominal X-ray	Small bowel obstruction, ileus, large bowel obstruction	Nonspecific
CT/CTA scan	All the above + inflammatory disease, mesenteric ischemia	Ionizing radiation, contrast allergy/reaction, expensive
MRI/MRA	Assessing the pregnant patient, chronic mesenteric ischemia, bile duct continuity	Slower, more time consumptive, expensive
Ultrasound	Cholecystitis, appendicitis	Operator dependent, body habitus dependent, does not view the entire abdominal field

CT computed tomography, *CTA* computed tomography angiography, *MRI* magnetic resonance imaging, *MRA* magnetic resonance angiography

due to a lack of oral contrast [5]. The advantages of a CT scan are that it can visualize most structures well and can detect many acute surgical pathologies. Smaller droplets of air, particularly located at the mesentery root, are best imaged through a CT scan compared to abdominal X-ray. Bowel wall edema, bowel distention, and ischemia as well as transition point locations are all best imaged on CT scan [6].

Fluid radiodensity is of particular interest to emergency general surgeons as it allows the differentiation between simple fluid and blood. The radiodensity is measured by Hounsfield units (HU) where water is 0 HU and air is −1000 HU. Fluid can measure anywhere between 0 and 50 HU, whereas a hematoma may measure approximately 45–65 HU. Bile, blood, and other fluids have ranges where the radiologist or surgeon can make a reasonable differential regarding the fluid, in some reports finding that <43 HU is sensitive for bowel perforation in blunt trauma [7]. Infections cannot be reliably predicted in this manner, but the presence of gas, loculation, or rim enhancement around a collection can all be signs of an infection or abscess. The postoperative period may make free intraperitoneal fluid more or less concerning depending on the operation and scenario and characterization of this fluid.

Other imaging modalities can be sought if presented different clinical situations. As will be discussed in their respective sections, suspected appendicitis and cholecystitis warrant an ultrasound of the right lower or right upper quadrant as their initial imaging. Due to the poor specificity of abdominal plain films, KUB X-rays are not the recommended primary imaging modality. Kellow et al. reviewed a series of more than 800 patients and found that abdominal X-rays obviated follow-up imaging in as little as 4% of patients and aided in diagnosis in only 2–8% [8]. The pregnant patient should undergo ultrasound or MRI rather than a CT as to avoid radiation. However, recent literature as shown that CT scans in the pregnant patient are safe with limited use and after nonionizing studies are deemed inconclusive. If a patient exhibits ongoing sepsis with an unclear source on CT scan, nuclear imaging with a tagged WBC abdominal scan to locate infection and/or abscesses may be used. Neutropenic patients may benefit from immediate CT scan due to their unreliability to develop leukocytosis or peritonitis on physical exam. However, a CT in this patient population rarely alters nonoperative intentions as most patients will likely have a medically treated disease such as enterocolitis or typhlitis [9].

Due to the emergent nature of these surgical pathologies and patients, imaging can help stratify risk using the American Association for the Surgery of Trauma (AAST) grading system, allowing the emergency patient to be distinguished from the elective case [10].

Stomach and Duodenum

Radiological exams should focus on ruling in or out inflammation, perforation, volvulus, hernia, ischemia, and obstruction; however there are many pathologies which may cause pain from a gastric or duodenal source.

Gastroduodenal Perforation

The stomach may perforate from ulceration, cancer, ischemia, or post-chemotherapy treatment and other pathologies which present as pneumoperitoneum on imaging. The first step in evaluation of the upper GI tract is usually through upright chest X-ray (CXR) or a KUB (kidney, ureter, and bladder X-ray), most likely in the AP (anterior-posterior) view. Although this imaging modality tends to be of lower sensitivity and falsely enlarges structures closest to the X-ray source (such as the heart), it is ideal for critically ill patients who cannot stand upright for long periods of time required for the PA (posterior-anterior) view. The pathognomonic sign for a perforated viscus is pneumoperitoneum, commonly referred to as "free air," which is gas presumably from the intestinal tract within the peritoneal cavity. The presence of free air and peritonitis on abdominal exam is a surgical emergency, and one may proceed to the operating room with the suspicion of a perforated viscus; however, further imaging can aid with operative planning in the stable patient. Demonstration of a perforation can be achieved via CT scan with IV contrast if ischemia/ulceration is suspected, with the ability to enhance the bowel walls. In this setting, oral contrast can be omitted as it does not increase the sensitivity of demonstrating a leak (19–42%) and can mask nonopacification of the bowel wall. In a study of 85 patients with pathologically confirmed perforations, radiologists could accurately locate the perforation in 86% of the patients on preoperative CT scan without oral contrast [11].

Nonvariceal Upper Gastrointestinal Bleeding

Treatment for gastrointestinal hemorrhage centers around stabilizing the patient and locating the site of the active bleed. History, presentation, and gastric lavage can aid in locating the bleed. Esophagogastroduodenoscopy (EGD) within 24 h is recommended for both definitive diagnosis and simultaneous treatment [12]. Multiple randomized controlled and retrospective studies have shown no benefit to early (within 6 h) endoscopy compared to endoscopy before 24 h from diagnosis [13, 14]. These studies enroll different patients with discrepancies between their Rockall and Glasgow Blatchford scores but overall confirm this finding. Early endoscopy does however have a higher likelihood to finding an actively bleeding vessel and a high incidence of hemostatic intervention by the endoscopist [15]. If EGD is performed and upper GI blood is found but the exact location is not delineated, CT angiography (CTA) of the abdomen is useful. The advantage over conventional angiography is that CTA can detect multiple sites of bleeding simultaneously, even if they are anatomically distant from each other [16]. CTA can detect acutely bleeding sources at rates from 0.3 mL/min, whereas conventional angiography may be slightly less sensitive at 0.5 mL to 1 mL/min [17]. In the setting of a bleed which is definitively found by endoscopy, but cannot be controlled, angiography and transcatheter arterial embolization (TAE) is the preferred treatment.[9]

Gastric Volvulus

The stomach may rotate upon two different axes to cause a mechanical obstruction and ischemia. Urgent decompression and detorsion is needed and as such, recognition must occur rapidly. Given the constellation of symptoms such as retching, epigastric pain, and inability to pass a nasogastric tube (Borchardt's triad),

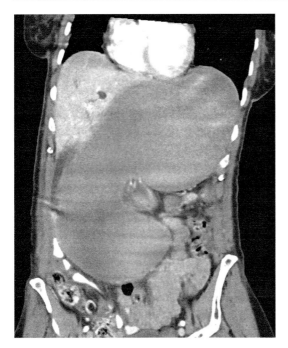

Fig. 3.1 CT scan showing organoaxial gastric volvulus with massive gastric distension

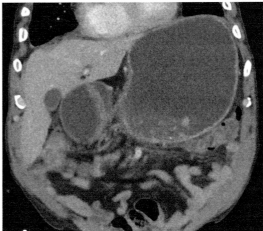

Fig. 3.2 CT scan showing gastric outlet obstruction with a distended stomach and decompressed small bowel

Along with an upright CXR, the absence of passage of oral contrast on either upper GI series or CT scan with PO contrast is indicative of gastric outlet obstruction (Fig. 3.2).

plain films can be ordered first. Gastric volvulus can be seen on chest X-ray and/or abdominal X-ray as a distended portion of the stomach with an air-fluid level and decompressed duodenum and small bowel. If necrosis or perforation is suspected, a CT scan with IV contrast may help visualize an under-perfused or frankly ischemic stomach wall as well as an abscess (Fig. 3.1). An upper GI fluoroscopic series can delineate the type and severity of volvulus: the twisting occurring upon the organoaxial or mesoenteroaxial axis as well as if contrast passes through the twisted portion. A volvulus may also be associated with paraesophageal hernia with herniated intrathoracic stomach, colon, or spleen.

Gastric Outlet Obstruction

This pathology had been a more prevalent etiology of upper abdominal pain and bloating; however since gastric acid suppression therapy, chronic strictures due to ulceration have declined.

Small Bowel

Small Bowel Obstruction

Suspected SBO is a frequent emergency surgical consultation. Most commonly caused by postoperative adhesions or hernias, a thorough physical exam is mandatory. Should a hernia be found, it can be rapidly dealt with; however in the absence of an overt hernia, radiologic exam is warranted. There is controversy with diagnosing an SBO on plain film X-rays vs immediately obtaining a CT scan. A CT with IV contrast can yield the most pertinent information as radiologists are able to adequately predict a need for surgery based on image characteristics [18]. If a high-grade SBO or an SBO with ischemia is suspected, oral contrast should *not* be given. Dilation of the small bowel >3 cm is concerning as well as the presence of a transition point, free fluid, and mesenteric edema. Small bowel fecalization ("small bowel feces sign") may represent functioning bowel, a reassuring sign; however this also portends slow transit through the small bowel [19].

Pathways requiring imaging to calculate the probability of an SBO requiring operative management have been proposed. Zielinski et al. found statistically significant features on CT scan were mesenteric edema, the lack of a small bowel feces sign, as well as a history of obstipation [20]. It is important to note most studies that use radiologic criteria to stratify risk for SBO exclude patients with peritonitis and/or findings of ischemia on CT. Also, a CT scan is not adequately sensitive for detecting early ischemia; however when the aforementioned signs are present, it is very specific for ischemia; one must rely on clinical judgment if findings are equivocal [21]. Only in the setting of a stable patient with an intermittent or low-grade SBO should oral contrast evaluate the bowel and/or be given as per a small bowel follow-through protocol or pathway [22]. In this setting, undiluted oral contrast can be followed with serial KUBs until it reaches the colon, usually within 8 h; however any time before 24 h is considered successful. This can be ~92% sensitive and specific for nonoperative resolution of the SBO [23]. The usage of oral contrast does have controversy within the literature, as most emergency surgical pathologies do not require opacification of the bowel lumen. However, there are still possible benefits of oral contrast as outlined by Kammerer et al., suggesting careful patient selection is required to obtain meaningful use. They argue that bowel edema, inflammation, and bowel delineation from surrounding structures, especially in thinner patients without much mesenteric fat, may benefit from oral contrast [24]. Oral contrast used as a cathartic is also a therapeutic option in those without the suspicion of ischemic bowel or strangulation. A closed-loop bowel obstruction is an entity which should be recognized early and treated quickly. A segment of the bowel with two transition points, a lumen narrowing or "beak sign," a radial pattern of mesenteric vasculature, and a "U/C" shape of the bowel are characteristic of a closed-loop obstruction [25] (Fig. 3.3). In patients with diffusely dilated small bowel, a CT can differentiate between an ileus reliably, with a sensitivity and specificity approaching of 90%. An Ileus is radiologically defined as distention of both the small

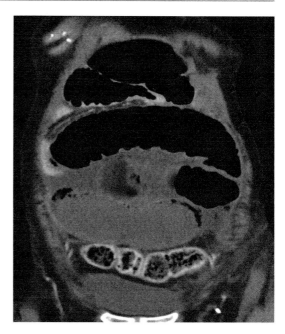

Fig. 3.3 Closed-loop SBO with free fluid

and large bowel without a clear transition point. Non-passage or oral contrast through the intestinal tract can also detect adynamic ileus. MRI for intestinal obstruction is reserved for the pediatric or pregnant population but should be pursued if all other tests are inconclusive.

CT enterography has questionable value in SBO, as some patients cannot tolerate large volumes of liquid [26].

Mesenteric Ischemia

One of the most worrisome pathologies which causes diffuse abdominal pain is acute mesenteric ischemia, commonly caused by embolism or thrombosis of the superior mesenteric artery. Nonocclusive mesenteric ischemia is caused by a generalized low-flow state to the intestines. In the clinical setting in which mesenteric ischemia is suspected, the recommended first-line imaging is a CTA of the abdomen and pelvis [27]. The CTA will reveal the site of embolism or thrombosis, stenosis, or dissection (Fig. 3.4). A venous phase CT will reveal mesenteric venous thrombosis as well. Bowel characteristics of ischemia can

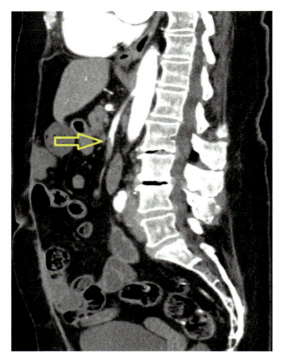

Fig. 3.4 Superior mesenteric artery embolism (arrow) causing acute mesenteric ischemia

include wall thickening, hypoattenuation, portal-venous gas, pneumatosis, and mesenteric strand-ing. With the findings of vessel abnormalities and the latter findings of bowel ischemia, the sensitiv-ity and specificity of a CTA reach 94% and 96%, respectively [27]. Conventional angiography is considered if preoperative planning is needed; however given the acuity of the ischemia, this is usually forgone to allow for rapid operative treat-ment. Magnetic resonance angiography is gener-ally not recommended as it has a poor sensitivity to detect distal thrombus or emboli [28].

Large Bowel

Appendicitis

Along with a compelling history and physical, imaging can diagnose appendicitis in the vast majority of cases with an acceptable negative exploration rate. In the setting of an unclear exam, imaging becomes the underpinning of diagnosis – in some reports cutting the negative appendectomy rate from 16% to 8% [29]. The current guidelines for imaging a patient with sus-pected appendicitis begins with a right lower quadrant ultrasound. Ultrasound is a very useful technique but is highly operator dependent and relies on favorable anatomy and anatomic win-dows. In combination with a high Alvarado score, findings such as a dilated and noncompressible appendix, hyperemia, and free fluid on ultra-sound can approach sensitivity and specificity of CT scan [30]. It is reserved as the sole modality for those who wish to avoid radiation such as the pediatric and pregnant population before an MRI. If the ultrasound is inconclusive, a CT with IV contrast is recommended as the sensitivity is near 90% and specificity is about 95% [31]. Evaluation by a surgeon should be carried out before ordering a CT scan in children or young adults due to the relatively benign nature of diag-nostic laparoscopy and availability of MRI. PO contrast should only be given if IV contrast can-not be used. CT is also beneficial in that perfora-tion, phlegmon, typhlitis, or a fecalith can be visualized and alter the treatment plan from sur-gery to medical management or vice versa. The anatomic position of the appendix can also be seen, facilitating surgical planning (retrocecal, malrotation). MRI is reserved for pregnant patients; however it should be noted that appendi-citis in the pregnant patient is an emergency, mandating a STAT MRI. If an MRI cannot be obtained, a CT scan while pregnant is thought to be safe, as previously stated in the Generalized Abdominal Pain section.

Diverticulitis

Diagnosing and staging the severity of diverticu-litis depends on radiographic evidence of inflam-mation of the colon and any associated abscesses, free fluid, or air. Thus, a CT scan with IV contrast should be ordered in this scenario. The IV con-trast is used to delineate the bowel wall and any abscess cavities. If used, PO contrast can differ-entiate diverticular pockets from adjacent abscesses – in some cases aiding in percutaneous drainage [32]. Rectal contrast is not suggested as the sensitivity and specificity are matched by conventional IV or PO contrast. Findings on CT scan can be suggestive of simple inflammation or an underlying malignant process. Classification of diverticulitis centers around the degree of inflammation and the presence of perforation. Hinchey et al. [33] originally described four stages: Stage 1, pericolic abscess; Stage 2, pelvic intra-abdominal/retroperitoneal abscess; Stage 3, generalized purulent peritonitis; and Stage 4, generalized fecal peritonitis. Since then, multiple attempts to better stratify the severity of diverticulitis has evolved, all centering around CT evidence of perforation and abscess as well as hemodynamic and perfusion status [34]. Lymphadenopathy and limited inflammation of the colon can be visualized and may portend a high risk of cancer-associated perforation. Following CT scan in the acute setting, patients should be evaluated with colonoscopy when diverticulitis has resolved.

Involvement of interventional radiology is recommended when abscesses are large enough to drain and percutaneously accessible. CT-guided aspiration and/or drain placement is warranted for stable patients.

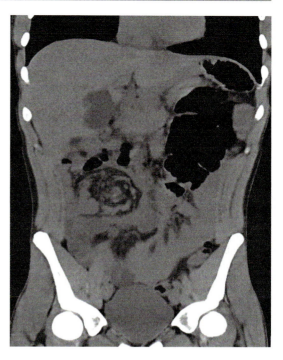

Fig. 3.5 Cecal volvulus with a prominent mesenteric swirl in the right lower quadrant and the cecum displaced into the left upper quadrant

Cecal and Sigmoid Volvulus

The most common site of colonic volvulus is the sigmoid (~90%) and the cecum (<20%). A cecal volvulus is a surgical emergency as the bowel twists along the ileocolic pedicle, its blood supply, and should be reported to the surgeon immediately (Fig. 3.5). An abdominal plain film can be diagnostic if a pathognomonic finding is seen, that being a twisted loop in the right lower quadrant "pointing to the left upper quadrant. A cecal "bascule" can also cause obstruction and a distended large loop of the bowel; however this is not a rotation around the ileocolic pedicle, but rather a folding of the cecum anteriorly and superiorly. A sigmoid volvulus is created when a redundant descending colon twists along the mesenteric root (Fig. 3.6). The pathognomonic finding in this case is a left lower quadrant obstruction with

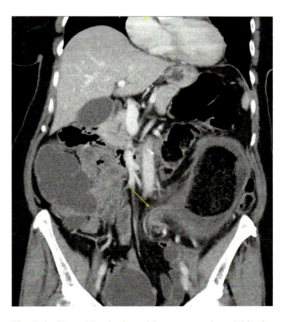

Fig. 3.6 Sigmoid volvulus with a mesenteric swirl in the left lower quadrant and distended colon with a transition point distally. *Arrow* denotes mesenteric swirl in the left lower quadrant

a distended loop pointing to the right upper quadrant given the appearance of a "coffee bean" shape. A bird's-beak narrowing is seen in the left lower quadrant if a gastrografin enema is performed. Although confirmed through history, physical, and abdominal X-ray, a CT scan with IV contrast can aid in decision-making if a cecal bascule is suspected rather than volvulus. A sigmoid volvulus would also be preferentially imaged with CT with IV contrast if a plain X-ray is insufficient. CT scan can display a whirling pattern of the tapering bowel, twisted mesentery, and a focal point at the fixated root. For a sigmoid volvulus, urgent decompression through colonoscopy is warranted, whereas immediate operative intervention is needed for cecal volvulus.

Lower GI Bleeding

Acute gastrointestinal bleeding suspected to be of lower GI source follows the principle of resuscitation and stabilization of the patient which then allows the localization of the source. If the patient is too unstable for imaging, urgent operative or in some cases, interventional radiologic, procedures are indicated.

In the stable or transient responder, localization of the bleeding source can be achieved through multiple avenues. The first appropriate modality should be through colonoscopy which is both diagnostic and therapeutic. If the lesion is not amenable to endoscopic hemostasis, conventional angiography and embolization can be employed. Angiography can detect bleeding rates between 0.5 and 1.5 ml/min. If the patient is stable and a source still not found, a CT angiogram (rate, 0.3–0.5 ml/min) can be obtained to localize the bleed. If persistent, low-volume bleeding occurs and colonoscopy nor CT angiogram reveals the source, a tagged RBC scan may pick up minute amounts of extravasating blood (0.1–0.5 ml/min). This is a poor exam to localize the exact location but can aid in the management choices. Demonstrated by Bentley et al., Tc-99 m-labeled RBC scan can detect rates of bleeding from 0.1 mL/min and may be used in patients with an obscure GI bleed, but it has an inferior sensitivity compared to angiography [35, 36]. Also, nuclear imaging is not always immediately available and may require extended time to scan. For these reasons, nuclear imagine is not recommended in the acute setting. For patients who are stable or display an intermittently bleeding pathology, a video capsule endoscopy may be useful [37].

Ischemic Colitis

Low-flow states to the bowel produce transient inflammation and injury to the target end organ. Ischemic colitis is thus best evaluated through CT with IV contrast [38, 39]. This allows the detection of bowel wall enhancement and arterial phase option of vessel inflow and runoff. Watershed areas of the bowel are most prone to low-flow states, and the presence or absence of collateral blood can be shown via CTA [40]. Concerning findings would be bowel wall edema, pneumatosis, free fluid, free air, or bowel wall discontinuity. Oral contrast should not be administered as it may obscure the character of the bowel wall. Defining the vasculature, CTA is ideal for evaluating the take of the aortic SMA and IMA roots. MRA can be used but is not as sensitive as CTA for more distal, small arteries as stated in the Mesenteric Ischemia section.

Postsurgical Anastomotic Leak

The nature of the operation and surgical anatomy must be known prior to evaluating patients with a suspicion for a postsurgical leak. As with generalized abdominal pain, A CT with IV contrast is usually sufficient as PO contrast has not shown an appreciable increase in the detection of small bowel or gastric discontinuity. A low anorectal anastomosis is at a significant risk for postoperative leak. To evaluate for postoperative leaks in patients who are status post low anterior resection or any variant of colectomy, CT w/ IV contrast is preferable with some exceptions. The caveat in postoperative patients is that the surgeon would want to demonstrate an actual leak, thus PO and rectal contrast should be given in these cases [41]. Creating a pressure column within the low-pressure reservoir which is the colon will allow interrogation of the staple line [42]. Once a leak is demonstrated, appropriate management via percutaneous drainage, endoscopic clipping, or operative repair can be pursued.

Hepatobiliary System

Cholecystitis

Right upper quadrant pain has a long differential and accounts for a myriad number of complaints and presentations. One of the most common causes for right upper quadrant pain is cholecystitis. Along with a compatible history, physical, and lab tests, imaging is required for diagnosis. For cholecystitis, a right upper quadrant ultrasound is the most cost effective [43] and quickest way to visualize the gallbladder [44]. The presence of a thickened gallbladder wall (>3 mm), pericholecystic fluid, and a positive Murphy's sign are diagnostic of cholecystitis. Acute calculus cholecystitis is diagnosed if imaging reveals the previous findings plus gallstones or sludge

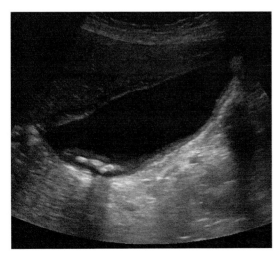

Fig. 3.7 Abdominal ultrasound revealing pericholecystic fluid, a thickened gallbladder wall, and sludge confirming cholecystitis

(Fig. 3.7). The sensitivity of ultrasound ranges from 80% to 90% and an 80–85% specificity for cholecystitis. It is important to note that gallstones are best seen with ultrasound rather than CT with sensitivities of ~95% and 80%, respectively, for cholelithiasis. The most sensitive imaging technique for cholecystitis is HIDA (hepatobiliary iminodiacetic acid) cholescintigraphy with a sensitivity of ~ 96% and specificity of 90%. Although more sensitive, a HIDA scan cannot visualize anatomic structures as well and cannot provide information such as common bile duct size and stone visualization which is why ultrasound is still the recommended first test. HIDA may also be falsely negative in severe gallbladder inflammation that produces intermittent or incomplete cystic duct occlusion. A CT scan can also be useful for operative planning and in ruling out other co-existing pathologies. Evidence of gallbladder perforation, extensive inflammation, polyps, masses, pancreatitis, or other challenging surgical scenarios can be ascertained via CT scan, but is not first-line imaging. MRI for cholecystitis is recommended in the pregnant patient if an ultrasound is inconclusive [45].

Choledocholithiasis and Cholangitis

Similar to cholecystitis, choledocholithiasis should be imaged through ultrasound to delineate the cause of obstruction, site, and severity. The sensitivity and specificity are often quoted at 73% and 91%, respectively, for common bile duct stones [46]. Reliable measurements of the biliary ducts can be ascertained with ultrasound in a quick manner. On average, the common bile duct is noted to be between 5 and 10 mm with an increase of ~1 mm per decade expected; however this assumption is questionable. Some studies reflect a normal upper limit of 6 mm with post-cholecystectomy patients having a 1 mm increase in size. In conjunction with laboratory tests, this can guide patient care toward further tests or interventions such as magnetic resonance cholangiopancreatography (MRCP), EUS, or ERCP. For stones >3 mm, MRCP sensitivity and specificity are 93–94% and 95–100%, respectively. EUS is similarly capable at 95% and 97%, respectively [47]. It is important to note that a CT scan is not recommended because of the inferiority of a CT scan to visualize gallstones; however multidetector CT cholangiography may rival MRCP and EUS. The American Society for Gastrointestinal Endoscopy (ASGE) has stratified those with right upper quadrant pain, jaundice, and fever into high (likely to have cholangitis), intermediate, or low probability of having choledocholithiasis. Based on these criteria, immediate ERCP or further imaging of the ducts with EUS or MRCP is pursued. If the suspicion is low, immediate cholecystectomy with IOC is offered. Post-cholecystectomy patients with new onset RUQ pain and elevated liver enzymes or bilirubin should be evaluated through immediate MRCP or ERCP. Intraoperative cholangiogram (IOC) can be completed if the patency of the duct has not been studied and the patient displays intermediate risk stratification criteria. Routine use of IOC is debatable but still commonly practiced. American Society for Gastrointestinal Endoscopy (ASGE) guidelines help risk stratify patient in regard to ruling out biliary obstruction (Table 3.2).

Pancreatitis

Diffuse, band-like upper abdominal pain is a common complaint and can be initial signs of pancreatitis. Within the United States, gallstones and alcohol are leading causes [48]; however gallstone pancreatitis requires general surgical admission or surgical consultation. The diagnosis of pancreatitis is made through history, physical exam, and elevated lipase and/or amylase levels. A right upper quadrant ultrasound should be performed to identify the presence of gallstones/sludge or choledocholithiasis. This information alone is sufficient to diagnose uncomplicated acute pancreatitis. In those that recover rapidly within the first few days of admission, it is reasonable to forgo a CT scan. However, those that have persistent pain or deteriorate clinically should be imaged to assess for progressing/necrotizing pancreatitis with or without superimposed infection. A prominent scoring classification of pancreatitis based on imaging is the Balthazar criteria, which utilizes a standardized CT grading system. Combining the points accrued from the grade of pancreatic inflammation and the percent necrosis relays a relative clinical severity known as the CT severity index (CTSI) score which is shown in Table 3.3 [49]. There are many clinical severity-stratifying clas-

Table 3.2 American Society for Gastrointestinal Endoscopy (ASGE) management algorithm

High risk (>50% chance of having CBD obstruction) – should receive preoperative ERCP	Any of the following Confirmed choledocholithiasis, clinically evident cholangitis, bilirubin >4 mg/dL Both CBD >6 mm and bilirubin >1.8–4 mg/dL
Intermediate risk (10–50% chance of having CBD obstruction) – should receive pre-op MRCP, EUS, or intraoperative cholangiogram	Any of the following Dilated CBD, age > 55, gallstone pancreatitis Any abnormal LFT
Low risk (<10% chance of having CBD obstruction) – no further imaging	None of the above with symptomatic cholelithiasis

Table 3.3 CT severity index (CTSI) score

Grade A	Normal	0 points
Grade B	Focal or diffuse enlargement or peripancreatic inflammation	1 point
Grade C	Pancreatic gland abnormalities	2 points
Grade D	Fluid collection	3 points
Grade E	Two or more fluid collections, gas adjacent to the pancreas	4 points

No necrosis	0 points
0–30% necrosis	2 points
30–50% necrosis	4 points
Over 50% necrosis	6 points

0–3 points	Mild acute pancreatitis
4–6 points	Moderate acute pancreatitis
7–10 points	Severe acute pancreatitis

sifications available, including Modified Marshall score, Ranson's criteria, POPS, BISAPS, APACHE II, and SOFA criteria, and in all severe or persistent cases, imaging should be obtained in conjunction. The Atlanta Criteria sums these findings up to portend a prognosis and clinical course [50]. Further management regarding peripancreatic fluid collections/abscesses which appear infected should be treated first medically and then, as clinically relevant, be drained via interventional radiologic methods. Drainage can later be augmented via up-sizing drains allowing for eventual video-assisted retroperitoneal pancreatic debridement (VARD) if warranted.

If still the etiology is still unclear or the pancreatitis is persistent/recurrent, an MRCP can be obtained to further aid in the detection of alternate causes such as malignancies or duct/liver pathology. MRCP can be limited due to the intense inflammation of acute pancreatitis, however.

Cellulitis and Necrotizing Soft Tissue Infection (NSTI)

The diagnosis of soft tissue infection relies heavily on clinical suspicion. Utilization of ultrasound to delineate an abscess cavity can be used for surgical planning. A CT scan with IV contrast is helpful in finding foreign bodies if a history of puncture wound or local trauma is obtained. IV contrast-enhanced CT scans can show obliterated end arterial thrombosis which may portend a higher risk of compartment syndrome associated necrotizing fasciitis. Classically, the presence of gas within the soft tissues, which is reported to be ~48% in positive cases, can be detected via CT [51]. More subtle signs such as inflammatory changes beneath the fascia and the presence of fluid collections can both point toward a higher likelihood of NSTI. In a study conducted by Zacharias et al., CT provided a 100% sensitivity and 81% specificity in a review of 67 patients, reflecting the possible utility of ruling out NSTI via CT [52]. In a further investigation of 167 patients, investigators found a sensitivity and specificity of 100% and 98%, respectively, with a

positive predictive value of 76% and a negative predictive value of 100% [53]. MRI with and without contrast for suspected extremity infection can add information such as determining underlying myositis, necrosis, or collection and has a historically slightly higher sensitivity and specificity than CT [54].

References

1. Stoker J, van Randen A, Laméris W, Boermeester MA. Imaging patients with acute abdominal pain. Radiology. 2009;253:31–46.
2. Abujudeh HH, Kaewlai R, McMahon PM, et al. Abdominopelvic CT increases diagnostic certainty and guides management decisions: a prospective investigation of 584 patients in a large academic medical center. AJR Am J Roentgenol. 2011;196:238–43. https://doi.org/10.2214/AJR.10.4467.
3. Hill BC, Johnson SC, Owens EK, Gerber JL, Senagore AJ. CT scan for suspected acute abdominal process: impact of combinations of IV, oral, and rectal contrast. World J Surg. 2010;34:699–703.
4. Kessner R, Barnes S, Halpern P, Makrin V, Blachar A. CT for acute nontraumatic abdominal pain – is oral contrast really required? Acad Radiol. 2017;24(7):840–5.
5. Levenson RB, Camacho MA, Horn E, Saghir A, McGillicuddy SLD. Eliminating routine oral contrast use for CT in the emergency department: impact on patient throughput and diagnosis. Emerg Radiol. 2012;19(6):513–7.
6. Menke J. Diagnostic accuracy of multidetector CT in acute mesenteric ischemia: systematic review and metaanalysis. Radiology. 2010;256(1):93–101.
7. Wong YC, Wang LJ, Wu CH, Chen HW, Lin BC, Hsu YP. Peritoneal fluid of low CT Hounsfield units as a screening criterion for traumatic bowel perforation. Jpn J Radiol. 2017;4:145–50.
8. Kellow ZS, MacInnes M, Kurzencwyg D, et al. The role of abdominal radiography in the evaluation of the nontrauma emergency patient. Radiology. 2008;248:887–93.
9. Badgwell BD, Cormier JN, Wray CJ, Borthakur G, Qiao W, Rolston KV, et al. Challenges in surgical management of abdominal pain in the neutropenic cancer patient. Ann Surg. 2008;248(1):104–9.
10. Tominaga GT, Staudenmayer KL, Shafi S, Schuster KM, Savage SA, Ross S, Muskat P, Mowery NT, Miller P, Inaba K. The American Association for the Surgery of Trauma grading scale for 16 emergency general surgery conditions: disease-specific criteria characterizing anatomic severity grading. J Trauma Acute Care Surg. 2016;81(3):593–602.
11. Hainaux B, Bertinotti E, Maertelaer V, Rubesova E, Capellutoe E. Accuracy of MDCT in predict-

ing site of gastrointestinal tract perforation. AJR. 2006;187:1179–83.

12. Gralnek IM, Dumonceau JM, Kuipers EJ, et al. Diagnosis and management of nonvariceal upper gastrointestinal hemorrhage: European Society of Gastrointestinal Endoscopy (ESGE) guideline. Endoscopy. 2015;47(10):a1–46.

13. Barkun AN, Bardou M, Kuipers EJ, Sung J, Hunt RH, Martel M, Sinclair P, International Consensus Upper Gastrointestinal Bleeding Conference Group. International consensus recommendations on the management of patients with nonvariceal upper gastrointestinal bleeding. Ann Intern Med. 2010;152:101–13.

14. Bjorkman DJ, Zaman A, Fennerty MB, Lieberman D, DiSario JA, Guest-Warnick G. Urgent vs. elective endoscopy for acute non-variceal upper-GI bleeding: an effectiveness study. Gastrointest Endosc. 2004;60(1):1–8. https://doi.org/10.1016/s0016-5107(04)01287-8.

15. Tai CM, Huang SP, Wang HP, et al. High-risk ED patients with nonvariceal upper gastrointestinal hemorrhage undergoing emergency or urgent endoscopy: a retrospective analysis. Am J Emerg Med. 2007;25(3):273–8. https://doi.org/10.1016/j.ajem.2006.07.014.

16. Wu LM, Xu JR, Yin Y, Qu XH. Usefulness of CT angiography in diagnosing acute gastrointestinal bleeding: a meta-analysis. World J Gastroenterol. 2010;16:3957–63.

17. Garcia-Blazquez V, Vicente-Bartulos A, Olavarria-Delgado A, et al. Accuracy of CT angiography in the diagnosis of acute gastrointestinal bleeding: systematic review and meta-analysis. Eur Radiol. 2013;23:1181–90.

18. Scrima A, Lubner MG, King S, Kennedy G, Pickhardt PJ. Abdominal multidetector computed tomography for suspected small-bowel obstruction: multicenter study comparing radiologists performance for predicting surgical outcomes. J Comput Assist Tomogr. 2017;41(3):388–93.

19. Khaled W, Millet I, Corno L, Bouley-Coletta I, Benadjaoud MA, Taourel P, Zins M. Clinical relevance of the feces sign in small-bowel onstruction due to adhesions depends on its location. AJR Am J Roentgenol. 2017;210:78.

20. Zielinski MD, Eiken PW, Heller SF, et al. Prospective, observational validation of a multivariate small-bowel obstruction model to predict the need for operative intervention. J Am Coll Surg. 2011;212:1068.

21. Sheedy SP, Earnest F 4th, Fletcher JG, et al. CT of small-bowel ischemia associated with obstruction in emergency department patients: diagnostic performance evaluation. Radiology. 2006;241:729–36.

22. Azagury D, Liu RC, Morgan A, Spain DA. Small bowel obstruction: a practical step-by-step evidence-based approach to evaluation, decision making, and management. J Trauma Acute Care Surg. 2015;79(4):661–8.

23. Ceresoli M, Coccolini F, Catena F, Montori G, Di Saverio S, Sartelli M. Water-soluble contrast agent in adhesive small bowel obstruction: a systematic review and meta-analysis of diagnostic and therapeutic value. Am J Surg. 2016;211(6):1114–25.

24. Kammerer S, Höink AJ, Wessling J, et al. Abdominal and pelvic CT: is positive enteric contrast still necessary? Results of a retrospective observational study. Eur Radiol. 2014;25(3):669–78.

25. Elsayes KM, Menias CO, Smullen TL, Platt JF. Closed-loop small-bowel obstruction: diagnostic patterns by multidetector computed tomography. J Comput Assist Tomogr. 2007;31(5):697–701.

26. Katz DS, Baker ME, Rosen MP, et al. ACR appropriateness criteria suspected small bowel obstruction. J Am Coll Radiol. 2013;10(6):402–9.

27. Acosta S, Wadman M, Syk I, et al. Epidemiology and prognostic factors in acute superior mesenteric artery occlusion. J Gastrointest Surg. 2010;14:628.

28. Shih MC, Hagspiel K. CTA and MRA in mesenteric ischemia: part 1, role in diagnosis and differential diagnosis. AJR Am J Roentgenol. 2007;188:452–61.

29. Howell JM, Eddy OL, Lukens TW, Thiessen ME, Weingart SD, Decker WW. American College of Emergency Physicians clinical policy: critical issues in the evaluation and management of emergency department patients with suspected appendicitis. Ann Emerg Med. 2010;55:71–116.

30. Reddy S, Kelleher M, et al. A highly sensitive and specific combined clinical and sonographic score to diagnose appendicitis. J Trauma Acute Care Surg. 2017;83(4):643–9.

31. Gorter R, Eker H, et al. Diagnosis and management of acute appendicitis. EAES consensus development conference 2015. Surg Endosc. 2016;30:4668–90.

32. Lorenz JM, Al-Refaie WB, Cash BD, Gaba RC, Gervais DA, Gipson MG, Kolbeck KJ, Kouri BE, Marshalleck FE, Nair AV, Ray CE Jr, Hohenwalter EJ. ACR appropriateness criteria radiologic management of infected fluid collections. J Am Coll Radiol. 2015;12(8):791–9.

33. Hinchey EJ, Schaal PG, Richards GK. Treatment of perforated diverticular disease of the colon. Adv Surg. 1978;12:85–109.

34. Sartelli M, Catena F, Abu-Zidan FM, Moore EE, et al. Management of intra-abdominal infections: recommendations by the WSES 2016 consensus conference. World J Emerg Surg. 2017;12:22. Published online 2017 May 4

35. Alavi A, Dann RW, Baum S, Biery DN. Scintigraphic detection of acute gastrointestinal bleeding. Radiology. 1977;124(3):753–6.

36. Bentley DE, Richardson JD. The role of tagged red blood cell imaging in the localization of gastrointestinal bleeding. Arch Surg. 1991;126(7):821–4.

37. Huprich JE, Fletcher JG, Fidler JL, Alexander JA, Guimaraes LS, Siddiki HA. Prospective blinded comparison of wireless capsule endoscopy and multiphase CT enterography in obscure gastrointestinal bleeding. Radiology. 2011;260:744–51.

38. Woodhams R, Nishimaki H, Fujii K, Kakita S, Hayakawa K. Usefulness of multidetector-row CT

(MDCT) for the diagnosis of non-occlusive mesenteric ischemia (NOMI): assessment of morphology and diameter of the superior mesenteric artery (SMA) on multi-planar reconstructed (MPR) images. Eur J Radiol. 2010;76(1):96–102.

39. Wiesner W, Hauser A, Steinbrich W. Accuracy of multidetector row computed tomography for the diagnosis of acute bowel ischemia in a non-selected study population. Eur Radiol. 2004;14(12):2347–56.

40. Menke J. Diagnostic accuracy of multidetector CT in acute mesenteric ischemia: systematic review and meta-analysis. Radiology. 2010;256:93–101.

41. Habib K, Gupta A, White D, Mazari FA, Wilson TR. Utility of contrast enema to assess anastomotic integrity and the natural history of radiological leaks after low rectal surgery: systematic review and meta-analysis. Int J Color Dis. 2015;30:1007–14.

42. Nicksa GA, Dring RV, Johnson KH, Sardella WV, Vignati PV, Cohen JL. Anastomotic leaks: what is the best diagnostic imaging study? Dis Colon Rectum. 2007;50:197–203.

43. Lalani T, Couto CA, Rosen MP, et al. ACR appropriateness criteria jaundice. J Am Coll Radiol. 2013;10(6):402–9.

44. Pasanen PA, Partanen KP, Pikkarainen PH, Alhava EM, Janatuinen EK, Pirinen AE. A comparison of ultrasound, computed tomography and endoscopic retrograde cholangiopancreatography in the differential diagnosis of benign and malignant jaundice and cholestasis. Eur J Surg. 1993;159(1):23–9.

45. Wallace GW, Davis MA, Semelka RC, Fielding JR. Imaging the pregnant patient with abdominal pain. Abdom Imaging. 2012;37(5):849–60.

46. Gurusamy KS, Giljaca V, Takwoingi Y, et al. Ultrasound versus liver function tests for diagnosis of common bile duct stones. Cochrane Database Syst Rev. 2015;(2):CD011548.

47. Giljaca V, Gurusamy KS, Takwoingi Y, Higgie D, Poropat G, Štimac D, Davidson BR. Endoscopic ultrasound versus magnetic resonance cholangiopancreatography for common bile duct stones. Cochrane Database Syst Rev. 2015;2:CD011549.

48. Whitcomb DC. Clinical practice: acute pancreatitis. N Engl J Med. 2006;354:2142–50.

49. Papachristou GI, Muddana V, Yadav D, O'Connell M, Sanders MK, Slivka A. Comparison of BISAP, Ranson's, APACHE-II, and CTSI scores in predicting organ failure, complications, and mortality in acute pancreatitis. Am J Gastroenterol. 2009;105:435–41.

50. Banks PA, Bollen TL, Dervenis C, et al. Classification of acute pancreatitis—2012: revision of the Atlanta classification and definitions by international consensus. Gut. 2013;62:102–11.

51. Leichtle SW, Tung L, Khan M, Inaba K, Demetriades D. The role of radiologic evaluation in necrotizing soft tissue infections. J Trauma Acute Care Surg. 2016;81(5):921–4.

52. Zacharias N. Diagnosis of necrotizing soft tissue infections by computed tomography. Arch Surg. 2010;145(5):452–5.

53. Martinez M, Peponis T, Hage A, Yeh DD, Kaafarani HMA, Fagenholz PJ, King DR, de Moya MA, Velmahos GC. The role of computed tomography in the diagnosis of necrotizing soft tissue infections. World J Surg. 2017;42:82.

54. Struk DW, Munk PL, Lee MJ, Ho SG, Worsley DF. Imaging of soft tissue infections. Radiol Clin N Am. 2001;39(2):277–303.

Antibiotics in Emergency General Surgery

4

Mitchell J. Daley, Emily K. Hodge, and Dusten T. Rose

Abbreviations

ADR	Adverse drug reaction
AMG	Aminoglycoside
AUC	Area under the curve
CDI	*Clostridium difficile* infection
Cmax	Peak drug concentration
CMS	Centers for Medicare and Medicaid Services
CNS	Central nervous system
CrCl	Creatinine clearance
CRE	Carbapenem-resistant *Enterobacteriaceae*
ESBL	Extended-spectrum beta-lactamase
FDA	Food and Drug Administration
FLQ	Fluoroquinolones
GI	Gastrointestinal
GNR	Gram-negative rod
ICU	Intensive care unit
IV	Intravenous
KPC	*Klebsiella pneumoniae* carbapenemase
MAOI	Monoamine oxidase inhibitor
MDRO	Multidrug-resistant organism
MIC	Minimum inhibitory concentration
MRSA	Methicillin-resistant *Staphylococcus aureus*
MSSA	Methicillin-susceptible *Staphylococcus aureus*
PAE	Post-antibiotic effect
PBP	Penicillin-binding protein
PCN	Penicillin
PCR	Polymerase chain reaction
PD	Pharmacodynamics
PK	Pharmacokinetics
SMX	Sulfamethoxazole
SrCr	Serum creatinine
T > MIC	Time above minimum inhibitory concentration
TMP	Trimethoprim
UA	Urinalysis
UTI	Urinary tract infection
Vd	Volume of distribution
VISA	Vancomycin-intermediate *Staphylococcus aureus*
VRE	Vancomycin-resistant *Enterococcus*

Introduction

Emergency general surgery patients are at risk for a variety of primary or secondary infectious complications. In noncardiac intensive care units (ICU), infectious-related mortality has been described as high as 60% [1]. Infectious disease is unique from most other disease processes encountered in surgery, given the underlying response to disease or treatment is influenced by

M. J. Daley (✉) · E. K. Hodge · D. T. Rose
Department of Pharmacy, Dell Seton Medical Center at the University of Texas, Austin, TX, USA
e-mail: mjDaley@ascension.org

© Springer International Publishing AG, part of Springer Nature 2019
C. V. R. Brown et al. (eds.), *Emergency General Surgery*, https://doi.org/10.1007/978-3-319-96286-3_4

the interplay of three independent factors: host, pathogen, and antimicrobial therapy. In the modern era, the medical community has increasingly described the benefit of prescribing the right antibiotics empirically in adjunct to appropriate source control procedures. However, broad-spectrum antibiotic use is a known risk factor in the development of multidrug-resistant bacteria, potentially rendering standard antibiotics ineffective. Therefore, clinicians must have a balanced approach to antibiotic therapy to ensure successful treatment of infections while minimizing the risk for propagating antibiotic resistance [2]. The purpose of this chapter is to review principles and recent advances for the diagnosis and treatment of bacterial infections. Relevant discussions of anti-infective agents for specific disease processes are discussed in other sections of this book.

Diagnosis of Infection

Fever is often the initial sign of possible infection. Depending on host factors and comorbid conditions, other nonspecific signs and symptoms may be present such as hypotension, tachycardia, tachypnea, confusion, rigors, lactic acidosis, leukopenia, leukocytosis, or thrombocytopenia. However, during the postoperative period, fever is nearly always noninfectious in the first 48–96 h [3]. Other noninfectious causes should also be considered during the diagnostic evaluation of fevers including central fever (cerebral infarction, hemorrhage, trauma), venous thromboembolism, and drug fever [4]. When an infection is strongly suspected, a systematic approach is favored over a "pan-culturing" strategy to identify the source of an infection. Specimens for cultures should be collected prior to the initiation of antibiotics unless doing so will result in substantial antibiotic delay, defined by the Surviving Sepsis Guidelines as 45 min [5].

High clinical suspicion of infection secondary to recent surgical procedures, indwelling devices, or signs/symptoms involving a single organ system should be prioritized during initial diagnostics. Surgical dressings should be removed to examine incisions. If incisions are opened, a culture should be obtained from a deep space. Superficial swabs are nonspecific and result in contamination. In patients who have been mechanically ventilated, a chest x-ray and sputum cultures should be obtained. It is important to distinguish aspiration pneumonia versus aspiration pneumonitis. The latter can often be distinguished by a rapid onset and offset of symptoms [6]. Lack of improvement in 48 h should raise the suspicion for bacterial pneumonia. Two peripheral sets (aerobic and anaerobic) of blood cultures are recommended for any patient with a suspected infection. One of these sets should be obtained from an intravascular catheter if in place ≥48 h. For patients at risk of endocarditis (intravenous drug user, known *Staphylococcus aureus* bacteremia), then multiple sets of blood cultures should be obtained. Urinary culture should only be obtained when high index of suspicion exists to decrease positive cultures secondary to Foley catheter colonization or asymptomatic bacteriuria. Potential strategies to prevent false-positive urine cultures include removing Foley catheters *prior* to urinalysis (UA) and only reflex culturing when pyuria (>10 WBC/hpf) exists on the UA, as this WBC/hpf threshold has demonstrated a high negative predictive value for a urinary tract infection (UTI) [7, 8].

Initial antibiotic therapy should be guided by local epidemiology and resistance patterns by utilizing the institution's antibiogram. Internal guidelines should be developed to prevent overprescribing of broad-spectrum antibiotics to ensure tailoring of indication-specific therapy. However, inappropriate initial therapy is an independent predictor of mortality. When broad-spectrum therapy is indicated, it is important to take an "antibiotic time-out" 48–72 h later to review culture data and clinical response to de-escalate antimicrobials as soon as possible [9].

Risk of increased morbidity and mortality with starting inappropriate empiric antibiotic therapy must be weighed with the consequences of antimicrobial resistance from careless prescribing of broad-spectrum antibiotics for extended durations. The use of rapid molecular testing not only decreases the turnaround time

Table 4.1 Rapid diagnostic test characteristics and detected pathogens

Test	Specimen(s)	Microorganism/targets detected
Polymerase chain reaction (PCR)	Stool Various (serum, nares)	*Clostridium difficile* *Staphylococcus aureus* (MRSA)
Multiplex PCR (simultaneous detection of multiple organisms) Nanoparticle probe technology (nucleic acid extraction and PCR amplification)	Serum Stool CSF Nasopharyngeal	Several bacteria Several viruses Resistance markers (*mecA*, *van* A/B, KPC)
Peptide nucleic acid fluorescence in situ hybridization (PNA-FISH)	Serum	*Staphylococcus* spp. *Enterococcus* spp. *Candida* spp. Gram-negative bacteria
Matrix-assisted laser desorption/ionization time-of-flight mass spectrometry (MALDI-TOF MS)	Direct from colony on many sample types	Gram-positive bacteria Gram-negative bacteria *Candida* spp. *Mycobacterium* spp.

KPC, Klebsiella pneumoniae carbapenemase

compared to conventional culturing methods but also increases sensitivity and specificity of the infecting pathogen. The use of rapid, multiplex polymerase chain reaction (PCR)-based testing has been shown to impact time to most effective antibiotic therapy, thereby decreasing mortality and de-escalating unnecessary anti-infectives. While a complete overview of these tests is outside the scope of this chapter, Table 4.1 below highlights some of the tests currently available and their characteristics [10]. Biomarkers, such as procalcitonin, may also be a useful tool to guide therapy de-escalation [9]. Because procalcitonin is a precursor of calcitonin, released in the presence of bacterial infections, it has been studied to initiate and discontinue antibiotics. It may be particularly helpful to differentiate an ongoing infection from a noninfectious process. While the procalcitonin cutoff for discontinuing therapy varies in the literature, there is a growing consensus to discontinue when the assay is ≤0.5 µg/L or decreased by ≥80% from the peak value [11].

Principles of Antibiotic Therapy

Effective eradication of an infection requires adequate source control and optimal use of antimicrobial therapy. A basic understanding of antimicrobial principles is essential to optimize antibiotic therapy. Pharmacokinetics (PK) refers to the patient's action toward a drug, including absorption, distribution, metabolism, and excretion [12]. The most clinically relevant PK concepts include bioavailability, volume of distribution (Vd), half-life, and clearance. Bioavailability, or the percent of drug absorbed, is influenced by route of administration. Intravenous antibiotics have 100% bioavailability, while oral antibiotics vary dependent on drug properties (e.g., absorption) or patient physiology (e.g., intestinal transit time) [13]. In shock states, intravenous routes are preferred to ensure adequate systemic exposure. Volume of distribution (Vd) is a theoretical estimate of the proportion of drug in the serum to tissues. In critical illness, fluid resuscitation, hypoalbuminemia, and capillary leak syndrome can result in fluid shift into the interstitial space [14]. For hydrophilic drugs, including beta-lactams, aminoglycosides (AMG), vancomycin, and colistin, this results in "dilution" with increased Vd and reduced plasma concentrations. Loading doses of hydrophilic antibiotics can be considered in an attempt to overcome expanded Vd and "fill the tank," independent of clearance [15]. Alternatively, lipophilic antimicrobials, including fluoroquinolones (FLQ), macrolides, linezolid, tigecycline, and clindamycin, have extensive Vd that are, therefore, less affected by resuscitation.

Half-life is the time required for the serum drug concentration to be reduced by half.

Three to five half-lives are used to estimate metabolism of 88–98% of total drug exposure. Half-life varies for each antibiotic, generally dependent on underlying hepatic function for hydrophobic antibiotics and renal function for hydrophilic antibiotics, determining total clearance. In critical illness, clearance can be either "impaired" with end-organ dysfunction or "augmented" with enhanced cardiac output due to physiologic response or resuscitation efforts [16]. The concern with altered clearance is risks of toxicity or suboptimal antibiotic exposure, respectively, both potentially leading to worse outcomes. Therefore, adjustment from standard antibiotic doses is appropriate to avoid the associated risks. Unfortunately, the commonly used surrogate for renal function, serum creatinine (SrCr), appears "normal" in those with augmented renal clearance. Therefore, direct measure with 8–24-h continuous urine creatinine collection is preferred if SrCr is normal and the patient demographics are less than 55 years, male, trauma, surgery, burns, or neurologic insult [16].

Pharmacodynamics (PD) is the physiologic or biochemical response to a drug. This is generally known as "what the drug does to the body or bug." The most clinically relevant and reported PD parameter is the minimum inhibitory concentration (MIC), defined as the lowest serum antimicrobial concentration required to inhibit visible growth of the microorganism [17]. The MIC is dependent on both the drug and bug combination, which the microbiology lab then interprets based on standardized MIC breakpoints. Clinically applied, susceptible organisms are likely to respond to treatment with standard antibiotic doses, whereas intermediate organisms may achieve clinical response, but higher than normal doses may be needed. If resistant, the infection is unlikely to respond to antimicrobial therapy, as doses required to overcome the resistance would likely cause toxicity to humans [18]. Of note, when selecting antibiotics, a clinician can compare MICs within an individual drug/bug relative to the known breakpoint to determine "degree of susceptibility." However, clinicians should not compare MIC values of different antibiotics; given the lowest MIC does not necessarily mean the most susceptible.

The PK-PD properties are integrated to describe the exposure-response relationship and determine the ability for an antibiotic to kill (bactericidal) or inhibit (bacteriostatic) the growth of a pathogen [14]. Beta-lactam antibiotics have "time-dependent" activity, where the percent of time the free drug concentration remains above the MIC (T > MIC) during a dosing interval exclusively determines bactericidal activity. Dose optimization techniques for "time-dependent" antibiotics include more frequent administration or extended infusions. Concentration-dependent antibiotics, such as AMGs, elicit kill activity based on the degree of peak concentration over the MIC (Cmax/MIC). Prescribing larger doses with less frequent administrations is a strategy to optimize peak concentrations, with a general target of ten times the MIC for aminoglycosides. Finally, certain antibiotics, such as vancomycin and FLQs, are reliant on both time and peak concentrations for bactericidal or static activity, known as concentration-dependent with time dependence. The ratio of area under the curve (AUC) to MIC (AUC/MIC) can be optimized by administering larger doses with either more frequent administration or prolonged infusions.

Antibacterial Agents

Once potential sources of infection have been identified and appropriate diagnostic tests have been performed, antimicrobial agents can then be selected based on national guideline recommendations and taking into consideration the antimicrobial activity, PK, and PD of each agent. The tables below describe the spectrum of activity and highlight some clinical pearls of commonly used antimicrobials in the acute care setting (Tables 4.2, 4.3, 4.4, and 4.5).

Table 4.2 General spectrum of activity for common intravenous beta-lactam antibiotics [19]

	Penicillin G	Ampicillin	Oxacillin/ Nafcillin	Ampicillin/ sulbactam	Piperacillin/ tazobactam	Cefazolin	Cefoxitin	Ceftriaxone	Cefepime	Imipenem Doripenem Meropenem	Ertapenem	Aztreonam
Gram-positive												
MSSA	–	–	+	+	+	+	±	±	+	+	+	–
MRSA	–	–	–	–	–	–	–	–	–	–	–	–
Coag - staph	–	–	±	–	–	–	–	–	–	–	–	–
Strep viridans	+	+	±	+	±	+	±	+	+	+	+	–
β-hemolytic strep	+	+	±	+	±	+	+	+	+	+	+	–
S. pneumoniae	+	+	±	+	±	–	±	+	+	+	+	–
E. faecalis	+	+	–	+	+	–	–	–	–	±	–	–
E. faecium	±	±	–	±	±	–	–	–	–	±	–	–
Gram-negative												
H. influenzae	–	±	–	+	+	–	+	+	+	+	+	+
E. coli	–	±	–	±	+	+	+	+	+	+	+	+
Klebsiella sp.	–	±	–	+	+	+	+	+	+	+	+	+
Enterobacter sp.	–	–	–	–	±	–	–	±	+	+	+	+
Serratia sp.	–	–	–	–	±	–	–	±	+	+	+	±
Proteus sp.	–	±	–	±	+	±	±	±	+	+	+	±
Citrobacter sp.	–	–	–	–	±	+	–	±	+	+	+	±
Aeromonas sp.	–	–	–	–	±	–	–	+	+	+	+	±
Acinetobacter sp.	–	–	–	±	±	–	–	–	±	±	–	–
Pseudomonas sp.	–	–	–	–	+	–	–	–	+	+	–	+
ESBL-positive	–	–	–	±	±	–	–	–	–	+	+	–
Anaerobes												
B. fragilis	–	–	–	+	+	–	±	–	–	+	+	–
Oral anaerobes	+	+	+	+	+	+	+	+	+	+	+	–

(+) = active; (−) = not active; (±) = less active to potential resistance

ESBL extended-spectrum beta-lactamase, *MSSA* methicillin-susceptible *Staphylococcus aureus*, *MRSA* methicillin-resistant *Staphylococcus aureus*, *sp,* species

Table 4.3 Beta-lactam antibiotics

Class	Drug example	Pearls
Penicillin: *Natural or semisynthetic compounds that display bactericidal activity by binding to penicillin (PCN)-binding proteins (PBP), inhibit peptidoglycan cross-linking, and result in bacterial cell lysis* [20]		
Natural PCN	Penicillin G	Drug of choice for *Streptococcus* species Inactivated by beta-lactamases produced by *S. aureus* and GNRs
Aminopenicillins	Ampicillin Ampicillin/sulbactam	Beta-lactamase inhibitor extends spectrum of ampicillin to GNRs and anaerobes Sulbactam has activity against *Acinetobacter baumannii* Resistance of *Escherichia coli* increasing, should not be used for empiric therapy in intra-abdominal sepsis
Penicillinase-resistant penicillins	Nafcillin Oxacillin	Drug of choice for methicillin-susceptible *Staphylococcus aureus* (MSSA)
Extended-spectrum penicillins	Piperacillin/tazobactam	Broadest antibacterial spectrum of this class, including *Pseudomonas aeruginosa (PSAR)* and anaerobes
Cephalosporins: *Mechanism of action of cephalosporins is identical to PCN* [21]		
First generation	Cefazolin	Alternative drug of choice for the treatment of MSSA Central nervous system penetration is poor No cephalosporin covers *Enterococcus* spp.
Second generation	Cefuroxime Cefoxitin	Enhanced activity against *E. coli, Klebsiella pneumoniae*, and some *Proteus* spp. Cefoxitin has anaerobic activity; however, *Bacteroides fragilis* resistance is increasing
Third generation	Ceftriaxone Ceftazidime Ceftazidime/avibactam Ceftolozane/tazobactam	Increased potency against GNRs resistant to extended-spectrum PCN or early generation cephalosporins May lack adequate empiric coverage of *S. aureus* Ceftriaxone is primarily hepatically metabolized and excreted Ceftazidime is considered to have activity against most GNRs, including PSAR Beta-lactamase inhibitor combinations are indicated for multidrug-resistant *Pseudomonas* spp.
Fourth generation	Cefepime	Broad spectrum of activity, including PSAR and *Aeromonas* spp. while maintaining activity against Gram-positive cocci
Fifth generation	Ceftaroline	First beta-lactam antibiotics to have activity against MRSA Similar Gram-negative coverage as ceftriaxone
Carbapenems: *Compact chemical structures readily diffuse through porin channels of Gram-negative bacilli and inhibit cell wall synthesis by binding PBP. Particularly resistant to beta-lactamases* [22]		
Carbapenems	Ertapenem	Inhibits most Gram-positive cocci, GNRs, including ESBL producers Does not have activity against PSAR or *Acinetobacter* spp. Its long half-life and extensive protein binding allow for once-daily administration
Antipseudomonal carbapenems	Meropenem Doripenem Imipenem	Broadest spectrum of activity of all beta-lactams, including PSAR Imipenem is coadministered with cilastatin to prevent deactivation within the renal brush boarder cells Meropenem and doripenem have enhanced activity against GNRs yet reduced *Enterococcus* activity
Monobactams: *High affinity for PBP3, causing bacterial cell wall lysis* [22]		
Monobactam	Aztreonam	No activity against any Gram-positive or anaerobic organisms Moderate activity against GNRs Synthetic and lacks the allergenic chemical structure Can be safely used in patients with significant PCN or cephalosporin allergies Consider double coverage of Gram-negative organisms if resistance exceeds 10–20%

ESBL extended-spectrum beta-lactamase, *GNR* Gram-negative rod, *MRSA* methicillin-resistant *Staphylococcus aureus*, *MSSA* methicillin-susceptible *Staphylococcus aureus*, *PBP* penicillin-binding protein, *PCN* penicillin, *PSAR* *Pseudomonas aeruginosa*

Table 4.4 General spectrum of activity for common non-beta-lactam antibiotics [23–35]

	Vancomycin	Daptomycin	Linezolid	Quinu/dalfo	Clindamycin	Cipro-floxacin	Levofloxacin	Moxi-floxacin	Aminoglyco-sides	TMP/SMX	Doxycycline	Tigecycline	Azithro-mycin	Poly-myxins	Metroni-dazole	Nitrofuran-toin
Gram-positive																
MSSA	+	+	+	+	+	–	+	+	–	+	+	+	+	–	–	+
MRSA	+	+	+	+	±	–	–	–	–	+	+	+	–	–	–	+
Coag - Staph	+	+	+	+	–	–	+	+	–	±	–	+	–	–	–	+
Strep viridans	+	+	+	+	±	–	+	+	–	+	+	+	+	–	–	–
β-hemolytic strep	+	+	+	+	±	–	+	+	–	±	±	+	+	–	–	–
S. pneumoniae	+	+	+	+	+	–	+	+	–	+	+	+	+	–	–	–
E. faecalis	+	+	+	–	–	+	+	+	–	–	±	+	–	–	–	+
E. faecium	+	+	+	+	–	–	+	+	–	–	±	+	–	–	–	+
VRE	–	+	+	+	–	–	–	–	–	–	±	±	–	–	–	+
Gram-negative																
H. influenzae	–	–	–	±	–	+	+	+	+	±	+	+	+	–	–	–
E. coli	–	–	–	–	–	+	+	+	+	±	±	+	–	+	–	+
Klebsiella sp.	–	–	–	–	–	+	+	+	+	±	±	+	–	+	–	+
Enterobacter sp.	–	–	–	–	–	+	+	+	+	+	–	+	–	+	–	+
Serratia sp.	–	–	–	–	–	+	+	+	+	+	–	+	–	–	–	–
Proteus sp.	–	–	–	–	–	+	+	+	+	+	–	–	–	–	–	–
Citrobacter sp.	–	–	–	–	–	+	+	+	+	+	–	+	–	+	–	+
Aeromonas sp.	–	–	–	–	–	+	+	+	–	+	+	+	–	–	–	–
Acinetobacter sp.	–	–	–	–	–	+	+	–	+	+	–	±	–	+	–	–
Pseudomonas sp.	–	–	–	–	–	+	+	–	+	–	–	–	–	+	–	–
ESBL-positive	–	–	–	–	–	±	+	–	±	±	–	+	–	+	–	±
Anaerobes																
B. fragilis	–	–	–	–	±	–	–	±	–	–	–	+	–	–	+	–
Oral anaerobes	+	–	–	+	+	–	–	+	–	+	+	+	–	–	+	–
Atypicals	–	–	–	–	–	+	+	+	–	+	+	+	+	–	–	–

ESBL extended-spectrum beta-lactamase, *MRSA* methicillin-resistant *Staphylococcus aureus*, *MSSA* methicillin-susceptible *Staphylococcus aureus*, *sp*. species, *quinu/dalfo* quinupristin/dalfopristin, *TMP/SMX* trimethoprim/sulfamethoxazole, *VRE* vancomycin-resistant *Enterococcus*

Table 4.5 Non-beta-lactam antibiotics

Class	Drug example	Pearls
Gram-positive agents [23–25]		
Glycopeptides	Vancomycin	Inhibits bacterial cell wall synthesis Broad activity against Gram-positive bacteria, drug of choice for MRSA Oral formulation used for *C. difficile* Therapeutic drug monitoring should be considered; target trough concentrations of 15–20 mcg/mL used as a surrogate to achieve AUC/MIC ratio $\geq$ 400 Toxicity: red man syndrome, nephrotoxicity
Lipopeptides	Daptomycin	Bactericidal antibiotic typically reserved for MRSA infections failing vancomycin therapy, vancomycin-intermediate *Staphylococcus aureus* (VISA), and VRE No clinical utility for pneumonia, inactivated by lung surfactant Muscle toxicity most common, monitor creatinine phosphokinase levels
Oxazolidinones	Linezolid Tedizolid	Typically reserved for MRSA infections failing vancomycin therapy, VISA, and VRE Bacteriostatic, protein synthesis inhibitor Generally well tolerated; caution drug-drug interactions due to monoamine oxidase inhibitor (MAOI) properties Available in both IV and PO formulations (100% bioavailable)
Lipoglycopeptide	Telavancin	Concentration-dependent, bactericidal antibiotic with activity against Gram-positive organisms, including MRSA and VISA Once-daily dosing Caution with CrCl $\leq$50 mL/min
Streptogramins	Quinupristin/dalfopristin	Streptogramin antibiotic with activity against many Gram-positive organisms, except *E. faecalis* Typically reserved for multidrug-resistant VRE due to side effects
Lincosamide	Clindamycin	Bacterial protein synthesis inhibitor May be used in combination with a beta-lactam agent to inhibit toxin production in clostridial and streptococcal toxic shock syndrome Increasing resistance among *S. aureus*, streptococci, and *Bacteroides* spp. may limit use Available IV and PO with great oral bioavailability Use associated with increased risk of *C. difficile* infection
Fluoroquinolones [26]		
Fluoroquinolones	Ciprofloxacin Levofloxacin Moxifloxacin	Concentration-dependent, bactericidal antibiotics that interfere with DNA synthesis Available IV and PO Excellent oral bioavailability; coadministration with cations or enteral tube feeds can decrease absorption Increasing resistance to nosocomial pathogens May be used to cover *Vibrio* or *Aeromonas* spp. following injuries in salt or fresh water, respectively [27] Toxicity: QT interval prolongation, CNS effects, arthropathy and tendinitis, risk factor for *C. difficile* diarrhea Risks of FQ use may outweigh benefits for treating certain uncomplicated infections (e.g., sinusitis, bronchitis, uncomplicated UTIs) [28]
Aminoglycosides [29]		

4 Antibiotics in Emergency General Surgery

Table 4.5 (continued)

Class	Drug example	Pearls
Aminoglycosides	Gentamicin Tobramycin Amikacin	Bactericidal antibiotics that inhibit protein synthesis Primarily reserved in combination with beta-lactams for resistant Gram-negative infections due to toxicities (e.g., nephrotoxicity, ototoxicity) and synergy with some Gram-positive infections No anaerobe activity Concentration-dependent activity and post-antibiotic effect (PAE) allow for once-daily dosing with many infections Therapeutic drug monitoring required
Sulfonamides [30]		
Sulfonamides	Trimethoprim/ sulfamethoxazole (TMP-SMX)	Fixed combination of two antimicrobials that synergistically inhibit bacterial folate synthesis Available IV and PO Drug of choice for *Stenotrophomonas maltophilia* and *Pneumocystis jirovecii* pneumonia Toxicity: GI upset, hypersensitivity reactions, renal dysfunction
Tetracyclines [31]		
Tetracyclines	Doxycycline/minocycline	Bacteriostatic antibiotics that inhibit protein synthesis Oral formulations most commonly used due to excellent bioavailability; absorption decreased with cations and enteral tube feeds Provides synergy with beta-lactam antibiotics for *Vibrio* species Caution: GI upset, photosensitivity, avoid use during pregnancy
Macrolides [25]		
Macrolides	Azithromycin	Bacteriostatic via inhibition of protein synthesis Most commonly used for treating community-acquired upper and lower respiratory tract infections Increasing *S. pneumonia* resistance my limit use Other uses: treatment of *Chlamydia trachomatis* and *Neisseria gonorrhoeae* infections Available IV and PO QT interval prolongation: monitor electrolytes and for concomitant QT prolonging medications, particularly in patients with underlying cardiac disease
	Erythromycin	Modernly, most commonly used to promote GI motility (motilin receptor agonist) in patients with gastroparesis or acute colonic pseudo-obstruction Caution: QT interval prolongation, drug interactions
Miscellaneous		
Polymyxins [32]	Polymyxin B Colistin	Systemic use primarily reserved for multidrug-resistant PSAR, *Acinetobacter baumannii*, and carbapenem-resistant *Enterobacteriaceae* (CRE)
Rifamycins [33]	Rifampin Rifaximin	Inhibit bacterial protein synthesis Activity against Gram-positive bacteria, but used in combination with other agents due to rapid development of resistance with monotherapy Rifampin: caution drug-drug interactions Rifaximin: primarily used for treatment of *C. difficile* and hepatic encephalopathy. Minimal adverse effects

(continued)

Table 4.5 (continued)

Class	Drug example	Pearls
Glycylcycline [31]	Tigecycline	Broad spectrum of antimicrobial activity, but reserved for multidrug-resistant organisms Mechanism of action similar to tetracyclines Black box warning: increased risk of death as compared with other antibiotics used to treat similar infections [34] Severe nausea
Nitroimidazoles [35]	Metronidazole	Concentration-dependent, bactericidal activity via inhibiting DNA synthesis Only provides anaerobic coverage Available IV and PO; excellent oral bioavailability Caution: disulfiram-like reactions with alcohol consumption, drug-drug interaction with warfarin, avoid in pregnancy
Others [36]	Nitrofurantoin	Oral antibiotic for the treatment and prophylaxis of acute cystitis without pyelonephritis Resistance rare, mechanism of action includes inhibition of multiple bacterial enzymes Avoid use with CrCl <60 mL/min (alternative <30 mL/min if limited duration)

AUC/MIC area under the curve/minimum inhibitory concentration, *CNS* central nervous system, *CRE* carbapenem-resistant *Enterobacteriaceae*, *CrCl* creatinine clearance, *GI* gastrointestinal, *IV* intravenous, *MAOI* monoamine oxidase inhibitor, *MRSA* methicillin-resistant *Staphylococcus aureus*, *PAE* post-antibiotic effect, *PO* oral, *TMP-SMX* trimethoprim-sulfamethoxazole, *VISA* vancomycin-intermediate *Staphylococcus aureus*, *VRE* vancomycin-resistant *Enterococcus*

Approach to Antibiotic Therapy

In the absence of definitive microbiologic pathogen identification, empiric antibiotic therapy should be selected to target the most likely organism for the suspected source of infection. Considerations should include pathogen, host, and antibiotic factors including common microbiology for a specific infection source, regional susceptibility patterns (e.g., antibiogram), patient's culture and antibiotic exposure history, patient comorbidities and immune defects, antibiotic penetration, and toxicity. Timely administration of appropriate, broad-spectrum antibiotics has consistently been associated with improved mortality [37]. In 2015, the Centers for Medicare and Medicaid Services (CMS) implemented the SEP-1 core measure, which specifies which broad-spectrum antibiotics are "appropriate" for either monotherapy or dual therapy criteria. Antibiotic therapy should be administered as soon as possible after recognition of an infection. The SEP-1 core measure assesses for administration within 3 h of the recognition of sepsis and septic shock, given incremental increases in mortality with measurable delays [5]. Table 4.6 is an

example of recommendations for empiric antibiotic selection consistent with current national guidelines while meeting the SEP-1 criteria [38]. More detailed and alternative recommendations can be found in the referenced guidelines. Beta-lactams listed in Table 4.6 meet the criteria for monotherapy to be compliant with the SEP-1 core measure. If, however, a patient has a beta-lactam allergy and aztreonam is used, the addition of vancomycin would be needed to achieve SEP-1 compliance. Expanded Gram-negative coverage (e.g., dual coverage with a beta-lactam and AMG) may be indicated if a patient has known risk factors for multidrug resistance (discussed below) or in the presence of septic shock to increase the likelihood that at least one active agent is present. Following pathogen identification and known susceptibilities, empiric antibiotic therapy should be de-escalated to the antibiotic with the narrowest spectrum of activity needed to cover the identified organism. Although recommended antibiotic duration varies by source, most serious infections associated with sepsis can be treated with 7–10 days of therapy, where more recent guidelines favor shorter durations (Table 4.6). Duration may be extended if initial therapy was not active against the identified

Table 4.6 Recommended empiric antibiotic selection and duration for common infections in emergency general surgery [IDSA]

Infectious source	Standard therapy (example)
Central nervous system (CNS) Healthcare-associated [39]	Empiric: cefepime* (CNS dose) + vancomycin Duration: 10–14 days, up to 21 days for GNR
Pneumonia Community-acquired (CAP) [40]	Empiric: ceftriaxone* + azithromycin Duration: 5 days
Pneumonia Hospital-acquired (HAP) Ventilator-associated (VAP) [41]	Empiric: cefepime* ± vancomycin Duration: 7 days (all organisms)
Intra-abdominal [42]	Empiric: piperacillin/tazobactam* ± vancomycin Duration: 4 days following source control
Bloodstream Catheter-related [43]	Empiric: cefepime* + vancomycin Duration: 7–14 days from first negative blood culture
Skin and soft tissue [44]	Empiric: piperacillin/tazobactam* + vancomycin ± clindamycin (toxic shock) Duration: 7–14 days
Urinary tract infection Catheter-related [45]	Empiric: cefepime* Duration: 7 days

*Antibiotics labeled with a * meet the CMS Sepsis Core Measure for monotherapy. Unless clear sequencing of antibiotics indicated, suggest giving antibiotic that meets the monotherapy criteria first.*
CAP community-acquired pneumonia, *CNS* central nervous system, *GNR* Gram-negative rod, *HAP* hospital-acquired pneumonia, *VAP* ventilator-associated pneumonia

pathogen, slow clinical improvement, concurrent bacteremia (e.g., *S. aureus*), or lack of timely source control [5]. De-escalation and minimization of duration are critical strategies to prevent superinfections (e.g., *C. difficile*), bacterial resistance, drug toxicity, and minimize costs.

Antibiotic Toxicity

Beta-Lactam Allergy Approximately 15–20% of patients "self-report" an allergy to beta-lactams, most commonly to PCN but also with cephalosporins and carbapenems [46, 47]. This is, however, an overestimate as only 5 percent of patients with a reported allergy to beta-lactams have a positive confirmatory skin test [48]. There are likely two driving forces that explain the inflated incidence. First, adverse drug reactions (ADRs; e.g., rash, upset stomach) are often misinterpreted as hypersensitivity reactions (e.g., hives, airway swelling, anaphylaxis). Second, IgE-mediated reactions diminish with time, effecting less than 20% of patients 10 years later [49]. It is imperative that the healthcare practitioner critically evaluate "self-reported" allergies to discriminate ADRs from true allergic reactions. This includes obtaining a medication history of prior beta-lactam use and tolerance. If a

patient does have a true PCN allergy, approximately 2% of patients may react to a cephalosporin and < 1% to a carbapenem [50–52]. Management strategies include challenge with an alternative beta-lactam class (e.g., use cephalosporin or aztreonam with PCN or cephalosporin allergy, respectively), choose a different antimicrobial class (consider dual coverage if more than 10–20% local resistance), or beta-lactam desensitization.

Nephrotoxicity Nephrotoxicity is a concern with several classes of commonly prescribed antibiotics. Reported rates of vancomycin-induced nephrotoxicity vary widely from 5% to 40% [53]. Vancomycin trough concentrations ≥15 mcg/mL, doses >4 g/day, and duration of therapy are all potential risk factors for developing vancomycin-induced nephrotoxicity [53, 54]. Patient-specific risk factors such as preexisting renal disease, obesity, severity of illness, and delivery of concurrent nephrotoxins may also influence risk [53, 55]. The combination of piperacillin-tazobactam and vancomycin has received increasing attention due to at least three times higher rates of nephrotoxicity reported in the literature compared with vancomycin monotherapy or vancomycin ± other beta-lactams [55–57]. Furthermore, the incidence of AKI may have a positive linear relationship with duration of the combination, thus reinforcing the importance of a 48–72-h "antibiotic time-out" and timely de-escalation of unnecessary broad-spectrum antibiotics. Nephrotoxicity due to AMGs is attributed to significant accumulation of drug in the renal cortex [29]. Fortunately, once-daily AMG dosing can be used to minimize neph-rotoxicity (saturable uptake into renal tubular cells) while simultaneously capitalizing on Cmax>MIC and PAE pharmacology. Polymyxin antibiotics have largely fallen out of favor due to significant nephrotoxicity associated with their use (30–60%); unfortunately, due to emergence of resistant Gram-negative bacteria, their use is being relied upon again in modern clinical prac-tice [32].

Neurotoxicity Seizures may occur with all beta-lactam antibiotics but most commonly following exposure to penicillin G, carbapenems, and cefepime (e.g., nonconvulsive status epilepticus) [58]. Although all carbapenems can cause seizures due to gamma-aminobutyric acid receptor antago-nism, risk is highest with imipenem (1–2% vs. 0.1–0.3%) [22]. Generally, risk of seizures is related to preexisting neurologic disease, advanced age, and renal insufficiency. Appropriate dose reduction based on corresponding renal function is the best strategy to avoid this risk. The FQ class is also known to cause neurotoxicity, including hal-lucinations, delirium, psychosis, and seizures [26]. The Food and Drug Administration (FDA) has issued a safety announcement that FQs may lead to disabling and potentially permanent serious side effects to the central nervous system, including neuropathy and seizures [28].

Superinfection Antibiotic exposure is an important, modifiable risk factor for *C. difficile* infection (CDI). Virtually any class of antibiotics can increase the risk of CDI due to disruption of normal intestinal flora; however clindamycin, FQs, and extended-spectrum cephalosporins have consistently been shown to confer the high-est risk of CDI in the community and hospital setting [59–61]. It is prudent for prescribers to

consider this risk when selecting antimicrobial agents especially when equally effective alterna-tive agents are available.

Bacterial Resistance

Gram-Positive Resistance

Methicillin-resistant *Staphylococcus aureus* is the most common Gram-positive resistant organism encountered in the US hospital setting with approximately 80,000 infections and over 11,000 deaths occurring in 2011 [62]. However, healthcare-associated rates appear to be decreas-ing secondary to preventative measures around central line-associated bloodstream infections (CDC Antimicrobial Stewardship). It is impor-tant to recognize patient risk factors that justify empiric vancomycin therapy. There is an increasing concern with vancomycin failure for MRSA bacteremia with MICs ≥1.5 mcg/mL [63]. Alternative anti-MRSA therapy should be considered for these isolates if clinical failure is suspected on appropriate vancomycin doses (troughs 15–20 mcg/mL).

Vancomycin-resistant *Enterococcus*, either *E. faecalis* or *faecium*, is associated with increased morbidity and mortality. This is related to their predilection for causing infections in immuno-compromised hosts with significant exposure to antibiotics. Vancomycin-resistant *Enterococcus* can be treated with daptomycin, linezolid, or tigecycline. Combination therapy with daptomy-cin plus beta-lactam antibiotics should be con-sidered for persistent infections in critically ill patients (Table 4.7). Antibiotic treatment options for cystitis include doxycycline, fosfomycin, and nitrofurantoin. Linezolid and daptomycin should be reserved for pyelonephritis [64].

Gram-Negative Resistance

Although some resistance is mediated through efflux pumps or porin channel modifications, the vast majority of Gram-negative bacterial resis-tance for beta-lactam antibiotics is enzymatic hydrolysis by beta-lactamases [65]. The most clinically relevant beta-lactamase enzymes encountered in the ICU include AmpC, ESBL, and CRE-producing carbapenemases.

Many *Enterobacteriaceae* have AmpC-encoding genes within their chromosomes including the SPACEM (*Serratia*, *Pseudomonas aeruginosa*, *Acinetobacter*, *Citrobacter* and *Enterobacter*, and *Morganella*) organisms [58]. Among these patho-

Table 4.7 Risk factors for multidrug-resistant organisms and MRSA

Risk factors for multidrug-resistant organisms (MDRO)
Recent antibiotic (e.g., fluoroquinolones) exposure (90 days)
High severity of illness/care in ICU
Chronic renal replacement therapy
Chronic indwelling catheters (vascular or urinary)
Recent surgery
Organ transplantation (solid and bone marrow)
Residence in skilled-nursing or extended-care facility
Known colonization or documented infection with MDRO in the past
Risk factors for methicillin-resistant Staphylococcus aureus (MRSA)
Purulent cellulitis or abscesses
Intravenous drug user (IVDU)
MRSA nasal colonization
Penetrating trauma
Recent viral illness
Same as above

ICU intensive care unit, *IVDU* intravenous drug user, *MDRO* multidrug-resistant organism, *MRSA* methicillin-resistant *Staphylococcus aureus*

gens, production of AmpC beta-lactamase occurs either "all the time" or following exposure to specific antibiotics with perceived in vitro susceptibility, such as third-generation cephalosporins (e.g., ceftriaxone), leading to the concept of "inducible resistance." Once produced, AmpC beta-lactamase confers resistance to most PCNs (including piperacillin/tazobactam) through third-generation cephalosporins and monobactams, necessitating treatment with cefepime or carbapenems. ESBLs, although originally common among *E. coli* and *K. pneumoniae*, are plasmid-mediated genes that can be easily transferred from one organism to the next. ESBLs hydrolyze most cephalosporins, with the exception of cefoxitin, most PCNs, and monobactams. The treatment of choice remains carbapenems; however, because some beta-lactamase inhibitors are stable to certain ESBLs, literature is accumulating suggesting that piperacillin/tazobactam may be a potential treatment option [66]. *E. coli* and *Klebsiella* spp. producing carbapenemases have gained more attention as these confer resistance to nearly all beta-lactams. Ceftazidime/avibactam is an option for non-New Delhi metallo-beta-lactamase (NDM)—producing carbapenemases and safer than traditional alternatives such as polymyxins. Given a lack of novel antibiotics in development, optimization of current antibiotics by applying antimicrobial stewardship principles with good infection control practices is key to combat antibiotic resistance [65] (Table 4.8).

Table 4.8 Treatment strategies for common multidrug-resistant organisms

Organism/patient presentation	Antibiotic(s)

MRSA
Persistent bacteremia
Vancomycin failure (MIC ≥ 1.5 μg/mL)
Clinical failure of deep-seated infection (epidural abscess, endocarditis, osteomyelitis)
	High-dose daptomycin (8–12 mg/kg) every 24 h, with or without
	  Beta-lactam
	  TMP-SMX
	Ceftaroline 600 mg every 8 h
	Linezolid 600 mg every 12 h

Carbapenem-resistant *Enterobacteriaceae* (CRE)	High-dose, prolonged infusion carbapenem with
	  Polymyxins (polymyxin B, colistin)
	  Nebulized antibiotics (tobramycin, colistin)[a]
	Ceftazidime-avibactam 2.5 grams every 8 h

Multidrug-resistant *Pseudomonas aeruginosa* (resistant to all beta-lactams, monobactams, and fluoroquinolones)	Ceftazidime-avibactam 2.5 grams every 8 h Ceftolozane-tazobactam 1.5–3 grams every 8 h Polymyxins (polymyxin B, colistin)
Extended-spectrum beta-lactamases (ESBL) producing *Enterobacteriaceae*	Ceftazidime-avibactam 2.5 grams every 8 h Ceftolozane-tazobactam 1.5–3 grams every 8 h Carbapenems Tigecycline (salvage therapy)

CRE carbapenem-resistant *Enterobacteriaceae*, *ESBL* extended-spectrum beta-lactamase, *MIC* minimum inhibitory concentration, *MRSA* methicillin-resistant *Staphylococcus aureus*, *TMX-SMX* trimethoprim-sulfamethoxazole
[a]Ventilator-associated pneumonia

References

1. Angus DC, Linde-Zwirble WT, Lidicker J, et al. Epidemiology of severe sepsis in the United States: analysis of incidence, outcome, and associated costs of care. Crit Care Med. 2001;29:1303–10.
2. Ho VP, Barie PS. Antibiotics for critically ill patients. In: Current surgical therapy., 11th edition. Philadelphia: Elsevier Saunders; 2014. p. 1271–8.
3. Narayan M, Medinilla SP. Fever in the postoperative patient. Emerg Med Clin N Am. 2013;31:1045–58.
4. Marik PE. Fever in the ICU. Chest. 2000;117:855–69.
5. Rhodes A, Evans LE, Alhazzani W, et al. Surviving sepsis campaign: international guidelines for Management of Sepsis and Septic Shock: 2016. Crit Care Med. 2016;45:486–552.
6. Joundi RA, Wong BM, Leis JA. Antibiotics "just in case" in a patent with aspiration pneumonitis. JAMA Intern Med. 2015;175:489–90.
7. Semeniuk H, Church D. Evaluation of the leukocyte esterase and nitrite dipstick screening tests for detection of bacteriuria in women with suspected uncomplicated urinary tract infections. J Clin Microbiol. 1999;37:3051–2.
8. Stovall RT, Haenal JB, Jenkins TC, et al. A negative urinalysis rules out catheter-associated urinary tract infection in trauma patients in the intensive care unit. J Am Coll Surg. 2013;217:162–6.
9. Barlam TF, Cosgrove SE, Abbo LM, et al. Implementing an antibiotic stewardship program: guidelines by the infectious diseases society of America and the society for healthcare epidemiology of America. Clin Infect Dis. 2016;62:1197–202.
10. Bauer KA, Perez KK, Forrest GN, et al. Review of rapid diagnostic tests used by antimicrobial stewardship programs. Clin Infect Dis. 2015;59(S3):S134–45.
11. Rhee C. Using procalcitonin to guide antibiotic therapy. Open Forum Infect Dis. 2016;4:ofw249.
12. Blumenthal DK, Garrison JC. Pharmacodynamics: molecular mechanisms of drug action. In: Brunton LL, Chabner BA, Knollman BC, editors. Goodman and Gilman's the pharmacological basis of therapeutics. 12th ed. New York: McGraw-Hill; 2011. p. 97–146.
13. Ho VP, Barie PS. Antibiotics for critically ill patients. In: Current surgical therapy., 11th edition. Philadelphia, PA: Elsevier Saunders; 2014. p. 1271–8.
14. Roberts JA, Lipman J. Pharmacokinetic issues for antibiotics in the critically ill patient. Crit Care Med. 2009;37:840–51.
15. Tsai D, Lipman J, Roberts JA. Pharmacokinetic/pharmacodynamics considerations for the optimization of antimicrobial delivery in the critically ill. Curr Opin Crit Care. 2015;21:412–20.
16. Hobbs ALV, Shea KM, Roberts KM, et al. Implications of augmented renal clearance on drug dosing in critically ill patients: a focus on antibiotics. Pharmacotherapy. 2015;35:1063–75.
17. Craig WA. Basic pharmacodynamics of antibacterials with clinical applications to the use of β-lactams, glycopeptides, and linezolid. Infect Dis Clin N Am. 2003;17:479–501.
18. Kuper KM, Boles DM, Mohr J, et al. Antimicrobial susceptibility testing: a primer for clinicians. Pharmacotherapy. 2009;29:1326–43.
19. Cosgrove SE, Avdic E, Dzintars K, et al (2015). Johns Hopkins Antibiotic Guideline 2015–2016. Available at: https://www.hopkinsmedicine.org/amp/guidelines/antibiotic_guidelines.pdf. Accessed 10 Oct 2017.
20. Doi Y, Chambers HF. Penicillin and beta-lactamase inhibitors. In: Bennett JE, editor. Mandell, Douglas, and Bennett's principles and practice of infectious diseases. 8th ed. Philadelphia: Saunders; 2015. p. 263–77.
21. Craig WA, Andes DR. Cephalosporins. In: Bennett JE, editor. Mandell, Douglas, and Bennett's principles and practice of infectious diseases. 8th ed. Philadelphia: Saunders; 2015. p. 278–92.
22. Doi Y, Chambers HF. Other β-lactams. In: Bennett JE, editor. Mandell, Douglas, and Bennett's principles and practice of infectious diseases. 8th ed. Philadelphia: Saunders; 2015. p. 293–7.
23. Murray BE, Arias CA, Nannini EC. Glycopeptides (vancomycin and teicoplanin), streptogramins (Quinupristin-dalfopristin), lipopeptides (daptomycin), and lipoglycopeptides (telavancin). In: Bennett JE, editor. Mandell, Douglas, and Bennett's principles and practice of infectious diseases. 8th ed. Philadelphia: Saunders; 2015. p. 377–400.
24. Cox HL, Donowitz GR. Linezolid and other oxazolidinones. In: Bennett JE, editor. Mandell, Douglas, and Bennett's principles and practice of infectious diseases. 8th ed. Philadelphia: Saunders; 2015. p. 406–9.
25. Sivapalasingam S, Steigbigel NH. Macrolides, clindamycin, and ketolides. In: Bennett JE, editor. Mandell, Douglas, and Bennett's principles and practice of infectious diseases. 8th ed. Philadelphia: Saunders; 2015. p. 358–75.
26. Hooper DC, Strahilevitz J. Quinolones. In: Bennett JE, editor. Mandell, Douglas, and Bennett's principles and practice of infectious diseases. 8th ed. Philadelphia: Saunders; 2015. p. 419–39.
27. Noonburg GE. Management of extremity trauma and related infections occurring in the aquatic environment. J Am Acad Orthop Surg. 2005;13:243–53.
28. U.S. Food and Drug Administration. FDA Drug Safety Communication: FDA advises restricting fluoroquinolone antibiotic use for certain uncomplicated infections; wars about disabling side effects that can occur together. Available at: http://www.fda.gov/Drugs/DrugSafety/ucm500143.htm. Accessed 10 Jan 2017.
29. Leggett JE. Aminoglycosides. In: Bennett JE, editor. Mandell, Douglas, and Bennett's principles and practice of infectious diseases. 8th ed. Philadelphia: Saunders; 2015. p. 310–21.
30. Zinner SH, Mayer KH. Sulfonamides and trimethoprim. In: Bennett JE, editor. Mandell, Douglas, and Bennett's principles and practice of infectious diseases. 8th ed. Philadelphia: Saunders; 2015. p. 410–8.

31. Moffa M, Brook I. Tetracyclines, glycylcyclines, and chloramphenicol. In: Bennett JE, editor. Mandell, Douglas, and Bennett's principles and practice of infectious diseases. 8th ed. Philadelphia: Saunders; 2015. p. 322–38.

32. Kaye KS, Pogue JM, Kaye D. Polymyxins (Polymyxin B and Colistin). In: Bennett JE, editor. Mandell, Douglas, and Bennett's principles and practice of infectious diseases. 8th ed. Philadelphia: Saunders; 2015. p. 401–5.

33. Maslow MJ, Portal-Celhay C. Rifamycins. In: Bennett JE, editor. Mandell, Douglas, and Bennett's principles and practice of infectious diseases. 8th ed. Philadelphia: Saunders; 2015. p. 339–49.

34. U.S. Food and Drug Administration. FDA drug safety communication: FDA warns of increased risk of death with IV antibacterial Tygacil (tigecycline) and approves new boxed warning. Available at: https://www.fda.gov/Drugs/DrugSafety/ucm369580.htm. Accessed 10 Oct 2017.

35. Nagel JL, Aronoff DM. Metronidazole. In: Bennett JE, editor. Mandell, Douglas, and Bennett's principles and practice of infectious diseases. 8th ed. Philadelphia: Saunders; 2015. p. 350–7.

36. Horton JM. Urinary tract agents: Nitrofurantoin, fosfomycin, and methenamine. In: Bennett JE, editor. Mandell, Douglas, and Bennett's principles and practice of infectious diseases. 8th ed. Philadelphia: Saunders; 2015. p. 339–49.

37. Seymour CW, Gesten F, Prescott HC, et al. Time to treatment and mortality during mandated emergency care for sepsis. N Engl J Med. 2017;376:2235–44.

38. Septimus EJ, Coopersmith CM, Whittle J, et al. Sepsis national hospital quality measure (SEP-1): multistakeholder work group recommendations for appropriate antibiotics for the treatment of sepsis. Clin Infect Dis. 2017;65:1565–9.

39. Tunkel AR, Hasbun R, Bhimraj A, et al. IDSA practice guidelines for healthcare-associated ventriculitis and meningitis. Clin Infect Dis. 2017;64:34–65.

40. Mandell LA, Wunderink RG, Anzueto A, et al. Infectious Diseases Society of America guidelines on community-acquired pneumonia in adults. Clin Infect Dis. 2007;44:27–72.

41. Kalil AC, Metersky ML, Klompas M, et al. Management of adults with hospital-acquired and ventilator associated pneumonia: 2016 clinical practice guidelines by the Infectious Diseases Society of America. Clin Infect Dis. 2016;63:1–51.

42. Mazuski JE, Tessier JM, May AK, et al. The Surgical Infection Society revised guidelines on the management of intra-abdominal infection. Surg Infect. 2017;18:1–75.

43. Mermel LA, Allon M, Bouza E, et al. Clinical practice guidelines for the diagnosis and management of intravascular catheter-related infection. Clin Infect Dis. 2009;49:1–45.

44. Stevens DL, Bisno AL, Chambers HF, et al. Practice guidelines for the diagnosis and management of skin and soft tissue infections. Clin Infect Dis. 2014;59:10–52.

45. Hooton TM, Bradley SF, Cardenas DD, et al. Diagnosis, prevention, and treatment of catheter-associated urinary tract infection in adults. Clin Infect Dis. 2010;50:625–63.

46. Barlam TF, Cosgrove SE, Abbo LM, et al. Implementing an antibiotic stewardship program: guidelines by the IDSA and SHEA. Clin Infect Dis. 2016;62:51–77.

47. Kuruvilla ME, Khan DA. Antibiotic allergy. In: Bennett JE, editor. Mandell, Douglas, and Bennett's principles and practice of infectious diseases. 8th ed. Philadelphia: Saunders; 2015. p. 298–303.

48. Salkind AR, Cuddy PG, Foxworth JW. The rational clinical examination; is this patient allergic to penicillin? JAMA. 2001;285:2498–505.

49. Sullivan T, Wedner HJ, Shatz GS, et al. Skin testing to detect penicillin allergy. J Allergy Clin Immunol. 1981;68:171–80.

50. Frumin J, Gallagher JC. Allergic cross-sensitivity between penicillin, carbapenem and monobactam antibiotics: what are the chances? Ann Pharmacother. 2009;43:304–15.

51. Solensky R, Khan DA. Drug allergy: an updated practice parameter. Ann Allergy Asthma Immunol. 2010;105:e1–78.

52. Kula B, Djordjevic G, Robinson JL. A systematic review: can one prescribe carbapenems to patients with IgE-mediated allergy to penicillins or cephalosporins? Clin Infect Dis. 2014;59:1113–22.

53. van Hal SJ, Paterson DL, Lodise TP. Systematic review and meta-analysis of vancomycin-induced nephrotoxicity associated with dosing schedules that maintain troughs between 15 and 20 milligrams per liter. Antimicrob Agents Chemother. 2013;57:734–44.

54. Lodise TP, Lomaestro B, Graves J, et al. Larger vancomycin doses (at least four grams per day) are associated with an increased incidence of nephrotoxicity. Antimicrob Agents Chemother. 2008;52:1330–6.

55. Giuliano CA, Patel CR, Kale-Pradhan PB. Is the combination of piperacillin-tazobactam and vancomycin associated with development of acute kidney injury? A meta-analysis. Pharmacotherapy. 2016;36:1217–28.

56. Luther MK, Timbrook TT, Caffrey AR, et al. Vancomycin plus piperacillin-tazobactam and acute kidney injury in adults: a systematic review and meta-analysis. Crit Care Med. 2017.; Epub ahead of print

57. Hammond DA, Smith MN, Li C, et al. Systematic review and metaanalysis of acute kidney injury associated with concomitant vancomycin and piperacillin/tazobactam. Clin Infec Dis. 2017;64:666–74.

58. Oki FY. Principles of critical care. 3rd ed. New York: The McGraw-Hill Companies; 2005. p. 641–97.

59. Brown KA, Khanafer N, Daneman N, et al. Meta-analysis of antibiotics and the risk of community-acquired Clostridium difficile infection. Antimicrob Agents Chemother. 2013;57:2326–32.

60. Deshpande A, Pasupuleti V, Thota P, et al. Community-associated Clostridium difficile infection and antibiotics: a meta-analysis. J Antimicrob Chemother. 2013;68:1951–61.

61. Loo VG, Am B, Poirier L, et al. Host and pathogen factors for Clostridium difficile infection and colonization. N Engl J Med. 2011;365:1693–703.
62. U.S. Department of Health and Human Services Centers for disease control and prevention. (2013) Antibiotic resistance threats in the United States, 2013. Available at: https://www.cdc.gov/drugresistance/threat-report-2013/pdf/ar-threats-2013-508.pdf. Accessed 26 October 2017.
63. van Hal SJ, Lodise TP, Paterson DL. The clinical significance of vancomycin minimum inhibitory concentration in Staphylococcus aureus infections: a systemic review and meta-analysis. Clin Infect Dis. 2012;54:755–71.
64. Heintz BH, Halilovic J, Christensen CL. Vancomycin-resistant Enterococcal urinary tract infections. Pharmacotherapy. 2010;30:1136–49.
65. Jacoby GA, Munoz-Price LS. The new β-lactamases. N Engl J Med. 2005;352:380–91.
66. Gutiérrez-Gutiérrez B, Pérez-Galera S, Salamanca E, et al. A multinational, preregistered cohort study of beta-lactam/beta-lactamase inhibitor combinations for treatment of bloodstream infections due to extended-spectrum-beta-lactamase-producing Enterobacteriaceae. Antimicrob Agents Chemother. 2016;20:4159–69.

Esophageal Perforation

5

Jared L. Antevil and Philip S. Mullenix

Introduction

The rapid evolution of nonsurgical treatment alternatives and the relatively low incidence of this condition have precluded the development of a unified, widely accepted approach. The available evidence suggests that dynamic management will drive the highest likelihood of clinical success. This chapter will provide recommendations for the initial diagnosis and management of patients with esophageal perforation, review its standard surgical management, and examine nonsurgical options. An evidence-based algorithm for the practical management of the condition is proposed. Anastomotic leaks and fistulae of the foregut are unique clinical scenarios that are outside the scope of this discussion. Likewise, the special considerations regarding pediatric patients are well described elsewhere.

One of the key tenets of successful management of esophageal perforation is early involvement of a multidisciplinary team, including physicians with expertise in surgical management, endoscopic techniques, and invasive radiological procedures. The optimal management of patients with esophageal perforation generally requires the services of more than one specialist, and early collaboration facilitates improved communication and care.

The reported mortality of esophageal perforation is between 18% and 30% [1, 2]. Factors demonstrated to correlate with increased mortality include thoracic-level perforation, spontaneous perforation, and delay in diagnosis [1]. The most consistent finding is that irrespective of etiology or time to diagnosis, most patients who present with established contamination or sepsis do poorly. Furthermore, patients who perforate in the context of an underlying esophageal malignancy have high mortality regardless of therapeutic approach.

Etiology

The three major etiologies of esophageal perforation are iatrogenic, "spontaneous" (Boerhaave syndrome), and traumatic. Less common causes include caustic ingestion and perforation associated with advanced malignancy.

Iatrogenic perforation is most often from endoscopic intervention such as dilation for achalasia or stricture. It can also occur from procedures such as transesophageal echocardiography or enteral feeding tube insertion or rarely from surgical procedures on structures in close anatomic proximity to the esophagus. Perforation

J. L. Antevil (✉) · P. S. Mullenix
Cardiothoracic Surgery Service, Department of Surgery, Uniformed Services University of the Health Sciences and the Walter Reed National Military Medical Center, Bethesda, MD, USA
e-mail: Jared.L.Antevil.mil@mail.mil

© Springer International Publishing AG, part of Springer Nature 2019
C. V. R. Brown et al. (eds.), *Emergency General Surgery*, https://doi.org/10.1007/978-3-319-96286-3_5

from endoscopy most often occurs at sites of physiologic luminal narrowing, such as at the cricopharyngeus, aortic knob, or gastroesophageal junction. Pathologic sites such as tumors or strictures are also high risk for injury. In most series, iatrogenic perforation has surpassed spontaneous perforation as the most common etiology, comprising up to 60% in some series [3]. Presumably this is the result of more frequent endoscopic inventions among the population at large.

Spontaneous perforation classically occurs following forceful vomiting or retching, typically in the distal esophagus with variable extension beyond the gastroesophageal junction. Compared to other etiologies, patients with spontaneous perforation tend to present later after time of symptom onset and often present a greater diagnostic dilemma and delay. This situation is often associated with massive contamination [4]. As a result, compared to those with iatrogenic perforation, these patients more often present with sepsis or systemic inflammatory response, require longer hospital stays, and have higher rates of morbidity and mortality [3, 5].

Esophageal perforation due to non-iatrogenic trauma is uncommon relative to iatrogenic etiology. It is most often the result of a penetrating mechanism of injury and is generally associated with injury to adjacent structures. Because these structures include the major airways and blood vessels of the cervical and thoracic regions, many patients may not survive to treatment [6].

Diagnosis

Clinical findings in esophageal perforation may include fever, subcutaneous emphysema, and chest or neck pain that can radiate to the back. In advanced cases, patients may present with respiratory failure and/or shock. Plain chest radiography (CXR) may reveal pleural effusion, pneumomediastinum, air in soft tissues of the chest or neck, free intra-abdominal air, or pneumomediastinum. The gold standard for diagnosis is a fluoroscopic swallow (contrast esophagram) study [7]. Computed tomography (CT) and endoscopic assessment are valuable adjuncts, but can-

not provide critical information ascertained from a dynamic swallow study, which allows characterization in a functional context of the exact location of perforation, size, degree of leakage, and presence of associated obstruction or mass. Multiple swallow views may be obtained in the absence of conclusive findings in any of these respects, and follow-on plain films can determine whether leaked contrast has subsequently drained back into the esophagus.

The false-negative rate for a swallow study with water-soluble contrast utilizing diatrizoate meglumine and diatrizoate sodium solution USP (Gastrograffin, Bracco Diagnostics Inc., Monroe Township, NJ, USA) may be as high as 30% [8]. Thin barium has a higher sensitivity for leak but is preceded by water-soluble contrast swallow at most institutions as barium can cause an intensive inflammatory response in the event of mediastinal extravasation [8]. Gastrografin must be used with extreme caution (or not at all) in patients at high risk for aspiration, as it can induce severe pulmonary injury [9].

When a conventional swallow study is not feasible, such as in intubated or noncooperative patients, a "CT swallow" can be performed with installation of contrast via a carefully placed nasogastric (NG) tube immediately prior to the study [10]. This study is also appropriate for patients with negative barium swallows in whom high clinical suspicion for perforation remains. Relative to a fluoroscopic swallow study, a CT swallow is less likely to localize the site of a perforation, classify the degree of containment, or quantify the return of contrast into the esophagus. A CT scan *can* provide useful information when performed following a fluoroscopic study. In the event of a negative fluoroscopic swallow, a CT indicating fluid or air outside the esophagus suggests a perforation that may have anatomically sealed or been contained. After a positive swallow, CT can characterize the degree of mediastinal and pleural space contamination and direct the optimal means and route for drainage procedures [8]. Many centers now perform a combined "swallow CT" where the fluoroscopic swallow study is immediately followed by a CT scan to maximize the anatomic information as well as the sensitivity for detecting even small leaks.

In general, endoscopy has little role in the acute diagnosis of esophageal perforation. It is invasive and cannot reliably determine an injury's anatomic extent (mucosal versus full thickness). A cautious endoscopic exam may be valuable for planning purposes if endoscopic treatment is being considered and may have a role in situations involving perforation related to suspected malignancy [7]. Flexible endoscopy does have a high rate of accuracy in assessment of traumatic injuries [11] (Fig. 5.1).

Historical Treatment

From Dr. Barrett's first successful surgical repair of esophageal perforation in 1947 through the late 1990s, surgical intervention was widely considered the only reliably effective therapy for this condition [12]. Surgical treatment for esophageal perforation has a reported mortality of 7–26% [3, 13], and mortality may exceed 60% in patients with underlying malignancy [14].

Historically, repair was discouraged in patients presenting greater than 24 h from time of symptom onset or injury, with worse outcomes cited for attempted repair in this context [15]. In situations where presentation was late, the standard solution was temporary esophageal diversion with drainage or in some cases (such as malignancy or advanced tissue destruction) resection and diversion. In such situations,

delayed restoration of continuity was planned for most patients surviving this initial insult.

The concept that primary repair was an ineffective surgical option beyond 24 h was challenged by reports in the late 1990s to early 2000s [2, 13, 14, 16]. Authors cited the high morbidity associated with diversion and the complex nature of subsequent reoperative reconstruction. In addition, it was observed that patients who presented later following the inciting event may have a more contained perforation and therefore may not manifest sepsis or acute toxicity at presentation [14, 17]. Few disputed the increased risk of complications and mortality in the context of established advanced contamination or sepsis. Indeed, it was felt that the degree of tissue contamination and destruction combined with the patient's clinical status was more important than timing in choosing between primary repair and other options [13, 14, 16]. In the absence of extensive tissue necrosis or malignancy, many believed primary surgical repair was the optimal strategy.

In parallel with these discussions, reports arose of "conservative" management for this condition. Arguably, the term conservative is misleading, given that it describes a treatment predicated on noninvasive management, and delay in surgery for patients with this condition has the potential for increased morbidity and mortality. Nevertheless, multiple contemporary reports described low mortality and surgical conversion rates with this nonoperative approach for highly selected patients [18, 19]. The most successful results of conservative management

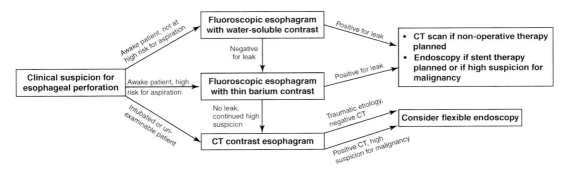

Fig. 5.1 Diagnostic algorithm

appeared to be associated with aggressive drainage, including nasogastric tube placement, tube thoracostomy, image-guided drainage of fluid collections, and frequent reimaging to confirm complete resolution.

The surgical repair of esophageal perforation continued to be plagued by high morbidity, with rates of post-repair leak approaching 39% [20]. There were long durations of inpatient and outpatient care. Thus, the morbidity of surgery, combined with the observation that some patients recover without it, led to the exploration of new treatment modalities.

Endoscopic Therapy

Stents for esophageal perforation were first attempted primarily in patients with high operative risk or those with persistent leak after repair. One report of stent placement in 32 patients with esophageal leak after attempted perforation repair described a 93% success rate, with only two patients requiring additional surgery [20]. Encouraging results such as these were the basis for introduction of endoscopic stenting for the primary management of perforation in patients otherwise fit for surgery – despite lack of approval from the US Food and Drug Administration for this indication. Although prospective data are scarce and heterogeneous, endoscopic stent placement is currently widely used in benign esophageal perforation.

Stents for esophageal perforation are either covered or partially covered and constructed of plastic or metal (nickel/titanium). Compared to plastic stents, metal stents have greater stent flexibility and generate less radial force. Fully covered stents provide optimal leak occlusion and are relatively easy to remove but are prone to migration, prompting many centers to primarily use partially covered stents. Partially covered stents allow some degree of tissue purchase to minimize migration and yet still provide an occlusive seal. Their removal is more challenging than that of fully covered stents, however still generally associated with low complication rates [21, 22]. The ideal stent type for esophageal per-

foration has not been standardized and remains dependent on local experience and availability.

Stents for the treatment of esophageal perforation are placed by experienced gastroenterologists or surgical endoscopists under general anesthesia or intravenous sedation. A contrast study is repeated at 24–72 h after placement to confirm leak exclusion, and an oral diet is resumed if there is no ongoing leak. Stents are generally removed at an interval of 4–6 weeks, with a repeat swallow study after removal [22, 23]. Leaving stents in place beyond 6 weeks increases the risk of complications such as stent erosion, impaction, or bleeding. In cases where a leak persists after stenting for 6 weeks, options include surgical treatment or repeat stenting.

The actual success rate of endoscopic stents for benign perforation is difficult to ascertain because most reports include patients stented for indications other than perforation, such as postoperative anastomotic leaks. Overall, however, the results are encouraging, with reported clinical success rates of 76–97% [5, 23, 24]. Stent therapy seems to be particularly successful for iatrogenic esophageal perforation, especially when combined with aggressive drainage [25]. A recent propensity-matched study comparing stent placement for esophageal perforation (combined with enteral nutrition and aggressive drainage) to transthoracic operative repair suggested shorter intensive care unit and hospital stays and lower overall costs with stents [26].

Stent migration remains a common occurrence after stenting for benign perforation, with reported rates of 17–40% [5, 23, 27, 28]. This problem occurs more frequently with fully covered stents compared to the partially covered devices. Migration is generally detected based on radiographic surveillance and can usually be managed with endoscopic re-intervention.

While early literature on esophageal stenting for perforation did not emphasize the importance of drainage procedures, more recent studies clearly demonstrate the importance of aggressive drainage, which often includes multiple drainage procedures [4, 21, 27]. For patients with esophageal perforation and thoracic sepsis, stent placement must be combined with chest tube placement, video-assisted thoracoscopic surgery (VATS), or open surgical drainage [4, 29, 30]. Other key adjuncts include enteral nutrition (via oral or enteric tube) and appropriate antibiotics [5].

Multiple authors have reported high rates of stent failure when attempted in patients with perforations involving the gastroesophageal junction. This appears to relate to technical difficulties associated with reliably visualizing and excluding the distal aspect of the perforation at this location [4, 5, 27, 28]. Perforation into the abdominal cavity generally contraindicates stent therapy, as in this setting leakage will remain uncontained. Furthermore, percutaneous drainage options are limited for the abdominal cavity, and surgical repair (laparoscopic or open) of intra-abdominal esophageal perforation is associated with significantly less morbidity and mortality than that of thoracic perforation [5, 28]. Failure of stents is also associated with those placed in proximal/cervical locations and in situations involving extensive injury >6 cm [5, 28].

When stenting is unsuccessful, morbidity rates are very high. In one cohort of patients with failed stents, 85% went on to require esophagectomy, and the mortality was 43% [27]. Multiple additional series have demonstrated that persistent leak or clinical deterioration after stent therapy for perforation is associated with high rates of diversion and/or resection and high mortality [4, 29]. In contrast, one group reported an 89% clinical success rate for esophageal stenting for selected cases of perforation, with no patients requiring esophagectomy or diversion, and zero mortality [5]. The authors emphasized the critical importance of aggressive drainage and enteral nutrition and advocated early conversion to surgical repair when initial stent therapy is not successful.

In addition to endoscopic stents, endoscopic clip application, suturing, and "vacuum therapy" techniques have all been described in small series [22]. These new modalities may ultimately find some limited therapeutic role, particularly among patients with iatrogenic perforation.

Treatment Algorithm

After the diagnosis of any esophageal perforation, therapy should begin with fluid resuscitation and the initiation of broad-spectrum antibiotics. Subsequent treatment for cervical or abdominal perforation is relatively straightforward. Because (1) surgical therapy is associated with significantly lower morbidity and mortality in these patients compared to those with intrathoracic perforation and (2) stent therapy has a much lower success rate in these locations [5, 28], stents have little role in extra-thoracic perforation.

For cervical perforation, nonsurgical treatment is a reasonable option in those patients with small, contained leaks and no evidence of systemic infection [7]. Therapy involves broad-spectrum antibiotics, bowel rest, and close clinical and radiographic surveillance, with surgical conversion for clinical decline or failure to resolve over 1–2 weeks. For cervical perforations with uncontained leakage or evidence of systemic inflammatory response or sepsis, surgical drainage and selective repair are indicated. This should be combined with establishment of enteral feeding access in nearly all cases. Because stenting across the upper esophageal sphincter is poorly tolerated by most patients, stents for cervical perforation are generally considered only in the setting of failure following surgical intervention, particularly for distal perforations [21, 28]. Techniques for the surgical management of cervical perforation are outlined later in this chapter (Fig. 5.2).

For intra-abdominal perforation, primary reinforced surgical repair is almost always indicated and should be combined with surgical enteral feeding access in essentially all cases [31]. Exceptions to this approach may include patients who are otherwise unfit for surgery or who present with known advanced malignancy. In these patients, attempted stent therapy may be more reasonable (albeit with a lower likelihood of success).

For thoracic perforation, the gold standard of surgical treatment has been challenged by proponents of stent therapy over the last decade.

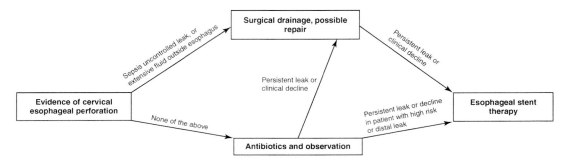

Fig. 5.2 Treatment algorithm for cervical perforation

In highly selected cases of intrathoracic perforation, therapy without surgical or stent repair ("conservative" treatment) may be appropriate [3]. Conservative treatment is rarely appropriate for patients with spontaneous perforation. These situations typically involve significant mediastinal and/or pleural contamination and thus mandate thoracoscopic or open thoracic surgical drainage. Conservative therapy should only be considered in cases where the perforation is localized/contained, there is no significant underlying esophageal pathology, and no clinical evidence of sepsis or systemic inflammatory response. These criteria are most often met in the setting of iatrogenic injury and early diagnosis [3, 19]. This approach may be particularly appropriate among patients who meet these criteria who have swallow studies demonstrating the return of all extravasated contrast back into the esophagus. This strategy may also be reasonable in those patients with air or fluid outside the esophagus on X-ray or CT imaging and no evidence of contrast extravasation on thorough swallow studies (sealed or microperforation).

Although mortality rates as high as 15% have been reported with conservative management [19], more recent studies suggest that when this strategy is combined with aggressive image-guided drainage and nutritional support, a mortality as low as 4% without surgical or stent repair is possible [18]. Patients are generally maintained strict nothing by mouth for at least 1 week, with a carefully positioned nasogastric tube in place, after which time a fluoroscopic

swallow study is repeated. In cases of clinical deterioration, repeat CT imaging is indicated. If this study demonstrates mediastinal or pleural space fluid collections amenable to percutaneous drainage, this should be pursued, with close monitoring for appropriate clinical response. In the case of extensive undrained pleural or mediastinal fluid, surgical drainage combined with either repair, stent placement, or diversion is indicated [1].

For patients not meeting criteria for the consideration of conservative therapy for thoracic esophageal perforation, a decision must be made between initial surgical and stent therapy. This decision must involve a surgeon with experience in thoracic surgery, who will serve as the primary operator for open repair or stent placement or drive the determination of the optimal route of drainage in the case of primary stent placement [5, 21]. Stents are generally inappropriate when a perforation extends beyond the gastroesophageal junction or with injuries greater than 6 cm – two situations associated with a high rate of stent failure [4, 5, 28, 32].

In patients with early perforation and extensive mediastinal or pleural space contamination, most advocate for primary surgical intervention [32]. When deciding between initial surgical management and stent therapy, it is important to consider that patients who present severely ill will likely have more favorable outcomes with surgery [1]. In cases of extensive delay to presentation, treatment must be individualized. In situations involving extensive esophageal tissue necrosis, surgical diversion may be the only viable option, as attempted primary repair in this setting is associated with high failure and mortality rates [15]. It is important to recognize, however, that some cases of delayed presentation involve only a contained perforation that may still be safely managed with stenting and drainage or primary surgical repair.

In the absence of extension across the gastroesophageal junction, long perforation, or advanced contamination, stent therapy is an option for most patients with intrathoracic perforation. The correct choice between primary stents and surgery remains controversial [12]. Stenting offers the advantage of decreased invasiveness and procedural morbidity when effective. Failure after initial stenting can also be followed by subsequent stent procedures in the absence of clinical sepsis [31]. However, if control of an esophageal leak is not achieved with primary stenting, current evidence suggests that the best results are achieved with rapid transition to an aggressive surgical approach [25].

There are conflicting reports on the success of stenting for spontaneous perforation, as this subset of patients generally presents with later diagnosis and more advanced infection. In one contemporary study of spontaneous perforation, mortality was three times higher in patients initially managed with stenting versus surgery, and nearly 85% of stent patients eventually required surgery [12]. Other studies suggest that the etiology of perforation does not affect the success or failure of any particular treatment modality [1, 12], decisions which instead should be driven by anatomic factors and the condition of the patient.

When stent therapy is pursued for thoracic esophageal perforation, therapy must include complete drainage by percutaneous, thoracoscopic, or open routes [12, 18, 21, 31]. Furthermore, it is important to recognize that many of these patients will require multiple drainage procedures. Most patients should have an NG tube in place for several days until a repeat swallow study is performed that confirms exclusion, at which point oral intake may be resumed

[5]. Others advocate for percutaneous endoscopic gastrostomy (PEG) tube placement concurrently with stenting, to provide for aggressive nutritional supplementation and obviate the need for NG tube drainage [21]. Patients with initial success after stent placement, confirmed by the lack of active contrast extravasation on subsequent swallow study (one to 3 days after stent placement) and absence of systemic infection, must be under close serial exams and periodic X-ray surveillance for stent migration [5, 21, 31]. These patients must also be monitored for undrained collections [21], as most will require multiple open or percutaneous drainage procedures [18, 31].

The surgical management of intrathoracic esophageal perforation generally entails primary two-layer closure combined with buttress of the repair with vascularized tissue and feeding tube placement [3]. In cases of underlying malignancy, mega-esophagus, non-dilatable stricture, or massive tissue damage, esophagectomy should be undertaken [3]. In a stable patient, primary reconstruction with a gastric conduit is appropriate. Otherwise, resection and diversion with delayed reconstruction are appropriate. Esophagectomy with primary anastomosis in the setting of esophageal perforation has a higher leak rate compared to elective esophagectomy, but the morbidity and lifestyle impediment associated with temporary diversion must also be considered. Patients with achalasia deserve special consideration as they are at risk for endoscopic perforation during therapeutic dilations or injections. In the setting of advanced achalasia with mega-esophagus, esophagectomy should be considered after perforation. Otherwise, esophageal myotomy (contralateral to the side of the perforation, extending well onto the stomach) after primary repair of intrathoracic perforation should be pursued.

The management of thoracic esophageal perforation is complex and requires individualized decisions by a multi-specialty care team. In this context, Fig. 5.3 outlines a proposed algorithm with general treatment guidelines.

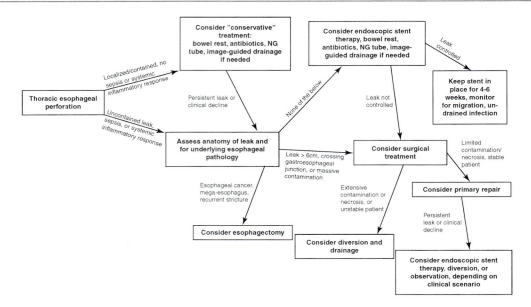

Fig. 5.3 Treatment algorithm for thoracic perforation

Surgical Technique: Cervical Perforation

Surgery is indicated in the majority of cases of cervical esophageal perforation. A minority of patients with iatrogenic perforation, no evidence of sepsis, and minimal contamination may be managed with observation, bowel rest, and antibiotics. When surgery is pursued, it should include drainage via a left cervical incision and repair in cases where the edges of the injury are clearly visible and viable after exposure. Although the midline cervical esophagus is accessible from the right or left neck, the recurrent laryngeal nerve is more closely associated with the esophagus on the right, and therefore a left-sided approach may be less likely to cause injury.

The patient should be placed in supine position with a bump behind the shoulder blades, neck gently hyperextended, and head tilted to the right. An NG tube should be in place, and the abdomen should be prepared for potential surgical feeding tube placement upon completion of the cervical procedure. Maximal exposure is obtained via incision from left earlobe to suprasternal notch, but a limited incision along the

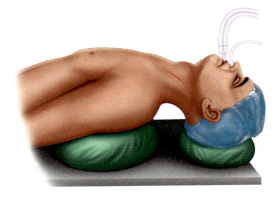

Fig. 5.4 Line for cervical incision

lower half to two-thirds of this line is generally adequate (Fig. 5.4). The incision is carried down onto the belly of the sternocleidomastoid muscle, which in turn is retracted laterally to expose the transverse course of the omohyoid muscle. The division of this muscle is critical to exposing the cervical esophagus. The carotid sheath is exposed following omohyoid division, and the sheath and its contents are retracted laterally, away from the trachea and thyroid gland. Blunt dissection in the plane between the carotid sheath and the thyroid will expose the middle thyroid vein, which should be ligated and divided. In some cases, the inferior thyroid artery will require division to provide safe exposure, without clinical consequence. The esophagus should be visible and palpable at this point if the NG tube is properly placed (Fig. 5.5).

Progressive blunt digital dissection lateral to the esophagus, down to the easily palpable cervical spine (and overlying prevertebral fascia), is fairly straightforward. In cases involving significant extra-luminal fluid or abscess, this dissection will generally enter the plane of the fluid collection. If tissue planes are severely effaced due to advanced or late infection, attempts to encircle the esophagus and primarily repair the injury should be avoided. Instead, careful blunt and sharp dissection should continue until there is wide drainage of all peri-esophageal fluid. In the absence of distal obstruction, the vast majority of cervical esophageal perforations will heal with drainage alone. In cases of drainage, treatment must also include debridement of all nonviable tissue, followed by extensive irrigation. There exist multiple options for wound management, but loose closure of the deep tissues over multiple passive rubber ("Penrose" type) drains, and placement of a wound vacuum dressing in lieu of skin closure is straightforward, reproduc-

ible, and effective. This approach facilitates adequate drainage, and the Penrose drains can be gradually backed out over the following week.

In cases where tissue quality is acceptable, the esophagus is mobilized circumferentially with careful digital dissection and encircled with a Penrose drain (Fig. 5.6). The recurrent laryngeal nerve, which runs in the tracheoesophageal groove, is vulnerable to injury during cervical esophageal procedures. Damage to this nerve is best avoided by maintaining surgical dissection directly on the muscular wall of the esophagus. Appropriate esophageal mobilization should provide for clear identification and exposure of the site of the injury, which is often located posteriorly at the level of the thyroid tracheal cartilage, just above the cricopharyngeus. After delineating the extent of the mucosal perforation by mobilizing overlying muscle fibers and debriding any nonviable tissue (Fig. 5.7), the mucosal defect should be closed with interrupted absorbable 3–0 or 4–0 sutures, with loose tissue approximation. Although not mandatory, some advocate esophageal bougie dilator placement to prevent narrowing during repair. Transverse closure theoretically leads to less luminal compromise, but with the exception of very large injuries, the injury can generally be closed longitudinally with minimal chance of stenosis. The esophageal muscle

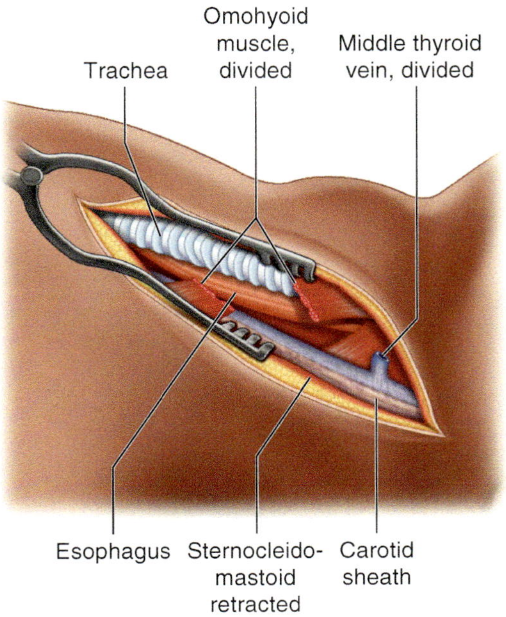

Omohyoid
muscle,   Middle thyroid
Trachea   divided   vein, divided

Esophagus Sternocleido- Carotid
            mastoid   sheath
            retracted

Fig. 5.5 Esophagus exposed via cervical incision

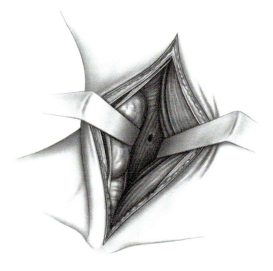

Fig. 5.6 Esophagus encircled via cervical incision

should be closed over the mucosal repair with absorbable suture, followed by advancement of an NG tube under direct palpation distal to the site. Digital palpation along the prevertebral fascia into the posterior mediastinum ensures adequate drainage of this space (Fig. 5.8). Finally, the wound bed should be copiously irrigated, and the cervical wound closed in layers over a drain. If there is extension of fluid below the level of the aortic arch on preoperative CT imaging, supplemental right thoracoscopic mediastinal drainage

should be considered. In situations involving extensive cervical esophageal injury and/or complex repair, surgical feeding tube placement (gastrostomy or jejunostomy) is prudent.

Surgical Technique: Repair of Intrathoracic Perforation

Prior to thoracic surgical intervention, it is important to ensure adequate fluid resuscitation and initiate broad-spectrum intravenous antibiotic therapy. Flexible endoscopy should be performed in cases concerning for esophageal malignancy or high-grade distal esophageal stricture; two situations that may be more optimally managed with resection versus repair. In stable patients, thoracic epidural placement is a reasonable preoperative consideration. The patient should have double-lumen endotracheal and NG tubes in place and should be placed in the lateral decubitus position. Following this, the operating room table should be flexed at the level of the iliac crest to facilitate maximal exposure.

For intrathoracic perforation and leak, the appropriate incision is determined by the level of injury. It is important to recognize that there is limited access to the distal esophagus and

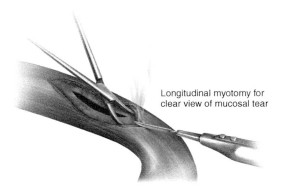

Longitudinal myotomy for clear view of mucosal tear

Fig. 5.7 Delineation of esophageal perforation (drawing needed). (With permission from Cooke and Lau [34]. Elsevier)

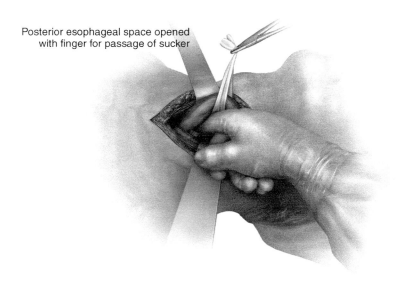

Posterior esophageal space opened with finger for passage of sucker

Fig. 5.8 Ensuring adequate mediastinal drainage. (With permission from Cooke and Lau [34]. Elsevier)

Level of Perforation	Surgical Approach(es)	Rationale
Cervical	Left Cervical	Avoidance of recurrent laryngeal nerve
Upper Thoracic	Right thoracotomy, 4th or 5th interspace (or thoracoscopy)	Aortic arch limits exposure from left chest
Lower Thoracic	Left thoracotomy, 7th or 8th interspace (or thoracoscopy)	Optimal exposure to esophageal hiatus
Gastroesophageal junction	Laparotomy (or laparoscopy)	Allows for repair and reinforcing fundoplication

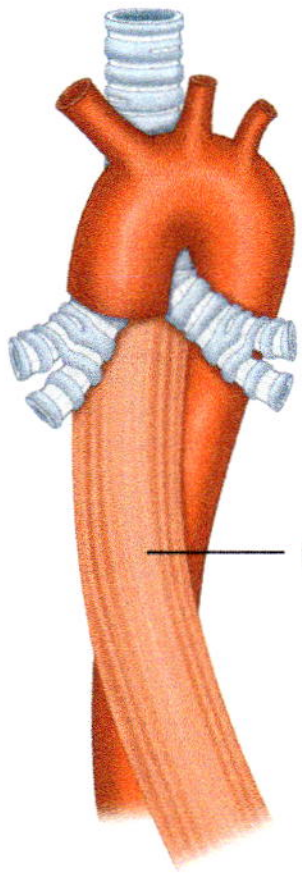

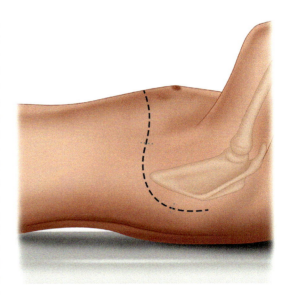

Esophagus

Fig. 5.9 Incisions for esophageal perforation

gastroesophageal junction from the right chest, and proximal esophageal access from the left chest is limited by the aortic arch and great vessels (Fig. 5.9). To access the proximal thoracic esophagus, a right lateral or posterolateral thoracotomy is appropriate, with a goal of entering the chest in the fourth or fifth intercostal space. To access the distal half of the thoracic esophagus, a left lateral or posterolateral seventh or 8th interspace thoracotomy is pursued. The landmarks for a posterolateral thoracotomy incision are shown in Fig. 5.10. Although muscle-sparing thoracotomy approaches (and even thoracoscopic approaches) are described for the management of a variety of intrathoracic conditions, a thoracotomy that involves division of the latissimus dorsi muscle and preservation of the serratus anterior muscle will provide adequate exposure with low incisional morbidity.

After incision of the skin and subcutaneous fat, the latissimus dorsi fascia and muscle are visible and should be divided with slow electrocautery exposing the underlying serratus anterior muscle and fascia. The serratus fascia should be incised to allow the elevation of the muscle anteriorly and off the chest wall, with division of loose areolar tissues and small perforating blood vessels deep to this muscle. This will allow for elevation of the scapula and the counting of ribs beneath the scapula to identify the appropriate level for entry. The first rib, palpable only with

Fig. 5.10 Line of incision for posterolateral thoracotomy; posteriorly, line begins midway between thoracic spine and medial scapula and extends to one fingerbreadth below scapular tip, before being extended anteriorly as needed for additional exposure

careful blunt dissection, is broad and flat. The second interspace is distinctly wider than either the first or third space. In general, the tip of the scapula overlies the sixth rib – this relatively constant anatomic finding proves generally adequate for planned incisional level for the surgical management of esophageal perforation. After dividing the intercostal muscle directly over the rib to access the pleural space, the intercostal incision is extended to the transverse process posteriorly and within several centimeters of the sternum anteriorly. Removing a small portion of the inferior rib reduces the likelihood of inducing a rib fracture with retraction.

If the surgical intent is a primary repair, the surgeon should consider harvesting an intercostal muscle flap at the time of thoracotomy, as this becomes impossible after a traditional thoracotomy has been completed. To harvest an intercostal flap, the intercostal muscle is gently dissected from the interspace at the level of the planned incision. The dissection should be cautious at the cephalad aspect of the muscle, where the neurovascular bundle must be meticulously dissected free from the overlying rib. The muscular pedicle should be mobilized to within several centimeters of the internal mammary artery medially (within several centimeters of the sternum), after which the muscle pedicle is divided anteriorly, mobilized posteriorly as far as possible, and then packed in a moist gauze prior to placement of a rib spreading retractor. The intercostal muscle flap can eventually be utilized as vascularized tissue to buttress an esophageal repair.

After thoracotomy is completed, perpendicular rib-spreading retractors should be placed and the lung retracted and packed anteriorly (Fig. 5.11). In the case of left thoracotomy for distal thoracic esophageal perforation, division of the inferior pulmonary ligament (fibro-fatty tissue between the left lower lobe and mediastinum) up to the level of the inferior pulmonary vein will aid exposure of the esophagus. For mid-esophageal perforation, which is accessed via right thoracotomy, encircling the azygous vein and dividing it with a vascular stapler will improve exposure. This maneuver is not associated with any clinical effects as long as careful hemostasis is confirmed. The NG tube should allow esophageal palpation, which is preceded by longitudinally opening the mediastinal pleura over the entire length of the exposed esophagus. For primary repair, the esophagus should be mobilized and encircled near the region of the perforation (Fig. 5.12). After encircling the esophagus with a Penrose drain, the site of injury should be examined by longitudinally dividing the esophageal muscle fibers above and below the site of perforation until the extent of the mucosal rent is clearly visible. In cases where the distal extent of a perforation cannot be visualized adequately via low left thoracotomy, the left diaphragm can be partially opened to facilitate exposure, with subsequent closure with permanent, interrupted mattress suture following completion of repair.

The decision to proceed with repair should be predicated on reasonable tissue quality and absence of extensive tissue devitalization or underlying pathology. If repair is deemed appropriate, the mucosal defect should be closed with interrupted absorbable 3-0 or 4-0 sutures, fol-

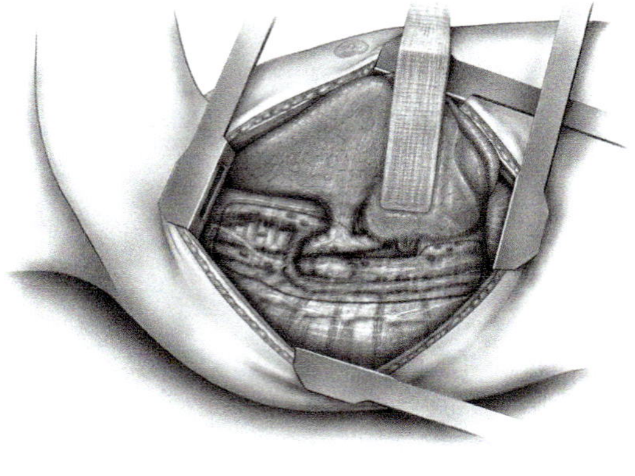

Fig. 5.11 Right thoracotomy for esophageal exposure, perpendicular rib-spreading retractors in place, lung retracted anteriorly

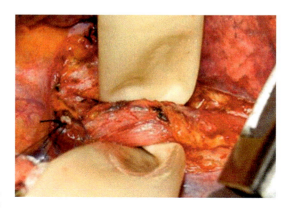

Fig. 5.12 Esophagus encircled in the thorax

lowed by closure of the overlying muscle with absorbable or silk sutures. An NG tube should be passed into the stomach with surgical guidance. Closure should be buttressed with an intercostal muscle flap, a vascularized pedicle of adjacent mediastinal pleura, or a partial fundoplication for repairs near the gastroesophageal junction. In cases of advanced pleural space contamination, pulmonary decortication may be required to facilitate complete lung expansion. After extensive pleural space irrigation, multiple chest tubes should be placed, the thoracotomy is closed in standard fashion, and a surgical feeding tube is placed.

After esophageal repair, the NG tube should be maintained for several days at a minimum, and at least one dependent pleural drain should remain in place until safe dietary advancement is confirmed. A fluoroscopic study should be completed 5–7 days following closure. If there is no leak, the NG can be removed (if still in place), and oral input gradually resumed. If advancement of diet does not lead to a change in the character or volume of pleural drain output (concerning for either recurrent leak or chylothorax), the remaining drain can be removed. If a swallow study suggests the existence of a persistent leak, most authors advocate endoscopic stent placement [20, 33] unless (1) there is evidence of extensive tissue necrosis, which would mandate additional surgical debridement and generally necessitate temporary diversion, or (2) a small, adequately drained leak is present, which may require no additional intervention.

Surgical Technique: Repair of Intra-abdominal Perforation

Again, an NG tube is left in place, and flexible endoscopy should be completed if there is any concern for esophageal malignancy or high-grade distal stricture. Intra-abdominal esophageal perforation typically involves an injury in the region of the gastroesophageal junction. After an upper midline laparotomy and placement of a retractor system, mobilizing the avascular attachments between the left liver lobe and the diaphragm facilitates

lateral liver retraction and improved access to the esophageal hiatus. Mobilization of the upper greater curvature of the stomach by division of the short gastric vessels in this region provides additional exposure and facilitates subsequent fundoplication (Fig. 5.13). The distal esophagus can be palpated using the NG tube and then mobilized bluntly from the underling aorta, eventually encircling it with a Penrose drain (Fig. 5.14).

As with thoracic repair, the extent of the mucosal perforation should be clearly delineated, all devitalized tissue debrided, and a two layer repair completed. The NG tube should be advanced into the stomach, followed by a fundoplication to reinforce the repair. For most patients, a partial fundoplication is appropriate, although

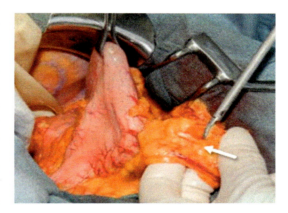

Fig. 5.13 Abdominal exposure of the esophagus; liver mobilized/retracted, short gastric arteries divided

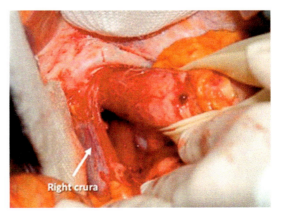

Fig. 5.14 Abdominal exposure, the esophagus encircled below diaphragmatic hiatus with Penrose drain

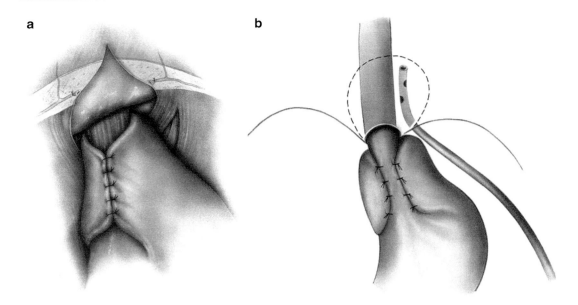

Fig. 5.15 Abdominal fundoplications; (**a**) complete (Nissen) fundoplication; (**b**) partial posterior fundoplication

complete (360°) fundoplication is a reasonable option for a patient with pre-existing gastro-esophageal reflux and no evidence of a motility disorder (Fig. 5.15). After copious irrigation and placement of a surgical feeding jejunostomy tube, the abdomen is closed in standard fashion. Most surgeons do not routinely leave drains following abdominal repairs. After fascial closure, the skin and soft tissues are managed with loose stapled closure, wound vacuum placement, or planned delayed primary closure.

Surgical Technique: Drainage for Intrathoracic Perforation

Selected cases of intrathoracic esophageal perforation may be managed with surgical drainage alone without repair. This may accompany esophageal stent placement or a trial of conservative therapy, when there are pleural or mediastinal fluid collections not amenable to drainage via tube thoracostomy or percutaneous image-guided drainage. Adequate drainage of the mediastinum and pleural space, and decortication of the lung, can generally be achieved with a thoracoscopic approach with single-lung ventilation. That said,

patients should always be counseled on the potential need to convert to open thoracotomy. The decision between a left and right thoracoscopy should be guided by preoperative imaging. In cases where there is contained mediastinal fluid, the posterior mediastinum is best accessed from the right pleural space in most cases. This is achieved by tilting the operating room table steeply to the left with the patient in a well-secured left lateral decubitus position, retracting the deflated lung anteriorly, and opening the mediastinal pleural between the azygous vein and the lung in layers until the fluid collection is encountered and drained. Priorities at surgery include the evacuation of all debris, drainage of all fluid collections, breaking up any loculations to create a unified pleural space, and lung decortication to ensure complete lung expansion. The pleural space should be irrigated copiously, with the placement of at least two dependent drains.

Surgical Technique: Esophageal Diversion

For patients who present with extensive mediastinal contamination, esophageal necrosis, or septic shock, esophageal diversion may be the only viable option. Diversion may also be needed after the failure of stent or surgical repair or may be the treatment of choice in a patient with underlying pathology that would otherwise indicate resection but does not possess the physiologic reserve to tolerate such a major procedure. Esophageal diversion entails the creation of a cervical esophagostomy with decompressive gastrostomy and feeding jejunostomy and is usually combined with transection of the gastroesophageal junction ("exclusion") to minimize the potential for retrograde mediastinal contamination.

The cervical esophagus is exposed and encircled as described earlier via a generous left neck incision. The esophagus should be mobilized into the posterior mediastinum with blunt dissection along the prevertebral fascia posteriorly, the membranous trachea anteriorly, and fibroareolar attachments laterally. After mobilizing the esophagus as far distally as safely possible, the NG tube is backed up to above the incision and the esophagus divided as distally as possible with an endoscopic stapler. Preserving maximal length will facilitate the creation of a stoma below the clavicle (much more manageable than a cervical stoma) and facilitate later reconstruction. A 2 cm counter-incision is created on the left upper anterior chest wall, just below the medial left clavicle. After creating a generous tunnel between the cervical incision and the upper chest wound, the proximal blind end of the esophagus is passed through this tract and delivered onto the chest wall. The stapled end is excised and the stoma matured in standard fashion. An upper midline laparotomy is then performed, and the esophagus is exposed at the hiatus as previously described. The esophagus is encircled at this level and transected with an endoscopic stapler, followed by placement of a decompressive gastrostomy and feeding jejunostomy. Bilateral tube thoracostomy is performed at the conclusion of the procedure. Reconstruction is planned for a later date and generally involves retrosternal placement of a gastric conduit.

Esophageal Resection

Esophagectomy is rarely indicated in the setting of esophageal perforation, as this is a major undertaking for an acutely ill patient. In more stable cases of perforation with underlying pathology such as early-stage esophageal malignancy, achalasia with mega-esophagus, or refractory stricture, esophagectomy can be considered. The technical details of this procedure are outside the scope of this chapter.

Summary

Esophageal perforation is an uncommon condition that continues to be associated with high levels of morbidity and mortality. Endoscopic stent therapy is being used with greater frequency for perforation and seems to offer advantages over a traditional surgical approach in select cases. Recognizing the limitations of the available evidence and considering the multiple therapeutic options, there exist several clear principles which must guide treatment. These include adequate resuscitation, aggressive drainage of associated fluid, satisfactory nutritional support, debridement of any nonviable tissue, and vigilance in monitoring a patient's response to therapy. Treatment must be individualized and driven by a team of experts with the intent of dynamic adjustment based on a patient's clinical course.

References

1. Abbas G, Schuchert MJ, Pettiford BL, Pennathur A, Landreneau J, Landreneau J, et al. Contemporaneous management of esophageal perforation. Surgery. 2009;146:749–55.
2. Brinster CJ, Singhal S, Lee L, Marshall MB, Kaiser LR, Kucharczuk JC. Evolving options in the management of esophageal perforation. Ann Thorac Surg. 2004;77:1475–83.
3. Sudarshan M, Elharram M, Spicer J, Mulder D, Ferri LE. Management of esophageal perforation in the endoscopic era: is operative repair still relevant? Surgery. 2016;160(4):1104–10.
4. Koivukangas V, Biancari F, Merilainen S, Ala-Kokko T, Saarnio J. Esophageal stenting for spontaneous

esophageal perforation. J Trauma Acute Care Surg. 2012;73:1011–3.

5. Freeman RK, Van Woerkorn JM, Vyverberg A, Ascioti AJ. Esophageal stent placement for the treatment of spontaneous esophageal perforations. Ann Thorac Surg. 2009;88:194–8.

6. Bryant AS, Cerfolio RJ. Esophageal trauma. Thorac Surg Clin. 2007;17:63–72.

7. Sancheti MS, Fernandez FG. Surgical management of esophageal perforation. Oper Tech Thoracic Cardiovasc Surg. 2016;2:234–50.

8. Kaman L, Iqbal B, Kochhar R. Management of esophageal perforation in adults. Gastroenterol Res. 2010;3:235–44.

9. Mohajer P, Annan E, Ahuja J, Sharif M, Sung A. Acute respiratory failure from aspiration pneumonitis: a complication of Gastrograffin contrast media. Chest. 2012;142:1017A.

10. Fadoo F, Ruiz DE, Dawn SK, Webb WR, Gotway MB. Helical CT esophagography for the evaluation of suspected esophageal perforation or rupture. Am J Roentgenol. 2004;182:1177–9.

11. Arantes V, Campolina C, Valerio SH, de Sa RN, Toledo C, Ferrari TA, Coelho LG. Flexible esophagoscopy as a diagnostic tool for traumatic esophageal injuries. J Trauma. 2009;66:1677–82.

12. Schweigert M, Beattie R, Solymosi N, Booth K, Dubecz A, Muir A, et al. Endoscopic stent insertion versus primary operative management for spontaneous rupture of the esophagus (Boerhaave syndrome): an international study. Am Surg. 2013;739:634–40.

13. Wang N, Razzouk AJ, Safavi A, Gan K, Van Ardsell GS, Burton PM, Fandrich BL, et al. Delayed primary repair of intrathoracic esophageal perforation: is it safe? J Thoracic Cardiovasc Surg. 1996;111:114–21.

14. Bhatia P, Fortin D, Inculet RI, Malthaner RA. Current concepts in the management of esophageal perforations: a twenty-seven year Canadian experience. Ann Thorac Surg. 2011;92:209–15.

15. Salo JA, Isolauri JO, Hiekkila LJ, Markkula HT, Heikkinen LO, Kivilaakso EO, et al. Management of delayed esophageal perforation with mediastinal sepsis. Esophagectomy or primary repair? J Thoracic Cardiovasc Surg. 1993;106:1088–91.

16. Jougon J, Mc Bride T, Delcambre F, Minniti A, Velly JF. Primary esophageal repair for Boerhaave's syndrome whatever the free interval between perforation and treatment. Eur J Cardiothorac Surg. 2004;25:475–9.

17. Kuppusamy MK, Hubka M, Felisky CD, Carrott P, Kline EM, Koehler RP, et al. Evolving management strategies in esophageal perforation: surgeons using nonoperative techniques to improve outcomes. J Am Coll Surg. 2011;213:164–71.

18. Vogel SB, Rout R, Martin TD, Abbitt PL. Esophageal perforation in adults: aggressive, conservative treatment lowers morbidity and mortality. Ann Surg. 2005;241:1016–23.

19. Hasan S, Jilaihawi AN, Prakash D. Conservative management of iatrogenic oesophageal perforation – a viable option. Eur J Cardiothorac Surg. 2005;28:7–10.

20. Keeling WB, Miller DL, Lam GT, Kilgo P, Miller JI, Mansour KA, et al. Low mortality after treatment for esophageal perforation: a single-center experience. Ann Thorac Surg. 2010;90:1669–73.

21. Herrera A, Freeman RK. The evolution and current utility of esophageal stent placement for the treatment of acute esophageal perforation. Thorac Surg Clin. 2016;26:305–14.

22. Romero RV, Khean-Lee G. Esophageal perforation: continuing challenge to treatment. Gastrointest Interv. 2013;2:1–6.

23. Hajj II, Imperiale TF, Rex DK, Ballard D, Kesler KA, Birdas TJ, et al. Treatment of esophageal leaks, fistulae, and perforations with temporary stents: evaluation of efficacy, adverse events, and factors associated with successful outcomes. Gastrointest Endosc. 2014;79:589–98.

24. Dasari BV, Neely D, Kennedy A, Spence G, Rice P, Mackle E, et al. The role of esophageal stents in the management of esophageal anastomotic leaks and benign esophageal perforations. Ann Surg. 2014;259:852–60.

25. Nason KS. Is open surgery for iatrogenic esophageal perforation now a surgical relic, like bloodletting and trepanation? J Thoracic Cardiovasc Surg. 2015;149:1556–7.

26. Freeman RK, Herrera A, Ascioti AJ, Dake M, Mahidhara RS. A propensity-matched comparison of cost and outcomes after esophageal stent placement or primary surgical repair for iatrogenic esophageal perfusion. J Thorac Cardiovasc Surg. 2015;149:1550–5.

27. Persson S, Elbe P, Rouvelas I, Lindblad M, Kumagai K, Lundell L, et al. Predictors for failure of stent treatment for benign esophageal perforations – a single center 10-year experience. World J Gastroenterol. 2014;20:10613–9.

28. Freeman RK, Acioti AJ, Giannini T, Mahidhara RJ. Analysis of unsuccessful esophageal stent placements for esophageal perforation, fistula, or anastomotic leak. Ann Thorac Surg. 2012;94:959–65.

29. Liang DH, Hwang E, Meisenback LM, Kim MP, Chan EY, Khaitan PG. Clinical outcomes following self-expanding metal stent placement for esophageal salvage. J Thorac Cardiovasc Surg. 2017;154:1145–50.

30. Wu G, Zhao YS, Fang Y, Qi Y, Li X, Jiao D, Ren K, Han X. Treatment of spontaneous esophageal rupture with transnasal thoracic drainage and temporary esophageal stent and jejunal feeding tube placement. J Trauma Acute Care Surg. 2017;82:141–9.

31. Ben-David K, Behrns K, Hochwald S, Rossidis G, Caban A, Crippen C, et al. Esophageal perforation management using a multidisciplinary minimally invasive treatment algorithm. J Am Coll Surg. 2014;218:768–74.

32. Nirula R. Esophageal perforation. Surg Clin N Am. 2014;94:35–41.
33. Freeman RK, Ascioti AJ, Dake M, Mahidhara RS. An analysis of esophageal stent placement for persistent leak after the operative repair of intratho-

racic esophageal perforations. Ann Thorac Surg. 2014;97:1715–20.
34. Cooke DT, Lau CL. Primary repair of esophageal perforation. Oper Tech Thoracic Cardiovasc Surg. 2008;5:126–37.

Variceal Hemorrhage for the Acute Care Surgeon

6

Paul J. Deramo and Michael S. Truitt

Background

Variceal hemorrhage accounts for one-third of cirrhosis-related deaths and represents the leading life-threatening complication of portal hypertension [1–3]. Esophageal varices are the most common cause of persistent, severe upper gastrointestinal hemorrhage, and in cirrhotic patients, are responsible for over 70% of acute bleeding episodes [4]. Furthermore, nearly 50% of patients with a diagnosis of cirrhosis have documented gastroesophageal varices so knowledge of the medical and surgical treatment of these patients is of interest to the Acute Care Surgeon [5].

While not the most common cause of upper gastrointestinal (GI) hemorrhage overall, esophageal varices account for 14% of hospitalizations for upper GI bleeding. Over the past 30 years, there have been significant advances in the management of variceal bleeding. Beginning in the late 1980s, when endovascular stent technology gave rise to transjugular intrahepatic portosystemic shunt (TIPS), the surgical management of esophageal variceal bleeding has largely been replaced by percutaneous intervention. During this time, the 6-week mortality has fallen from

40% to 15% [6, 7]. While a significant improvement, variceal bleeding is still highly lethal compared to other causes of GI bleeding which usually resolve with conservative or endoscopic therapies and carry reported mortality of 3%. In patients who are not suitable candidates for TIPS placement, emergency surgical therapy may be required as a life-saving measure. This underscores the importance of a multidisciplinary approach for patients with variceal bleeding and the need for the Acute Care Surgeon to understand the physiology and the various treatment modalities at their disposal.

History

In 1543, the famous physician anatomist Vesalius first drew detailed pictures of the portal venous system [8]. Over 200 years later, Morgagni described a patient who developed upper abdominal pain and upper GI hemorrhage and died in short order [8]. At autopsy, the stomach had several dark patches, and he wondered whether small but dilated vessels had oozed into the gastric wall. In 1841, Raciborski first recognized that collaterals could form between the systemic and portal venous systems, and a decade later, Sappey would go on to discover esophageal varices [8]. In the early 1900s, Banti recognized that diseased spleens could lead to varices, and others identified elevated portal pressures in many patients with

P. J. Deramo
Methodist Dallas Medical Center, Dallas, TX, USA

M. S. Truitt (✉)
Department of Surgery, Methodist Dallas Medical Center, Dallas, TX, USA
e-mail: michaeltruitt@mhd.com

© Springer International Publishing AG, part of Springer Nature 2019
C. V. R. Brown et al. (eds.), *Emergency General Surgery*, https://doi.org/10.1007/978-3-319-96286-3_6

esophageal varices and cirrhosis [9]. Finally, in 1928, Sir Archibald McIndoe concluded that portal pressures are increased in cirrhotic patients – what he coined "portal hypertension" [9].

As the pathophysiology of ascites and esophageal varices was elucidated, surgeons looked for ways to combat the increased portal pressures. In 1877, Nikolai Eck, a Russian military surgeon who was studying liver perfusion in dogs, successfully anastomosed the portal vein to the side of the vena cava, and Pavlov would later describe the "meat intoxication" known as hepatic encephalopathy that developed in dogs with Eck's fistula [9]. Whipple would later attempt to decompress the portal system by anastomosing mesenteric venous branches with the systemic circulation and, after clotting several of these shunts, experimented with anastomosing the splenic and renal veins [9]. This laid the groundwork for future surgical therapies in the management of esophageal varices.

Simultaneously, there was a push to develop nonsurgical therapies for esophageal bleeding. In 1868, Kussmaul utilized a modified lighted tube originally used for urologic procedures to examine the inside of a human stomach, and Mikulicz, in 1881, created the first "gastroscope" to examine the upper gastrointestinal tract [8]. In the following years, flexible and rigid gastroscopes were developed, and by the 1930s, sclerotherapy with quinine-urethane solutions was possible [8]. In the 1950s, well after balloon tamponade was found to be a useful strategy, Sengstaken and Blakemore created the first nasogastric tube with a balloon to control variceal hemorrhage, though patients frequently developed severe aspiration or life-threatening airway obstruction [9]. Stiegmann then took the concept of rectal hemorrhoid banding and developed the first esophageal variceal ligation device, later demonstrating superiority to sclerotherapy in a multicenter trial [9].

Over the next three decades, a variety of surgical shunt procedures were developed and refined to deal with portal hypertension and variceal bleeding. But the most significant advance occurred with the introduction of TIPS which has revolutionized the care of patients with variceal

bleeding and has slowly turned surgical shunts into legacy operations.

Pathophysiology of Variceal Hemorrhage

At the most basic level, variceal bleeding is the result of any process that increases the pressure gradient between the portal venous and systemic venous systems. In the case of cirrhosis, hepatic fibrosis and regenerative nodules impede portal venous blood flow. This increased resistance, by Ohm's law (pressure = flow × resistance), leads to an increased portosystemic pressure gradient. Though not fully understood, splanchnic hormones and other humoral mediators – particularly nitric oxide – facilitate hyperdynamic augmentation of blood flow from systemic to portal circulation. This increase blood flow – hepatic autoregulation – causes engorgement of normally small venous collaterals leading to an increased risk of spontaneous hemorrhage [10]. Coagulopathy and thrombocytopenia, hallmarks of advanced cirrhosis, only intensify the bleeding as does concurrent bacterial infection. On endoscopy, these dilated submucosal veins appear to bulge out above the surrounding mucosa. These can appear necrotic or ulcerated after recent hemorrhage or intervention (Fig. 6.1).

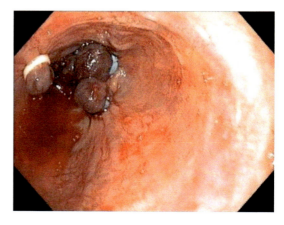

Fig. 6.1 Esophageal varices after recent banding with necrotic appearance, slight ulceration. (Ref: http://fromnewtoicu.com/tips/)

Table 6.1 Causes of portal hypertension by category

Common etiologies of portal hypertension
Prehepatic
1. Portal vein thrombosis
2. Splenic vein thrombosis
Hepatic
1. Pre-sinusoidal – Schistosomiasis, chronic viral hepatitis, Wilson's disease, hemochromatosis, amyloidosis, sarcoidosis, tuberculosis
2. Sinusoidal – Cirrhosis (all etiologies)
3. Post-sinusoidal – Veno-occlusive disease
Post-hepatic
1. Budd-Chiari disease (hepatic vein thrombosis)
2. Inferior caval occlusion/thrombosis

Familiarity with the causes of portal hypertension (Table 6.1) is essential for the proper management of variceal hemorrhage. Prehepatic portal hypertension is usually the result of portal vein thrombosis, the most common cause in children. Esophageal varices develop as the result of increased portal pressures, and routine screening for varices plays a role in the management of these patients. In adults, idiopathic non-cirrhotic portal hypertension has emerged as a diagnosis of exclusion once major causes of portal hypertension have been ruled out [11]. These patients often present with esophageal and gastric variceal bleeding and splenomegaly. The decision to anticoagulate patients with chronic portal vein thrombosis must be weighed against the possibility of gastrointestinal hemorrhage and the risk of endoscopic or surgical intervention.

In contrast, isolated gastric variceal hemorrhage is a different clinical entity associated with left-sided portal hypertension. Usually secondary to pancreatic pathology, the splenic venous pressures increase though portal venous pressures remain unchanged [12]. The resulting gradient leads to gastroepiploic venous hypertension and, ultimately, bleeding from gastric varices characteristic of this disease. Splenectomy eliminates the splenic and gastroepiploic venous hypertension and prevents future variceal bleeding.

Intrahepatic causes of portal hypertension include most etiologies of cirrhosis as well as schistosomiasis. These increased portal pressure gradients typically occur at the level of the sinusoids from hepatic fibrosis or immediately post-sinusoidal from regenerative nodules – both increasing resistance to portal venous outflow leading to the classic esophageal variceal hemorrhage common for these patients. Management with well-studied medical, endoscopic, and percutaneous interventions is the mainstay of therapy though surgical shunts and devascularization procedures are effective for select patients.

Finally, post-hepatic portal hypertension occurs as a result of Budd-Chiari syndrome or hepatic vein thrombosis as well as some cardiac pathologies [13]. Most cases are secondary to inherited thrombophilia, and patients often present with ascites and abdominal pain though less likely gastrointestinal bleeding from gastric and esophageal varices. In these patients, anticoagulation is the mainstay of therapy with angioplasty, thrombolysis, or stenting reserved for refractory cases. TIPS and liver transplantation are downline therapies [13].

Ultimately, the goals of care with portal hypertension and associated gastroesophageal varices are threefold: *prevent* bleeding, *stop* bleeding when it occurs, and *prevent recurrent* bleeding. We will focus on the management of acute bleeding and the prevention of recurrent bleeding.

Acute Bleeding

Diagnosis

The definitive diagnosis of esophageal variceal bleeding in the acute setting can usually be inferred from the patient history and constellation of physical exam findings. Patients with a history of liver disease who present with hematemesis or other signs of upper gastrointestinal bleeding should be presumed to have variceal bleeding until proven otherwise. Full laboratory workup including frequent complete blood count, complete metabolic profile, coagulation studies, and lactate should be obtained rapidly to determine physiologic baseline and guide resuscitation. Type and cross-match of 4–6 units of packed red blood cells – and the liberal use of a massive transfusion – are mandatory given the possibility of rapid and profuse hemorrhage. Thromboelastography may also be helpful

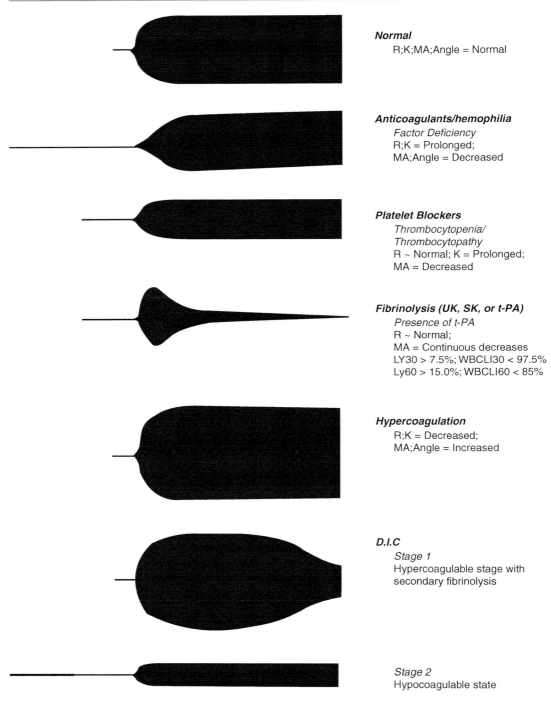

Normal
R;K;MA;Angle = Normal

Anticoagulants/hemophilia
Factor Deficiency
R;K = Prolonged;
MA;Angle = Decreased

Platelet Blockers
Thrombocytopenia/
Thrombocytopathy
R ~ Normal; K = Prolonged;
MA = Decreased

Fibrinolysis (UK, SK, or t-PA)
Presence of t-PA
R ~ Normal;
MA = Continuous decreases
LY30 > 7.5%; WBCLI30 < 97.5%
Ly60 > 15.0%; WBCLI60 < 85%

Hypercoagulation
R;K = Decreased;
MA;Angle = Increased

D.I.C
Stage 1
Hypercoagulable stage with
secondary fibrinolysis

Stage 2
Hypocoagulable state

Fig. 6.2 Common TEG patterns, hypocoagulable state often seen in patients with high risk of early rebleeding

in guiding a targeted resuscitation (Fig. 6.2). This may be of particular benefit as the goal of resuscitation without volume overload is particularly salient in the cirrhotic patient.

Nasogastric lavage can help confirm bleeding proximal to the duodenum and may improve endoscopic visualization. Ultimately, prompt endoscopic evaluation remains the gold standard for diagnosis and early initial management of gastroesophageal variceal hemorrhage.

Management

Variceal hemorrhage has defined time points and terminology which have been simplified for comparing therapies and applying clinical algorithms. *Time zero* starts at the admission to a medical facility for variceal bleeding. *Acute bleeding episodes* encompass the first 5 days from *time zero*. During the acute bleeding episode, bleeding is considered *clinically significant* if the patient has hypotension and tachycardia and requires two or more units of packed red blood cells in the first 24 h after time zero. *Failed treatment* occurs with development of hemorrhagic shock, recurrent bleeding, or 4-point drop of hemoglobin during the acute bleeding episode. The goals of initial management include stopping variceal hemorrhage and enacting measures to prevent *early* (up to 6 weeks) and late *rebleeding* (after 6 weeks) (Fig. 6.3).

Compared to other forms of upper gastrointestinal bleeding – where roughly 90%

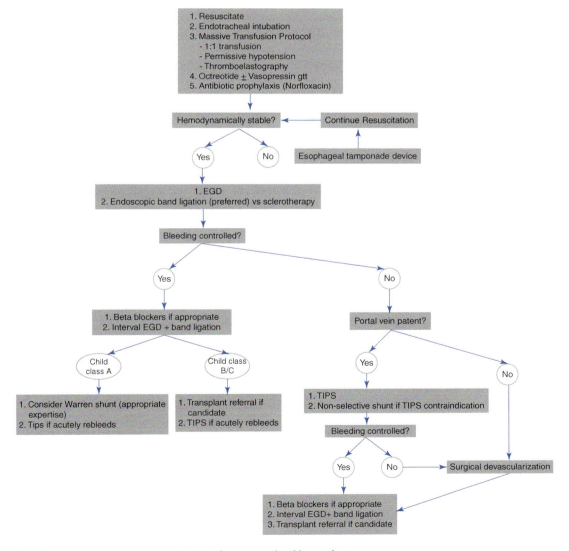

Fig. 6.3 Suggested management algorithm for acute variceal hemorrhage

spontaneously resolve – variceal bleeding spontaneously ceases only 50% of the time. Most early rebleeding occurs within 72 h of initial hemorrhage control, and patients remain at risk during the early rebleeding period. Beyond 6 weeks, the risk of recurrent rebleeding and associated mortality are the same as in cirrhotics who never had a bleeding episode. The goals of long-term management include prophylaxis and minimizing risk factors of variceal hemorrhage.

Initial Management

Given the possibility of fatal hemorrhage, management of esophageal variceal bleeding starts with the ABCs – airway, breathing, and circulation. Early endotracheal intubation is vital to minimize the risk of aspiration and allows for controlled endoscopic intervention. Placement of two large-bore IVs and a Foley catheter allow for the expeditious administration of blood products and careful monitoring of resuscitation. This is of paramount importance as patients with a hemoglobin <10 or hemodynamic instability have been demonstrated to have poorer prognosis. Early ICU admission and endoscopic evaluation are important for quickly addressing changes in hemodynamic status.

In patients with variceal hemorrhage as a result of cirrhosis, correction of hemorrhagic shock with blood products must be carefully balanced against the risk of over-resuscitation. Any precipitous increase in blood volume may increase portal venous pressure and thus further exacerbate variceal hemorrhage. This has led to the adoption of a permissive hypotension strategy often utilized in trauma patients, emphasizing mentation rather than systolic blood pressure as a marker for adequate perfusion. More importantly, the resuscitation should be balanced with blood, platelets, and plasma products. Several algorithms include recombinant factor VIIa and prothrombin complex concentrate for rapid correction of coagulopathy though these agents are expensive and randomized control trials have failed to show a significant decrease in early rebleeding or mortality with their use.

Pharmacologic Agents

Once the patient has become hemodynamically stable, pharmacologic therapies are then indicated to slow the rate of variceal bleeding [14]. Vasoactive medications such as somatostatin and vasopressin affect splanchnic blood flow by constricting mesenteric arterioles and thus diminishing portal venous inflow. Octreotide is given as a bolus of 50 mcg and then given infused continuously at 50mcg/hr for 3–5 days. In severe variceal hemorrhage, continuous vasopressin infusion may be added which has a 60% success rate of achieving variceal hemostasis. However, the systemic effects of vasopressin must be considered as well as the need for simultaneous nitroglycerin. Terlipressin is initiated at 2 mg and titrated every few hours until hemorrhage abates.

Terlipressin is the only agent with a proven mortality benefit but is not currently available in the United States, and sodium levels must be monitored given the risk of hyponatremia [15]. Octreotide has been shown to decrease rebleeding and is more effective when combined with sclerotherapy or endoscopic variceal ligation. Octreotide is also superior to vasopressin for initial control of bleeding with far fewer side effects. Vasopressin should be avoided as a first-line agent to control bleeding.

While continuous proton pump inhibitor (PPI) infusions are commonly started for patients with upper GI bleeding, there are no prospective trials demonstrating a benefit of PPI in the management of esophageal variceal bleeding.

Antibiotics/Prokinetics

Of cirrhotic patients hospitalized with GI bleeding, roughly 20% have a bacterial infection on admission, and roughly 50% will develop a nosocomial infection during the hospital stay [16, 17]. Various hypotheses regarding an increased risk of aspiration, spontaneous bacterial peritonitis, endoscopic or percutaneous instrumentation, and bacterial translocation have been proposed to explain the correlation of bleeding with increased infection risk. Most bacterial isolates are gram-negative bacilli originating from the GI tract.

Nevertheless, no study has proven causation of an increased risk of bleeding with infection.

The preponderance of guidelines supports a short course of prophylactic antibiotics, classically norfloxacin 400 mg or ciprofloxacin 400 mg twice daily. In advanced cirrhosis or centers with known quinolone resistance, ceftriaxone 1 g daily is preferred [16, 17]. Most advocate for 7 days of treatment.

Prokinetic agents such as erythromycin and metoclopramide have been studied extensively in upper GI bleeding to help clear the stomach before endoscopic intervention. Most conclude that there is a small decrease in duration of the initial endoscopic procedure and improved visualization though no mortality benefit has been identified.

Finally, lactulose can be helpful as a cathartic to combat the hepatic encephalopathy present and to expel blood products from the GI tract while limiting azotemia.

Balloon Tamponade

For patients with torrential esophageal variceal hemorrhage, variceal balloon tamponade is a helpful temporizing measure until more definitive therapy can be arranged [18]. The three common tamponade balloons are the Linton-Nachlas tube (gastric balloon, gastric suction port), the Sengstaken-Blakemore tube (gastric balloon, esophageal balloon, gastric suction port), and the Minnesota tube (modified Sengstaken-Blakemore tube with proximal esophageal suction port). The Sengstaken-Blakemore tube is widely available but requires an additional nasogastric tube with the tip secured proximal to the esophageal balloon to suction proximal secretions (Fig. 6.4).

A patient should undergo endotracheal intubation before placement of a balloon tamponade device to secure the airway and minimize the risk of aspiration. When available, portable x-ray imaging or fluoroscopy should be used to help with placement and ensure proper placement of the gastric balloon. Use of water mixed with iodinated contrast may help identify the balloons on imaging. Frequently, inflation of the gastric balloon and gentle traction will result in the ces-

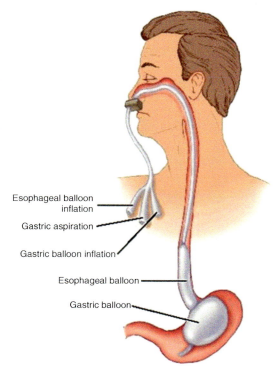

Fig. 6.4 Sengstaken-Blakemore tube placement with description of different ports; esophageal tube (not pictured) proximal to the esophageal balloon necessary to minimize aspiration

sation of bleeding. If this is unsuccessful, the esophageal balloon should also be inflated to control more proximal varices. This balloon must be let down for a few minutes every 1–2 h to prevent esophageal mucosal pressure necrosis.

While trials have demonstrated that variceal tamponade is comparable to pharmacologic and endoscopic therapy during the acute bleeding episode (up to 90% success), variceal tamponade is associated with significant risks – especially in the hands of inexperienced providers. Complication rates are roughly 30% and include aspiration, mucosal injury, and potential airway obstruction. Esophageal rupture is nearly uniformly fatal in advanced cirrhotics but rare in contemporary series. While initial hemorrhage control is excellent, there is a 50% early rebleeding rate [18]. Thus, a balloon tamponade device should only be removed once the definitive therapy is immediately available.

Endoscopic Management

After intubation and hemodynamic stabilization during the acute bleeding episode, prompt endoscopic evaluation is paramount and should be carried out within 12 h of time zero. Sclerotherapy and endoscopic variceal band ligation (EVL) are the two major endoscopic options available to control variceal bleeding. While both are highly effective (90% success in large meta-analyses), EVL has lower rates of early rebleeding, stricture, and decreased mortality and is the recommended first-line treatment [19, 20].

Newer clinical trials favor EVL as the best treatment for early rebleeding and suggest the lower complication rate is explained by more superficial tissue injury as compared to sclerotherapy [19, 20]. Sclerotherapy is also more likely than EVL to increase portal pressures, thus increasing the likelihood of early rebleeding.

For the 10% of patients who fail endoscopic therapy, repeat endoscopy is indicated. Balloon tamponade is a useful adjunct while awaiting more definitive therapy such as TIPS or surgical shunts.

Percutaneous Management

Paracentesis

Cirrhotic patients with large abdominal ascites have higher variceal pressure gradients between the portal and systemic venous systems than patients without ascites. This has led some to hypothesize that large volume ascites may increase risk of variceal hemorrhage. While no studies have demonstrated a decreased risk of variceal bleeding after paracentesis, large volume paracentesis has been shown to decrease variceal pressures [21, 22]. Thus, in patients with ascites and esophageal variceal hemorrhage, early paracentesis may be a useful adjunct to limit blood loss.

Transjugular Intrahepatic Portosystemic Shunt (TIPS)

TIPS is perhaps the most significant advance in the management of variceal hemorrhage over the past 30 years and has largely replaced surgery as first-line intervention after the failure of pharmacologic and endoscopic therapies. Interventional radiologists pass a needle catheter via the transjugular route which is wedged in a branch of the right hepatic vein. A needle is passed through the liver parenchyma into the intrahepatic portal vein, dilated until the portosystemic pressure gradient falls below 12, over which a stent (usually PTFE covered) is deployed creating a functional side-to-side portacaval anastomosis (Fig. 6.5). This is comparable to a nonselective surgical shunt.

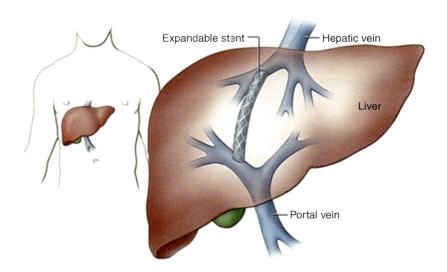

Fig. 6.5 TIPS stent, shunt from portal to hepatic venous system. (Ref: http://virclinic.com/varicose-veins/portal-hypertension-cirrhosis/)

Though common in many interventional radiology suites, emergency TIPS demands taking hemodynamically unstable patients to a noncritical environment potentially during active resuscitation. Emergency TIPS has a procedural mortality of around 2% with a 30-day mortality around 25% [23, 24]. Patients uniformly develop worsening of hepatic encephalopathy as a result of portal decompression though this can be managed with pharmacologic agents [25].

TIPS has a 90–100% success rate in achieving hemostasis and, compared to emergently placed surgical shunts, significantly lower mortality – especially in poor surgical candidates. Indications include refractory variceal hemorrhage for all portal hypertensive etiologies as well as refractory ascites. Contraindications to placement include severe heart failure or pulmonary hypertension, uncontrolled sepsis, and portal vein thrombosis though some centers report success with recanalizing the portal vein for TIPS creation. An important consideration prior to TIPS placement is the ability to interrogate the shunt given the risk of stenosis though this has been less of an issue with new covered stents.

When deciding upon emergency TIPS or surgical shunting, operative risk, transplant candidacy, and patient factors must be considered. While TIPS is the obvious choice for poor surgical patients with no hope of transplant, patients who are good surgical candidates and may be transplanted more than 12 months later or live in a remote area with poor access for shunt surveillance may be served well by surgical shunts which have similar rebleeding rates and significantly lower stenosis rates.

Surgical Procedures

Variceal hemorrhage from portal hypertension can be addressed surgically either directly or indirectly. Direct control of hemorrhage involves either transgastric direct variceal suture ligation or esophagogastric devascularization procedures. Indirect control of hemorrhage can be achieved with portosystemic shunt procedures (Table 6.2).

Table 6.2 Common surgical portosystemic shunt procedures

Portosystemic shunt types
Nonselective shunts
1. End-to-side portocaval shunt
2. Side-to-side portocaval shunt
3. Mesocaval shunt
4. Central splenorenal shunt
Selective shunts
1. Distal splenorenal (Warren) shunt
2. Small-diameter portacaval graft shunt

Shunts

For acute esophageal variceal bleeding, emergency surgical shunting has largely been supplanted by TIPS placement given the much lower complication and mortality rate. However, surgical shunting has proven effectiveness in stopping hemorrhage and decreasing rebleeding and has a lower stenosis rate.

Nonselective shunts decompress the entire portal venous system by diverting flow from the portal to caval system. Examples include portacaval shunts (side-to-side, end-to-side), mescal shunts, and central splenorenal shunts. Higher rates of hepatic encephalopathy are traded for lower rate of ascites accumulation. ***Selective*** shunts decompress a portion of the portal venous system while maintaining portal sinusoidal perfusion. The two most popular types include the distal splenorenal (Warren) shunt and the portacaval H-graft shunt.

For patients in whom emergency TIPS is unavailable, is contraindicated, or has failed, surgical shunts should be pursued based on available expertise. Portacaval shunts are the most common and technically straightforward, with nonselective portacaval shunts having sustained benefit in the prevention of rebleeding [4]. If portal vein thrombosis is present, an *end-to-side* portacaval shunt is technically feasible and will decompress the portal system though ascites may be exacerbated as the sinusoid vessels are not decompressed. In contrast, a *side-to-side* portacaval shunt is a more technically demanding procedure, as pancreatic collateral vessel hemorrhage and caudate lobe hypertrophy can limit exposure for anastomosis [4]. Finally, *large-diameter interposition mesocaval shunts* or *central spleno-renal shunts* avoid dissection near the portal vein, thus limiting the complications of future liver transplantation. Mortality for emergency shunt operations ranges from 25 to 50% though, if patients survive, surgical shunts lead to over 70% long-term survival rates [4].

At laparotomy, nonselective portacaval shunts are best performed from a right lateral approach where control of the portal vein and vena cava is achieved while circumventing dense retroperitoneal or omental varices [4]. Regardless of perceived risk or benefit of each shunt, comfort and available expertise should guide the choice of surgical shunt though, in general, nonselective shunts are best in the emergent setting (quickest decompression of the portal system) and selective shunts should be reserved for the elective setting where slower decompression of varices may be accomplished.

Devascularization

For patients with extrahepatic portal vein thrombosis or extensive splanchnic venous thrombosis, shunt procedures are not indicated or beneficial to control bleeding [26]. In patients who have failed portosystemic shunt therapy, esophagogastric variceal devascularization procedures are useful to directly stop variceal hemorrhage. The key to success with devascularization procedures involves separating the azygous venous system from the intramucosal venous plexus.

The Sugiura procedure, originally described in the 1970s in Japan, was developed to address esophageal variceal hemorrhage in Child class A and B patients [27]. The original two-stage procedure – an abdominal and thoracic approach which included para-gastroesophageal devascularization, esophageal transection and reanastomosis, splenectomy, vagotomy, and pyloroplasty – had high morbidity and mortality rates outside of Japan prompting several modifications. Today, a common modified Sugiura procedure is performed through an abdominal approach with upper gastric devascularization, 6–7 cm of esophageal devascularization, splenectomy, and direct esophageal variceal ligation [28]. The esophageal transection step has been

largely abandoned given the near 100% mortality associated with an anastomotic leak.

Mortality for emergency devascularization procedure ranges from 13 to 32% though there is <5% rate of recurrent bleeding [27, 28].

Prevention of Recurrent Bleeding

After acute variceal hemorrhage, one-third of patients will develop recurrent hemorrhage within 6 weeks (early rebleeding) and 70% will recur over time. Thus, acute care surgeons need to be well versed on common preventive strategies. Following stabilization of an acute variceal bleed, secondary prophylaxis therapies include medical, endoscopic, shunt, and even devascularization procedures as previously described.

For the compensated cirrhotic, nonselective beta-blockers (e.g., propranolol) started upon hospital discharge have demonstrated a marked improvement in rebleeding rates though most studies fail to show a mortality benefit. Several studies have compared propranolol, sclerotherapy, EVL, or a blend of these therapies, and propranolol combined with EVL produces the greatest reduction in rebleeding rate. Decompensated patients appear to have a higher mortality with beta-blocker therapy but may benefit from aggressive EVL therapy.

Despite the demonstrated decreased mortality and complication rate of emergency TIPS as compared to surgery for acute hemorrhage, the data is less clear for prevention of recurrent bleeding. TIPS increases encephalopathy, and studies have demonstrated either no change or worsening of mortality when compared to standard medical therapy. In addition, TIPS stents may complicate future liver transplantation if stents occupy the superior vena cava or right atrium.

Similarly, selective portosystemic surgical shunts such as the small-diameter portocaval H-graft shunt or distal splenorenal (Warren) shunt have proven benefit in reducing recurrent bleeding though surgeons with experience in these procedures are increasingly rare [29]. A small-diameter (8-mm) portacaval H-graft (ringed Gore-Tex) shunt is a technically straightforward selective shunt. Approaching from the right lateral side, the porta and cava are exposed, and the graft is anastomosed to each vein in end-to-side fashion [4]. These shunts are 90% successful in the prevention of rebleeding, with 80% long-term patency rates [4]. In the case of the Warren shunt, the procedure involves ligating the gastroepiploic arcade from the pylorus to the first short gastric, ligating distal splenic venous tributaries from the pancreas, detaching the splenic vein near the superior mesenteric venous confluence, exposing the left renal vein to perform an end-to-side splenorenal anastomosis, and finally ligating the left gastric and right gastroepiploic veins. Compared to nonselective shunts, this produces a slower decompression of varices but is also associated with lower rates of encephalopathy. Some studies have shown the Warren shunt is more cost-effective and less prone to dysfunction and encephalopathy when compared to TIPS [30]. Moreover, compared to sclerotherapy, the Warren shunt achieves superior hemorrhage control but fails to demonstrate survival benefit. In centers with appropriate surgical expertise, the Warren shunt provides the best bridge to transplant in Child class A patients.

Ultimately, given the mixed results of surgical shunts, the vanishing number of centers with surgical expertise, and the advent of coated TIPS stents (markedly decreasing stent thrombosis), TIPS should be considered the gold standard for medical and endoscopic failures.

Conclusion

Variceal hemorrhage is the leading fatal complication of portal hypertension and responsible for most acute bleeding episodes in the cirrhotic patient. Despite advances in medical, endoscopic, and percutaneous approaches to hemorrhage control, emergency surgical intervention may occasionally be indicated. The acute care surgeon should be well versed in critical care, the principles of 1:1 resuscitation, and endoscopic/surgical options available to combat this difficult problem. TIPS has largely replaced surgical shunts, though the Warren shunt should be considered in the elective setting for the prevention of recurrent bleeding.

References

1. Brunner F, Berzigotti A, Bosch J. Prevention and treatment of variceal haemorrhage in 2017. Liver Int. 2017;37(Suppl 1):104–15.
2. Abraldes JG, Bosch J. The treatment of acute variceal bleeding. J Clin Gastroenterol. 2007;41(3):S312–7.
3. Gav P, Chapman R. Modern management of oesophageal varices. Postgrad Med J. 2001;77:75–81.
4. Townsend C, Beauchamp RD. The liver. Sabiston textbook of surgery. 19th ed. Philadelphia, PA: Elsevier Saunders; 2012.
5. Garcia-Tsao G, et al. Prevention and management of gastroesophageal varices and variceal hemorrhage in cirrhosis. Hepatology. 2007;46(3):922–38.
6. Peter DJ, Dougherty JM. Evaluation of the patient with gastrointestinal bleeding. Emerg Med Clin North Am. 1999;17(1):239–61.
7. Bendtsen F, et al. Treatment of acute variceal bleeding. Dig Liver Dis. 2008;40:328–36.
8. Philips CA, Sahney A. Oesophageal and gastric varices: historical aspects, classification and grading: everything in one place. Gastroenterol Rep (Oxf). 2016;4(3):186–95.
9. Dzeletovic I, Baron TH. History of portal hypertension and endoscopic treatment of esophageal varices. Gastrointest Endosc. 2012;75(6):1244–9.
10. Eipel C, Abshagen K, Vollmar B. Regulation of hepatic blood flow: the hepatic arterial buffer response revisited. World J Gastroenterol. 2010;16(48):6046–57.
11. Schouten J, Verheij J, Seijo S. Idiopathic non-cirrhotic portal hypertension: a review. Orphanet J Rare Dis. 2015;10:67.
12. Thompson RJ, Taylor MA, McKie LD, Diamond T. Sinistral portal hypertension. Ulster Med J. 2006;75(3):175–7.
13. Darwish MS, Plessier A, Hernandez-Guerra M, Fabris F, Eapen CE, Bahr MJ, Trebicka J, Morard I, Lasser L, Heller J, Hadengue A, Langlet P, Miranda H, Primignani M, Elias E, Leebeek FW, Rosendaal FR, Garcia-Pagan JC, Valla DC, Janssen HL. EN-Vie (European Network for Vascular Disorders of the Liver). Etiology, management, and outcome of the Budd-Chiari syndrome. Ann Intern Med. 2009;151(3):167–75.
14. Wells M, Chande N, Adams P, Beaton M, Levstik M, Boyce E, Mrkobrada M. Meta-analysis: vasoactive medications for the management of acute variceal bleeds. Aliment Pharmacol Ther. 2012;35(11):1267–78.
15. Ioannou G, Doust J, Rockey DC. Terlipressin for acute esophageal variceal hemorrhage. Cochrane Database Syst Rev. 2003; (1):CD002147.
16. de Franchis R, Baveno V. Revising consensus in portal hypertension: report of the Baveno V consensus workshop on methodology of diagnosis and therapy in portal hypertension. J Hepatol. 2010;53(4):762–8.
17. Lee YY, Tee H, Mahadeva S. Role of prophylactic antibiotics in cirrhotic patients with variceal bleeding. World J Gastroenterol. 2014;20(7):1790–6.

18. Chojkier M, Conn HO. Esophageal tamponade in the treatment of bleeding varices. A decade progress report. Dig Dis Sci. 1980;25(4):267–72.
19. Stiegmann GV, Goff JS, Michaletz-Onody PA, Korula J, Lieberman D, Saeed ZA, Reveille RM, Sun JH, Lowenstein SR. Endoscopic sclerotherapy as compared with endoscopic ligation for bleeding esophageal varices. N Engl J Med. 1992;326:1527–32.
20. Laine L, Cook D. Endoscopic ligation compared with sclerotherapy for treatment of esophageal variceal bleeding. A meta-analysis. Ann Intern Med. 1995;123(4):280–7.
21. Kravetz D, Romero G, Argonz J, Guevara M, Suarez A, Abecasis R, Bildozola M, Valero J, Terg R. Total volume paracentesis decreases variceal pressure, size, and variceal wall tension in cirrhotic patients. Hepatology. 1997;25(1):59–62.
22. Kravetz D, Bildozola M, Argonz J, Romero G, Korula J, Muñoz A, Suarez A, Terg R. Patients with ascites have higher variceal pressure and wall tension than patients without ascites. Am J Gastroenterol. 2000;95(7):1770–5.
23. Freedman AM, Sanyal AJ, Tisnado J, Cole PE, Shiffman ML, Luketic VA, Purdum PP, Darcy MD, Posner MP. Complications of transjugular intrahepatic portosystemic shunt: a comprehensive review. Radiographics. 1993;13(6):1185–210.
24. Bañares R, Casado M, Rodríguez-Láiz JM, Camúñez F, Matilla A, Echenagusía A, Simó G, Piqueras B, Clemente G, Cos E. Urgent transjugular intrahepatic portosystemic shunt for control of acute variceal bleeding. Am J Gastroenterol. 1998;93(1):75–9.
25. Gazzera C, Righi D, Doriguzzi Breatta A, Rossato D, Camerano F, Valle F, Gandini G. Emergency transjugular intrahepatic portosystemic shunt (TIPS): results, complications and predictors of mortality in the first month of follow-up. Radiol Med. 2012;117(1):46–53.
26. Selzner M, Tuttle-Newhall JE, Dahm F, Suhocki P, Clavien PA. Current indication of a modified Sugiura procedure in the management of variceal bleeding. J Am Coll Surg. 2001;193(2):166–73.
27. Sugiura M, Futagawa S. Esophageal transection with paraesophagogastric devascularizations (the Sugiura procedure) in the treatment of esophageal varices. World J Surg. 1984;8(5):673–9.
28. Voros D, Polydorou A, Polymeneas G, Vassiliou I, Melemeni A, Chondrogiannis K, Arapoglou V, Fragulidis GP. Long-term results with the modified Sugiura procedure for the management of variceal bleeding: standing the test of time in the treatment of bleeding esophageal varices. World J Surg. 2012;36(3):659–66.
29. Boyer TD, Kokenes DD, Hertzler G, Kutner MH, Henderson JM. Effect of distal splenorenal shunt on survival of patients with primary biliary cirrhosis. Hepatology. 1994;20(6):1482–6.
30. Zacks SL, Sandler RS, Biddle AK, Mauro MA, Brown RS. Decision-analysis of transjugular intrahepatic portosystemic shunt versus distal splenorenal shunt for portal hypertension. Hepatology. 1999 May;29(5):1399–405.

Upper Gastrointestinal Bleeding

7

Marcel Tafen and Steven C. Stain

Description of the Problem

Bleeding from the GI tract is a common, life-threatening condition, with more than 500,000 hospital discharges in the United States for gastrointestinal bleeding [1]. The mortality of UGIB is between 2.2% and 10% [2, 3]. Elderly populations are disproportionally affected: patients >65 years and older account for 65% of hospitalizations for GIB, and only 10% of hospitalized patients are younger than 45 years of age [1]. Patients admitted with UGIB utilize significant hospital resources as 20–30% of hospitalized patients require six or more units of blood, but surgical intervention is required in only 4–15% of patients. However, when patients require an operation, 69% of operations are done emergently [2, 4, 5].

Upper gastrointestinal bleeding (UGIB) (Table 7.1) has various causes and is defined as any bleeding originating proximal to the ligament of Treitz which is the most common site of bleeding (45%), with lower gastrointestinal bleeding (24%) being less common and the source being unspecified in 31% [1]. The incidence of UGIB appears to be decreasing, with an estimated annual incidence of UGIB reported as 108/100,000 hospitalizations per population in 1995 compared to 78/100,000 in 2015 [6, 7].

The care of patients with upper GI bleeding is multidisciplinary and requires a team approach. Teams involved include gastroenterologists, emergency medicine physicians, interventional radiologist, critical care physicians, and surgeons. Acute care surgeons have the unique potential to manage these patients from beginning to end and may be involved at any stage of the disease process.

Approaching the UGIB Patient

History and Physical Exam

Upon presentation, vital signs should be evaluated and simultaneous resuscitation initiated in the case of instability. A quick history should be taken with special focus on the events surrounding the current UGIB, prior episodes, comorbid conditions, medications, and past surgical history. This approach will focus the diagnostic strategy and may guide initial therapy. A history of epigastric postprandial abdominal pain occurring between half an hour and 3.5 h after a meal, or pain which wakes up the patient at night, or pain relieved by food, vomiting, or antacids is suggestive of peptic ulcer disease. A history of liver disease would suggest a likely variceal bleeding source. Elements in the past surgical

M. Tafen · S. C. Stain (✉)
Department of Surgery, Albany Medical College,
Albany, NY, USA
e-mail: stains@amc.edu

© Springer International Publishing AG, part of Springer Nature 2019
C. V. R. Brown et al. (eds.), *Emergency General Surgery*, https://doi.org/10.1007/978-3-319-96286-3_7

Table 7.1 Classification of UGIB based on pathophysiology and anatomy

Variceal	Non-variceal
Bleeding varices Portal hypertensive gastropathy	

	Ulcerative
	  Gastric ulcer
	  Duodenal ulcer
	  Gastroduodenal
	  Cameron lesions
	  Stress-induced ulcer
	  Marginal ulcer

	Erosive (caustic, infectious,
	peptic, iatrogenic)
	  Gastritis
	  Duodenitis
	  Gastroduodenitis

	Tumors
	  Adenocarcinoma
	  Squamous cell carcinoma
	  GIST
	  Metastasis
	  Lymphoma
	  Benign

	Iatrogenic/traumatic/foreign body

	Vascular
	  Arteriovascular
	  malformation
	  Dieulafoy's lesions

	Miscellaneous
	  Hemobilia
	  Hemosuccus pancreaticus
	  Aortoenteric fistula

history such as placement of aortic graft, recent hepatic procedures, trauma, and pancreatitis, among others, will provide valuable clues as well. Medication list should stress the use of anticoagulants, antiplatelet agents, beta-blockers, calcium channel blockers, and other vasoactive medications.

The assessment should be quick and borrowed from the Advanced Trauma Life Support "ABCDE" principles. The safety of the patient's airway should be ensured. Vomiting patients and those with altered mental status should be intubated to secure the airway and expedite upcoming endoscopic evaluation. Chest roentgenogram (CXR) should be obtained if aspiration is of concern. Oxygen should be supplemented to guarantee normal oxygen saturation and to optimize

oxygen-carrying capacity in the setting of acute blood loss anemia. Evaluation for shock includes baseline vital signs, orthostatic determination of postural hypotension, pallor, and mental status changes. Reliable IV access should be obtained with at least two large-bore IVs. Initial laboratory tests include complete blood counts, coagulation studies, liver function tests, and type and cross-match to have blood available if needed. Most importantly, infusion of warm fluids should be started and the response to volume resuscitation monitored. "Responders" will stabilize after the initial bolus of fluid. "Transient responders" will decompensate once the infusion is completed, while "non-responders" fail to respond all together.

The patient should be exposed and examined for peritonitis, stigmata of liver disease, abdominal distension, and melena. Rectal examination should be done to look for easily accessible pathology such as hemorrhoids and rectal masses. Foley catheter should be placed for monitoring. Temperature should be checked and hypothermia anticipated especially in the setting of massive transfusion.

Nasogastric lavage can help rule out an UGIB source as bilious aspirates in the absence of blood significantly decrease the likelihood of UGIB. Coffee-ground aspirates will suggest subacute bleeding, while bright red blood suggests ongoing hemorrhage, particularly when that blood fails to clear with lavage.

GI bleeding patients should be treated at or transferred to a facility with critical care capability and sufficient resources to support massive transfusion protocol, advanced interventional endoscopy, and a surgeon capable of managing UGIB. On presentation, surgical consultation should be obtained even though the vast majority of patients stop bleeding after resuscitation and medical management. This ensures that the surgical team learns about the patient, follows the response to resuscitation, and tracks the results of endoscopic therapy along with the admitting team.

Resuscitation

Once the fact of UGIB is established, high-dose proton pump inhibitors (PPI) like omeprazole should be administered as an intravenous bolus of 80 mg followed by a continuous infusion at 8 mg/h. High-dose PPI administration is cost-effective and decreases the incidence of high stigmata of bleeding at endoscopy as well as the need for endoscopic hemostasis [8] albeit without effect on rebleeding, surgery, or mortality rates [9]. However, high-dose intravenous PPI after endoscopic therapy decreases the rate of rebleeding. Therefore, double-dose oral PPI for 11 days following 72 h of intravenous PPI is recommended for high-risk patients [10].

Volume resuscitation should be initiated as soon as IV access is obtained. This can be achieved using crystalloids and colloids initially while waiting for blood products, or blood products can be started immediately if they are available. In hemorrhagic shock, multiple endpoints are pursued to assess adequate resuscitation and the patient's overall response to therapy. Hemodynamic parameters such as central venous pressure (CVP), mean arterial pressure (MAP), and cardiac output/index along with lactate, central venous oxygen saturation (ScvO$_2$), urine output, and normalization of coagulation studies should be considered. The goals of resuscitation need not be the restoration of normal blood pressure. Until definitive hemorrhage control, principles of "hypotensive resuscitation" should be followed, allowing mean arterial pressures as low as 50 mmHg as long as there is evidence of adequate end-organ perfusion. This strategy has been shown to be safe and may reduce the risk of postoperative coagulopathy and death in trauma patients with hemorrhagic shock [11].

Unstable patients, transient responders, nonresponders, symptomatic patients, or patients with massive hemorrhage should receive blood transfusion as soon as possible. For that purpose, crossmatched, type-specific, or type O packed red blood cells should be used in decreasing order of preference based on availability from the blood bank. Exsanguinating patients should receive type O PRBC initially and until crossmatched products are available. Any existing or developing coagulopathy should be aggressively treated via infusion of plasma, platelets, and factor concentrates as needed.

Stable UGIB in intermediate- to low-risk patients, in whom intravascular volume has been restored, will benefit from a restrictive transfusion strategy where it is recommended to transfuse for hgb < 7 [12]. This strategy has been validated among critical care patients across the board, and it was shown in a randomized controlled trial that in UGIB, patients on the restrictive transfusion strategy had a higher 6-week survival, lower adverse event, and lower rebleeding rates as opposed to patients in a more liberal transfusion strategy. Early aggressive resuscitation decreased organ failure and mortality. The abovementioned benefits were shown in both NVUGIB and VUGIB [13] (Fig. 7.1).

If the UGIB is related to portal hypertension, it is important not to over-resuscitate. Medical therapy should be instituted along with judicious resuscitation. Specifically, somatostatin or its analog (octreotide) should be started for portal pressure reduction through decrease of splanchnic blood flow.

In patients with VUGIB, besides the multisystem organ failure resulting from acute blood loss, encephalopathy, hepatorenal syndrome, and systemic infections contribute to mortality. Therefore, prophylactic antibiotics should be given because cirrhotic patients have high rate of infections from the GI tract due to bacterial translocation. Antibiotic prophylaxis in VUGIB improves survival and decreases infectious complications [14]. During resuscitation, patients with VUGIB often will require endotracheal intubation to protect airways in the setting of vomiting, encephalopathy or hemodynamic instability.

Laboratory Studies

Every patient should receive a complete metabolic panel, a complete blood count, coagulation studies and a type and crossmatch. Unstable patients should have their hemoglobin, platelets, PTT, PT, fibrinogen measured serially. Hemoglobin levels can be misleading in acutely bleeding patients because of insufficient time for the cardiovascular system to equilibrate with extravascular volume and reflect the true concentration of hemoglobin. All patients

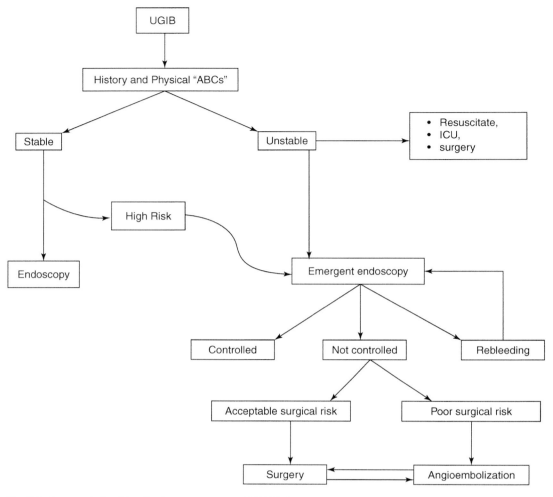

Fig. 7.1 Proposed algorithm for the management of NVUGIB

receiving large amount of transfusions could benefit from thromboelastography (TEG) if available. TEG is increasingly used as a point of care test as it simultaneously studies the integrated effects of different blood components involved in the coagulation cascade including thrombolysis [15]. Laboratory data can assist in risk stratification, bleeding localization, and guide therapy. The blood urea nitrogen (BUN) is elevated in GI bleeding [16] in general, and this is attributed to the digestion of blood in the GI tract [17] and its subsequent absorption. Furthermore, BUN to creatinine (Cr) ratio (BUN/Cr) >30 is 90% specific for UGIB with a positive likelihood ratio of 7.5 [18]. This test,

nonetheless, has a low sensitivity of 39% [19]. EKG and cardiac enzymes should be sent to evaluate for myocardial ischemia.

Restoration of Coagulation

Patients with UGIB are often coagulopathic due to anticoagulant administration, consumption of coagulation factors during hemorrhage, underlying liver disease or as an effect of transfusion itself. Aggressive correction of coagulopathy decreases mortality [20]; therefore, it should be aggressively pursued. The following values should be targeted: international normalized ratio (INR) <1.5 and platelets $>50 \times 10^9$ per liter [21].

Anticoagulation should be discontinued for patients on Coumadin, and INR should be reversed with vitamin K and FFP. Alternatively, prothrombin complex concentrate (PCC) should be used in conjunction with vitamin K for cases where rapid reversal is necessary or circulatory volume overload is a risk [22, 23] and for all direct oral anticoagulant (DOAC) reversal [14, 24]. For patients on Pradaxa, the specific reversal agent idarucizumab (Praxbind) is now available. If this agent is not available, then emergent hemodialysis is indicated to reverse the effects of Pradaxa. Low-dose aspirin for secondary cardiovascular prophylaxis in select patients may be continued [25].

Endoscopy

Endoscopy is essential for patients with UGIB to establish definitive diagnosis and guide therapy as early endoscopy improves outcomes in acute UGIB [26]. An important decision to be made is whether endoscopy needs to be done emergently or can wait for 12–24 h. For patients with severe UGIB, early upper endoscopy is recommended after hemodynamic resuscitation [25]. It is important that the endoscopist has the capability of performing the full range of therapeutic options, based on the endoscopic findings. Based on the timing of endoscopy from the time of presentation, there is *early endoscopy* which comprises (1) *very early* or *emergent* endoscopy (<8–12 h), (2) *urgent endoscopy* (12–24 h), and (3) *delayed endoscopy* (> 24 h) [25, 27]. This approach was shown to decrease mortality [28] and length of stay [29]. Very early endoscopy is indicated for "non-responders" and "transient responders" or in patients with evidence of ongoing bleeding (hematemesis, non-clearing bright red aspirates) or for patients for whom reversal of anticoagulation is not possible [25]. The advantage of second-look endoscopy is controversial and not routinely recommended. However, it may decrease the rebleeding rate of peptic ulcer bleeding in patients with unsatisfactory first endoscopic hemostasis, NSAID use, or massive transfusion [30].

Presentation and Management of Specific UGIB Etiologies

Non-variceal UGIB: Peptic Ulcers

Gastroduodenal peptic ulcers are the most frequent cause of UGIB and constitute more than 1/3 of patients with UGIB (Table 7.2). The underlying etiologies include *H. pylori* infection, NSAID use, gastrinoma, and stress. UGIB due to peptic ulcers stops spontaneously in 80% of the cases [35]. Peptic ulcers can cause eruptive bleeding when the ulcer base erodes into a blood vessel, usually the gastroduodenal artery [36]. Important risk factors include high levels of acid secretion and NSAID use, but interestingly, patients with bleeding ulcers have a lower prevalence of *Helicobacter pylori* than non-bleeding ulcers [36].

Bleeding peptic ulcers present with melena (20%), hematemesis (30%), or both (50%) [37]. Bright red blood per rectum can be from an upper gastrointestinal source when there is at least 1000 ml of blood entering the GI tract from an upper source. Bright red blood hematochezia occurring concomitantly with fresh blood

Table 7.2 Most frequent causes of UGIB

Diagnosis	Frequency of occurrence (%)
Peptic ulcer disease	32–60
Duodenal	20–36
Gastric	12–24
Mucosal erosive disease[a]	13–38
Esophagitis	4–10
Gastroesophageal varices	4–33
Mallory-Weiss tear	3–7
Neoplasm	1–5
Angiodysplasia	1–3
Dieulafoy's lesions	1
Aortoenteric fistula	<1
Cameron lesion	<1
Hemobilia	<1
Not localized or unknown	5–25

References [7, 31–34]
[a]Mucosal erosive disease includes esophagitis, gastritis, duodenitis, and gastroduodenitis

hematemesis implies brisk UGIB and has a mortality rate of 30% [2].

Zollinger-Ellison syndrome (ZES) causes less than 1% of peptic ulcer disease, and it is the constellation of excessive gastric acid production causing severe peptic ulcer disease and diarrhea. Gastrinoma, the neuroendocrine tumor responsible for the hypersecretion of gastrin, most commonly arises sporadically or less commonly is associated with multiple endocrine neoplasia syndrome type 1 (MEN-1). The excessive amount of gastrin secreted by gastrinoma leads to hyperplasia of the parietal cells and increased basal gastric acid output, which breach the gastric and duodenal mucosal defenses leading to ulceration. Clinically, ZES is characterized by the presence of abdominal pain and diarrhea which both improve after administration of proton pump inhibitors [38].

Endoscopic Therapy for Non-variceal UGIB

Following endoscopy therapy, about 10–30% of patients have clinical evidence of rebleeding [5]. Among patients with stigmata of recent hemorrhage who rebleed after therapeutic endoscopy,

19% go on to require surgery or interventional radiology, and 27% of those patients die [26].

The timing of endoscopy depends on the risk of mortality and rebleeding. Therefore, it becomes important to identify high-risk patients. High-risk UGIB patients require higher level of care, aggressive resuscitation, earlier consultant's involvement, and more prompt procedures (endoscopy). Prior to endoscopic evaluation, patients are risk-stratified based on clinical and laboratory data. The Forrest Classification [39] (Fig. 7.2) standardizes the description of peptic ulcer and is used to identify the patients at risk of persistent ulcer bleeding, rebleeding, and mortality [25]. Other endoscopic features that predict adverse outcome and treatment failure include (1) large ulcer (> 2 cm), (2) visible vessel, (3) blood in the gastric lumen, and (4) ulcer in the posterior duodenal wall [40]. Three-quarters of the UGIB patients have *H. pylori* infection; therefore, vigorous attempts should be made to detect the presence of *H. pylori* acutely and retest the patient later to increase the diagnostic yield [25, 41]. When *H. pylori* is found, eradication with antibiotics should be pursued, and successful eradication should be documented [36].

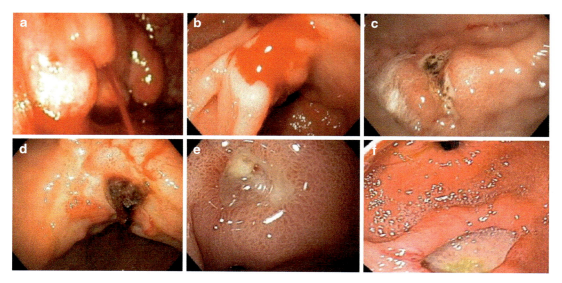

Fig. 7.2 Appearance of ulcers at endoscopy according to Forrest. Forrest Classification of ulcers: (**a**) *Forrest Ia*: ulcer spurting blood. (**b**) *Forrest Ib*: ulcer oozing blood. (**c**) *Forrest IIa*: ulcer with visible ves-sel. (**d**) *Forrest IIb*: ulcer with adherent clot. (**e**) *Forrest IIc*: ulcer with flat pigmented spot. (**f**) *Forrest III*: ulcer with clean base. (Pictures courtesy of Sven Hida, MD)

Once the bleeding is located, endoscopic therapeutic measures are taken for high-risk ulcers. Endoscopic therapies include:

(a) Injection therapy, with saline or vasoconstricting agents like epinephrine, sclerosing agents like ethanolamine.
(b) Thermal therapy is achieved by contact using a heater probe, a bipolar electrocautery, or argon plasma coagulator.
(c) Mechanical therapy involves using band ligation, clipping.
(d) Newer technologies include endoscopic spraying of topical hemostatic agents [42].

Surgical Management for NVUGIB

Indications for Surgical Intervention

Indications for surgery for UGIB are (1) hemorrhage not amenable to endoscopic control, (2) hemorrhage with post-endoscopy transfusion requirements >4 units [43, 44], (3) lack of endoscopic capacity, (4) recurrent bleeding after two attempts at endoscopic control, (5) lack of transfusion capabilities or limited supply, (6) absence of consent to transfuse as in the case of Jehovah's Witnesses, (7) repeated hospitalization for UGIB, and (8) concurrent indication of laparotomy such as perforation or obstruction [45, 46].

Surgical Management of Bleeding Gastric Ulcer

Options for surgical management of bleeding gastric ulcer include (1) oversewing of the bleeding ulcer through a surgical gastrostomy. Biopsy of the ulcer should be performed at the time of the surgery. Other options include (2) gastric resection for giant ulcers located on the lesser curvature (Pauchet procedure) and (3) partial gastrectomy for ulcer at the antrum. Other maneuvers to control the bleeding gastric ulcer are (4) simple ulcer excision [46] and (5) total gastrectomy for massively bleeding erosive gastritis. In the situation of diffusely, massively bleeding gastric erosions in an unstable patient, damage control principles can be utilized. It could require gastrostomy with packing the stomach with or without hemostatic agents and tem-

porarily closing the gastrostomy. After resuscitation and rewarming, the patient is taken back for a second-look procedure where the packs are removed [47, 48]. Another option is to perform catheter-directed intra-arterial delivery of vasopressin [49].

Surgical Management of Bleeding Duodenal Ulcers

First of all, the surgeon needs to have a confirmation of the location of the ulcer from the endoscopist report or be present for the esophagogastroduodenoscopy (EGD). This will avoid the mistake of performing an unnecessary duodenostomy and extending it into a gastroduodenostomy. Surgical options for bleeding duodenal ulcers include (1) simple suture ligation, (2) suture ligation with drainage procedure and truncal vagotomy, (3) suture ligation and antrectomy, and (4) suture ligation and highly selective vagotomy. The ulcer is usually located at the first portion of the duodenum and sometimes at the proximal second portion of the duodenum. Kocher maneuver is necessary to mobilize the duodenum. A 3 cm pyloromyotomy should be performed, and if the ulcer is not in the duodenum, that incision should be extended to get more exposure in either direction. Intraoperative gastroscopy should be considered to look for a gastric source if not identified after duodenotomy.

Bleeding is initially controlled by applying direct pressure. Using a heavy braided suture on a non-cutting needle, three U-sutures should be placed around the gastroduodenal artery (GDA) proximally and distally at the 12 and 6 o'clock positions and around the transverse pancreatic branch at the 3 o'clock position to control the bleeding from the transverse pancreaticoduodenal artery (Fig. 7.3). If the ulcer is found and there is no active bleeding, suture ligation should still be performed. Care should be taken to avoid the common bile duct which runs deeper.

The longitudinally oriented incision should be closed transversely with a standard Heineke-Mikulicz pyloroplasty. Historically, a vagotomy has been used to reduce acid secretion; however, with the availability of proton pump

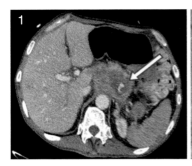 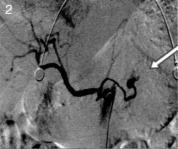 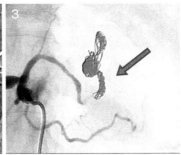

Fig. 7.3 Transcatheter angioembolization of bleeding gastric ulcer. 1. Computed tomography scan showing bleeding originating from the left gastric artery. 2. Angiogram showing pseudoaneurysm arising from the left gastric artery. 3. Coils in the artery

inhibitors and *H. pylori* treatment, vagotomy is not indicated unless the patient is noncompliant, will likely require NSAID treatment or has recurrent bleeding. There is evidence that a more extensive procedure, such as ligation with antrectomy, may have a lower incidence of rebleeding, but the higher morbidity associated with resection hence the advent of effective medical treatment make this approach rarely necessary [50].

Other Causes of NVUGIB and Their Managements

Mucosal Erosive Disease

Mucosal erosive disease of the upper gastrointestinal tract is the second most common cause of UGIB [33]. Esophagitis, gastritis, and duodenitis arise from alterations resulting in a break in the mucosa that does not extend to the muscularis mucosae and that may be infiltrated by inflammatory cells on histology. On endoscopy, mucosal erosive disease has the appearance of diffuse erythema, without significant depth erosions and mucosal hemorrhages.

Esophagitis accounts for approximately 10% of UGIB, but typically it is self-limited and carries a low morbidity and mortality [7, 31–34, 51]. Elderly and critically ill patients are at higher risk [52]. Reflux esophagitis is the most common cause, but another important subtype is infectious esophagitis, which includes viral (herpes simplex virus or CMV) or fungal or bacterial infections, all affecting immunocompromised hosts.

Gastritis and duodenitis most commonly cause bleeding in the setting of coagulopathy and are diagnosed by endoscopy which has the benefit of excluding other causes of bleeding. Causes of gastritis and duodenitis [53] include NSAID use, alcohol intake, portal gastropathy, and stress. Nearly all patients (>80%) with critical illness develop gastroduodenal erosions [54, 55]. Among patients admitted to the intensive care unit (ICU), 16% will still develop UGIB, despite receiving stress ulcer prophylaxis. Fortunately significant bleeding will develop in only 6% of these patients. Stress gastritis occurs in critically ill patients after stress events such as trauma, shock, sepsis, severe head trauma (Cushing's ulcers), and burns (Curling's ulcers). The pathogenesis is multifactorial and includes mucosal ischemia and reperfusion caused by fluctuation of splanchnic blood flow and perhaps an overactive parasympathetic system (vagus) causing hypersecretion of acid and pepsin [56, 57]. About 50–77% of ICU patients with UGIB may die of other causes, such as multiple system organ failure or underlying disease [58–60]. Risk factors for bleeding due to stress ulcers include respiratory failure, coagulopathy, older age, repair of abdominal aortic aneurysm, severe burns, multiple organ failure, neurological trauma, sepsis or septic shock, and high-dose corticosteroid. Respiratory failure requiring mechanical ventilation for more than 48 h or coagulopathy is a very strong risk factor for clinically relevant UGIB [61].

The treatment for mucosal erosive disease is supportive along with acid suppressive therapy using proton pump inhibitors (PPI). Provocating agents such anticoagulation and nasogastric tube should be eliminated. For infectious esophagitis, antibiotics should be added.

Mallory-Weiss Lesions

Mallory-Weiss lesions are longitudinal lacerations in the gastric and/or esophageal mucosa near the gastroesophageal junction caused by mechanical forces of increasing intra-abdominal pressure like in forceful vomiting or retching. Other causes of these lacerations have been described and include coughing, hiccups, CPR, and colonoscopic preparation. Diagnosis is made with endoscopy. The bleeding is self-limiting in 90% of the cases [62]. Endoscopic therapies mostly used are epinephrine injection, heater probe, and band ligation. Surgery may be required for oversewing the laceration [62].

Dieulafoy's Lesions

Dieulafoy's lesions are large submucosal arteries close to the surface usually found in the proximal stomach along the lesser curvature but can be found anywhere else in the GI tract, with the duodenum being the next most common location [63]. Hemorrhage usually occurs after the vessel perforates. It is thought to be a pressure ulceration of the epithelium overlying a dilated artery [64]. Patients present with melena, hematemesis, followed by recurrent intermittent bleeding without a prior history or classic risk factors for GIB. The diagnosis is made by endoscopy, but unfortunately multiple endoscopies may be required to locate the bleed. Endoscopic therapy, usually with sclerotherapy, is curative in 95% of the cases [65]. Surgery is indicated if endoscopic treatment fails, but the lesion should be marked, and the location should be known, and operative therapy will consist of underrunning the blood vessel. In the case where the lesion cannot be found intraoperatively, endoscopic ultrasound can be used.

Hemobilia

Hemobilia is a gastrointestinal bleeding emanating from the biliary tree that comes through the ampulla of Vater [66]. Common causes include

biliary tract procedures, trauma, biliary obstruction, cholangitis, cholecystitis, and pancreatitis. Classically, hemobilia presents with right upper quadrant abdominal pain, GI bleeding, and jaundice, with or without melena and/or hematemesis. CT scan and MRI are the diagnostic tools of choice, and blood from the papilla can be seen with endoscopy using a side-viewing scope. Treatment is by angiography with percutaneous trans-arterial catheter embolization. Surgery may be necessary (rarely) for failed angiography, and depending on the situation, options will include cholecystectomy with ligation of the relevant hepatic artery branch or resection by hepatectomy.

Hemosuccus Pancreaticus

Hemosuccus pancreaticus is another rare form of GI bleeding where there is transpapillary pouring of blood into the GI tract. In this situation, the gastrointestinal hemorrhage results from the erosion of the blood vessel into a pancreatic pseudocyst that communicates with the pancreatic duct. Like in hemobilia, the diagnosis can be made by CT scan and MRI with bleeding from the pancreatic duct which can be visible from the ampulla of Vater at endoscopy with a side-viewing scope. The preferred treatment is angiographic embolization.

Aortoenteric Fistula

Aortoenteric fistula constitutes the majority of the fistula between an artery and the GI system. Other communications have been described with the esophagus, the stomach and the small bowel, and the artery including the aorta. But the most common is aortoenteric fistula between the duodenum and the aorta. It can form from pressure necrosis of the bowel caused by the aortic aneurysm for primary aortoenteric fistula or the aortic graft for secondary aortoenteric fistula (most often due to fistula formation secondary to aortic infection). Patients present with back pain, fever, and hematemesis with or without hematochezia. These are "herald bleeds" before the ultimate massive GI bleed. A pulsatile mass may be present on physical examination. In the presence of a previous aortic graft, and an UGIB, aortoenteric fistula should be suspected. Endoscopy is primarily performed to rule out other causes of GI bleeding and may visualize the fistula, adherent clot, or the aortic graft. The diagnostic test of choice is CT scan which will demonstrate signs of inflammation between the aorta or the graft and the duodenum. The treatment consists of antibiotics, emergent graft explantation with extra-anatomical bypass, and closure of the enterotomy.

Cameron Lesions

Cameron lesions are erosions or ulcerations of the gastric mucosa found within a hiatal hernia. Cameron lesions exist in up to 5% of hiatal hernias and are responsible for about 0.2% and 3.8% of overt and occult UGIB, respectively [67]. The incidence of these lesions is proportional to the size of the hernia [68].

Variceal Upper Gastrointestinal Bleeding

In patients with liver cirrhosis (90%) or hepatic vein obstruction (non-cirrhotics), portal hypertension worsens over time, leading to the formation of esophageal and gastric varices. Further increase in portal pressure causes the rupture of varices and subsequent bleeding [69]. Risk factors for variceal bleeding include variceal size, presence of red marks on varices, and high Child classification [70]. Patients with variceal UGIB have a mortality three times higher than that of non-variceal VUGIB [2, 3], and it could be as high as 15–30% [71]. For variceal UGIB, the Model for End-Stage Liver Disease (MELD) score is accurate in predicting risk of mortality [72]. Management of VUGIB along with ressucitation includes vasoactive drug therapy (nitrates, beta-blockers, somatostatin/octreotide) antibiotic prophylaxis endoscopy.

Endoscopic Therapy for Variceal Bleeding

In general, emergent EGD is required for VUGIB, both for diagnosis and therapy. Endoscopic therapy for VUGIB consists primar-

ily of endoscopic sclerotherapy (EST) or endoscopic band ligation (EBL). The therapies work by interrupting the flow through the esophageal or gastric system of venous collaterals. EBL is the treatment of choice due to lower complication profile, rebleeding rates, and number of treatments required to eradicate varices as compared to EST [73]. These therapies are less successful with gastric varices due to the profound depth of varices. Complications include ulceration, perforation, stricture formation, dysphagia, chest pain, worsening of the portal hypertensive gastropathy, and systemic embolization of sclerosing agent. EST and EBL have shown the ability to control active bleeding at the first treatment in 77% and 86% of the time [73] with a 21% and 12% rebleeding rate, respectively [74]. Overall, a 10–20% failure of medical and endoscopic treatment is expected. EBL should be repeated if the patient is stable and the bleeding is mild. For refractory bleeding varices in an unstable patient's balloon, tamponade may be achieved with the Sengstaken-Blakemore tube [75] or self-expanding metal stent (SEMS) [76]. In the past, the use of Sengstaken-Blakemore tube was 60–90% effective at controlling variceal bleeding [77] but should be used for less than 24 h. It should be used as a bridge to definitive treatment, because bleeding will recur after the release of tamponade in half of the patients. Major complications of balloon tamponade occur in 10–20% of cases and include aspiration, esophageal rupture, and airway obstruction [78, 79].

Surgical Therapy for Variceal Bleeding

Following endoscopic therapy or temporizing measure with balloon tamponade, definitive control should be achieved by decompressing the varices. This is achieved by diverting the flow of blood away from the portal toward the systemic circulation using a shunt. Operative portosystemic shunts are now of historic interest, and the shunt of choice today is the transjugular intrahepatic portosystemic shunt (TIPS). TIPS is less invasive and consists of placing fluoroscopically a large-bore stent

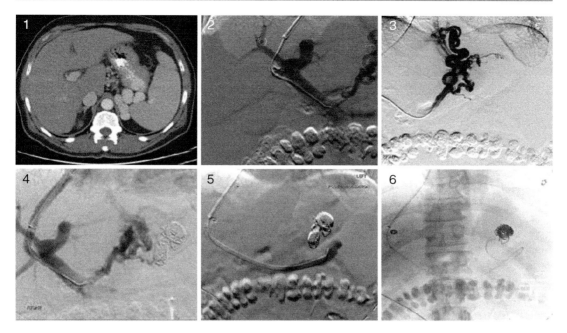

Fig. 7.4 Diagnostic and therapeutic angiography for variceal bleeding. 1. Multiple gastroesophageal varices secondary to portal HTN. 2. 3. Access gained into the portal venous system through the hepatic vein, liver parenchyma. 4. 5. Varices catheterized and embolized. 6. Transjugular intrahepatic portosystemic shunt (TIPS) placed. (Images courtesy of Gary Siskin, MD)

between the hepatic veins and the portal veins within the liver (Fig. 7.4). In VUGIB, TIPS is indicated for (1) *salvage TIPS*, refractory active variceal hemorrhage despite medical and endoscopic therapy, (2) recurrent variceal hemorrhage despite medical and endoscopic therapy, and (3) *early TIPS*, now proposed after the initial variceal bleeding episode for Child B cirrhotics and selected Child C patients. Significant reductions in treatment failure (97% vs 50%) and mortality were shown when compared to medical therapy plus endoscopy [80]. Unfortunately, TIPS can worsen encephalopathy due to impaired hepatic protein metabolism and ensuing hyperammonemia. Operative portocaval shunting (end-to-side or splenorenal shunt) is rarely needed. In esophageal devascularization and transection, "Sugiura procedure" is a last-ditch treatment for refractory bleeding when shunting is not possible. The mortality for the Sugiura procedure is extremely high [78].

Patients with refractory VUGIB with encephalopathy along with refractory ascites or hepatorenal syndrome should be referred to a transplant center for consideration for liver transplant.

In non-cirrhotic patients, sinistral portal hypertension (SPH) should be suspected. SPH manifests as bleeding gastric varices in the setting of patent portal vein, normal hepatic function, and splenic vein thrombosis caused by pancreatic pathology. Causes include trauma, pancreatitis, or cancer. Splanchnic arteriography is necessary for accurate diagnosis. Splenectomy is curative [81].

Diagnostic and Interventional Radiology for UGIB

Endoscopy is nondiagnostic in 10–15% and non-therapeutic in 20% of cases, respectively [4]. Where traditional surgery was the logical next step, angioembolization has been used particularly when patients are too sick to undergo a surgical intervention. The use of radiology for the localization of bleeding and achieving hemostasis in UGIB has increased.

Although rarely used, nuclear medicine studies may have a role in detecting intermittent bleeding and can detect bleeding with as little as 0.1 ml/min. Technetium-99m-labeled erythrocyte scan is preferred over the technetium-99m-labeled colloid because it remains in the intravascular space for 24 h allowing for repeated scanning [82].

Hemodynamically stable patients in the appropriate clinical setting (pancreatitis, following percutaneous hepatobiliary procedures, tumor) can have their UGIB localized by contrast-enhanced computed tomography angiography (CTA) scan. CTA scan detects bleeding as slow as 0.3 ml/h [83] (Fig. 7.3), and it has the advantage of localizing the source and defining the etiology at the same time. Angiographic examination for suspected UGIB source requires celiac trunk angiography and selective angiography of the gastroduodenal artery and left gastric artery. The key is to get the patient to the angiography suite as soon as possible when ongoing bleeding is suspected even if the patient is coagulopathic as a bleeding rate of at least 0.5 ml/h is required for the bleeding to be detected.

Portography not only permits TIPS creation to decrease portal venous pressures but will allow the visualization of gastric varices and potential embolization of bleeding varices [84] (Fig. 7.4). Angiographic therapy is indicated for severe, persistent bleeding after failure of endoscopic therapy in patients for whom surgery is not an option either because of the high risk of surgery or its unavailability [85]. The use of angiography and radiography-guided angioembolization is required in 1% of admissions or less [3, 86] (Figs. 7.5 and 7.6). There are case series of positive experience with transcatheter angioembolization (TAE) used to treat refractory massive UGIB with a technical success ranging from 52% to 98% [85]. One of those groups reports complications and 1-month mortality rates of 10% and 26.7%, respectively, with a rebleeding rate of 28% and an 11.6% rate of surgery. Although the rebleeding rates are high, these patients could avoid the higher mortality of surgery [5]. Complications of TAE include access site hematoma, arterial dissection, contrast nephrotoxicity, and bowel ischemia [88].

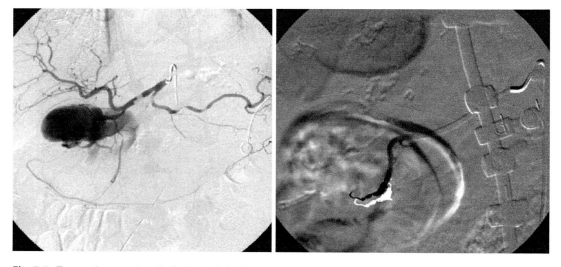

Fig. 7.5 Transcatheter angioembolization of bleeding duodenal ulcer. 1. Angiogram showing bleeding duodenal ulcer through gastroduodenal artery. 2. Coils placed in the gastroduodenal artery

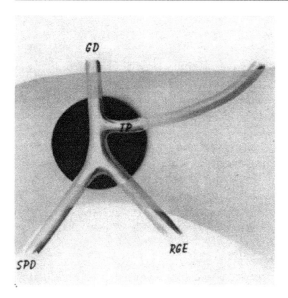

Fig. 7.6 Gastroduodenal artery complex. The two major types of "T" intersections are illustrated. Arteries: GD gastroduodenal, TP transverse pancreatic, SPD superior pancreaticoduodenal, RGE right gastroepiploic. (Reproduced from Berne and Tosoff [87])

References

1. Zhao Y, Encinosa W. Hospitalizations for gastrointestinal bleeding in 1998 and 2006: statistical brief #65. Healthcare Cost and Utilization Project (HCUP) statistical briefs [Internet]. Rockville: Agency for Healthcare Research and Quality (US); 2006-2008.
2. Silverstein FE, Gilbert DA, Tedesco FJ, Buenger NK, Persing J. The national ASGE survey on upper gastrointestinal bleeding. I. Study design and baseline data. Gastrointest Endosc. 1981;27(2):73–9. No abstract available.
3. Abougergi MS, Travis AC, Saltzman JR. Impact of day of admission on mortality and other outcomes in upper GI hemorrhage: a nationwide analysis. Gastrointest Endosc. 2014;80(2):228–35.
4. Rosenstock SJ, Moller MH, Larsson H, Johnsen SP, Madsen AH, Bendix J, et al. Improving quality of care in peptic ulcer bleeding: nationwide cohort study of 13,498 consecutive patients in the Danish Clinical Register of Emergency Surgery. Am J Gastroenterol. 2013;108(9):1449–57.
5. Loffroy R, Estivalet L, Cherblanc V, Sottier D, Guiu B, Cercueil JP, et al. Transcatheter embolization as the new reference standard for endoscopically unmanageable upper gastrointestinal bleeding. World J Gastrointest Surg. 2012;4(10):223–7.
6. Abougergi MS, Travis AC, Saltzman JR. The in-hospital mortality rate for upper GI hemorrhage has decreased over 2 decades in the United States: a nationwide analysis. Gastrointest Endosc. 2015;81(4):882–8.
7. Longstreth GF. Epidemiology of hospitalization for acute upper gastrointestinal hemorrhage: a population-based study. Am J Gastroenterol. 1995;90(2):206–10.
8. Sreedharan A, Martin J, Leontiadis G, Doward S, Howden CW, Forman D, et al. Proton pump inhibitor treatment initiated prior to endoscopic diagnosis in upper gastrointestinal bleeding. Cochrane Database Syst Rev. 2010;7:CD005415.
9. Al-Sabah S, Barkun AN, Herba K, Adam V, Fallone C, Mayrand S, et al. Cost-effectiveness of Proton-pump inhibition before endoscopt in upper gastrointestinal bleeding. Clin Gastroenterol Hepatol. 2008;6(4):418–25.
10. Cheng HC, Wu CT, Chang WL, Cheng WC, Chen WY, Sheu BS. Double oral esomeprazole after a 3-day intravenous esomeprazole infusion reduces recurrent peptic ulcer bleeding in high-risk patients: a randomised controlled study. Gut. 2014;63(12):1864–72.
11. Morrison CA, Carrick MM, Norman MA, Scott BG, Welsh FJ, Tsai P, et al. Hypotensive resuscitation strategy reduces transfusion requirements and severe postoperative coagulopathy in trauma patients with hemorrhagic shock: preliminary results of a randomized controlled trial. J Trauma. 2011;70(3):652–63.
12. Laine L, Jensen DM. Management of patients with ulcer bleeding. Am J Gastroenterol. 2012;107(3):345–60; quiz 361.
13. Baradarian R, Ramdhaney S, Chapalamadugu R, Skoczylas L, Wang K, Rivilis S, et al. Early intensive resuscitation of patients with upper gastrointestinal bleeding decreases mortality. J Gastroenterol. 2004;99(4):619–22.
14. Siegal DM, Konkle BA. What is the effect of rivaroxaban on routine coagulation tests? Hematology Am Soc Hematol Educ Program. 2014;2014(1):334–6.
15. Blasi A, Beltran J, Pereira A, Martinez-Palli G, Torrents A, Balust J, et al. An assessment of thromboelastometry to monitor blood coagulation and guide transfusion support in liver transplantation. Transfusion. 2012;52(9):1989–98.
16. Black DAK, Powell JF. Absorption of haemoglobin iron. Biochem J. 1942;36(1-2):110–2.
17. Ernst AA, Haynes ML, Nick TG, Weiss SJ. Usefulness of the blood urea nitrogen/creatinine ratio in gastrointestinal bleeding. Am J Emerg Med. 1999;17(1):70–2.
18. Richards RJ, Donica MB, Grayer D. Can the blood urea nitrogen/creatinine ratio distinguish upper from lower gastrointestinal bleeding? J Clin Gastroenterol. 1990;12(5):500–4.
19. Witting MD, Magder L, Heins AE, Mattu A, Granja CA, Baumgarten M. ED predictors of upper gastrointestinal tract bleeding in patients without hematemesis. Am J Emerg Med. 2006;24(3):280–5.
20. Jairath V, Kahan BC, Stanworth SJ, Logan RF, Hearnshaw SA, Travis SP, Palmer KR, Murphy MF. Prevalence, management, and outcomes of patients with coagulopathy after acute nonvariceal upper gastrointestinal bleeding in the United Kingdom Transfusion. 2013;53(5):1069–76. doi: https://doi.org/10.1111/j.1537-2995.2012.03849.x. Epub 2012 Aug 15.

21. Razzaghi A, Barkun AN. Platelet transfusion threshold in patients with upper gastrointestinal bleeding: a systematic review. J Clin Gastroenterol. 2012;46(6):482–6.

22. Hickey M, Gatien M, Taljaard M, Aujnarain A, Giulivi A, Perry JJ. Outcomes of urgent warfarin reversal with frozen plasma versus prothrombin complex concentrate in the emergency department. Circulation. 2013;128(4):360–4.

23. Refaai MA, Goldstein JN, Lee ML, Durn BL, Milling TJ Jr, Sarode R. Increased risk of volume overload with plasma compared with four-factor prothrombin complex concentrate for urgent vitamin K antagonist reversal. Transfusion. 2015;55(11):2722–9.

24. Fawole A, Daw HA, Crowther MA. Practical management of bleeding due to anticoagulants dabigatran, rivaroxaban, and apixaban. Cleve Clin J Med. 2013;80(7):443–51.

25. Gralnek IM, Dumonceau JM, Kuipers EJ, Lanas A, Sanders DS, Kurien M, et al. Diagnosis and management of nonvariceal upper gastrointestinal hemorrhage: European Society of Gastrointestinal Endoscopy (ESGE) Guideline. Endoscopy. 2015;47(10):a1–46.

26. Hearnshaw SA, Logan RF, Lowe D, Travis SP, Murphy MF, Palmer KR. Use of endoscopy for management of acute upper gastrointestinal bleeding in the UK: results of a nationwide audit. Gut. 2010;59(8):1022–9.

27. Bethea ED, Travis AC, Saltzman JR. Initial assessment and management of patients with nonvariceal upper gastrointestinal bleeding. J Clin Gastroenterol. 2014;48(10):823–9.

28. Wysocki JD, Srivastav S, Winstead NS. A nationwide analysis of risk factors for mortality and time to endoscopy in upper gastrointestinal haemorrhage. Aliment Pharmacol Ther. 2012;36:30–6.

29. Tsoi KKF, Ma TKW, Sung JJY. Endoscopy for upper gastrointestinal bleeding: how urgent is it? Nat Rev Gastroenterol Hepatol. 2009;6:463–9.

30. Park SJ, Park H, Lee YC, Choi CH, Jeon TJ, Park JC, et al. Effect of scheduled second-look endoscopy on peptic ulcer bleeding: a prospective randomized multicenter trial. Gastrointest Endosc. 2017. pii: S0016-5107(17)32117-X. doi: https://doi.org/10.1016/j.gie.2017.07.024. [Epub ahead of print].

31. Rockall TA, Logan RF, Devlin HB, Northfield TC. Incidence of and mortality from acute upper gastrointestinal haemorrhage in the United Kingdom. Steering Committee and members of the National Audit of Acute Upper Gastrointestinal Haemorrhage. BMJ. 1995;311:222–6.

32. Vreeburg EM, Snel P, de Bruijne JW, Bartelsman JF, Rauws EA, Tytgat GN. Acute upper gastrointestinal bleeding in the Amsterdam area: incidence, diagnosis, and clinical outcome. Am J Gastroenterol. 1997;92:236–43.

33. Enestvedt BK, Graknek IM, Mattek N, Lieberman DA, Eisen G. An evaluation of endoscopic indications and findings related to nonvariceal upper-GI hemorrhage in a large multicenter consortium. Gastrointest Endosc. 2008;67(3):422–9.

34. Kim JJ, Sheibani S, Park S, Buxbaum J, Laine L. Causes of bleeding and outcomes in patients hospitalized with upper gastrointestinal bleeding. J Clin Gastroenterol. 2014;48(2):113–8.

35. Freeman ML. Stigmata of hemorrhage in bleeding ulcers. Gastrointest Endosc Clin N Am. 1997;7(4):559–74.

36. Laine L, Peterson WL. Bleeding peptic ulcer. N Engl J Med. 1994;331(11):717–27.

37. Wara P. Endoscopic prediction of major rebleeding—a prospective study of stigmata of hemorrhage in bleeding ulcer. Gastroenterology. 1985;88(5 Pt 1):1209–14.

38. Mendelson AH, Donowitz M. Catching the zebra: clinical pearls and pitfalls for the successful diagnosis of Zollinger-Ellison syndrome. Dig Dis Sci. 2017;62(9):2258–65. https://doi.org/10.1007/s10620-017-4695-7. Epub 2017 Aug 3.

39. Forrest JA, Finlayson ND, Shearman DJ. Endoscopy in gastrointestinal bleeding. Lancet. 1974;2(7877):394–7.

40. Bratanic A, Puljiz Z, Ljubicicz N, Caric T, Jelicic I, Pulkiz M, et al. Predictive factors of rebleeding and mortality following endoscopic hemostasis in bleeding peptic ulcers. Hepatogastroenterology. 2013;60:112–7.

41. Sánchez-Delgado J, Gené E, Suárez D, et al. Has H. pylori prevalence in bleeding peptic ulcer been underestimated? A meta-regression. Am J Gastroenterol. 2011;106:398–405.

42. Barkun AN, Moosavi S, Martel M. Topical hemostatic agents: a systematic review with particular emphasis on endoscopic application in GI bleeding. Gastrointest Endosc. 2013;77:692–700.

43. Prachayakul V, Aswakul P, Chantarojanasiri T, Leelakusolvong S. Factors influencing clinical outcomes of Histoacryl® glue injection-treated gastric variceal hemorrhage. World J Gastroenterol. 2013;19(15):2379–87. https://doi.org/10.3748/wjg.v19.i15.2379. Published online 2013 Apr 21.

44. Lee YJ, Min BR, Kim ES, Park KS, Cho KB, Jang BK, et al. Predictive factors of mortality within 30 days in patients with nonvariceal upper gastrointestinal bleeding. Korean J Intern Med. 2016;31(1):54–64. https://doi.org/10.3904/kjim.2016.31.1.54. Published online 2015 Dec 28.

45. Napolitano L. Refractory peptic ulcer disease. Gastroenterol Clin North Am. 2009;38(2):267–88.

46. Lee CW, Sarosi GA Jr. Emergency ulcer surgery. Surg Clin North Am. 2011;91(5):1001–13.

47. Brown DP. Gastric packing in the control of massive gastroduodenal hemorrhage. Am J Gastroenterol. 1970;54(1):49–51.

48. Cortese F, Colozzi S, Marcello R, Muttillo IA, Giacovazzo F, Nardi M, et al. Gastroduodenal major haemorrhages in critical patients: an original surgical technique. Am Ital Chir. 2013;84(6):671–9.

49. White RI Jr, Harrington DP, Novak G, Miller FJ Jr, Giargiana FA Jr, Sheff RN. Pharmacologic control

of hemorrhagic gastritis: clinical and experimental results. Radiology. 1974;111(3):549–57.

50. Millat B, Hay JM, Valleur P, et al. Emergency surgical treatment for bleeding duodenal ulcer: oversewing plus vagotomy versus gastric resection, a controlled randomized trial. French Associations for Surgical Research. World J Surg. 1993;17(5):568–73. discussion 574.

51. Sugawa C, Steffes CP, Nakamura R, Sferra JJ, Sferra CS, Sugimura Y, et al. Upper GI bleeding in an urban hospital. Etiology, recurrence, and prognosis. Ann Surg. 1990;212(4):521–6; discussion 526-7.

52. Zimmerman J, Shohat V, Tsvang E, Arnon R, Safadi R, Wengrower D. Esophagitis is a major cause of upper gastrointestinal hemorrhage in the elderly. Scand J Gastroenterol. 1997;32(9):906–9.

53. Owen DA. Gastritis and carditis. Mod Pathol. 2003;16(4):325–41.

54. Czaja AJ, McAlhany JC, Pruitt BA Jr. Acute gastroduodenal disease after thermal injury. An endoscopic evaluation of incidence and natural history. N Engl J Med. 1974;291(18):925–9.

55. Martin LF. Gastrointestinal bleeding in critically ill patients. N Engl J Med. 1994;331(1):51–2; author reply 52-3.

56. Goldman MS Jr, Rasch JR, Wiltsie DS, Finkel M. The incidence of esophagitis in peptic ulcer disease. Am J Dig Dis. 1967;12(10):994–9.

57. Barletta JF, Mangram AJ, Sucher JF, Zach V. Stress ulcer prophylaxis in neurocritical care. Neurocrit Care. 2017; https://doi.org/10.1007/s12028-017-0447-y. [Epub ahead of print].

58. Peura DA, Johnson LF. Cimetidine for prevention and treatment of gastroduidenalmuscosal lesions in patients in an intensive care unit. Ann Intern Med. 1985;103(2):173–7.

59. Schuster DP, Rowley H, Feinstein S, McGue MK, Zuckerman GR. Prospective evaluation of the risk of upper gastrointestinal bleeding after admissions to a medical intensive care unit. Am J Med. 1984;76(4):623–30.

60. Zuckerman GR, Shuman R. Therapeutic goals and treatment options for prevention of stress ulcer syndrome. Am J Med. 1987;83(6A):29–35.

61. Cook DJ, Reeve BK, Scholes LC. Histamine-2-receptor antagonists and antacids in the critically ill population: stress ulceration versus nosocomial pheumonia. Infect Control Hosp Epidemiol. 1994;15(7):437–42.

62. Sugawa C, Benishek D, Walt AJ. Mallory-Weiss syndrome. A study of 224 patients. Am J Surg. 1983;145(1):30–3.

63. Lee YT, Walmsley RS, Leong RW, Sung JJ. Dieulafoy's lesion. GastrointestvEndosc. 2003;58(2):236–43.

64. Juler GL, Labitzke HG, Lamb R, Allen R. The pathogenesis of Dieulafoy's gastric erosion. Am J Gastroenterol. 1984;79(3):195–200.

65. Norton ID, Petersen BT, Sorbi D, Balm RK, Alexander GL, Gostout CJ. Management and long-term prognosis of Dieulafoylesion. Gastrointest Endosc. 1999;50(6):762–7.

66. Cathcart S, Birk JW, Tadros M, Schuster MJ. Hemobilia: an uncommon but notable cause of upper gastrointestinal bleeding. Clin Gastroenterol. 2017;51(9):796–804.

67. Camus M, Jensen DM, Ohning GV, Kovacs TO, Ghassemi KA, Jutabha R, et al. Severe upper gastrointentestinal hemorrhage from linear gastric ulcers in large hiatal hernias: a large prospective case series of Cameron ulcers. Endoscopy. 2013;45(5):397–400.

68. Gray DM, Kushnir V, Kalra G, Rosenstock A, Alsakka MA, Patel A, et al. Cameron lesions in patients with hiatal hernias: prevalence, presentation, and treatment outcome. Dis Esophagus. 2015;28(5):448–52.

69. Berzigotti A, Bosch J, Boyer TD. Use of noninvasive markers of portal hypertension and timing of screening endoscopy for gastroesophageal varices in patients with chronic liver disease. Hepatology. 2014;59(2):729–31.

70. Merli M, Nicolini G, Angeloni S, et al. Incidence and natural history of small esophageal varices in cirrhotic patients. J Hepatol. 2003;38:266–72.

71. Carbonell N, Pauwels A, Serfaty L, Fourdan O, Lévy VG, Poupon R. Improved survival after variceal bleeding in patients with cirrhosis over the past two decades. Hepatology. 2004;40(3):652–9.

72. Reverter E, Tandon P, Augustin S, Turon F, Casu S, Bastiampillai R, et al. A MELD-based model to determine risk of mortality among patients with acute variceal bleeding. Gastroenterology. 2014;146(2):412–9. e3.

73. Stiegmann GV, Goff JS, Michaletz-Onody PA, Korula J, Lieberman D, Saeed ZA, et al. Endoscopic sclerotherapy as compared with endoscopic ligation for bleeding esophageal varices. N Engl J Med. 1992;326(23):1527–32.

74. Villanueva C, Piqueras M, Aracil C, et al. A randomized controlled trial comparing ligation and sclerotherapy as emergency endoscopic treatment added to somatostatin in acute variceal bleeding. J Hepatol. 2006;45:560–7.

75. Sengstaken RW, Blakemore AH. Balloon tamponage for the control of hemorrhage from esophageal varices. Ann Surg. 1950;131:781–9.

76. Wright G, Lewis H, Hogan B, et al. A self-expanding metal stent for complicated variceal hemorrhage: experience at a single center. Gastrointest Endosc. 2010;71:71–8.

77. D'Amico G, Pagliaro L, Bosch J. The treatment of portal hypertension: a meta-analytic review. Hepatology. 1995;22(1):332–54.

78. Yoshida H, Mamada Y, Taniai N, Yoshioka M, Hirakata A, Kawano Y, et al. Treatment modalities for bleeding esophagogastric varices. J Nippon Med Sch. 2012;79(1):19–30.

79. Lin CT, Huang TW, Lee SC, et al. Sengstaken-Blakemore tube related esophageal rupture. Rev Esp Enferm Dig. 2010;102:395–6.

80. García-Pagán JC, Caca K, Bureau C, Laleman W, Appenrodt B, Luca A, et al.; Early TIPS (Transjugular Intrahepatic Portosystemic Shunt) Cooperative Study Group. Early use of TIPS in patients with cirrhosis and variceal bleeding. Am Surg. 1990;56(12):758–63.

81. Evans GR1, Yellin AE, Weaver FA, Stain SC. Sinistral (left-sided) portal hypertension. N Engl J Med. 2010;362(25):2370–9.

82. Grady E. Gastrointestinal bleeding scintigraphy in the early 21st century. J Nucl Med. 2016;57(2):252–9. https://doi.org/10.2967/jnumed.115.157289. Epub 2015 Dec 17.

83. Chua AE, Ridley LJ. Diagnostic accuracy of CT angiography in acute gastrointestinal bleeding. J Med Imaging Radiat Oncol. 2008;52(4):333–8.

84. Gaba RC. Transjugular intrahepatic portosystemic shunt creation with embolization or obliteration for variceal bleeding. Tech Vasc Interv Radiol. 2016;19(1):21–35.

85. Barkun AN, Bardou M, Kuipers EJ, Sung J, Hunt RH, Martel M, et al.; International Consensus Upper Gastrointestinal Bleeding Conference Group. International consensus recommendations on the management of patients with nonvariceal upper gastrointestinal bleeding. Ann Intern Med. 2010;152(2):101–13.

86. Abougergi MS, Avila P, Saltzman JR. Impact of insurance status and race on outcomes in nonvariceal upper gastrointestinal hemorrhage: a nationwide analysis. J Clin Gastroenterol. 2017; https://doi.org/10.1097/MCG.0000000000000909. [Epub ahead of print].

87. Berne CJ, Tosoff L. Peptic ulcer perforation of the gastroduodenal artery complex: clinical features and operative control. Ann Surg. 1969;169(1):141–4.

88. Shin JH. Recent update of embolization of upper gastrointestinal tract bleeding. Korean J Radiol. 2012;13(Suppl1):S31–9.

Gastroduodenal Perforations

8

Elisa Furay and W. Drew Fielder

Introduction

Gastroduodenal perforation management has changed over the past several decades as a result of a better understanding of its common etiologies. The most clinically significant and leading cause of these perforations is peptic ulcer disease. Other less common causes include trauma, malignancy, chronic steroid use, and iatrogenic injury during endoscopic procedures [1]. While treatment of gastroduodenal perforations remains surgical, the number of patients presenting with this problem has declined over the past decade due to improved medical management of peptic ulcer disease [2]. This shift in care is largely due to the advent of H2 receptor antagonists, proton pump inhibitors, and therapies targeted at *Helicobacter pylori* (*H. pylori*) eradication. The change in treatment of peptic ulcer disease has resulted in an overall decrease in hospitalizations, but the occurrence of emergent surgery related to its acute complications has remained steady [3, 4]. Therefore, even with a decline in peptic ulcer-driven hospitalizations, an acute care surgeon on call will likely encounter a critically ill patient needing an emergent surgical intervention, with the surgeon having only minimal experience with elective peptic ulcer surgery.

E. Furay · W. D. Fielder (✉)
University of Texas at Austin, Dell Medical School,
Austin, TX, USA
e-mail: DFielder@ascension.org

Pathophysiology

Historically, the pathogenesis of peptic ulcer disease was thought to be caused by excessive acid secretion, but it is now known that the most common causes are *H. pylori* and chronic nonsteroidal anti-inflammatory drug (NSAID) use. This knowledge implies that the vast majority of peptic ulcer disease, and its complications, are due to modifiable risk factors.

H. pylori is more commonly found in duodenal ulcers than gastric ulcers, and our complete understanding of how *H. pylori* produces ulcers is still being investigated. However, it is clear that infection of the gastric mucosa affects gastric acid secretion which leads to peptic ulcers [4, 5]. *H. pylori* is diagnosed by noninvasive measures such as urea breath tests, stool antigen studies, or serology testing. Since its discovery, many trials have demonstrated the importance of eradication of *H. pylori* infections in order to prevent ulcer recurrence [4]. By 1994, the National Institutes of Health consensus conference recommended *H. pylori* eradication as a primary goal of ulcer treatment [6]. This therapy most commonly includes "triple therapy" with lansoprazole, amoxicillin, and clarithromycin.

The use of NSAIDs and aspirin has also been determined to play a significant role in peptic ulcer disease by inhibiting prostaglandins, which are essential in the stomach's protective mucosal barrier [5, 7]. Currently, our understanding of peptic ulcer disease suggests that NSAIDs, either

C. V. R. Brown et al. (eds.), *Emergency General Surgery*, https://doi.org/10.1007/978-3-319-96286-3_8

alone or in combination with *H. pylori*, cause the vast majority of ulcers and associated complications [8]. Individuals taking NSAIDs and aspirin reportedly have a four- and twofold increase in complications related to peptic ulcer disease, respectively [5, 7, 9].

Epidemiology

The incidence of perforation in peptic ulcer disease is 2–10% [10]. Once common in all age groups, peptic ulcer disease has become a disease of the elderly. Lifetime prevalence of peptic ulcer disease in the general population has been estimated to be about 5–10% with an incidence of 0.1–0.3% per year [5]. Patients are most commonly over 70 years old with a male predominance of 1.5:1 [4]. The increased age predominance can be attributed to longer life expectancies and the relation between age and NSAID dependence. For the surgeon, this means surgical interventions will most likely occur with older and more fragile individuals, making expedient and well-planned operations paramount.

Endoscopic interventions such as endoscopic retrograde cholangiopancreatography (ERCP), esophageal dilation, and endoscopic biopsy have replaced invasive procedures which have been associated with higher patient morbidity. Although this shift has improved overall patient outcomes, iatrogenic injury causing perforation remains a common surgical complication. Perforations have been reported in 0.5–2.1% of sphincterotomies associated with ERCP [11] and 3–5% during pneumatic dilation for achalasia [12]. Because these complications require prompt surgical evaluation, it is essential for the on-call surgeon to be familiar with their management.

Diagnosis and Management

Perforation significantly increases mortality. In the elderly, mortality associated with perforation may be as high as 50% [10]. Therefore, both early perforation detection and prompt resuscitation are crucial. Patients usually present with an acute onset of epigastric pain which, given enough time, can progress to diffuse peritonitis as well as signs and symptoms of sepsis. Diagnosis can be made with an upright chest x-ray or computed tomography (CT) scan showing free intraperitoneal air or extravasated contrast material. Intraoperative methylene blue dye injected via a nasogastric tube can be used to assist with intraoperative identification of the area of perforation [13].

Initial management in all patients with perforations is aimed at fluid resuscitation and initiation of antibiotic therapy. If the perforation is secondary to ulcer disease, acid suppression is also an important step in management. A perioperative care protocol based on the Surviving Sepsis guideline, including goal-directed resuscitation, has been shown to improve 30-day survival in these patients [14]. Once initial resuscitation is begun, surgical intervention must be undertaken promptly as research has shown every hour of surgical delay is associated with a 2.4% decrease in 30-day survival [15]. Efforts should be taken to minimize delays beyond 12 h as delays beyond this time frame are associated with significant increases in morbidity, operative times, hospital length of stays, and mortality [16]. It is important to consider biopsies during these operative interventions as about 4–5% of benign-appearing ulcers are malignant [4]. If the ulcer is not biopsied or excised at the time of the original operation, the patient should eventually undergo an upper endoscopy and biopsy to rule out malignancy.

The site of perforation dictates the operative approach. The primary goals of surgical management in gastroduodenal perforations are to repair the perforation and minimize the degree of contamination. If there are viable edges at the site of perforation, a primary repair should be attempted in addition to an omental buttress. This is most commonly the approach with endoscopic-related or traumatic perforations. In peptic ulcer disease, the tissue surrounding a perforation can be friable making primary repair difficult and, when attempted, may actually worsen the perforation. In this case, a Graham patch closure is the most common and simplistic procedure to perform.

This repair involves omentopexy of the area of perforation without primary closure.

Duodenal ulcers are more commonly seen in *H. pylori*-positive patients. Postoperative eradication of *H. pylori* is associated with a lower rate of symptomatic ulcer recurrence, including ulcer pain, bleeding, obstruction, and reperforation [17]. This makes knowledge of a patient's *H. pylori* status important as it influences postoperative therapy. As mentioned previously, tissue biopsy of the ulcer should be obtained either at the time of the procedure or postoperatively as 4–5% of even benign uncomplicated duodenal ulcers are deemed malignant [18].

Prepyloric gastric ulcers may be managed in the same fashion as duodenal ulcers. For perforated gastric ulcers located along the greater curvature, antrum, or body, the surgeon should perform a stapled wedge excision of the ulcer [19]. This repair may also be covered with an omental buttress. Ulcers along the lesser curvature, both distal and proximal, pose difficulties. Ulcers located along the distal lesser curvature and are unable to be excised and closed should be treated with a distal gastrectomy [20] and

combined with a Billroth I or II gastrojejunostomy or Roux-en-Y gastrojejunostomy (Fig. 8.1). Ulcers that are located along the proximal lesser curvature (near the GE junction) and are unable to be excised and closed should be treated with a subtotal gastrectomy combined with a Roux-en-Y gastrojejunostomy. Other options for resections are the Pauchet procedure (extension of distal gastrectomy to include the site of perforation) or a Csendes procedure (distal gastrectomy with excision of a tongue-shaped extension and subsequent Roux-en-Y esophagogastrojejunostomy) (Fig. 8.2) [4].

The initial management of Iatrogenic injuries associated with endoscopic procedures, specifically ERCP, should mimic the aforementioned interventions involving fluid resuscitation, antibiotic therapy, and possible nasogastric decompression. The location of these injuries dictates the management strategy. Stapfer, a commonly used classification system, utilizes the anatomic location of injury as well as the mechanism and severity of injury. Stapfer type I are free bowel wall perforations, usually from the endoscope, and these tend to be larger and require immediate operative repair. Type II are retroperitoneal duodenal perforations and are secondary to periampullary injury. These are the most commonly encountered type of perforation and require surgical intervention depending on severity [21]. Type III perforations involve the pancreatic or distal common bile duct and are usually secondary to wire, basket, or balloon instrumentation. Type IV perforations occur when only retroperitoneal air is seen and may not represent true perforation. Some authors suggest that in the absence of physical exam findings, retroperitoneal air can be a result of insufflation used to maintain lumen

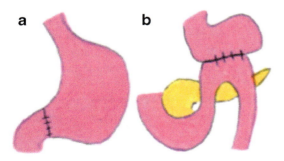

Fig. 8.1 Billroth reconstruction options. (**a**) Type I – gastroduodenostomy. (**b**) Type II – gastrojejunostomy. (Courtesy of Ann Sullivan)

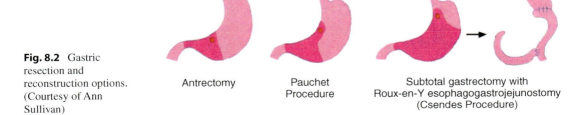

Fig. 8.2 Gastric resection and reconstruction options. (Courtesy of Ann Sullivan)

Antrectomy   Pauchet Procedure   Subtotal gastrectomy with Roux-en-Y esophagogastrojejunostomy (Csendes Procedure)

patency during endoscopic procedures [22, 23]. Medical management can be attempted in patients with retroperitoneal perforations who are hemodynamically stable and who exhibit no evidence of peritonitis [23–25]. Surgery should be reserved for patients with hemodynamic instability, exam findings consistent with peritonitis, a large free perforation, and a biliary obstruction or for those who do not improve after a trial of nonoperative management [26].

The size of the perforation should also be considered. Giant perforated ulcers are those greater than 2 cm. Data suggest that gastric resection with reconstruction is a better treatment option as these larger perforations have been linked to higher incidences of malignancy and have increased leak rates [27]. Such ulcers are more commonly found in the distal stomach, so distal gastrectomy with gastrojejunostomy would be the surgery of choice. In an emergent setting, this operative approach is not always feasible making an omental patch a reasonable option. A variation of the omental patch that has been used for more extensive defects is the pedicled omental plug. This has been described as a pedicle of omentum that is sutured to a nasogastric tube and pulled through the perforation to plug the hole [28].

Patients presenting with complicated duodenal ulcers in close proximity to the pancreaticobiliary system pose a technically difficult situation for the surgeon as these ulcers are unable to be resected and can be difficult to close primarily or patch. In this setting surgeons should consider adjunctive diversion and decompression of enteric contents to assist with healing. The use of "triple tube therapy" or pyloric exclusion accomplishes these goals. Triple tube ostomy approach includes placement of a tube gastrostomy, retrograde tube duodenostomy, and feeding jejunostomy [29, 30] (Fig. 8.3). This option isolates a duodenal repair from gastric, biliary, and pancreatic secretions as well as provides a way to provide enteral nutrition.

Another option for enteric diversion to assist with healing is pyloric exclusion. This refers to making a gastrotomy, oversewing or stapling off the pylorus to allow diversion of enteric contents from the duodenum, and re-establishing bowel

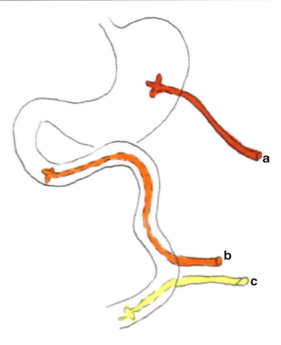

Fig. 8.3 Triple tube therapy for complex duodenal perforations. (A) Tube gastrostomy, (B) retrograde tube duodenostomy, (C) feeding jejunostomy tube. (Courtesy of Ann Sullivan)

continuity with a gastrojejunostomy. The pylorus usually reopens in 3–6 weeks [29, 31]. One benefit of this approach is that the patient maintains their ability to continue oral enteral feeding. Currently, no studies have demonstrated a survival benefit associated with the use of pyloric exclusion. Some authors do suggest a lower fistula rate when pyloric exclusion is combined with primary repair [32]. Other studies have consistently demonstrated prolonged hospital stays associated with the use of pyloric exclusion [33]. Given the limited evidence for and against its utilization, pyloric exclusion should be used in a limited fashion and at the discretion of the surgeon.

The indications for acid-reducing surgery in patients with perforation are limited as proton pump inhibitors (PPIs) and *H. pylori* eradication have been successful in decreasing ulcer recurrence. The only patients that may benefit from surgical intervention are those with a high risk of recurrence. These patients are those with significant complications despite optimal medical therapy and allergies to medical treatment or ones unable to change modifiable risk factors (NSAID/aspirin abusers). The addition of a vagotomy should not be considered in patients who are hemodynamically unstable or have a significant amount of intraperitoneal contamination. When the surgeon believes a vagotomy is indicated, the easiest procedure to perform is a truncal vagotomy and pyloroplasty. A truncal vagotomy involves transection of the right and left vagal trunks. Dividing these trunks sacrifices innervation to the pancreas, stomach, small intestine, proximal colon, and hepatobiliary tree; therefore, a truncal vagotomy must be combined with a gastric-emptying procedure like pyloroplasty. Highly selective vagotomy involves denervation of branches supplying the lower esophagus and stomach, with preservation of the posterior nerve on the lesser curvature of the stomach, the nerve of Latarjet. This decreases the incidence of dumping syndrome that is associated with truncal vagotomy. Although this is a described operative approach, it is technically more difficult and is associated with higher ulcer recurrence rates [34]; for this reason we do not advocate its use in the acute care surgery setting. When compared to other definitive ulcer operations, truncal vagotomy is associated with the highest rates of dumping syndrome and with recurrence rates ranging from 10% to 15% [10, 35]. The most effective surgery to manage peptic ulcer disease is antrectomy combined with vagotomy. This technique best controls acid secretion and has the lowest ulcer recurrence rate, ~5% [10]. It is associated with a higher mortality rate than vagotomy and pyloroplasty and has the potential to result in a difficult duodenal stump or anastomotic leak [4].

In recent years there has been a significant shift toward minimally invasive surgery. Studies have shown that laparoscopic repair is safe and effective if patients are properly selected. Laparoscopic repair has been shown to have shorter operative times, earlier ambulation, reduced hospital stays, earlier return to activity, and decreased pain requirements postoperatively. Most patients that are having laparoscopic repairs performed are relatively healthy with minimal amounts of peritoneal contamination. Patients with risk factors for increased mortality at presentation should not be considered for laparoscopic intervention.

These include individuals who present in shock, have delayed presentation >24 h, have a major medical illness, or are >70 years old [18, 19, 36]. As always, the operative plan must take into consideration the operating surgeon's experience as well as the patient's clinical picture.

Although not commonly utilized, nonoperative management may be reasonable in a small subset of patients with a perforated peptic ulcer. This subset includes those who are young, healthy, and hemodynamically stable and have no signs of diffuse peritonitis. The decision to pursue nonoperative management must be weighed against the risk of increased morbidity and mortality associated with surgical delay [14]. The only prospective randomized trial that compared operative and nonoperative management for perforated peptic ulcer disease found is that an initial period of nonoperative treatment of 12 h and close observation did not lead to increased morbidity or mortality [37]. In patients older than 70, nonoperative management should be avoided as this age group is less likely to seal the perforation spontaneously [37]. In order to pursue nonoperative management, the following should be demonstrated on a Gastrografin upper GI series: an ulcer, filling of the duodenum, and lack of spillage of the contrast into the peritoneal cavity [37]. These patients must show clinical improvement during this 12-h observation period; if no improvement is appreciated or a clinical decline is seen during this time, then patients should undergo operative intervention.

Conclusion

Although gastroduodenal perforations continue to be primarily a surgical problem, the number of these surgical interventions is decreasing. This is due to an improvement in medical management aimed at common etiologies of gastroduodenal perforations [38]. The discovery of *H. pylori*, the advent of antacid medications, and the known relationship of NSAID use to peptic ulcer disease have been instrumental in reducing the complications associated with peptic ulcer disease as well as almost eliminating the role of elective ulcer surgery and vagotomies. This transition in treatment has put today's acute care surgeon in the unique position of having little to no experience in electively caring for these patients but being called to emergently manage their complications, primarily gastroduodenal perforations.

The goal in all patients with gastroduodenal perforations is early diagnosis, hemodynamic stabilization, followed by antibiotic therapy and most often surgical intervention. Location of the perforation should help guide the surgeon in their operative planning. Resectional therapies are often more challenging, and the majority of cases can be managed by simple repair and patch procedures. There is a limited role for nonoperative management, but successful outcomes can only be achieved in a small subset of patients including those with iatrogenic perforations.

Overall, it is essential for today's acute care surgeons to be familiar with the management, both medical and surgical, for gastroduodenal perforations as efficient decision making and interventions ultimately improve patient outcomes.

References

1. Nirula R. Gastroduodenal perforation. Surg Clin North Am. 2014;94(1):31–4.
2. Lanas A, García-Rodríguez LA, Polo-Tomás M, Ponce M, Quintero E, Perez-Aisa MA, et al. The changing face of hospitalisation due to gastrointestinal bleeding and perforation. Aliment Pharmacol Ther. 2011;33(5):585–91.
3. Wang YR, Richard Wang Y, Richter JE, Dempsey DT. Trends and outcomes of hospitalizations for peptic ulcer disease in the United States, 1993 to 2006. Ann Surg. 2010;251(1):51–8.
4. Lee CW, Sarosi GA Jr. Emergency ulcer surgery. Surg Clin North Am. 2011;91(5):1001–13.
5. Lanas A, Chan FKL. Peptic ulcer disease. Lancet. 2017;390(10094):613–24.
6. NIH consensus conference. Helicobacter pylori in peptic ulcer disease. NIH consensus development panel on helicobacter pylori in peptic ulcer disease. JAMA. 1994;272(1):65–9.
7. Lanas A, García-Rodríguez LA, Arroyo MT, Gomollón F, Feu F, González-Pérez A, et al. Risk of upper gastrointestinal ulcer bleeding associated with selective cyclo-oxygenase-2 inhibitors, traditional non-aspirin non-steroidal anti-inflammatory drugs, aspirin and combinations. Gut. 2006;55(12):1731–8.
8. Huang J-Q, Sridhar S, Hunt RH. Role of helicobacter pylori infection and non-steroidal anti-inflammatory drugs in peptic-ulcer disease: a meta-analysis. Lancet. 2002;359(9300):14–22.
9. Lanas Á, Carrera-Lasfuentes P, Arguedas Y, García S, Bujanda L, Calvet X, et al. Risk of upper and lower gastrointestinal bleeding in patients taking nonsteroidal anti-inflammatory drugs, antiplatelet agents, or anticoagulants. Clin Gastroenterol Hepatol. 2015;13(5):906–12. e2.
10. Lagoo J, Pappas TN, Perez A. A relic or still relevant: the narrowing role for vagotomy in the treatment of peptic ulcer disease. Am J Surg. 2014;207(1):120–6.
11. Cotton PB, Lehman G, Vennes J, Geenen JE, Russell RC, Meyers WC, et al. Endoscopic sphincterotomy complications and their management: an attempt at consensus. Gastrointest Endosc. 1991;37(3):383–93.
12. Andriulli A, Loperfido S, Napolitano G, Niro G, Valvano MR, Spirito F, et al. Incidence rates of post-ERCP complications: a systematic survey of prospective studies. Am J Gastroenterol. 2007;102(8):1781–8.
13. Laforgia R, Balducci G, Carbotta G, Prestera A, Sederino MG, Casamassima G, et al. Laparoscopic and open surgical treatment in gastroduodenal perforations: our experience. Surg Laparosc Endosc Percutan Tech. 2017;27(2):113–5.
14. Møller MH, Adamsen S, Thomsen RW, Møller AM, Peptic Ulcer Perforation (PULP) trial group. Multicentre trial of a perioperative protocol to reduce mortality in patients with peptic ulcer perforation. Br J Surg. 2011;98(6):802–10.
15. Buck DL, Vester-Andersen M, Møller MH, Danish Clinical Register of Emergency Surgery. Surgical delay is a critical determinant of survival in perforated peptic ulcer. Br J Surg. 2013;100(8):1045–9.
16. Svanes C, Lie RT, Svanes K, Lie SA, Søreide O. Adverse effects of delayed treatment for perforated peptic ulcer. Ann Surg. 1994;220(2):168–75.
17. Wong C-S, Chia C-F, Lee H-C, Wei P-L, Ma H-P, Tsai S-H, et al. Eradication of helicobacter pylori for prevention of ulcer recurrence after simple closure of perforated peptic ulcer: a meta-analysis of randomized controlled trials. J Surg Res. 2013;182(2):219–26.
18. Siu WT, Leong HT, Law BKB, Chau CH, Li ACN, Fung KH, et al. Laparoscopic repair for perforated peptic ulcer: a randomized controlled trial. Ann Surg. 2002;235(3):313–9.
19. Lagoo SA. Laparoscopic repair for perforated peptic ulcer. Ann Surg. 2002;235(3):320–1.
20. McGee GS, Sawyers JL. Perforated gastric ulcers. A plea for management by primary gastric resection. Arch Surg. 1987;122(5):555–61.
21. Polydorou A, Vezakis A, Fragulidis G, Katsarelias D, Vagianos C, Polymeneas G. A tailored approach to the management of perforations following endoscopic retrograde cholangiopancreatography and sphincterotomy. J Gastrointest Surg. 2011;15(12):2211–7.

22. Stapfer M, Selby RR, Stain SC, Katkhouda N, Parekh D, Jabbour N, et al. Management of duodenal perforation after endoscopic retrograde cholangiopancreatography and sphincterotomy. Ann Surg. 2000;232(2):191–8.

23. Genzlinger JL, McPhee MS, Fisher JK, Jacob KM, Helzberg JH. Significance of retroperitoneal air after endoscopic retrograde cholangiopancreatography with sphincterotomy. Am J Gastroenterol. 1999;94(5):1267–70.

24. Kumbhari V, Sinha A, Reddy A, Afghani E, Cotsalas D, Patel YA, et al. Algorithm for the management of ERCP-related perforations. Gastrointest Endosc. 2016;83(5):934–43.

25. Fatima J, Baron TH, Topazian MD, Houghton SG, Iqbal CW, Ott BJ, et al. Pancreaticobiliary and duodenal perforations after periampullary endoscopic procedures: diagnosis and management. Arch Surg. 2007;142(5):448–54; discussion 454–5.

26. Chung RS, Sivak MV, Ferguson DR. Surgical decisions in the management of duodenal perforation complicating endoscopic sphincterotomy. Am J Surg. 1993;165(6):700–3.

27. Kumar P. Treatment of perforated giant gastric ulcer in an emergency setting. World J Gastrointest Surg. 2014;6(1):5.

28. Jani K, Saxena AK, Vaghasia R. Omental plugging for large-sized duodenal peptic perforations: a prospective randomized study of 100 patients. South Med J. 2006;99(5):467–71.

29. Ho VP, Patel NJ, Bokhari F, Madbak FG, Hambley JE, Yon JR, et al. Management of adult pancreatic injuries. J Trauma Acute Care Surg. 2017;82(1):185–99.

30. Agarwal N, Malviya NK, Gupta N, Singh I, Gupta S. Triple tube drainage for "difficult" gastroduodenal perforations: a prospective study. World J Gastrointest Surg. 2017;9(1):19.

31. Seamon MJ, Pieri PG, Fisher CA, Gaughan J, Santora TA, Pathak AS, et al. A ten-year retrospective review: does pyloric exclusion improve clinical outcome after penetrating duodenal and combined pancreaticoduodenal injuries? J Trauma. 2007;62(4):829–33.

32. Degiannis E, Krawczykowski D, Velmahos GC, Levy RD, Souter I, Saadia R. Pyloric exclusion in severe penetrating injuries of the duodenum. World J Surg. 1993;17(6):751–4.

33. DuBose JJ, Inaba K, Teixeira PGR, Shiflett A, Putty B, Green DJ, et al. Pyloric exclusion in the treatment of severe duodenal injuries: results from the National Trauma Data Bank. Am Surg. 2008;74(10):925–9.

34. Salam IM, Doorly T, Hegarty JH, McMullin JP. Highly selective vagotomy versus truncal vagotomy and drainage for chronic duodenal ulceration: a ten year retrospective study (1972-1982). Ir J Med Sci. 1984;153(2):60–4.

35. Emås S, Eriksson B. Twelve-year follow-up of a prospective, randomized trial of selective vagotomy with pyloroplasty and selective proximal vagotomy with and without pyloroplasty for the treatment of duodenal, pyloric, and prepyloric ulcers. Am J Surg. 1992;164(1):4–12.

36. Boey J, Choi SK, Poon A, Alagaratnam TT. Risk stratification in perforated duodenal ulcers. A prospective validation of predictive factors. Ann Surg. 1987;205(1):22–6.

37. Crofts TJ, Park KG, Steele RJ, Chung SS, Li AK. A randomized trial of nonoperative treatment for perforated peptic ulcer. N Engl J Med. 1989;320(15):970–3.

38. Bashinskaya B, Nahed BV, Redjal N, Kahle KT, Walcott BP. Trends in peptic ulcer disease and the identification of helicobacter pylori as a causative organism: population-based estimates from the US nationwide inpatient sample. J Glob Infect Dis. 2011;3(4):366–70.

Benign and Malignant Gastric Outlet Obstruction

9

John Saydi and S. Rob Todd

List of Abbreviations

BUN	Blood urea nitrogen
CA	Cancer antigen
CEA	Carcinoembryonic antigen
CT	Computed tomography
DGE	Delayed gastric emptying
EUS	Endoscopic ultrasound
GOO	Gastric outlet obstruction
HSV	Highly selective vagotomy
IHPS	Idiopathic hypertrophic pyloric stenosis
PD	Pneumatic dilation
PSPGJ	Partial stomach partitioning gastrojejunostomy
PUD	Peptic ulcer disease
SV	Selective vagotomy
TV	Truncal vagotomy
UGI	Upper gastrointestinal imaging

Background

Gastric outlet obstruction (GOO) can be defined as any mechanical or functional blockage preventing adequate drainage and decompression of the stomach in the normal antegrade fashion. Because this can occur via multiple pathophysiologic processes, GOO cannot be defined as a single entity yet instead as a clinical syndrome caused by multiple etiologies. Despite its name, gastric pathology is not the lone culprit in this syndrome. The duodenum is a retroperitoneal structure that is intimately involved with the liver, gallbladder, and pancreas, and disease of these organs and others can lead to intraluminal, intrinsic, and extrinsic causes of GOO.

The precise incidence of GOO is unknown; however, it is estimated that approximately 2000 operations are performed annually for GOO in adults in the United States [1, 2]. There are both benign and malignant causes of GOO, and their prevalence has evolved over time as knowledge of the disease has increased and medical management has improved. Before the advent of antihistamines and proton pump inhibitors and the discovery and ability to treat *Helicobacter pylori*, benign disease was the leading cause of GOO, mostly secondary to peptic ulcer disease (PUD) [3]. With the decline in incidence of *Helicobacter pylori* and rates of PUD, it is thought that operative GOO related to PUD has also decreased [1, 2, 4]. In contrast, as it now stands, malignancy is the most common cause of gastric outlet obstruction in adults [5–7].

Etiology

Malignant GOO tends to be a late complication of advanced disease most often due to a delay

J. Saydi · S. R. Todd (✉)
Michael E. DeBakey Department of Surgery, Baylor College of Medicine, Houston, TX, USA
e-mail: srtodd@bcm.edu

© Springer International Publishing AG, part of Springer Nature 2019
C. V. R. Brown et al. (eds.), *Emergency General Surgery*, https://doi.org/10.1007/978-3-319-96286-3_9

in presentation. Various etiologies include gastric, duodenal, hepatic, gallbladder, biliary, pancreatic, and ampullary carcinomas, stromal tumors, carcinoids, lymphoma, and metastatic carcinoma. Pancreatic cancer is the most common malignant etiology, and up to 15–20% of patients with primary gastric, duodenal, or pancreatic carcinoma develop GOO [8, 9]. Malignancy can result in either intrinsic obstruction with luminal obliteration of the antrum, pylorus, or proximal duodenum or extrinsic compression, both of which prevent gastric emptying.

Peptic ulcer disease results in approximately 5–8% of all cases of GOO and is the most common benign etiology [2, 10]. Causes for PUD include excessive gastric acid secretion, *Helicobacter pylori* infection, and nonsteroidal anti-inflammatory drug use among others. Although the pathophysiology behind the development of PUD by these three etiologies varies, they can all result in a vicious cycle of gastric distention, gastrin release, and excessive acid production [2]. Over time, this results in pyloric and/or duodenal bulb edema, spasm, circumferential outflow scarring, and gastric distention with eventual atony [10].

Another important cause of benign GOO to be aware of is ingestion of caustic substances. Acidic and alkaline substances can result in gastric antral and/or pyloric scarring over time that can significantly reduce gastric emptying with roughly one third of caustic ingestions resulting in GOO [11]. Less common and rare etiologies of GOO include gastric polyps, gastric volvulus, and inflammatory conditions (Crohn's disease, pancreatitis, tuberculosis) (Table 9.1).

In the pediatric population, the incidence of GOO is approximately 2–4 cases per 1000 births in the Western population, with idiopathic hypertrophic pyloric stenosis (IHPS) being the leading cause [12, 13]. Other etiologies occur rarely but include similar causes as in adults such as PUD, volvulus, polyps, ingestion of caustic substances, and neoplasms [13].

Table 9.1 Etiologies of gastric outlet obstruction

Intraluminal causes
Bezoar
Foreign body
Gallstone
Polyp
Scarring secondary to caustic ingestion
Intrinsic causes
Peptic ulcer disease
Malignancy
Volvulus
Hematoma
Hypertrophic pyloric stenosis
Infiltrative disease (i.e., amyloidosis)
Inflammatory conditions (i.e., Crohn's disease, pancreatitis, tuberculosis)
Extraluminal causes
Malignancy
Annular pancreas
Superior mesenteric artery syndrome
Pancreatic pseudocyst

Clinical Manifestations

Symptoms of GOO can be severe and quite nonspecific. Common symptoms include nausea, vomiting, anorexia, reflux, abdominal pain, bloating/distention, dehydration, malnutrition, and weight loss. A telling sign often reported is nonbilious vomiting of previously consumed foods, as this signifies the inability of the stomach to empty, as well as the isolation of the stomach from the second portion of the duodenum [8]. In patients with underlying malignancy, their complaints may erroneously be attributed to chemotherapy and/or radiation therapy side effects. It is important to obtain a detailed history to establish a temporal understanding of when symptoms began, as this can help delineate between operative emergencies and more chronic etiologies. The stomach is a very distensible organ that has the ability to enlarge significantly and accommodate large volumes, especially with chronic disease, which can go unnoticed until the patient presents with a high-grade obstruction [14].

Physical examination findings are dictated by the patient's duration of obstruction and severity of the underlying etiology, especially in cases of malignancy. Exam findings of dehydration are not always reliable; however, severe dehydration can present as hypovolemic shock with tachycardia and hypotension, orthostatic hypotension, decreased urine output, dry mucous membranes, sunken eyes, decreased capillary refill, and poor skin turgor. Chronic obstruction can result in malnutrition and weight loss with temporal wasting, loss of fat and muscle bulk, and general weakness. A dilated stomach can be identified as a tympanic mass in the epigastrium and left upper quadrant upon percussion and can generate a succussion splash upon auscultation [8]. In cases of metastatic disease, it may be possible to palpate a gastric mass and/or identify supraclavicular or periumbilical lymphadenopathy. Malignancy may also result in jaundice in the setting of biliary compression and elevated bilirubin levels. Findings of peritonitis should raise concern for the possibility of perforation, and urgent intervention should take place. In infants presenting with pyloric stenosis, a palpable "olive-sized mass" can be appreciated in the epigastrium.

Diagnosis

Laboratory Studies

Similar to physical examination findings, the presence of laboratory abnormalities depends on the duration of obstruction and severity of symptoms. Hyperemesis can result in significant electrolyte abnormalities and resultant hypokalemic, hypochloremic metabolic alkalosis. Dehydration can cause renal hypoperfusion with acute kidney injury demonstrated by an elevated blood urea nitrogen (BUN) and creatinine. Anemia can be seen as the result of bleeding from PUD, malignancy, or polyps or from bone marrow suppression. A liver function panel, conjugated bilirubin level, and pancreatic amylase and lipase can be helpful in cases concerning for malignancy and biliary compression. Tumor markers such as cancer antigen (CA) 19-9 and carcinoembryonic

antigen (CEA) are generally nonspecific but may aid in diagnosing a malignant cause for obstruction when clinically correlated. Lastly, significantly elevated gastrin levels can be seen with GOO secondary to gastric antral distention stimulating hydrochloric acid secretion and downstream gastrin secretion [15]. This can often raise concern for Zollinger-Ellison syndrome and needs to be interpreted based on the clinical context.

Radiologic Studies

Plain radiographs of the abdomen in patients with GOO can demonstrate an enlarged gastric bubble with minimal small bowel air distal to the duodenum, although this finding is nonspecific and can be seen with gastroparesis [16]. In the rare occasion that GOO is caused by impaction of a radiopaque gallstone, such as with Bouveret's syndrome, it would be possible to identify the obstruction on plain imaging. The addition of barium or water-soluble contrast can aid in identifying the degree and location of obstruction and, in etiologies such as volvulus, may help to delineate the underlying cause. However, there is an increased risk of aspiration with the use of contrast in patients with an already distended stomach, and adequate decompression is important.

In the past, the use of a saline-load test allowed for the ability to obtain objective data used to establish a diagnosis of GOO and guide surgical intervention [10]. The stomach was adequately drained, a saline load was given, and residuals were checked 30 min later. Nowadays, CT imaging and endoscopy have supplanted previous means of evaluation. Computed tomography imaging is the most specific means of radiologic evaluation and can be used to confirm the presence of a mechanical obstruction versus gastroparesis, determine the level and cause of obstruction, and identify findings concerning for ischemia [16]. Generally, CT imaging includes the use of intravenous contrast, while oral contrast is not required as it unnecessarily increases the risk for aspiration. When intravenous contrast is contraindicated, such as in patients with acute kidney injury, chronic kidney disease, or allergy, unenhanced CT imaging can be obtained; however, this may result in an incomplete evaluation. Studies have indicated that unenhanced CT imaging can be useful for identifying possible areas of bowel ischemia. This has not been investigated in cases of GOO [16]. The use of CT imaging to obtain stereotactic biopsy samples is another useful technique that allows for specific tissue sampling in cases where malignancy is suspected (Fig. 9.1).

The evaluation of GOO in the pediatric population depends on the age of the patient and presenting symptoms. In infants, IHPS is the most common cause of GOO, and ultrasound is the preferred first-line imaging modality. Classically, fluoroscopic upper gastrointestinal imaging (UGI) had been the primary diagnostic method, but ultrasound has since become the mainstay evaluation tool as it avoids the need for ionizing radiation and has a greater than 95% sensitivity and specificity for IHPS [13]. By directly visualizing the pylorus and taking measurements related to muscle layer thickness and pylorus length, standardized criteria have been developed that support surgical intervention or lead to further testing [13]. Aside from IHPS in infants, the evaluation of GOO in all pediatric age groups generally begins with UGI or ultrasound studies. Although CT imaging provides the most complete means of evaluation in most cases, it requires a large dose of ionizing radiation and usually requires sedation for an adequate study to be obtained, increasing the risk of aspiration [13]. When choosing an imaging modality, one must consider the resources available to them. While ultrasound can provide for a diagnosis with minimal consequences to the patient, the examination is limited by the ultrasonographer's skill level and abilities, while CT imaging is a standard evaluation technique that has little variability.

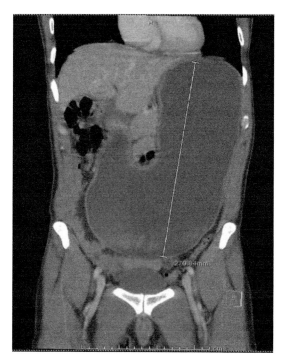

Fig. 9.1 Computed tomography scan with intravenous contrast demonstrating severe gastric distention up to 27 cm secondary to peptic ulcer disease in a 49-year-old Hispanic male

Endoscopic Evaluation

When GOO is suspected after obtaining an adequate history and physical examination along with imaging studies, endoscopy becomes the next step for further evaluation and management. Endoscopy is the gold standard for the diagnosis of GOO and can be both diagnostic and therapeutic [8]. Endoscopy can help to characterize obstructions as benign or malignant in unclear cases by obtaining biopsy samples. However, due to variations in biopsy techniques and random sampling, the sensitivity of endoscopic biopsy samples is poor and can be erroneously benign, especially in cases of high-grade obstruction with distal malignancy or extraluminal malignancy without mucosal penetration [5, 17]. As such, clinical findings, laboratory values, and imaging, in addition to endoscopic evaluation, should all be taken into consideration when attempting to diagnose a malignant cause of GOO.

Often, obstruction at the level of the pylorus or proximal duodenum is unable to be traversed using the adult-size endoscope, and a smaller-diameter scope or guide wires are required.

Direct visualization of the obstruction or stricture using contrast with fluoroscopy can allow for therapeutic procedures such as dilation or stent placement. Endoscopic ultrasound (EUS) is a technique allowing for biopsies and stent placement to be performed under direct visualization. Endoscopic ultrasound-guided procedures allow for further evaluation and management of GOO in a less invasive manner; however, it is highly technical and requires the services of a skilled endoscopist.

Surgical Therapy

Preoperative preparation includes gastric decompression with a large bore nasogastric tube and adequate fluid resuscitation. Optimization of nutritional status is pivotal in patients with GOO, especially in cases of chronic obstruction and malignancy, as these patients often present in a state of poor health. In non-acute cases, early intervention to improve a patient's nutritional status can aid postoperative healing and decrease complications. If endoscopic evaluation is performed and the obstruction able to be traversed, placement of a distal feeding tube allows for supplemental nutrition. Alternatively, TPN can be administered when a feeding tube cannot be placed or when oral feeds are not tolerated post intervention. Lastly, a surgical feeding jejunostomy can be placed intraoperatively distal to the obstruction or bypass procedure that would allow for immediate enteral feeding.

Management of Benign Causes of GOO

Surgical intervention for benign causes of GOO should be considered after conservative medical management has failed to improve obstructive symptoms. Roughly 2% of patients with PUD develop GOO, and in the 1970s and 1980s before the introduction of antacids, surgery was the preferred treatment option [18]. In the early 1980s, Weiland et al. retrospectively reviewed 87 patients with PUD complicated by GOO and found that, after initial medical management, 56% of patients required surgical intervention during their original hospital stay, while on late follow-up, 98% of chronic and 64% of acute disease eventually required surgical intervention [19]. The current initial management for GOO complicating PUD includes *Helicobacter pylori* treatment, antacid therapy, and pneumatic dilation (PD) [1]. Perng et al. prospectively evaluated 42 patients who underwent PD and found that while this provides for the initial relief of symptoms, one third of patients ultimately required surgery. The authors recommend surgical intervention for all patients who require more than two courses of PD [20].

When indicated, surgical intervention includes the combination of an acid reduction procedure along with an appropriate bypass procedure. There are many options, with much controversy as to which is best. Options for acid reduction include truncal vagotomy (TV), selective vagotomy (SV), or highly selective vagotomy (HSV). Truncal and selective vagotomy denervate the pylorus and must be paired with a pyloroplasty, an antrectomy, or pylorus exclusion with gastroenterostomy, while HSV can be paired with either a pyloroplasty or a gastroenterostomy [1, 21] (Table 9.2).

When deciding on an acid-reducing procedure, it is important to consider the side effects of each procedure and the concomitant bypass procedure necessary to preserve adequate gastric function and drainage. Popularized by Lester Dragstedt in the 1940s, TV was the first generation of acid-reducing surgery that was subsequently adapted and improved upon. While TV results in the total denervation of the gastric parietal cells to decrease acid production, it also results in dysfunction of the pylorus, gallbladder, and other splanchnic organs [22]. Post-vagotomy diarrhea can occur due to denervation of the biliary tree allowing for uncontrolled passage of unconjugated bile salts. While generally self-limiting, oral bile acid sequestrants such as cholestyramine can decrease symptoms making surgical intervention rare. In addition, TV results in delayed gastric emptying and must be combined with either a pyloroplasty or an antrectomy with Billroth reconstruction,

Table 9.2 Paired acid reduction and gastric emptying procedures

	Nerves divided	Results in…	Required paired procedure
Truncal vagotomy	Main trunk of the vagus nerve	Denervation of the pylorus and splanchnic organs (liver, biliary tree, pancreas, small and large bowel)	Pyloromyotomy, pyloroplasty, antrectomy with Billroth reconstruction, Roux-en-Y procedure, or gastrojejunostomy
Selective vagotomy	Anterior and posterior gastric nerves of Latarjet	Denervation of the pylorus but preservation of splanchnic innervation	Pyloromyotomy, pyloroplasty, antrectomy with Billroth reconstruction, Roux-en-Y procedure, or gastrojejunostomy
Highly selective vagotomy (parietal cell vagotomy)	Preganglionic vagal fibers of the gastric fundus and body	Denervation of gastric fundal and body acid-producing parietal cells but pylorus and gastric emptying intact	Pyloromyotomy, pyloroplasty, or gastrojejunostomy, however normally not required unless GOO also present

both of which are irreversible and the latter of which results in increased rates of dumping syndrome, alkaline reflux gastritis, and weight loss [23, 24]. However, when performed for uncomplicated ulcer disease, TV with antrectomy results in lower rates of recurrence of ulcer disease when compared to HSV [23]. Building upon the success of TV, SV requires the meticulous dissection of paraesophageal vagal nerve fibers and is generally more successful at treating gastric ulcers than TV while preserving gallbladder and splanchnic organ function [22]. Still requiring concomitant pyloroplasty, SV was never popularized in the United States due to the complex dissection needed to properly perform the procedure [22].

Parietal cell vagotomy, also known as HSV, results in the division of preganglionic vagal fibers that innervate the acid-producing gastric antral parietal cells. Discriminate denervation preserves antegrade antral propulsion and when performed for obstruction can be combined with either pyloroplasty or gastrojejunostomy, preserving normal gastric anatomy and effective gastric emptying. This limits alkaline reflux gastritis and, when it occurs, produces a more mild, transient, and self-limiting dumping syndrome [22]. A double-blinded randomized controlled trial was performed by Csendes et al. comparing three different surgical techniques for the treatment of GOO secondary to duodenal ulcer. Ninety patients were randomized to receive either HSV with gastrojejunostomy, HSV with Jaboulay gastroduodenostomy, or SV with antrectomy. For all three interventions, there were no differences in the

postoperative course, and gastric acid reduction was similar in all groups. However, at mean follow-up of 98 months, long-term reflux symptom improvement was better for HSV with gastrojejunostomy when compared to HSV with Jaboulay gastroduodenostomy, but was not significantly different when compared to SV with antrectomy [23]. The authors recommended a HSV with gastrojejunostomy as the surgical intervention of choice for GOO secondary to PUD as it provides similar long-term outcomes and symptom improvement, while avoiding the anatomic alteration and unwanted side effects of antrectomy [23].

Although gastrojejunostomy is reversible when compared to pyloroplasty, it can result in delayed gastric emptying that is generally self-limiting but can limit a patient's oral intake [23]. When compared to TV, HSV has higher rates of ulcer recurrence; however, this may be attributed to a technical failure to divide all antral parietal cell vagal branches as there are observed variations among surgeons [24]. While the merits of gastric acid reduction remain under debate, clearly there is no single, ideal operative approach. When performed for GOO, surgeons must be familiar with a variety of techniques as the proper acid reduction and bypass procedure is dictated by the patient's acuity in presentation, variation in anatomy, and overall stability [22].

When evaluating other benign causes of GOO, the necessary operative approach is dictated by the underlying cause. With caustic ingestion, acidic or alkaline solutions will pool in the gastric antrum as it is the most dependent portion, resulting in pyloric and antral scarring [25]. While pyloro-plasty may seem to be an adequate option, it is not recommended as scarring often extends beyond the pylorus into adjacent tissues and is not a suffi-cient long-term solution [25]. Definitive surgical therapy depends on the extent of scarring and tis-sues involved and may require stricturoplasty, antrectomy with a Billroth procedure or Roux-en-Y reconstruction, subtotal gastrectomy, or total gastrectomy [25]. When presented with a case of gastric volvulus, endoscopic or surgical interven-tion depends on the stability of the patient and presence of comorbid conditions that preclude sur-gical intervention. When able to be performed, surgical repair is preferred and includes detorsion of the stomach, resection of nonviable ischemic tissues, and gastric fixation with PEG placement or gastropexy to the anterior abdominal wall. Regardless of the etiology of obstruction, adequate treatment requires removal of the obstruction and reestablishing antegrade drainage or generating an alternative means for gastric decompression.

In the pediatric population, there is a signifi-cant amount of data supporting laparoscopic pylo-romyotomy for the treatment of GOO secondary to pyloric stenosis. As this is not a surgical emer-gency, it is important to evaluate and correct the patient's electrolytes preoperatively as repeated emesis can result in significant abnormalities and dehydration. With adequate resuscitation, laparo-scopic pyloromyotomy is a minimally invasive procedure that is generally well tolerated and results in immediate postoperative improvement in oral feeding. Technical considerations to be aware of include adequate release of the pyloric muscular fibers proximally and distally to prevent postoperative recurrence. Most often, recurrence occurs due to inadequate dissection proximally toward the stomach, while perforation occurs mostly with excessive distal dissection involving the first portion of the duodenum.

Management of Malignant Causes of GOO

Generally, by the time patients present with obstructive symptoms secondary to a malignant cause, they will already have advanced stage dis-ease at which point curative resection may no longer be an option. The decision to perform a potentially curative or palliative resection is one that requires careful evaluation of multiple fac-tors including the extent of disease, the prognosis and natural history of the tumor, the patient's functional status, and ability to tolerate a proce-dure, in addition to their individual desires and goals of care. If deemed a possibility, curative surgical intervention can range from performing a gastric wedge resection, subtotal gastrectomy with a Billroth procedure or Roux-en-Y recon-struction to a total gastrectomy.

In many cases, GOO from malignancy pre-cludes curative intervention, at which point pal-liation is pursued with goals of symptom relief and improving quality of life. Classically, surgi-cal gastrojejunostomy has been the standard of care for malignant GOO as it provides a reliable means for gastric drainage and allows for patients to eat orally [14]. However, improvements in endoscopic stenting have led to its increased use to provide gastric decompression in a minimally invasive manner when surgical intervention is deemed high risk. When deciding between endo-scopic or surgical care, patient selection is pivotal to provide the safest and most durable interven-tion. Endoscopic stenting of obstruction is con-sidered in patients who are poor surgical candidates due to short life expectancy and sig-nificant comorbidities or those with metastatic or heavy disease burden [8]. Self-expanding metal stents are a safe alternative that, when compared to surgical intervention, are less invasive, have fewer complications, and are more cost effective with quicker return of normal gastric function and decreased length of hospital stay [8, 14]. A systematic review by Dormann et al. evaluated 606 patients with malignant GOO and found that 97% of patients had successful endoscopic stent placement with 89% receiving relief of symp-toms and increased oral intake [26].

While there are advantages to a less invasive means of gastric decompression, endoscopic stenting should not be performed in patients with distant or multiple malignant intestinal obstruc-tions, in cases of gastric perforation, or in patients with a life expectancy of less than 1 month [8, 14]. The major stent-related complications include perforation, bleeding, infection, stent migration, stent occlusion from food, stricture or tumor burden, and biliary obstruction [8]. Dormann et al. identified an overall complication rate of 28%, with obstruction being the most common at 17.2% [26]. A systematic review by Jeurnink et al. identified 1046 patients who underwent gastroduodenal stent placement for malignant GOO, 18% of whom developed recurrent obstructive symptoms [27]. While the short-term benefits of endoscopic stenting are clear, it should be limited to patients with shorter life expectancies as it is not a long-term solution.

In contrast, surgical gastrojejunostomy is a more durable option for gastric decompression and drainage in the setting of malignant GOO for patients with a life expectancy greater than 2 months [28]. Jeurnink et al. performed a multi-center, prospective, randomized trial comparing open and laparoscopic gastrojejunostomy to endoscopic stent placement. While patients improved more rapidly with stent placement, they more often developed recurrent obstructive symptoms requiring repeat interventions, while long-term relief was sustained with gastrojejunostomy [28]. In select patients without significant malignant ascites who can tolerate insufflation, laparoscopic gastrojejunostomy provides a less invasive surgical option compared to an open procedure and has shown to decrease morbidity, blood loss, length of hospital stay, and time to oral intake [14, 29]. Malignancy causing GOO can also lead to biliary tree compression or invasion that inhibits adequate drainage. In patients with good functional status, a single procedure including gastrojejunostomy with biliary bypass may be the preferable intervention [30].

Variations in Technique and Alternative Surgical Options

To assure proper drainage of the stomach and function of the bypass, factors to consider when creating a gastrojejunostomy include stoma size and positioning. When mobilizing small bowel for stoma creation, the jejunal loop can be brought to the stomach in an antecolic or retro-colic manner in relation to the transverse colon. In a retrospective analysis by Umasankar et al., there were no differences comparing functional or long-term outcomes for antecolic or retrocolic gastrojejunostomies [31]. Both techniques have their advantages, with antecolic being easier and quicker to perform, while retrocolic has the benefit of a shorter afferent loop [31]. Major complications related to gastrojejunostomy include anastomotic leak, afferent loop syndrome, internal hernia, marginal ulcers, dumping syndrome, alkaline gastritis, and delayed gastric emptying (DGE). Of these, DGE is one of the most common and can be very troublesome to patients as it hinders their ability to eat. In patients undergoing pancreaticoduodenal resection and subsequent gastrojejunostomy creation, a reported 19–57% developed DGE, causes of which were probably multifactorial and include alterations in neuro-hormonal pathways in addition to general post-operative ileus [32, 33]. Meta-analysis of randomized control trials comparing rates of DGE after pancreaticoduodenectomy with antecolic versus retrocolic reconstruction demonstrates that the type of reconstruction has no significant effect on the subsequent development of DGE [33].

Multiple variants and modifications have been made to the conventional gastrojejunostomy in an attempt to decrease the incidence of postoperative DGE. One such variant is termed partial stomach partitioning gastrojejunostomy (PSPGJ). This involves dividing the distal portion of the stomach along the greater curvature in a vertical fashion, while maintaining a 2–3 cm tunnel along the lesser curvature, leaving a connection between the proximal and distal portions of the stomach [34]. Partitioning the stomach in this manner creates a smaller proximal portion to which a jejunal bypass can be created, facilitating gastric emptying [34]. This also keeps food or potentially irritating medications away from tumor in cases of malignant GOO while still maintaining a conduit through which endoscopic evaluation of the distal portion can be done [34]. Meta-analysis of several retrospective comparative studies observed a decrease in incidence of DGE and length of hospital stay when bypass was performed with a PSPGJ compared to conventional gastrojejunostomy [34]. Although promising, this technique has not been popularized in Western medicine as there is a lack of scientific data to support its use.

While a surgical gastrojejunostomy provides a durable and long-term treatment option for established cases of GOO, it may have benefit as a prophylactic means to prevent future GOO in cases of malignancy. Lillemoe et al. published a prospective, randomized trial evaluating the role of creating a prophylactic retrocolic gastrojejunostomy in patients with periampullary carcinoma. During the initial operation for resection, 87 patients were deemed to have unresectable disease and were randomized to receive a prophylactic retrocolic gastrojejunostomy versus no surgical bypass. At late follow-up, none of the 44 patients who underwent gastrojejunostomy developed GOO, while 8 out of 43 who did not undergo gastrojejunostomy creation at initial exploratory laparotomy went on to develop GOO requiring intervention at that time [35]. Review of randomized controlled trials evaluating the role of prophylactic gastrojejunostomy creation in patients with unresectable periampullary cancer revealed that although mean operating time was increased by 45 min, the incident of late GOO with prophylactic gastrojejunostomy creation was significantly decreased from 27.8% to 2.5% [36]. Although these studies are limited to cases of unresectable periampullary carcinoma and further studies applied to other causes of obstruction are warranted, there is a clear benefit for patients being able to avoid a potential complication requiring additional intervention.

Conclusion

Gastric outlet obstruction is a complex condition that has many possible etiologies. CT imaging provides a significant amount of data to evaluate the underlying cause and develop a treatment plan. Endoscopic evaluation and intervention options continue to improve and provide for minimally invasive treatments, especially in patients with advanced malig-

nancy and poor prognosis where quality of life is so important. Until endoscopic stenting techniques advance to provide for a more reliable and durable option, surgical gastrojejunostomy remains the gold standard for long-term gastric decompression. In select patients with good functional status, laparoscopic gastrojejunostomy is a safe option that minimizes morbidity and shortens recovery. Attempting to decrease postoperative complications, modifications to the conventional gastrojejunostomy have been attempted but will require more definitive data until they can be considered valid alternatives.

References

1. Gibson JB, Behrman SW, Fabian TC, Britt LG. Gastric outlet obstruction resulting from peptic ulcer disease requiring surgical intervention is infrequently associated with helicobacter pylori infection. J Am Coll Surg. 2000;191(1):32–7.
2. Behrman SW. Management of complicated peptic ulcer disease. Arch Surg. 2005;140(2):201–8.
3. Kreel L, Ellis H. Pyloric stenosis in adults: a clinical and radiological study of 100 consecutive patients. Gut. 1965;6(3):253–61.
4. el-Serag HB, Sonnenberg A. Opposing time trends of peptic ulcer and reflux disease. Gut. 1998;43:327.
5. Shone DN, Nikoomanesh P, Smith-Meek MM, Bender JS. Malignancy is the most common cause of gastric outlet obstruction in the era of H2 blockers. Am J Gastroenterol. 1995;90(10):1769–70.
6. Khullar SK, DiSario JA. Gastric outlet obstruction. Gastrointest Endosc Clin N Am. 1996;6(3):585–603.
7. Johnson CD. Gastric outlet obstruction malignant until proved otherwise. Am J Gastroenterol. 1995;90(10):1740.
8. Brimhall B, Adler DG. Enteral stents for malignant gastric outlet obstruction. Gastrointest Endosc Clin N Am. 2011;21(3):389–403, vii-viii.
9. Larssen L, Medhus AW, Hauge T. Treatment of malignant gastric outlet obstruction with stents: an evaluation of the reported variables for clinical outcome. BMC Gastroenterol. 2009;9:45.
10. Jaffin BW, Kaye MD. The prognosis of gastric outlet obstruction. Ann Surg. 1985;201(2):176–9.
11. Kochhar R, Kochhar S. Endoscopic balloon dilation for benign gastric outlet obstruction in adults. World J Gastrointest Endosc. 2010;2(1):29–35.
12. Pandya S, Heiss K. Pyloric stenosis in pediatric surgery: an evidence-based review. Surg Clin North Am. 2012;92(3):527–39, vii-viii.

13. Otjen JP, Iyer RS, Phillips GS, Parisi MT. Usual and unusual causes of pediatric gastric outlet obstruction. Pediatr Radiol. 2012;42(6):728–37.
14. Potz BA, Miner TJ. Surgical palliation of gastric outlet obstruction in advanced malignancy. World J Gastrointest Surg. 2016;8(8):545–55.
15. Dacha S, Razvi M, Massaad J, Cai Q, Wehbi M. Hypergastrinemia. Gastroenterol Rep. 2015;3(3):201–8.
16. Millet I, Doyon FC, Pages E, Faget C, Zins M, Taourel P. CT of gastro-duodenal obstruction. Abdom Imaging. 2015;40(8):3265–73.
17. Dada SA, Fuhrman GM. Miscellaneous disorders and their management in gastric surgery: volvulus, carcinoid, lymphoma, gastric varices, and gastric outlet obstruction. Surg Clin North Am. 2011;91(5):1123–30.
18. Baitchev G, Hristova P, Ivanov I. Surgical treatment of gastric outlet obstruction. Khirurgiia (Sofiia). 2009;(6):23–6.
19. Weiland D, Dunn DH, Humphrey EW, Schwartz ML. Gastric outlet obstruction in peptic ulcer disease: an indication for surgery. Am J Surg. 1982;143(1):90–3.
20. Perng CL, Lin HJ, Lo WC, Lai CR, Guo WS, Lee SD. Characteristics of patients with benign gastric outlet obstruction requiring surgery after endoscopic balloon dilation. Am J Gastroenterol. 1996;91(5):987–90.
21. Miller A, Schwaitzberg S. Surgical and endoscopic options for benign and malignant gastric outlet obstruction. Curr Surg Rep. 2014;2:48.
22. Donahue PE. Parietal cell vagotomy versus vagotomy-antrectomy: ulcer surgery in the modern era. World J Surg. 2000;24(3):264–9.
23. Csendes A, Maluenda F, Braghetto I, Schutte H, Burdiles P, Diaz JC. Prospective randomized study comparing three surgical techniques for the treatment of gastric outlet obstruction secondary to duodenal ulcer. Am J Surg. 1993;166(1):45–9.
24. Chan VMY, Reznick RK, O'Rourke K, Kitchens JM, et al. Meta-analysis of highly selective vagotomy versus truncal vagotomy and pyloroplasty in the surgical treatment of uncomplicated duodenal ulcer. Can J Surg. 1994;37(6):457–64.
25. Gupta V, Wig JD, Kochhar R, Sinha SK, Nagi B, Doley RP, Gupta R, Yadav TD. Surgical management of gastric cicatrisation resulting from corrosive ingestion. Int J Surg. 2009;7(3):257–61.
26. Dormann A, Meisner S, Verin N, Wenk Lang A. Self-expanding metal stents for gastroduodenal malignancies: systematic review of their clinical effectiveness. Endoscopy. 2004;36(6):543–50.
27. Jeurnink SM, van Eijck CH, Steyerberg EW, Kuipers EJ, Siersema PD. Stent versus gastrojejunostomy for the palliation of gastric outlet obstruction: a systematic review. BMC Gastroenterol. 2007;7:18.
28. Jeurnink SM, Steyerberg EW, van Hooft JE, van Eijck CH, Schwartz MP, Vleggaar FP, Kuipers EJ, Siersema PD, Dutch SUSTENT Study Group. Surgical gastrojejunostomy or endoscopic stent placement for the palliation of malignant gastric outlet obstruction (SUSTENT study): a multicenter randomized trial. Gastrointest Endosc. 2010;71(3):490–9.
29. Navarra G, Musolino C, Venneri A, De Marco ML, Bartolotta M. Palliative antecolic isoperistaltic gastrojejunostomy: a randomized controlled trial comparing open and laparoscopic approaches. Surg Endosc. 2006;20(12):1831–4.
30. Del Piano M, Ballare M, Montino F, Todesco A, Orsello M, Magnani C, Garello E. Endoscopy or surgery for malignant GI outlet obstruction? Gastrointest Endosc. 2005;61:421–6.
31. Umasankar A, Kate V, Ananthakrishnan N, Smile SR, Jagdish S, Srinivasan K. Anterior or posterior gastro-jejunostomy with truncal vagotomy for duodenal ulcer – are they functionally different? Trop Gastroenterol. 2003;24(4):202–4.
32. Nikfarjam M, Kimchi ET, Gusani NJ, Shah SM, Sehmbey M, Shereef S, Staveley-O'Carroll KF. A reduction in delayed gastric emptying by classic pancreaticoduodenectomy with an antecolic gastrojejunal anastomosis and a retrogastric omental patch. J Gastrointest Surg. 2009;13(9):1674–82.
33. Zhou Y, Lin J, Wu L, Li B, Li H. Effect of antecolic or retrocolic reconstruction of the gastro/duodenojejunostomy on delayed gastric emptying after pancreaticoduodenectomy: a meta-analysis. BMC Gastroenterol. 2015;15:68.
34. Kumagai K, Rouvelas I, Ernberg A, Persson S, Analatos A, Mariosa D, Lindblad M, Nilsson M, Ye W, Lundell L, Tsai JA. A systematic review and meta-analysis comparing partial stomach partitioning gastrojejunostomy versus conventional gastrojejunostomy for malignant gastroduodenal obstruction. Langenbeck's Arch Surg. 2016;401(6):777–85.
35. Lillemoe KD, Cameron JL, Hardacre JM, Sohn TA, Sauter PK, Coleman J, Pitt HA, Yeo CJ. Is prophylactic gastrojejunostomy indicated for unresectable periampullary cancer? A prospective randomized trial. Ann Surg. 1999;230(3):322–8.
36. Gurusamy KS, Kumar S, Davidson BR. Prophylactic gastrojejunostomy for unresectable periampullary carcinoma. Cochrane Database Syst Rev. 2013;2:CD008533.

Acute Cholecystitis

10

Aaron M. Williams, Ben E. Biesterveld, and Hasan B. Alam

Introduction

Acute cholecystitis is one of the most significant diseases of the Western world, and gallstone disease plays a key role in its development. Gallstone disease represents a significant global problem with 10–15% of the adult population being affected in developed countries [1–3]. Although the majority of patients are unaffected, 1–4% become symptomatic each year [4, 5]. Most individuals present with biliary colic; however, 10–35% of patients will eventually develop acute cholecystitis if left untreated [6, 7].

As acute cholecystitis usually requires intervention for management, it accounts for one-third of all emergency surgery hospital admissions [8]. As such, approximately 100,000 cholecystectomies are performed for acute cholecystitis in the United States annually. Without prompt intervention, it can result in significant morbidity and mortality. In severe cases or in high-risk patient populations, including the elderly, it can cause potentially life-threatening complications including gallbladder gangrene, perforation, or empy-

A. M. Williams · B. E. Biesterveld
Department of Surgery, Section of General Surgery,
University of Michigan Hospital,
Ann Arbor, MI, USA

H. B. Alam (✉)
Department of Surgery, University of Michigan
Hospital, Ann Arbor, MI, USA
e-mail: alamh@med.umich.edu

ema. As early cholecystectomy is advocated for acute cholecystitis, general and acute care surgeons should be well versed in its pathogenesis, clinical presentation, severity assessment, diagnostic workup, operative strategies, as well as alternative treatments in order to employ the most safe and effective patient care.

Pathogenesis

Acute cholecystitis is defined as acute inflammation of the gallbladder wall. The pathogenesis is primarily due to obstruction of biliary outflow, typically involving the infundibulum or cystic duct. Obstruction secondary to gallstones occurs in nearly 90–95% of cases and is often termed *acute calculous cholecystitis*. When gallstone impaction occurs, mucosal phospholipases cause hydrolysis of luminal lecithin, resulting in toxic lysolecithin production. Exposure of the biliary epithelium to these toxic agents results in disruption of the glycoprotein mucus layer of the gallbladder wall, allowing the detergent effects of bile salts to induce inflammation. Following inflammation and gallbladder wall damage, dysmotility ensues causing gallbladder distention. As the intraluminal pressure rises, serosal edema, mucosal sloughing, and venous and lymphatic congestion develop, which ultimately leads to cystic artery thrombosis where ischemia and gallbladder necrosis often follow. As the

© Springer International Publishing AG, part of Springer Nature 2019
C. V. R. Brown et al. (eds.), *Emergency General Surgery*, https://doi.org/10.1007/978-3-319-96286-3_10

gallbladder fundus is the most distal region from the cystic artery origin, it is often the most sensitive to ischemia and the most common location where gallbladder necrosis and perforation may occur.

Although the primary pathophysiologic mechanism of acute cholecystitis is an unresolved obstruction, secondary biliary infection may occur. Positive bile cultures, the most common of which include gram-negative bacteria, such as *Escherichia coli* and *Klebsiella* spp., have been found in 15–30% of patients undergoing cholecystectomy for acute cholecystitis [9]. Patients who have previously undergone biliary instrumentation, including endoscopic sphincterotomy, demonstrate an even greater incidence with rates as high as 60% [10].

Although the overwhelming majority of acute cholecystitis cases are secondary to gallstones, the remaining 5–10% are termed *acute acalculous cholecystitis*. This scenario typically occurs in critically ill patients following severe trauma, major burns, high-risk surgery, and severe sepsis or in patients with a history of poorly controlled diabetes or an acquired immunodeficiency syndrome. Patients who are on prolonged total parental nutrition (TPN), postpartum, or have received blood products are also at increased risk. The pathogenesis of acute acalculous cholecystitis is secondary to bile stasis or gallbladder ischemia/reperfusion injury. Bile stasis, which can be caused by prolonged TPN or mechanical ventilation, changes the composition of bile, resulting in highly concentrated bile salts contributing to gallbladder distention. As the intraluminal pressure rises, venous congestion with subsequent ischemia may occur similarly to the development of acute calculus cholecystitis. In contrast, when most critically ill trauma, burn, postoperative, and septic patients sustain shock, decreased splanchnic blood flow occurs, which can result in gallbladder wall ischemia. For patients with known intravascular depletion, bile viscosity may increase causing highly concentrated bile salts to form, ultimately resulting in stasis and subsequent biliary outflow obstruction leading to acute cholecystitis.

Clinical Presentation

For a patient with suspected acute cholecystitis, history should focus on abdominal pain onset, pattern, quality, as well as anything that relieves or worsens it. Most patients present with severe, constant right upper quadrant (RUQ) or epigastric pain with radiation to the right subscapular region. Presentation is often preceded by intermittent, less severe, shorter episodes, often characterized as biliary colic. Many patients will have a known history of gallstones, which have been identified during prior workup or discovered incidentally. Other presenting symptoms often include nausea, vomiting, and anorexia, while fever, chills, and night sweats are variably present.

On physical examination, the most common finding is RUQ abdominal tenderness, guarding, or rebound. However, one-third of patients exhibit the classic Murphy's sign, which is defined as inspiratory arrest upon palpation of the gallbladder secondary to pain induced by the gallbladder meeting the examiner's fingers.

Although most patients present in this manner, all of these signs and symptoms may be blunted or absent in patients who are immunosuppressed, are obese, have poorly controlled diabetes, or are critically ill with an altered sensorium. A high index of suspicion is required in these patients to avoid missing the diagnosis.

Differential Diagnosis

Differentiating acute cholecystitis from other biliary tract pathology is important as treatment strategies may vary significantly depending on pathology. These include biliary colic, choledocholithiasis, cholangitis, and gallstone pancreatitis. However, numerous other disease processes may present similarly to acute cholecystitis and must be included in the differential diagnosis as well. These include both intra-abdominal diseases such as peptic ulcer disease, gastritis, pancreatitis, mesenteric ischemia, hepatitis, and colitis, along with extra-abdominal diseases including pneumonia and myocardial infarction.

An appropriate history and physical examination should be utilized to help narrow the differential diagnosis and allow for appropriate laboratory and imaging studies to be conducted.

Laboratory Studies and Imaging

There are no laboratory studies that can conclusively diagnose acute cholecystitis. A mild to moderate degree of leukocytosis with a left shift is typically present. Total bilirubin and alkaline phosphatase levels are typically normal with acute cholecystitis; however, severe or complicated forms can sometimes result in mildly elevated bilirubin (>2.0 mg/dL) and alkaline phosphatase, secondary to liver bed inflammation, gallbladder perforation, or bile duct compression. In general, such elevations should also warrant consideration for alternative diagnoses including choledocholithiasis or cholangitis. Lipase and amylase are usually normal unless there is concomitant pancreatitis. Other laboratory studies including blood urea nitrogen, creatinine, prothrombin time (PT), and international normalized ratio (INR) may be elevated in severe disease with organ dysfunction reflecting systemic involvement.

Numerous imaging modalities exist and may play a role in aiding the diagnosis of acute cholecystitis. However, the optimal imaging method is dependent on the pretest probability of diagnosing acute cholecystitis when compared to other intra-abdominal processes. Ultrasonography (US), computed tomography (CT), hepatobiliary scintigraphy (HIDA), and magnetic resonance imaging (MRI) vary in cost and availability, along with sensitivity and specificity, for the detection of acute cholecystitis. Proper utilization of these imaging modalities is dependent on the specific clinical scenario and context.

Abdominal US is considered the first-line imaging choice for acute cholecystitis due to its widespread availability, lack of invasiveness, lack of ionizing radiation, short examination time, and its inexpensive nature. US findings of acute cholecystitis typically include gallstones and sludge, gallbladder wall thickening (>4 mm), gallbladder

distention, peri-cholecystic fluid, and possibly a gallstone lodged in the gallbladder neck or cystic duct (Fig. 10.1). The technician or radiologist may also detect a sonographic Murphy's sign. Although US has a sensitivity greater than 90% for detecting gallstones, it is only 70–80% sensitive for detecting signs of acute cholecystitis [11]. However, when such findings are combined with clinical suspicion and a positive sonographic Murphy's sign, an overall accuracy of greater than 90% can be achieved in diagnosing acute cholecystitis [12].

HIDA may be a useful study in patients with a high index of suspicion, but the diagnosis remains uncertain. Technetium-labeled derivate of iminodiacetic acid is injected intravenously and taken up by hepatocytes and secreted in bile, which allows for visualization of the biliary tree with scintigraphy. A normal study reveals full delineation of the biliary tree including the gallbladder along with prompt emptying of the radiolabeled agent into the duodenum. However, non-visualization of the gallbladder is reflective of cystic duct or gallbladder neck obstruction, which is consistent with acute cholecystitis. HIDA can be more accurate than US alone as it is able to reveal acute cholecystitis in approximately 95% of patients [11]. However, HIDA has several limitations. It is not useful in patients with hepatic dysfunction or cirrhosis, as it requires hepatic excretion of bile. Further,

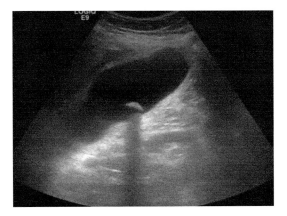

Fig. 10.1 Ultrasound revealing classic findings of acute cholecystitis including cholelithiasis, gallbladder sludge, thickened gallbladder wall, and peri-cholecystic fluid

HIDA is expensive, time-intensive, and only available at select centers. Thus, it should be reserved for selected cases only, where the diagnosis is unclear.

CT provides the most overall detailed anatomic evaluation and is most useful when evaluating for complications of acute cholecystitis or when alternative diagnoses are suspected. CT is generally less sensitive than US for the diagnosis of acute cholecystitis, especially early in the disease course [13, 14]; however, findings including gallbladder wall thickening, peri-cholecystic stranding or fluid, gallbladder distention, subserosal edema, and bile attenuation may be present (Fig. 10.2). Complicated forms of acute cholecystitis, including gangrenous and emphysematous cholecystitis, may be diagnosed by the presence of intraluminal or intramural gas and an irregular or discontinuous gallbladder wall. Other complications including empyema, Mirizzi's syndrome, and cholecystoenteric fistulae may also be observed.

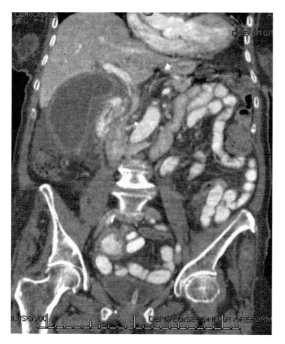

Fig. 10.2 Coronal CT section demonstrating a markedly distended and irregularly thickened gallbladder with peri-cholecystic fluid and stranding concerning for severe acute cholecystitis

Patients in the emergency department commonly undergo a CT scan for evaluation of abdominal pain prior to surgical consultation. Although not first-line imaging for acute cholecystitis and cholelithiasis, CT may aid in diagnosis. If clinical suspicion is high, CT signs of acute cholecystitis are present, and no other intra-abdominal pathology is noted, further imaging, including US, is generally not required.

MRI may also be a useful alternative for acute cholecystitis when US appears to be technically degraded. In recent years, it has become more widely available, less expensive, and faster. There is no significant difference between MRI and US in detecting acute cholecystitis, as sensitivity and specificity are as high as 85% and 81%, respectively [11]. Magnetic resonance cholangiopancreatography (MRCP) may also be a viable option when concomitant choledocholithiasis is a concern, as it has a negative predictive value of 100% and can help facilitate decision-making regarding the need for preoperative ERCP [15].

Although diffuse gallbladder wall thickening is commonly present in acute cholecystitis, it can be a non-specific sign observed in a wide variety of systemic diseases, including hypoalbuminemia, ascites, hepatitis, and chronic cholecystitis, along with liver, renal, and heart failure and other inflammatory diseases. Thus, the presence of gallbladder wall thickening alone is not diagnostic of acute cholecystitis, and the patient's overall clinical picture must be considered.

In addition to sensitivity and specificity, costs, radiation exposure, false-positive and false-negative findings, and delays in treatment must be taken into account when selecting the most appropriate diagnostic study. The American College of Radiology has developed evidence-based recommendations to guide this decision-making [16].

Complications of Cholecystitis

Complications of acute cholecystitis are common. The most relevant complications to emergency general surgery are listed below, although others exist including Mirizzi's syndrome, cholecystoenteric fistula, and gallstone ileus.

Gangrenous Cholecystitis

A common complication following acute cholecystitis is gangrenous cholecystitis, which may occur in 2–40% of cases [17–19]. Factors such as male sex, advanced age, diabetes mellitus, and delayed surgery contribute to its development [17]. Further, perforation in the setting of gangrene may be present in up to 10% of cases. Intraoperatively, focal transmural necrotic defects in the gallbladder wall may be observed. The presence of loculated or free-flowing intraperitoneal bile may further confirm the presence of gangrene with subsequent perforation.

Emphysematous Cholecystitis

When gas-forming organisms cause secondary infection of the gallbladder wall, emphysematous cholecystitis is present. Patients most affected include males, individuals between 40 and 60 years old, and poorly controlled diabetics. Plain film or CT imaging may help identify the presence of intramural gas; however, this may not be identifiable on US imaging and can even further degrade US study quality. Without early treatment, patients with emphysematous cholecystitis often develop gangrene, perforation, and abscess.

Peri-cholecystic Abscess

A peri-cholecystic abscess may be present in up to 20% of acute cholecystitis cases [20]. On imaging, these abscesses will typically appear as intramural or peri-cholecystic rim-enhancing fluid collections, which may be unilocular or have septations with irregular contours. Extension into the adjacent hepatic parenchyma usually present as a complex cystic mass with surrounding parenchymal edema.

Diagnosis and Severity of Disease

Although acute cholecystitis remains a common disease for the general and acute care surgeon, its diagnosis and management still remains a challenge in some settings. Within recent years, select diagnostic criteria, including the Tokyo Guidelines (TG13/18), have been constructed to help aid in diagnosis (Table 10.1) [21]. As there is no single clinical or laboratory finding with sufficient diagnostic accuracy to establish or exclude the diagnosis of acute cholecystitis, a combination of a detailed history, physical examination, laboratory data, and imaging studies is required. If there is a high index of suspicion despite a negative or non-diagnostic workup, further evaluation or consultation may be warranted.

To help stratify the severity of acute cholecystitis following diagnosis, the Tokyo Guidelines (TG13/18) group also constructed a severity grade scale ranging from local to systemic involvement (Table 10.2) [21]. Grade I represents mild disease with only minimal inflammatory changes in the gallbladder. Grade II represents moderate disease with associated elevated white blood cell count (>18,000/mm^3), a palpable RUQ mass, duration of complaints greater than 72 h, and marked local inflammation (biliary peritonitis, gangrenous cholecystitis, emphysematous cholecystitis, hepatic abscess, and peri-cholecystic

Table 10.1 Diagnosis of acute cholecystitis: Tokyo Guidelines 2013/2018

Criteria	
A. Local inflammation	1. Murphy's sign
	2. RUQ mass/pain/tenderness
B. Systemic inflammation	1. Fever and/or shaking chills
	2. Abnormal WBC count
	3. Elevated CRP
C. Imaging	Imaging findings characteristic of acute cholecystitis
Definite diagnosis	
Diagnosis of acute cholecystitis	One item in A + one item in B
	C confirms diagnosis when acute cholecystitis is suspected clinically

Adapted from Yokoe et al. [41]

Table 10.2 Assessment of acute cholecystitis severity: Tokyo Guidelines 2013/2018

Severity of acute cholecystitis	
Mild (Grade I)	Does not meet criteria of "moderate" or "severe" acute cholecystitis at time of initial diagnosis
Moderate (Grade II)	Acute cholecystitis associated with any one of the following conditions: 1. Elevated WBC count (>18,000/mm³) 2. Palpable tender RUQ mass 3. Symptoms greater than 72 h 4. Marked local inflammation (gangrenous or emphysematous cholecystitis; peri-cholecystic or hepatic abscess)
Severe (Grade III)	Acute cholecystitis associated by onset of dysfunction in at least one of the following organs/systems: 1. Neurologic dysfunction (disturbance of consciousness) 2. Cardiovascular dysfunction (hypotension requiring pressors) 3. Respiratory dysfunction (PaO_2/FiO_2 ratio < 300) 4. Renal dysfunction (oliguria, serum creatinine >2 mg/dL) 5. Hepatic dysfunction (elevated PT/INR >1.5) 6. Hematologic dysfunction (platelet count <100,000/mm³)

Adapted from Yokoe et al. [41]

abscess). Finally, Grade III represents severe acute cholecystitis with evidence of cardiovascular, neurological, respiratory, hepatic, or hematologic dysfunction. As disease courses are dynamic, the severity of acute cholecystitis should be reassessed frequently to determine the patient's response to appropriate treatment. If the patient cannot be treated appropriately, prompt transfer to a center with capabilities including acute care surgery, interventional radiology, and endoscopy should be facilitated.

Initial Management

Once a definitive diagnosis of acute cholecystitis has been reached, initial treatment includes intravenous fluids and antibiotic therapy with appropriate gram-negative and anaerobic coverage. Blood pressure, heart rate, and urine output should be monitored closely to assess for the development of septic shock or progression of acute cholecystitis. Although patients commonly present with RUQ pain, opioid analgesics, including morphine, should be administered selectively as they may cause sphincter of Oddi contraction, ultimately elevating intraluminal biliary pressure.

In general, the current recommendation in the treatment of acute cholecystitis involves early cholecystectomy whenever possible. This treatment strategy addresses the current episode of acute cholecystitis and prevents future bouts and subsequent complications related to gallstone disease. A patient's overall clinical status, including duration of symptoms and severity of disease, must be taken into account along with overall medical comorbidities. Patients with minimal comorbidities presenting with mild or moderate acute cholecystitis should undergo cholecystectomy. However, severe acute cholecystitis in patients who are critically ill or who have significant comorbidities may be better candidates for percutaneous cholecystostomy or endoscopic therapy, including transpapillary stenting or transmural drainage. A trial of conservative therapy with antibiotics may be reserved for patients with mild acute cholecystitis in the setting of significant comorbidities that make surgery unacceptably high risk. However, in the vast majority of patients, early laparoscopic cholecystectomy is the treatment of choice.

Timing of Cholecystectomy

Laparoscopic cholecystectomy is the treatment of choice for patients with acute cholecystitis. However, the optimal timing of surgery for acute cholecystitis has been controversial within the last decade. Two approaches exist including early surgery within 72 h of admission versus an initial trial of conservative therapy with antibiotics until inflammation subsides, followed by delayed cholecystectomy several weeks later. Within recent years, numerous studies have been conducted to provide further insight. The ACDC ("Acute Cholecystitis—early laparoscopic surgery versus antibiotic therapy and Delayed elective Cholecystectomy") study is a randomized, prospective, open-label, parallel group trial which compared immediate surgery within 24 h of admission to initial antibiotic therapy followed by delayed cholecystectomy 7–45 days later [22]. Morbidity rate was significantly lower in immediate surgery (11.8%) when compared to delayed surgery (34.4%), and conversion rate to open surgery was not significantly different. Further, hospital stay (5.4 vs. 10.0 days; $p < 0.001$) and total hospital costs were significantly less ($p < 0.05$) in immediate surgery when compared to delayed surgery [22]. Within recent years, other randomized trials have validated such findings and even demonstrated that early cholecystectomy for patients with over 72 h of symptoms have less morbidity (14% vs. 39%; $p < 0.05$), total length of stay (4 vs. 7 days; $p < 0.001$), duration of antibiotic therapy (2 vs. 10 days; $p < 0.001$), and total hospital costs ($p < 0.05$) with no differences in operative time and postoperative complications ($p > 0.05$) when compared to delayed cholecystectomy [23]. Such findings are in line with our practice, and we feel that immediate laparoscopic cholecystectomy should be the mainstay of treatment in operable patients. However, conservative management and alternative strategies may prove useful in those deemed inoperable.

Laparoscopic Cholecystectomy

The laparoscopic approach has become the standard for cholecystectomy in the setting of acute cholecystitis. Laparoscopy has demonstrated significant benefits including decreased morbidity, hospital stay, postoperative pain, time to return of normal function, and overall hospital costs. Although the conversion rate to open cholecystectomy is higher in acute cholecystitis than other elective biliary cases, patients with acute cholecystitis can undergo laparoscopic cholecystectomy in approximately 80% of cases [24]. However, patients with a hostile abdomen, severe inflammation, or known aberrant anatomy may be best served with an open approach.

The basic steps of the procedure include preoperative planning, patient positioning, equipment setup, abdominal access, exposure of the gallbladder and cystic structures, dissecting the gallbladder and cystic structures until the critical view of safety (CVS) is obtained, division of the cystic duct and artery, and dissection of the gallbladder off the liver parenchyma, followed by abdominal closure.

Following induction of general anesthesia, the patient should be positioned in the supine position. Some surgeons prefer the left arm tucked to help facilitate ease of intraoperative cholangiography (IOC) if required. A Foley catheter may be considered if the case is suspected to be difficult or if there is a high chance of conversion to an open approach.

Either an open Hassan or a closed Veress needle technique may be utilized to obtain access to the abdomen. Direct optical trocar insertion under continuous visualization is also a safe and rapid option for initial entry. Pneumoperitoneum should be established to 15 mmHg, and a 30-degree laparoscope should be inserted at the periumbilical port. Three additional ports should be placed in the subxiphoid epigastrium and the medial and lateral right subcostal regions. The patient should then be positioned in reverse Trendelenburg to facilitate displacement of the small bowel and omentum out of the operative field.

Initial exposure is obtained by grasping the gallbladder fundus and retracting it cephalad over the liver to expose the body of the gallbladder. An inflamed and distended gallbladder may be difficult to grasp and maneuver. Needle aspiration of gallbladder contents may be utilized to help ease in grasping the gallbladder for retraction. A 14-gauge angiocatheter may also be placed through a stab incision to help facilitate this maneuver.

Adjacent structures, including omentum, duodenum, and colon, should be identified as they may be adhered to the gallbladder secondary to inflammation. These structures should be visualized and their locations noted before proceeding with dissection to prevent injury. If involved, the plane between the gallbladder and adjacent structures should be identified, and peeling should occur downward and in parallel to the gallbladder wall as pulling outward may cause injury. Adhesions to the liver capsule should also be identified and be divided with scissors or electrocautery to prevent a liver capsular tear. Further, a dense, inflammatory rind encasing the gallbladder may be present, which requires careful dissection. A combination of blunt dissection utilizing a laparoscopic peanut dissector or suction irrigator may be required, as electrocautery tends to be less effective if substantial edema is present.

Once the gallbladder is exposed, the infundibulum is grasped and retracted laterally to open Calot's triangle, and the peritoneum is incised and opened. Dissection continues until the cystic duct and artery are exposed anteriorly and posteriorly and are the only structures entering the gallbladder, which constitutes the CVS (Fig. 10.3). Once the CVS has been achieved, the cystic duct and artery are then doubly clipped and divided.

Although not always discussed, gallbladder dissection off of the liver parenchyma is a key portion of the case. Gallbladder retraction must provide an appropriate amount of tension to allow for alveolar dissection in the correct plane. In the incorrect plane, bleeding from the liver

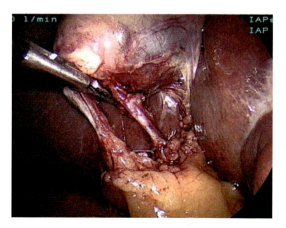

Fig. 10.3 Intraoperative demonstration of achieving the critical view of safety. (Adapted from SAGES, Image Category: Gallbladder; Critical View of Safety, 2014. https://www.sages.org/image-category/gallbladder)

parenchyma or bile leak, which occurs due to subvesical ducts coursing through the liver parenchyma deep to the gallbladder fossa, may occur. If bleeding from the liver parenchyma is noted, it may require electrocautery at elevated levels or even an argon laser. Following safe removal, the gallbladder is then placed into a specimen bag and removed from the abdomen. Hemostasis is then ensured, followed by closure of all port sites. The patient is then awakened from anesthesia.

Although the fundamental technique of laparoscopy in acute cholecystitis is the same as in elective cases, the substantial inflammation, gallbladder distention, and hypervascularity make the operation much more difficult. However, the same standards of proper visualization and anatomic definition must be applied in acute cholecystitis. If there is inability to discern anatomy or suspicion for aberrant anatomy exists, IOC may be utilized if the surgeon is comfortable with performing it. Some surgeons may utilize a "dome-down" laparoscopic dissection when substantial inflammation impairs the cystic dissection and isolation. Beginning at the fundus, the gallbladder is circumferentially dissected until the infundibulum and cystic duct conjoin. If not employed routinely, this technique may or may not prove helpful. The cystic duct may also appear thickened and/or foreshortened secondary to acute inflammation. If the duct is too wide for clip application, it must be ensured that it is the cystic duct rather than the common bile duct or aberrant anatomy. This can be achieved by further dissection or IOC. After the cystic duct has been verified, an endoloop or laparoscopic stapler may be utilized. Although these pearls may aid in a successful laparoscopic approach to cholecystectomy, conversion to an open approach may be required in 10–20% of cases. Surgeons should not hesitate to convert to open if anatomy cannot be clearly defined secondary to inflammation or other factors. The risks of a potentially devastating bile duct or vascular injury when persisting laparoscopically far outweigh the mildly increased morbidity of open cholecystectomy.

Intraoperative Cholangiography

The decision to perform IOC may aid in determining biliary anatomy, assessing for an obstructive process including gallstones, and evaluating for a potential biliary injury.

Briefly, the cystic duct approach entails placing a clip across the proximal cystic duct as close as possible to the infundibulum. A ductotomy is then performed leaving adequate length for double clip ligation distally. Prior to utilization, the 5F cholangiocatheter (Reddick, LeMaitre Vascular, Inc) should be flushed with saline to avoid air in the tubing, which if injected, could be misinterpreted as gallstones. The cholangiocatheter is then inserted through an introducer sheath via a separate incision along the right subcostal margin, and the tip is maneuvered through the ductotomy into the cystic duct distal to the ductotomy. The balloon is then inflated securing the catheter and occluding the cystic duct lumen.

An infundibular approach may also be utilized if significant scarring and inflammation of the porta hepatis is present. In this instance, a Kumar clamp may be applied to the infundibulum, and a needle tip cholangiocatheter may be inserted into the side channel. Other techniques include a fundal approach or a direct needle cholangiogram involving the common bile duct when exposed during open conversion.

Following appropriate cholangiocatheter insertion, C-arm fluoroscopy is positioned over the RUQ. A water-soluble contrast (25 cc of low osmolar radiopaque contrast) diluted in normal saline 1:1 is injected, delineating the biliary anatomy. The cystic duct, common bile duct, common hepatic duct, left hepatic ducts, right hepatic ducts, and passage of contrast into the duodenum must be visualized for a sufficient IOC (Fig. 10.4). If a filling defect is noted suggesting the presence of gallstones, glucagon may be administered to minimize contraction of the sphincter of Oddi. Some surgeons recommend a power flush of normal saline to aid in gallstone passage. However, we feel that it can cause reflux into the pancreatic duct and increase the chances of post-IOC pancreatitis. A choledochoscope may also be inserted and

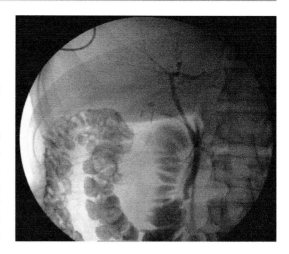

Fig. 10.4 Normal intraoperative cholangiogram. Note the visualization of the entire biliary tree including intrahepatic ducts, common hepatic duct, common bile duct, cystic duct, and contrast passage into the duodenum without filling defect

can provide various therapeutic options if the surgeon feels comfortable.

Open Cholecystectomy

Because laparoscopic cholecystectomy is the standard approach for acute cholecystitis, most open cholecystectomies occur in the setting of conversion, which occurs in up to 20% of cases. There are a number of risk factors, which may contribute to open conversion, including obesity, duration of symptoms, male sex, cirrhosis, and leukocytosis. The primary indication for conversion to open is inability to define relevant biliary or vascular anatomy. Other indications include suspected injury to the biliary tree, vasculature, or bowel, uncontrolled hemorrhage, failure to make sufficient surgical progress, intolerance of pneumoperitoneum, or concern for gallbladder cancer. Only a few conditions mandate open cholecystectomy without attempt at laparoscopy, which will be up to surgeon discretion and preference.

The gallbladder is most easily accessed through an oblique RUQ incision (Kocher), which should be placed two fingerbreadths below the costal margin. Alternatively, an upper midline laparotomy incision can also be used. If a previous attempt at laparoscopy was made, this incision can be made extended through laparoscopic port site incisions. After incising the anterior rectus sheath and dividing the rectus muscle with electrocautery, the superior epigastric vessels can be ligated or cauterized, facilitating abdominal access through the posterior rectus sheath.

Appropriate retraction is the key to the operation. A Bookwalter or other fixed-table retractor should be utilized to elevate the liver, expose the gallbladder, and keep bowel out of the operative field. We prefer a fundus-down approach. The gallbladder fundus is grasped with a Kelly clamp to aid in retraction, and the visceral peritoneum is incised with electrocautery separating the gallbladder from the anterior liver edge. The medial and lateral peritoneal attachments are then opened to aid in mobilization, and electrocautery is used to dissect the gallbladder free from the liver. Once the gallbladder is suspended from its pedicle, a combination of sharp and blunt dissection is performed until the cystic duct and artery are exposed. Simple ligation of the cystic duct and artery is performed with separate silk ties. If the gallbladder neck or cystic duct appears necrotic, a drain should be placed to control a bile leak should it occur.

Bailout Maneuvers

Even the most experienced surgeons will encounter gallbladders that cannot be removed safely. When early difficulty is encountered, the surgeon should consider conversion to an open approach or IOC as previously mentioned. However, if difficulty persists early in the intraoperative course or the patient becomes hemodynamically unstable, cholecystostomy tube placement should be considered as an early bailout maneuver. If there is significant difficulty dissecting the gallbladder wall off of the liver parenchyma, the anterior wall may be excised leaving the posterior wall partially or wholly intact, and the intact remaining mucosa may be cauterized to prevent mucocele formation. This strategy can prevent repeated

injury to the hepatic parenchyma, which could result in bleeding or bile leak.

If cystic structures are unable to be safely dissected and isolated, a subtotal cholecystectomy is preferred. Within recent years, much confusion has been present regarding what a subtotal cholecystectomy entails. Two subtypes of subtotal cholecystectomy have been well described— "fenestrating" and "reconstituting" [25]. A subtotal fenestrating cholecystectomy involves identifying the cystic duct orifice from within the lumen of the gallbladder and oversewing it without leaving a gallbladder remnant, while a subtotal reconstituting cholecystectomy leaves a small gallbladder remnant, which may be closed with suture or a laparoscopic stapler [25]. For a subtotal reconstituting cholecystectomy, all gallstones should be removed if possible to minimize the possibility of future cholelithiasis and cholecystitis episodes in the gallbladder remnant. Although the reconstituting approach results in a decreased incidence of bile fistulae, most fistulas appear to resolve spontaneously in the fenestrating approach [26, 27]. It is our general practice to perform a subtotal reconstituting cholecystectomy. In performing any of these bailout maneuvers, a closed suction drain should be placed to control the potential bile leak (Figs. 10.5 and 10.6).

Intraoperative and Postoperative Complications

Cholecystectomy for acute cholecystitis in the emergent/urgent setting is generally more difficult than elective cholecystectomy. Major bile duct injury is the most feared and morbid complication of cholecystectomy causing bile leak. If there is concern for an intraoperative bile duct injury, early recognition is key. The technical aspects of repair are well described in the literature [28–30]. However, if the surgeon recognizes such an injury and does not feel comfortable with repair, appropriate drainage and transfer to a center with hepatobiliary expertise can help decrease morbidity and improve patient outcomes.

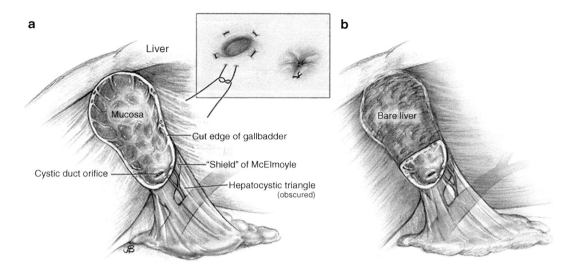

Fig. 10.5 Subtotal fenestrating cholecystectomy. The anterior peritonealized portion of the gallbladder is excised. The cystic duct is closed from the inside of the gallbladder lumen with a purse-string suture (inset). The posterior wall with mucosa (**a**) may be left intact but should be ablated. Further gallbladder wall excision may occur leaving only the lowest portion of the gallbladder wall remaining (**b**). (From Strasberg et al. [25])

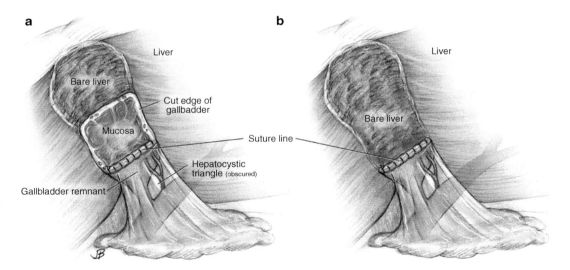

Fig. 10.6 Subtotal reconstituting cholecystectomy. The anterior peritonealized portion of the gallbladder wall is excised. The lowest portion of the gallbladder wall is closed with either suture or staples. The posterior wall with mucosa (**a**) may be left intact above the closure site, but should be ablated. Further wall excision may occur leaving only the lowest portion of the gallbladder wall remaining (**b**). (From Strasberg et al. [25])

The majority of postoperative bile leaks are secondary to cystic duct leakage or small subvesicular ducts. When cystic dissection and ligation are overly difficult, the gallbladder is extremely adherent to the liver, cystic tissue quality is poor, or a bailout method is utilized, suspicion should be higher for postoperative bile leak. A closed suction drain should be placed, as bile leaks may not necessarily be detected intraoperatively. If a low-volume bile leak is detected postoperatively, it will typically resolve with drainage alone. However, if a high-volume leak is detected, further evaluation with endoscopic retrograde cholangiopancreatography (ERCP) with sphincterotomy and stent placement is usually therapeutic. This may reduce the volume of bile leakage into the abdomen and decrease time to bile leak resolution. If no leak is detected postoperatively, the drain may be removed at the time of discharge.

Medical Management

All patients diagnosed with acute cholecystitis should receive appropriate antibiotic therapy, as it is the cornerstone of medical management [21, 31]. In general, select patient groups, including those with mild acute cholecystitis in the setting of moderate to severe comorbidities, may be treated conservatively [21]. However, in recent years, some controversy exists as studies suggest that antibiotics may not necessarily be indicated for conservative management or those scheduled for cholecystectomy [32]; however, this is not our institution's current practice. Antibiotic strategies vary in the literature and depend on community-acquired versus healthcare-associated etiologies, but focus on providing coverage for gram-negative (*Escherichia coli*, *Enterobacter* spp., *Klebsiella* spp.) and anaerobic (*Bacteroides* spp. and *Clostridium* spp.) bacteria. For patients who undergo cholecystectomy with adequate source control, antibiotics may be discontinued within 24 h. If source control is not achieved, an extended antibiotic duration may be warranted. If patients fail to improve within 72 h of initiation of medical

management, we strongly recommend consideration of surgical or alternative approaches.

Cholecystostomy

Cholecystostomy placement may be considered in patients who fail medical therapy, are high-risk for general anesthesia, such as those in the ICU or with extensive cardiopulmonary disease, or have severe acute cholecystitis with local complications. In these circumstances, an operation would be associated with increased morbidity, mortality, and high rates of open conversion. The advantage of cholecystostomy includes immediate biliary decompression and results in successful resolution of symptoms in approximately 90% of cases [33]. Further, cholecystostomy tubes can be placed percutaneously under ultrasound guidance with minimal to light sedation. Cholecystostomy can be a viable intraoperative bailout as well. Overall, it is associated with a low rate of serious complications but high rates of tube dysfunction (45%) and re-intervention (28%) [34].

After resolution of symptoms, cholecystography may be performed, which is typically 4–6 weeks following the episode. If contrast freely flows into the duodenum, a patent cystic duct and common bile duct are present, and the tube may be clamped and subsequently removed. However, if the cystic duct is not patent, the tube should remain in place until surgery.

Some studies demonstrate a wide range of recurrent biliary events following cholecystostomy, reporting 7–55% [33–35]. However, interval cholecystectomy appears to be associated with a decreased likelihood of recurrent biliary complications and increased successful laparoscopic completion of cholecystectomy [34]. Although this decision is based on patient age, functional status, comorbidities, and overall risk, we generally favor interval cholecystectomy when the patient is deemed an operable candidate. However, we recognize that cholecystostomy may be a terminal procedure in select patients.

Endoscopic Therapy

Within recent years, endoscopic gallbladder drainage (EGBD) has evolved as an alternative gallbladder drainage technique to percutaneous cholecystostomy. EGBD can be performed by two approaches, including transpapillary and transmural.

The transpapillary approach utilizes ERCP to facilitate gallbladder drainage via the cystic duct with plastic pigtail stents or a nasobiliary catheter across the papillae. Adequate drainage is achieved in 83–91% of cases and is as effective as percutaneous drainage [36, 37]. As with ERCP approaches, post-procedural pancreatitis and bleeding may occur following sphincter cannulation and sphincterotomy.

The transmural approach utilizes endoscopic ultrasound (EUS) to access the gallbladder through the gastric antrum or duodenum. Following puncture and tract dilation, a stent is then positioned with the proximal end in the gallbladder lumen and the distal end in the gastrointestinal lumen. EUS-guided approaches have higher technical success rates than ERCP approaches with success achieved in over 95% of cases [38].

Overall, endoscopic approaches show similar technical success to percutaneous methods and may appear to be a safer approach to inoperable patients with acute cholecystitis [38].

Postoperative Management

For patients who undergo uncomplicated cholecystectomy for acute cholecystitis, most are able to return home within 24 h. Regular diet may be resumed immediately and oral pain medications may provide sufficient analgesia. Antibiotics are not indicated beyond the immediate postoperative period if adequate source control was obtained.

Postoperative fever, abdominal pain, or jaundice should warrant further evaluation, and bile leak, bile injury, or a retained stone should be suspected. US should be the initial study of choice, and the presence of postoperative fluid collections and/or biliary tree dilation should be assessed. Postoperative fluid collections could represent biloma, hematoma, or abscess. US- or CT-guided aspiration or drain placement will help differentiate these and can provide adequate drainage. If biloma is suspected, ERCP with sphincterotomy and stent placement will help control bile flow into the biliary tree. If biliary dilatation is present, it may represent a retained common bile duct stone or bile duct injury causing obstruction. In these cases, ERCP should also be utilized for evaluation, and interventions such as stone extraction or stent placement may be performed.

Multi-specialty Management Protocols

Patients with biliary diseases such as cholelithiasis, cholecystitis, choledocholithiasis, and gallstone pancreatitis are often managed by physicians from very different backgrounds. Either the initial care or the treatment of complications may include physicians from emergency medicine, internal medicine, critical care, gastroenterology, radiology, and surgery. This can lead to a wide variability in ordering of diagnostic tests, timing of interventions, and other key decisions. In our experience, development of evidence-based consensus protocols can streamline the delivery of care, minimize conflicts, and optimize the use of institutional resources. The University of Michigan protocol is freely available, and it can be modified as needed to fit the needs of different institutions [39, 40].

References

1. Shaffer EA. Epidemiology and risk factors for gallstone disease: has the paradigm changed in the 21st century? Curr Gastroenterol Rep. 2005;7(2):132–40.
2. Stinton LM, Shaffer EA. Epidemiology of gallbladder disease: cholelithiasis and cancer. Gut Liver. 2012;6(2):172–87.

3. Tazuma S. Gallstone disease: epidemiology, pathogenesis, and classification of biliary stones (common bile duct and intrahepatic). Best Pract Res Clin Gastroenterol. 2006;20(6):1075–83.
4. McSherry CK, Ferstenberg H, Calhoun WF, Lahman E, Virshup M. The natural history of diagnosed gallstone disease in symptomatic and asymptomatic patients. Ann Surg. 1985;202(1):59–63.
5. Gracie WA, Ransohoff DF. The natural history of silent gallstones: the innocent gallstone is not a myth. N Engl J Med. 1982;307(13):798–800.
6. Carter HR, Cox RL, Polk HC Jr. Operative therapy for cholecystitis and cholelithiasis: trends over three decades. Am Surg. 1987;53(10):565–8.
7. Strasberg SM. Acute calculous cholecystitis. N Engl J Med. 2008;358(26):2804–11.
8. Gomes CA, Junior CS, Di Saveiro S, Sartelli M, Kelly MD, Gomes CC, et al. Acute calculous cholecystitis: review of current best practices. World J Gastrointest Surg. 2017;9(5):118–26.
9. den Hoed PT, Boelhouwer RU, Veen HF, Hop WC, Bruining HA. Infections and bacteriological data after laparoscopic and open gallbladder surgery. J Hosp Infect. 1998;39(1):27–37.
10. Reinders JS, Kortram K, Vlaminckx B, van Ramshorst B, Gouma DJ, Boerma D. Incidence of bactobilia increases over time after endoscopic sphincterotomy. Dig Surg. 2011;28(4):288–92.
11. Kiewiet JJ, Leeuwenburgh MM, Bipat S, Bossuyt PM, Stoker J, Boermeester MA. A systematic review and meta-analysis of diagnostic performance of imaging in acute cholecystitis. Radiology. 2012;264(3):708–20.
12. Pinto A, Reginelli A, Cagini L, Coppolino F, Stabile Ianora AA, Bracale R, et al. Accuracy of ultrasonography in the diagnosis of acute calculous cholecystitis: review of the literature. Crit Ultrasound J. 2013;5(Suppl 1):S11.
13. Harvey RT, Miller WT Jr. Acute biliary disease: initial CT and follow-up US versus initial US and follow-up CT. Radiology. 1999;213(3):831–6.
14. Fidler J, Paulson EK, Layfield L. CT evaluation of acute cholecystitis: findings and usefulness in diagnosis. AJR Am J Roentgenol. 1996;166(5):1085–8.
15. Chang JH, Lee IS, Lim YS, Jung SH, Paik CN, Kim HK, et al. Role of magnetic resonance cholangiopancreatography for choledocholithiasis: analysis of patients with negative MRCP. Scand J Gastroenterol. 2012;47(2):217–24.
16. Yarmish GM, Smith MP, Rosen MP, Baker ME, Blake MA, Cash BD, Hindman NM, Kamel IR, Kaur H, Nelson RC, Piorkowski RJ, Qayyum A, Tulchinsky M. ACR appropriateness criteria® right upper quadrant pain. Available at https://acsearch.acr.org/docs/69474/Narrative/. American College of Radiology. Accessed 5 Dec 2017.
17. Fagan SP, Awad SS, Rahwan K, Hira K, Aoki N, Itani KM, et al. Prognostic factors for the development of gangrenous cholecystitis. Am J Surg. 2003;186(5):481–5.
18. Nikfarjam M, Niumsawatt V, Sethu A, Fink MA, Muralidharan V, Starkey G, et al. Outcomes of contemporary management of gangrenous and nongangrenous acute cholecystitis. HPB Off J Int Hepato Pancreato Biliary Assoc. 2011;13(8):551–8.
19. Aydin C, Altaca G, Berber I, Tekin K, Kara M, Titiz I. Prognostic parameters for the prediction of acute gangrenous cholecystitis. J Hepato-Biliary-Pancreat Surg. 2006;13(2):155–9.
20. Takada T, Yasuda H, Uchiyama K, Hasegawa H, Asagoe T, Shikata J. Pericholecystic abscess: classification of US findings to determine the proper therapy. Radiology. 1989;172(3):693–7.
21. Miura F, Okamoto K, Takada T, Strasberg SM, Asbun HJ, Pitt HA, et al. Tokyo guidelines 2018: initial management of acute biliary infection and flowchart for acute cholangitis. J Hepatobiliary Pancreat Sci. 2018;25(1):31–40. https://doi.org/10.1002/jhbp.509. Epub 2018 Jan 8.
22. Gutt CN, Encke J, Koninger J, Harnoss JC, Weigand K, Kipfmuller K, et al. Acute cholecystitis: early versus delayed cholecystectomy, a multicenter randomized trial (ACDC study, NCT00447304). Ann Surg. 2013;258(3):385–93.
23. Roulin D, Saadi A, Di Mare L, Demartines N, Halkic N. Early versus delayed cholecystectomy for acute cholecystitis, are the 72 hours still the rule?: a randomized trial. Ann Surg. 2016;264(5):717–22.
24. Terho PM, Leppaniemi AK, Mentula PJ. Laparoscopic cholecystectomy for acute calculous cholecystitis: a retrospective study assessing risk factors for conversion and complications. World J Emerg Surg. 2016;11:54.
25. Strasberg SM, Pucci MJ, Brunt LM, Deziel DJ. Subtotal cholecystectomy-"fenestrating" vs "reconstituting" subtypes and the prevention of bile duct injury: definition of the optimal procedure in difficult operative conditions. J Am Coll Surg. 2016;222(1):89–96.
26. Henneman D, da Costa DW, Vrouenraets BC, van Wagensveld BA, Lagarde SM. Laparoscopic partial cholecystectomy for the difficult gallbladder: a systematic review. Surg Endosc. 2013;27(2):351–8.
27. Elshaer M, Gravante G, Thomas K, Sorge R, Al-Hamali S, Ebdewi H. Subtotal cholecystectomy for "difficult gallbladders": systematic review and meta-analysis. JAMA Surg. 2015;150(2):159–68.
28. Kaman L, Behera A, Singh R, Katariya RN. Management of major bile duct injuries after laparoscopic cholecystectomy. Surg Endosc. 2004;18(8):1196–9.
29. Mercado MA, Chan C, Salgado-Nesme N, Lopez-Rosales F. Intrahepatic repair of bile duct injuries. A comparative study. J Gastrointest Surg Off J Soc Surge Aliment Tract. 2008;12(2):364–8.
30. Winslow ER, Fialkowski EA, Linehan DC, Hawkins WG, Picus DD, Strasberg SM. "sideways": results of repair of biliary injuries using a policy of side-to-side hepatico-jejunostomy. Ann Surg. 2009;249(3):426–34.

31. Galili O, Eldar S Jr, Matter I, Madi H, Brodsky A, Galis I, et al. The effect of bactibilia on the course and outcome of laparoscopic cholecystectomy. Eur J Clin Microbiol Infect Dis Off Publ Eur Soc Clin Microbiol. 2008;27(9):797–803.

32. van Dijk AH, de Reuver PR, Tasma TN, van Dieren S, Hugh TJ, Boermeester MA. Systematic review of antibiotic treatment for acute calculous cholecystitis. Br J Surg. 2016;103(7):797–811.

33. Yeo CS, Tay VW, Low JK, Woon WW, Punamiya SJ, Shelat VG. Outcomes of percutaneous cholecystostomy and predictors of eventual cholecystectomy. J Hepatobiliary Pancreat Sci. 2016;23(1):65–73.

34. Alvino DML, Fong ZV, McCarthy CJ, Velmahos G, Lillemoe KD, Mueller PR, et al. Long-term outcomes following percutaneous cholecystostomy tube placement for treatment of acute calculous cholecystitis. J Gastrointest Surg Off J Soc Surg Aliment Tract. 2017;21(5):761–9.

35. Zarour S, Imam A, Kouniavsky G, Lin G, Zbar A, Mavor E. Percutaneous cholecystostomy in the management of high-risk patients presenting with acute cholecystitis: timing and outcome at a single institution. Am J Surg. 2017;214(3):456–61.

36. Widmer J, Alvarez P, Sharaiha RZ, Gossain S, Kedia P, Sarkaria S, et al. Endoscopic gallbladder drainage for acute cholecystitis. Clin Endosc. 2015;48(5):411–20.

37. Hamada T, Nakai Y, Isayama H, Koike K. Transpapillary versus transmural biliary drainage in patients with an indwelling duodenal stent: when is one indicated over the other? Gastrointest Endosc. 2013;77(4):670.

38. Khan MA, Atiq O, Kubiliun N, Ali B, Kamal F, Nollan R, et al. Efficacy and safety of endoscopic gallbladder drainage in acute cholecystitis: is it better than percutaneous gallbladder drainage? Gastrointest Endosc. 2017;85(1):76–87.e3.

39. Demehri FR, Alam HB. Evidence-based management of common gallstone-related emergencies. J Intensive Care Med. 2016;31(1):3–13.

40. Demehri FR, Alam HB. Evaluation and management of gallstone-related diseases in non-pregnant adults. Care. UoMGfIC. Available from http://www.med.umich.edu/1info/FHP/practiceguides/gallstone/Gallstonefinal.pdf. Accessed 5 Dec 2017.

41. Yokoe M, Takada T, Strasberg SM, Solomkin JS, Mayumi T, Gomi H, et al. Diagnostic criteria and severity assessment of acute cholecystitis in revised Tokyo Guidelines. J Hepatobiliary Pancreat Sci. 2012;19:578–86.

Choledocholithiasis

11

Morgan Schellenberg and Meghan Lewis

Epidemiology

The presence of gallstones in the common bile duct, termed choledocholithiasis, is a significant cause of surgical disease that affects millions of people worldwide. The incidence cannot be precisely determined, because it is not always symptomatic. However, symptomatic cholelithasis affects between 10% and 15% of the adult population in developed countries [1], and up to 25% of these patients are also found to have choledocholithiasis at the time of cholecystectomy [2]. The prevalence of choledocholithiasis has been rising with life expectancy. Its global burden is therefore increasing, with annual medical expenses exceeding $2.2 billion USD [2]. Morbidity and mortality from choledocholithiasis result from the many associated complications. These are classified as acute or chronic, either of which can be life-threatening.

Pathophysiology

The pathogenesis of choledocholithiasis is dependent on the type of stone. Primary bile duct stones form in the bile ducts, while secondary bile duct stones form in the gallbladder and are subsequently released into the biliary system.

Primary bile duct stones are usually brown or black pigment stones. These form from bacterial infection: hydrolysis of glucuronic acid from bilirubin occurs by bacterial beta-glucuronidase. This results in a decreased solubility of deconjugated bilirubin and the formation of stones. Brown pigment stones are, consequently, composed of calcium salts of unconjugated bilirubin, deconjugated bile acids, and varying amounts of cholesterol and saturated long-chain fatty acids.

Secondary bile duct stones are of mixed composition but are composed largely of cholesterol in the majority of cases. The minority of secondary bile duct stones are pigmented, also referred to as black pigment stones, and are composed primarily of bilirubin due to hemolytic disease.

Risk factors for choledocholithiasis include male sex (ratio of 1.2:0.9) and increasing age, with the average age of diagnosis being 67 years [2]. In addition, conditions leading to bile stasis, inflammation, and infection predispose to stone formation. Examples include biliary anatomic abnormalities, primary and secondary sclerosing cholangitis, parasites, or cholecystectomy at a young age, leading to common bile duct dilation.

M. Schellenberg
Division of Trauma and Surgical Critical Care, LAC+USC Medical Center, Los Angeles, CA, USA

M. Lewis (✉)
Division of Trauma and Surgical Critical Care, LAC+USC Medical Center, University of Southern California, Los Angeles, CA, USA
e-mail: Meghan.lewis@med.usc.edu

© Springer International Publishing AG, part of Springer Nature 2019
C. V. R. Brown et al. (eds.), *Emergency General Surgery*, https://doi.org/10.1007/978-3-319-96286-3_11

Dietary risk factors, such as malnutrition, and genetic risk factors have also been implicated.

Ethnic differences have also been observed. Secondary bile duct stones are more common in Native Americans and Hispanic populations than in Caucasians and are less common in African Americans. In addition, secondary bile duct stones predominate in Western countries and Japan, while primary bile stones occur more frequently in Southeast Asia.

Diagnosis

The first step in securing a diagnosis of choledocholithiasis is performing an appropriate history and physical examination. A proper history should take into consideration the known risk factors for biliary tract disease. Though cholelithiasis is more common in females, choledocholithiasis is more prevalent in males. Specific risk factors for choledocholithiasis include patients with known choledochal cysts and those with recurrent biliary tract inflammation (e.g., primary sclerosing cholangitis) or infection (which occurs most frequently among East Asian populations).

Choledocholithiasis should be suspected in patients with right upper quadrant pain, nausea, emesis, and signs or symptoms of cholestasis, such as acholic stools, dark urine, pruritus, jaundice, and scleral icterus. However, jaundice and scleral icterus are not generally observed until the serum bilirubin has risen to approximately 2.5 mg/dL. Therefore, these presenting symptoms are less common than may be expected. Patients with choledocholithiasis typically report an antecedent history of biliary colic, characterized by postprandial right upper quadrant pain that is precipitated by large or fatty meals. Less commonly, choledocholithiasis may be asymptomatic and found incidentally on imaging.

On physical examination, a general inspection of the patient can be informative. An obese body habitus is more suspicious for biliary tract disease. The eyes and skin should be inspected for icterus and jaundice, respectively. Vital signs are essential for differentiating choledocholithiasis from ascending cholangitis; fever and tachycardia favor the latter. Examination of the abdomen in choledocholithiasis typically reveals localized right upper quadrant or epigastric tenderness. Murphy's sign, the classic examination finding in acute cholecystitis, is generally absent in choledocholithiasis. If a patient's history and physical examination raise concern for choledocholithiasis, the clinician should proceed to laboratory investigations.

Laboratory Values

The laboratory findings most suggestive of choledocholithiasis include elevated cholestatic markers: hyperbilirubinemia, elevated alkaline phosphatase (ALP), and elevated gamma-glutamyl transpeptidase (GGT). A mild leukocytosis and transaminitis may also occur; however, a markedly elevated white blood cell count with a clinical picture suggestive of choledocholithiasis raises concern for the diagnosis of ascending cholangitis. Similarly, more than a moderate rise in transaminases (>800) is suspicious for alternate diagnoses, including viral hepatitis.

Bilirubin is typically elevated to a mean of 1.5–1.9 mg/dL [3, 4]. Bilirubin may be more useful than ALP in predicting choledocholithiasis, because bilirubin typically rises within hours of biliary obstruction. ALP, on the other hand, takes longer to rise because its synthesis from the biliary epithelium must be induced by the presence of cholestasis. ALP has also been shown to be less sensitive (57% vs. 69%) and less specific (86% vs. 88%) than bilirubin in the diagnosis of choledocholithiasis [5]. However, an elevated ALP is a more common finding than an elevated bilirubin among patients with choledocholithiasis (80% vs 60%) [6].

Non-cholestatic sources of ALP also exist, including bone and placenta. For this reason, measuring serum GGT can be useful to confirm a cholestatic source when a patient's ALP is elevated. A recently published study demonstrated that a GGT $\geq$ 300 units/L on admission was one of the most predictive factors of choledocholithiasis unlikely to resolve spontaneously [7].

In practice, transaminases, bilirubin, and ALP are routinely obtained at admission for all patients with suspected biliary tract disease. GGT, conversely, is ordered more selectively, in cases where there is clinical suspicion for extra-biliary sources of elevated ALP. All laboratory values are then used in conjunction with the clinical presentation to determine the need for imaging and to guide further decision-making.

Imaging

A variety of imaging modalities are available to assess the bile ducts for choledocholithiasis. Common options are transabdominal ultrasonography and various forms of cholangiography, including endoscopic retrograde cholangiopancreatography (ERCP), magnetic resonance cholangiopancreatography (MRCP), and intraoperative cholangiogram (IOC). Less frequently utilized modalities include CT cholangiography (CTC), endoscopic ultrasonography (EUS), intraductal ultrasonography (IDUS), and percutaneous transhepatic cholangiography (PTC).

Transabdominal ultrasound (US) is an excellent modality for assessment of the biliary tree and should be the first investigation performed in all patients with suspected biliary tract pathology. It is relatively inexpensive, widely available, and noninvasive. Its main disadvantage is operator dependency. US is especially useful in suspected choledocholithiasis, as visualization of a stone in the common bile duct (CBD) on ultrasound is the strongest predictor of choledocholithiasis confirmed on ERCP or surgically [5, 8, 9], with a specificity of 1.00 [5] (Fig. 11.1). Patients with a stone in the CBD demonstrated on US have such a high probability of having a final diagnosis of choledocholithiasis that no confirmatory test is required, and the patient can proceed directly to stone extraction [8]. A dilated (>6 mm) CBD on US is also a strong predictor of choledocholithiasis [8]. However, it is not considered diagnostic. For this reason, an additional confirmatory test in these patients may be indicated prior to proceeding with invasive attempts at stone extraction.

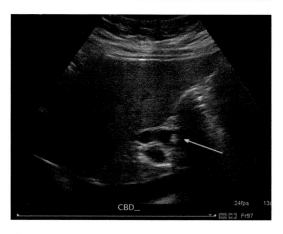

Fig. 11.1 Ultrasound of the right upper quadrant with evidence of choledocholithiasis (arrow)

In contrast to the high specificity of US at detecting stones in the CBD, the sensitivity of US for choledocholithiasis is less than 60% in most studies [10]. Therefore, patients with clinical or laboratory evidence of biliary stasis but nondiagnostic ultrasonography benefit from confirmatory testing.

Confirmatory testing is accomplished with cholangiography, which is available in several modalities. ERCP has long been regarded as the gold standard for diagnosis of choledocholithiasis; however, it is also the most invasive form of cholangiography. It is performed with a sideviewing duodenoscope, with cannulation of the ampulla and injection of contrast into the biliary and pancreatic ducts. It is a very useful technique because it allows for stone extraction and therefore can be therapeutic in addition to diagnostic. However, its high-risk profile, significant-associated costs, and requirement for skilled personnel have relegated the primary role of ERCP to stone extraction if alternative diagnostic tests are available.

MRCP is a favored diagnostic modality by many centers because it is noninvasive and it does not require a physician to be present. MRCP is an MRI performed of enhanced T2-weighted sequences, emphasizing stationary fluid in the biliary and pancreatic ducts. It therefore does not require administration of contrast material. MRCP has a sensitivity of 83–92% and specificity of 91–97% [11–13], making it a very useful confirmatory test. Its main weakness is its inability to reliably detect small (<6 mm) stones [8]. It is also not available at all centers, and has several relative and absolute contraindications. Patients with surgical clips or air in the biliary system from bilioenteric anastomoses may have inconclusive results, and patients with implanted metal, pacemakers, or claustrophobia may not be able to safely undergo the examination.

IOC at the time of laparoscopic cholecystectomy is another viable option to interrogate the CBD for stones. IOC has a sensitivity of 97% and specificity of 95–100% [11, 14], making it an excellent test to rule in or out suspected choledocholithiasis. Major society guidelines recommend either IOC or MRCP as the diagnostic test of choice for patients with intermediate risk of choledocholithiasis [8]. In most centers, resource and personnel availability are the deciding factors between these two modalities. However, the available evidence suggests that IOC is more sensitive, specific, and cost-effective than MRCP [11]. Barriers to its use include added operative time (approximately 10–20 min) and the requirement by some states for a fluoroscopy license to perform IOC. In addition, the management of stones discovered at IOC can often be challenging.

Less common modalities for diagnosis of choledocholithiasis include CTC, EUS, IDUS, and PTC. CTC involves the administration of either oral or IV contrast agents and is a helical CT scan with 3D reconstructions. It has been used successfully in Europe for many years. Despite good results, it has not gained widespread use in North America, largely because of concerns about the safety of the contrast agents. The contrast agents have been associated with nausea and vomiting, hepatorenal toxicity, hypotension, cardiopulmonary symptoms, severe skin reactions, anaphylaxis, and, rarely, death. An additional limitation of CTC is that insufficient opacification of the bile ducts may occur in cases of hyperbilirubinemia or liver insufficiency. Finally, it exposes patients to a high level of radiation. CTC does have the benefits of operator independence, low level of invasiveness, and low technical failure rate. It may be especially useful in locations that lack an MRI scanner.

EUS has a sensitivity of 93–97% and specificity of 94–95% for diagnosing choledocholithiasis [10, 15]. It is performed transgastrically or transduodenally. Its advantage over other modalities is its ability to reliably detect very small stones. However, it is invasive, requires skilled personnel, and is not widely available, all of which are factors limiting its routine use. It is most frequently utilized to evaluate idiopathic pancreatitis for occult stones or to evaluate common bile duct dilatation prior to possible ERCP.

Similar to EUS, IDUS is an invasive form of ultrasonography that can be performed at the time of ERCP. It is performed with a thin probe, inserted through the working channel of a duodenoscope. IDUS is a relatively new technology and is not available at many centers. It is the most sensitive form of ultrasonography for detection of small stones and sludge. IDUS has been successfully utilized after ERCP to confirm duct clearance and prevent subsequent recurrence of choledocholithiasis.

Similar to ERCP, PTC is a more invasive form of cholangiography which allows for possible stone extraction. The liver is punctured percutaneously under fluoroscopic guidance, and contrast is injected into the intrahepatic biliary ductal system. PTC is more successful in patients with dilated biliary ducts. Like ERCP, PTC is used primarily for stone extraction and not for diagnosis of choledocholithiasis, unless other less invasive methods have failed or are unavailable. Additionally, ERCP has been demonstrated to be superior to PTC in terms of complication and success rates, so PTC is generally reserved for situations when ERCP is unsuccessful or not possible, such as in altered biliary anatomy.

Although national society guidelines recommend that the choice of confirmatory test be made according to both cost and local expertise [8], in-depth analyses of cost-effectiveness of these strategies are limited. Therefore, the decision-making in most centers is guided by resource availability. Ultimately, patients with choledocholithiasis demonstrated on any of the above modalities require stone extraction by one of several methods.

Management

After the diagnosis of choledocholithiasis has been secured, there are a number of management decisions that follow. These include the administration of antibiotics, the method of stone retrieval, and the timing of cholecystectomy.

Antibiotics for Choledocholithiasis

The use of routine antibiotics in choledocholithiasis as prophylaxis against cholangitis is not well studied and remains controversial. Antibiotics are clearly indicated for patients with cholangitis. Most clinicians would also consider initiating antibiotics for patients with choledocholithiasis who present with fever or leukocytosis, despite not meeting all diagnostic criteria for cholangitis. At our center, we administer antibiotics to patients with choledocholithiasis for prophylaxis against cholangitis if the patient is febrile ($\geq$38.5 C) or has a marked leukocytosis (generally $\geq$15,000). We also consider antibiotic proxphylaxis for patients with certain high-risk comorbidities, including diabetes mellitus and immunosuppression.

In selecting an appropriate antibiotic, the clinician must factor in both the typical causative agents as well as the local antibiogram. Blood cultures should be sent on all patients with concern for cholangitis. Biliary samples taken during ERCP or CBDE should also be collected. A positive biliary culture can be expected in most patients with cholangitis (93% in one study), but blood cultures are infrequently positive (26%) [16]. The most common agent isolated from biliary cultures is *E. coli*, followed by *Enterococcus* species, *Klebsiella pneumoniae*, and *Pseudomonas aeruginosa* [16]. Appropriate regimens include a third-generation cephalosporin, penicillin derivative, or fluoroquinolone, with no need for routine anaerobic coverage unless the patient has had a previous bilioenteric anastomosis [17]. At our institution, we commonly use ceftriaxone as the empiric agent of choice and subsequently tailor therapy according to culture results.

Method of Stone Retrieval

The options for stone retrieval include ERCP, either preoperatively or postoperatively, PTC, and CBD exploration (CBDE), performed either open or laparoscopically. Practically, the method selected must take into account patient factors, local expertise and equipment, cost, and the available evidence on successful stone clearance rates for each method.

ERCP

ERCP is considered by most to be the standard approach to stone retrieval for cases of choledocholithiasis. In ERCP, an experienced endoscopist passes a side-viewing endoscope through the mouth and upper GI tract until the second stage of the duodenum is encountered. The ampulla of Vater is cannulated through the sphincter of Oddi in order to gain access to the biliary tree. A cholangiogram is then obtained, and the presence of choledocholithiasis is established or confirmed, depending on the extent of the pre-procedure investigations. Next, deep cannulation of the biliary tree and attempts at stone removal are performed, using baskets and/or extraction balloons to sweep stones antegrade into the duodenum. After stone removal, a sphincterotomy is typically performed, using electrocautery to cut through the sphincter of Oddi to widen it and facilitate passage of stones.

Due to concern for long-term complications after sphincterotomy, papillary balloon dilation of the sphincter was developed as an alternative to sphincterotomy. It is a common practice in Asia but is infrequently used in North America [18]. Available high-quality evidence comparing sphincterotomy to balloon dilation is limited, although one RCT and a subsequent study with 6.5 years of follow-up data showed significantly more post-ERCP pancreatitis but fewer long-term complications among patients who underwent balloon dilation as compared to sphincterotomy [19, 20]. In the absence of further evidence in support of balloon dilation, most consider sphincterotomy to be the standard approach. If stone extraction cannot be accomplished before sphincterotomy or balloon dilation, management of the sphincter can precede stone extraction and may facilitate stone removal.

Laser lithotripsy for choledocholithiasis involves the application of a laser to a stone in the biliary tree, which aids in its removal by fragmenting it. It can be accomplished during a standard ERCP through the endoscope, and it is an especially helpful adjunct for extracting large stones after removal attempts with conventional methods have failed. It is successful in approximately 90% of cases [21]. However, high costs limit the widespread use of this technology.

The success rates of ERCP depend upon the size of the stone, with success rates of roughly 85% in stones <2 cm and 60% in stones >2 cm [22]. ERCP also requires an experienced endoscopist and the availability of fluoroscopy. Additionally, the use of ERCP is limited to patients with appropriate anatomy. Patients who have undergone previous gastric bypass with either Billroth II or Roux-en-Y reconstruction typically cannot undergo conventional ERCP. After Billroth II, ERCP can be attempted through the mouth but requires the endoscopist to pass the scope through the gastrojejunostomy and retrograde up into the duodenum, which is technically challenging and can be a prohibitively long route for the endoscope. In patients with a previous Roux-en-Y gastric bypass, ERCP cannot be performed through the mouth because of the distance that must be traversed through the reconstructed GI tract to access the duodenum. These patients can undergo laparoscopic-assisted ERCP, in which a surgeon accesses the gastric remnant laparoscopically and passes the endoscope into it, from which point a relatively conventional ERCP can ensue. Post-gastric bypass patients

frequently require operative management of their choledocholithiasis due to their anatomic reconfigurations.

Although ERCP is a preferred method of stone extraction, it carries well-described risks which must be considered. There is 5% risk of post-ERCP pancreatitis and a 2% risk of bleeding after a sphincterotomy [23]. There is also a risk of duodenal perforation, either from the endoscopy or sphincterotomy. Post-ERCP perforation may require operative intervention and can be fatal in rare cases. Patients must therefore be appropriately consented for the procedure.

ERCP is typically performed preoperatively and followed by cholecystectomy at the same hospital admission. Preoperative timing was historically preferred due to concerns about cystic duct stump leak induced by postoperative ERCP [24]. More recent evidence suggests that postoperative ERCP is safe and does not increase the rate of cystic duct stump leaks [25]; therefore, laparoscopic cholecystectomy followed by postoperative ERCP is an option for choledocholithiasis. However, there is also evidence that this approach increases hospital length of stay, costs, and healthcare utilization [25], making it potentially not the preferred management strategy. Instead, postoperative ERCP may be better reserved for instances of retained CBD stones.

Percutaneous Transhepatic Cholangiography (PTC)

As discussed previously, PTC is both diagnostic and therapeutic in the management of choledocholithiasis. After percutaneous transhepatic cannulation of the biliary tree, many of the methods used for stone extraction parallel the techniques used in ERCP. These include balloons, baskets, and laser lithotripsy via the PTC catheter. Although PTC can play an important role in the diagnosis, treatment, and palliation of biliary tract malignancies, its use in choledocholithiasis is generally reserved for stone extraction among patients with anatomy that is unfavorable for extraction with ERCP.

CBDE

When other methods of stone retrieval have failed or are impossible, CBDE is indicated for stone extraction. CBDE can be performed open or laparoscopically. While an open CBDE should be within the skill set of any general surgeon, laparoscopic CBDE may require more advanced training in laparoscopy and/or hepatobiliary surgery.

Laparoscopic CBDE is an attractive management strategy because it can be performed concurrently with laparoscopic cholecystectomy, thereby allowing a one-stage procedure. Prior to performing a CBDE, the surgeon performs laparoscopic dissection of Calot's triangle, identifies the cystic duct, and performs an intraoperative cholangiogram through the cystic duct. If choledocholithiasis is confirmed, the surgeon may flush the duct with normal saline. Often, intravenous glucagon is administered to relax the sphincter of Oddi. If the stone does not clear from the duct with flushing, the surgeon can proceed with a laparoscopic bile duct exploration, convert to an open procedure for common bile duct exploration, or finish the laparoscopic cholecystectomy and proceed with postoperative ERCP, as described above. An important disadvantage of the last option is that unsuccessful postoperative ERCP would then mandate a second operation for common bile duct exploration.

Laparoscopic CBDE can be accomplished by one of two routes: transcystic or transductal. In the transcystic approach, access to the cystic duct is achieved during the intraoperative cholangiogram. Stone extraction is then accomplished by the use of balloons, Fogarty catheters, baskets, or forceps, with or without the aid of a choledochoscope. The transcystic approach is preferred over the transductal approach when feasible, as it allows for shorter operative time and hospital length of stay [26]. However, it is most successful for relatively small stones (<10 mm) that are located distal to the cystic duct/common hepatic duct confluence. If the transductal approach is required, the CBD is identified laparoscopically as described above, and stone extraction proceeds through a choledochotomy. Both transcystic and

transductal laparoscopic CBDE carry a success rate of greater than 90% [27–29].

An open CBDE is typically performed through a right subcostal incision, but can also be approached through an upper midline laparotomy. A Kocher maneuver is performed, and the hepatoduodenal ligament is identified. The peritoneum overlying the portal triad is opened carefully, and the CBD is then distinguished from the proper hepatic artery and the portal vein based on anatomic position (Fig. 11.2a). The CBD is located anteriorly and on the patient's right within the hepatoduodenal ligament, while the proper hepatic artery is located more medially, and the portal vein is posterior. If the anatomy is unclear, a seeker needle can be used prior to suture placement or choledochotomy, with the aspiration of bile confirming the identity of the CBD.

Once the CBD has been identified, a longitudinal choledochotomy, approximately 1.5–2 cm in length, is planned distally on the CBD near the duodenum. Stay sutures are placed at the apices of the planned choledochotomy (Fig. 11.2b). An 11-blade scalpel is then used to begin the choledochotomy, which is completed with Potts scissors (Fig. 11.2c–d). Once the lumen of the CBD is accessed, a variety of methods can be employed for stone extraction. The surgeon should begin by flushing normal saline into the bile duct lumen to see if this will allow for stone passage. If it does not, balloon dilators, Fogarty catheters, baskets, forceps, or a choledochoscope can be used to facilitate stone removal (Fig. 11.2e). In cases of impacted stones that cannot be retrieved, a choledochoduodenostomy or Roux-en-Y choledochojejunostomy can be created proximal to the site of impaction to allow for biliary drainage.

After stone extraction, a completion cholangiogram is obtained to confirm biliary tract clearance, and the choledochotomy is closed. Although choledochotomies were classically closed over a T-tube, the contemporary management does not include routine T-tube placement. A recent meta-analysis showed that T-tube placement after laparoscopic CBDE had no effect on the rates of postoperative biliary complications or the need for re-intervention, and therefore the authors argue against the routine use of T-tubes [30].

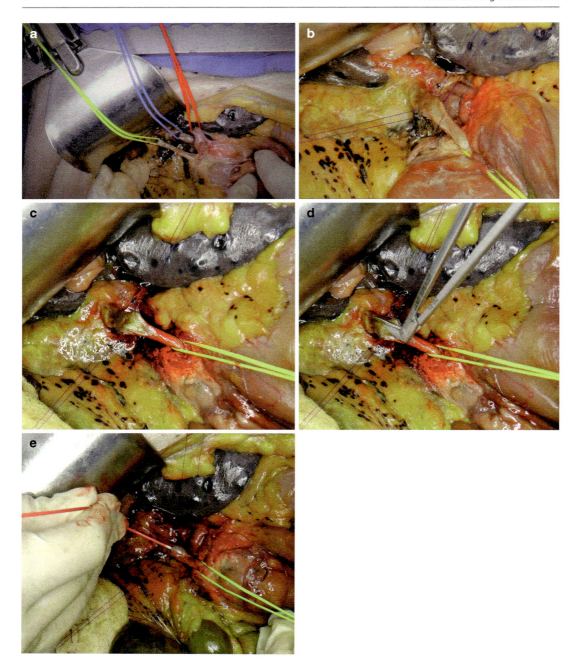

Fig. 11.2 (a–e) Common Bile Duct Exploration. (**a**) After Kocherization, the structures in the portal triad are identified based on anatomical location. Yellow, common bile duct. Red, proper hepatic artery. Blue, portal vein. (**b**) Stay sutures are placed at the 3 o'clock and 9 o'clock positions around the planned choledochotomy. (**c–d**) An 11-blade is used to begin the longitudinal choledochotomy between stay sutures. Potts scissors are used to complete it. (**e**) A Fogarty catheter can be used to attempt stone retrieval through the choledochotomy

Another recent meta-analysis showed that primary duct closure after laparoscopic CBDE resulted in fewer complications, shorter duration of surgery, lower hospital costs, and a shorter postoperative length of stay [31]. The evidence for the role of T-tube placement after open CBDE parallels the literature after laparoscopic CBDE. A Cochrane review of six randomized studies ($n = 359$) showed that T-tube placement after open CBDE resulted in longer operative time and hospital length of stay without any improvement in other clinical outcomes [32]. These authors advocate for future study on the long-term effects of T-tube drainage prior to dismissing the routine use of T-tubes entirely; however in the interim, T-tube drainage should be restricted to RCTs.

After closure of the choledochotomy, the final step in CBDE is to perform a cholecystectomy.

Timing of Cholecystectomy

There are multiple studies, including one large ($n = 266$), multicenter, randomized controlled trial [33], confirming the utility of cholecystectomy at the index admission for complicated biliary tract disease after duct clearance. Although these studies principally evaluated same-admission cholecystectomy after gallstone pancreatitis, the literature is often extrapolated to the patient population with choledocholithiasis due to similarities in pathophysiology. These well-designed studies have demonstrated that index admission cholecystectomy is more cost-effective than delayed elective cholecystectomy [34] and prevents readmission for gallstone-related complications [33, 34]. It is our practice to perform same-admission cholecystectomy for patients with choledocholithiasis after clearing the ducts.

Summary

There are many management options and sequences which can be used to clear the bile

ducts of stones and remove the gallbladder. All methods are relatively effective, with ≥85% rates of successful stone extraction for most stones. Local expertise often dictates the preferred management strategy. Although cost must be considered, available cost data comparing strategies for stone retrieval are limited. One recent study showed that one-stage management with laparoscopic cholecystectomy and transcystic laparoscopic CBDE was the most cost-effective strategy when compared to ERCP and laparoscopic cholecystectomy or laparoscopic cholecystectomy and transductal laparoscopic CBDE [35]. This took into consideration successful CBD clearance, number of procedures required, hospital length of stay, and overall costs. However, the expertise required to effectively and safely perform laparoscopic CBDE significantly limits the widespread implementation of this as the preferred method of stone clearance.

In patients with conventional anatomy (i.e., without previous gastric bypass), the approach preferred in most centers [36], including our own, is for patients with diagnosed choledocholithiasis to undergo preoperative ERCP. If the completion cholangiogram demonstrates duct clearance, it is followed by laparoscopic cholecystectomy at the same hospital admission. We reserve CBDE for patients in whom ERCP is not technically possible. Although postoperative ERCP appears to be a safe alternative, we typically reserve this approach for patients in whom a retained CBD stone is discovered postoperatively.

Complications

Important complications of choledocholithiasis can be either acute, such as ascending cholangitis and gallstone pancreatitis (GSP), or chronic, including biliary stricture formation, intrahepatic stones, recurrent pyogenic cholangitis, hepatic abscesses, secondary biliary cirrhosis, and bile duct carcinomas.

Acute

Ascending Cholangitis

Ascending cholangitis, which can range from mild to life-threatening, is defined as infection of the biliary tree resulting from cholestasis. The clinical presentation of ascending cholangitis is classically described as Charcot's triad: fever, jaundice, and right upper quadrant pain. This constellation of symptoms is observed in up to 75% of patients with ascending cholangitis [37]. Although choledocholithiasis also frequently presents with pain and jaundice, fever is not typically present unless ascending cholangitis is developing. Reynold's pentad describes the presence of all three components of Charcot's triad, and also mental status changes and hypotension, suggesting life-threatening cholangitis.

Although both Charcot's triad and Reynolds' pentad are highly specific for ascending cholangitis, neither is sufficiently sensitive for screening for the diagnosis. The 2013 Tokyo Guidelines therefore set forth criteria for diagnosing ascending cholangitis [38]. The diagnosis of ascending cholangitis should be suspected if fever, shaking chills, or laboratory evidence of inflammation is present, in addition to evidence of cholestasis or imaging suggestive of the diagnosis. Cholestasis is demonstrated by the clinical presence of jaundice or with elevated bilirubin or ALP. Suggestive imaging is qualified in the guidelines as biliary dilatation or the demonstration of a precipitating factor, such as a gallstone or stricture. If fever, shaking chills, or laboratory evidence of inflammation is present in addition to both cholestasis and suggestive imaging, the diagnosis of cholangitis is said to be definite [38].

Management of cholangitis consists of fluid resuscitation, antibiotic therapy, close clinical monitoring, and urgent decompression of the biliary tree.

Gallstone Pancreatitis (GSP)

Gallstones are the most common cause of pancreatitis worldwide, accounting for nearly half of all cases [39]. The pathophysiology of GSP is incompletely understood but involves the tran-

sient passage of stones from the CBD. The proposed mechanisms by which choledocholithiasis induces pancreatitis include bile reflux from partial occlusion of the ampulla and edema of the pancreatic duct induced by the transient presence of the stone.

Gallstone pancreatitis is managed initially with fluid resuscitation, close clinical monitoring, and a brief period of bowel rest. Patients with mild pancreatitis only require bowel rest until the inflammation begins to subside, typically not lasting more than 24–48 h. The resolution is heralded by a decrease in epigastric pain and the downtrending of the white blood cell count or serum lipase. More severe cases of pancreatitis may result in ileus and intolerance of oral nutrition. Enteral nutrition should be initiated in these patients through an nasogastric or nasojejunal feeding tube, with parenteral nutrition reserved only for those patients who cannot tolerate enteral feeding.

Clinicians should maintain a high suspicion for concomitant choledocholithiasis in patients with gallstone pancreatitis, so laboratory biomarkers should be followed serially. Also, once the pancreatitis has resolved, patients should be managed with cholecystectomy at the index hospital admission [40]. This is recommended to prevent recurrence, and the associated morbidity and mortality. For patients who cannot tolerate cholecystectomy, ERCP with sphincterotomy is a suitable alternative [40].

Chronic

Biliary Strictures

Biliary strictures result from the inflammatory response of bile ducts to choledocholithiasis, characterized by collagen deposition, fibrosis, and narrowing of the lumen of the ducts. When strictures become symptomatic, patients present with features of biliary stasis, similar to the typical acute presentation of choledocholithiasis. Although MRCP is an excellent imaging modality for biliary strictures, ERCP has the additional diagnostic advantage of allowing for endoscopic brushings to exclude malignancy, and also the therapeutic advantage of endoscopic interventions, such as dilation of the stricture or placement of a biliary stent. However, symptomatic biliary strictures, even if found to be benign, often require surgery with resection and reconstruction.

Intrahepatic Stones

Intrahepatic stones are found in the hepatic bile ducts. Similar to common bile duct stones, these stones can be primary or secondary. In general, intrahepatic stones will be primary in populations at risk for primary choledocholithiasis and secondary in populations at risk for secondary choledocholithiasis. Intrahepatic stones are also noted to occur at a higher incidence in malnutrition and low socioeconomic class. Intrahepatic stones can be challenging to manage because there is a high rate of recurrence. ERCP and PTC can be used for stone extraction; however, surgical resection of the involved lobe may be required due to high rates of recurrence with stone extraction alone [41].

Recurrent Pyogenic Cholangitis

Recurrent pyogenic cholangitis can develop in patients with intrahepatic stones, wherein the presence of intrahepatic stones causes repeated cycles of inflammation and infection in the intrahepatic bile ducts. It is marked by biliary stricturing and obstruction, leading to recurrent episodes of bacterial cholangitis. It is especially prevalent among people of Southeastern Asian origin. In the acute phases of the disease, when cholangitis is present, the management principles are the same as in ascending cholangitis, with emphasis on fluid resuscitation, early antibiotic therapy, and prompt biliary drainage. Over the long term, these patients require either repeated stone extraction using PTC or ERCP or surgical resection of the involved lobe with reconstruction by hepaticojejunostomy.

Hepatic Abscesses

Infections in the biliary tree related to choledocholithiasis can spread to the liver hematogenously, via the portal vein or hepatic artery, or directly through the biliary system. Both routes of spread can result in pyogenic hepatic abscesses. Patients present with right upper quadrant pain and infectious signs and symptoms. US and CT are the most useful diagnostic modalities and can also be used for image-guided drainage, which in conjunction with antibiotic therapy is the recommended treatment for this complication.

Secondary Biliary Cirrhosis and Portal Hypertension

Secondary biliary cirrhosis develops when repeated episodes of infection and inflammation from biliary stasis and strictures of the bile ducts cause injury to the liver over time, which can progress to cirrhosis. This is an unusual complication of choledocholithiasis but does rarely occur. Secondary biliary cirrhosis carries the same risks and complications as other types of cirrhosis, including the development of portal hypertension. Prompt treatment of choledocholithiasis is recommended to prevent this severe complication. Once cirrhosis occurs, early involvement of a hepatologist is prudent, because liver transplantation may ultimately be necessary.

Bile Duct Carcinomas

Hepatolithiasis, recurrent pyogenic cholangitis, and (to a lesser degree) choledocholithiasis are established risk factors for bile duct carcinomas, likely due to chronic inflammation and repeated mechanical manipulation. Although these patients do not necessarily warrant routine screening for cholangiocarcinoma, a retrospective cohort study of patients with hepatolithiasis showed that age >40, weight loss, elevated ALP (mean 426 u/L), and CEA > 4.2 ng/mL were associated with an increased risk of cholangiocarcinoma [42].

Conclusions

Choledocholithiasis is a common condition whose diagnosis is secured using a combination of clinical history, physical examination, laboratory values, and imaging investigations. US is the initial imaging modality of choice. Patients with US findings that include a stone visualized within the CBD do not require confirmatory imaging and should go directly for stone extraction. Patients with US findings suggestive of choledocholithiasis or laboratory values concerning for cholestasis should undergo MRCP or IOC before attempts at stone extraction. Options for stone extraction include ERCP, PTC, and laparoscopic or open common bile duct exploration, the choice of which depends upon local expertise and cost considerations. Stone extraction should precede same-admission cholecystectomy when feasible. When available, a one-step procedure consisting of laparoscopic transcystic common bile duct exploration and laparoscopic cholecystectomy appears to be the most cost-efficient approach to choledocholithiasis; however, this option may not be widely available.

References

1. Stinton L, Shaffer E. Epidemiology of gallbladder disease: cholelithaisis and cancer. Gut Liver. 2012;6(2):172–87.
2. Krawczyk M, Stoeks C, Lammert F. Genetics and treatment of bile duct stones: new approaches. Curr Opin Gastroenterol. 2013;29(3):329–35.
3. Peng WK, Sheikh Z, Paterson-Brown S, et al. Role of liver function tests in predicting common bile duct stones in patients with acute calculous cholecystitis. Br J Surg. 2005;92:1241–7.
4. Onken JE, Brazer SR, Eisen GM, et al. Predicting the presence of choledocholithiasis in patients with symptomatic cholelithiasis. Am J Gastroenterol. 1996;91:762–7.
5. Abboud PAC, Malet PF, Berlin JA, Staroscik R, Cabana MDC, Clarke JR, Shea JA, Schwartz JS, Williams SV. Predictors of common bile duct stones prior to cholecystectomy: a meta-analysis. Gastrointest Endosc. 1996;44:450–9.
6. Padda MS, Singh S, Tang SJ, Rockey DC. Liver test patterns in patients with acute calculous cholecystitis and/or choledocholithiasis. Aliment Pharmacol Ther. 2009;29:1011–8.
7. Bourgouin S, Truchet X, Lamblin G, De Roulhae J, Platel JP, Balandraud P. Dynamic analysis of commonly used biochemical parameters to predict common bile duct stones in patients undergoing laparoscopic cholecystectomy. Surg Endosc. 2017;31(11):4725–34. Epub ahead of print.
8. American Society for Gastrointestinal Endoscopy. The role of endoscopy in the evaluation of suspected choledocholithiasis. Gastrointest Endosc. 2010;71(1):1–9.
9. Barkun AN, Barkun JS, Fried GM, et al. Useful predictors of bile duct stones in patients undergoing laparoscopic cholecystectomy. Ann Surg. 1994;220:32–9.
10. Tse F, Barkun JS, Barkun AN. The elective evaluation of patients with suspected choledocholithiasis undergoing laparoscopic cholecystectomy. Gastrointest Endosc. 2004;60(3):437–48.
11. Epelboym I, Winner M, Allendorf JD. MRCP is not a cost-effective strategy in the management of silent common bile duct stones. J Gastrointest Surg. 2013;17:863–71.
12. Verma D, Kapadia A, Eisen GM, et al. EUS vs MRCP for detection of choledocholithiasis. Gastrointest Endosc. 2006;64:248–54.
13. Romagnuolo J, Bardou M, Rahme E, et al. Magnetic resonance cholangiopancreatography: a meta-analysis of test performance in suspected biliary disease. Ann Intern Med. 2003;139:547–57.
14. Machi J, Tateishi T, Oishi AJ, et al. Laparoscopic ultrasonography versus operative cholangiography during laparoscopic cholecystectomy: review of the literature and a comparison with open intraoperative ultrasonography. J Am Coll Surg. 1999;188:361–7.
15. Garrow D, Miller S, Sinha D, et al. Endoscopic ultrasound: a meta-analysis of test performance in suspected biliary obstruction. Clin Gastroenterol Hepatol. 2007;6:616–23.
16. Sahu MJ, Chacko A, Dutta AK, Prakash JAJ. Microbial profile and antibiotic sensitivity pattern in acute bacterial cholangitis. Indian J Gastroenterol. 2011;30(5):204–8.
17. Solomkin JS, Mazuski JE, Baron EJ, Sawyer RG, Nathens AB, DiPiro JT, Buchman T, Dellinger EP, Jernigan J, Gorbach S, Chow AW, Bartlett J. Guidelines for the selection of anti-infective agents for complicated intra-abdominal infections. Clin Infect Dis. 2003;37:997–1005.
18. Lai KH, Chan HH, Tsai TJ, Cheng JS, Hsu PI. Reappraisal of endoscopic papillary balloon dilation for the management of common bile duct stones. World J Gastrointest Endosc. 2015;7:77–86.
19. Yasuda I, Fujita N, Maguchi H, Hasebe O, Igarashi Y, Murakami A, Mukai H, Fujii T, Yamao K, Maeshiro K, Tada T, Tsujino T, Komatsu Y. Long-term outcomes after endoscopic sphincterotomy versus endoscopic papillary balloon dilation for bile duct stones. Gastrointest Endosc. 2010;72(6):1185–91.
20. Fujita N, Maguchi H, Komatsu Y, Yasuda I, Hasebe O, Igarashi Y, Murakami A, Mukai H, Fujii T, Yamao K, Maeshiro K, JESED Study Group. Endoscopic sphincterotomy and endoscopic papillary balloon dilatation for bile duct stones: a prospective randomized controlled multicenter trial. Gastrointest Endosc. 2003;57(2):151–5.
21. Binmoeller KF, Bruckner M, Thonke F, Soehendra N. Treatment of difficult bile duct stones using mechanical, electrohydraulic, and extracorporeal shock wave lithotripsy. Endoscopy. 1993;25:201–6.
22. Wan XJ, Xu ZJ, Zhu F, Li L. Success rate and complications of endoscopic extraction of common bile duct

stones over 2 cm in diameter. Hepatobiliary Pancreat Dis Int. 2011;10(4):403–7.

23. Freeman ML, Nelson DB, Sherman S, Haber GB, Herman ME, Dorsher PJ, Moore JP, Fennerty MB, Ryan ME, Shaw MJ, Lande JD, Pheley AM. Complications of endoscopic biliary sphincterotomy. N Engl J Med. 1986;335:909–18.

24. Surick B, Washington M, Ghazi A. Endoscopic retrograde cholangiopancreatography in conjunction with laparoscopic cholecystectomy. Surg Endosc. 1993;7(5):388–92.

25. Cohen S, Bacon BR, Berlin JA, Fleischer D, Hecht GA, Loehrer PJ, McNair AE, Mulholland M, Norton NJ, Rabeneck L, Ransohoff DF, Sonnenberg A, Vannier MW. Gastrointest Endosc. 2002;56(6):803–9.

26. Topal B, Aerts R, Penninckx F. Laparoscopic common bile duct stone clearance with flexible choledochoscopy. Surg Endosc. 2007;21:2317–21.

27. Mellinger JD, MacFayden BD. Laparoscopic common bile duct exploration. In: Cameron JL, editor. Current surgical therapy. 9th ed. Philadelphia: Mosby; 2008.

28. Tinoco R, Tinoco A, El-Kadre L, Peres L, Sueth D. Laparoscopic common bile duct exploration. Ann Surg. 2008;247:674–9.

29. Petelin JB. Laparoscopic common bile duct exploration. Surg Endosc. 2003;17:1705–15.

30. Zhang W, Li G, Chen YL. Should T-tube drainage be performed for choledocholithiasis after laparoscopic common bile duct exploration? A systematic review and meta-analysis of randomized controlled trials. Surg Laparosc Endosc Percutan Tech. 2017.; Epub ahead of print.;27:415.

31. Podda M, Polignano FM, Luhmann A, Wilson MS, Kulli C, Tait IS. Systematic review with meta-analysis of studies comparing primary duct closure and T-tube drainage after laparoscopic common bile duct exploration for choledocholithiasis. Surg Endosc. 2016;30(3):845–61.

32. Gurusamy KS, Koti R, Davidson BR. T-tube drainage versus primary closure after open common bile duct exploration. Cochrane Database Syst Rev. 2013;21(6):CD005640.

33. da Costa DW, Bouwense SA, Schepers NJ, Besselink MG, van Santvoort HC, van Brunschot S, Bakker OJ, Bollen TL, Dejong CH, van Goor H, Boermeester MA, Bruno MJ, van Eijck CH, Timmer R, Weusten BL, Consten EC, Brink MA, Spanier BWM, Bilgen EJS, Nieuwenhuijs VB, Hofker HS, Rosman C, Voorburg AM, Bosscha K, Duijvendijk v, Gerritsen JJ, Heisterkamp J, de Hingh IH, Witteman BJ, Kruyt PM, Scheepers JJ, Molenaar IQ, Schaapherder AF, Manusama ER, van der Waaij LA, van Unen J, Dijkgraaf MG, van Ramshorst B, Gooszen HG, Boerma D, Dutch Pancreatitis Study Group. Same-admission versus interval cholecystectomy for mild gallstone pancreatitis (PONCHO): a multicenter randomised controlled trial. Lancet. 2015;386:1261–8.

34. da Costa DW, Dijksman LM, Bouwense SA, Schepers NJ, Besselink MG, van Santvoort HC, Boerma D, Gooszen HG, Dijkgraaf MG, Dutch Pancreatitis Study Group. Cost-effectiveness of same-admission versus interval cholecystectomy after mild gallstone pancreatitis in the PONCHO trial. Br J Surg. 2016;103(12):1695–703.

35. Mattila A, Mrena J, Kellokumpu I. Cost-analysis and effectiveness of one-stage laparoscopic versus two-stage endolaparoscopic mangement of cholecystocholedocholithiasis: a retrospective cohort study. BMC Surg. 2017;17:79–86.

36. Baucom RB, Feurer ID, Shelton JS, Kummerow K, Holzman MD, Poulose BK. Surgeons, ERCP, and laparoscopic common bile duct exploration: do we need a standard approach for common bile duct stones? Surg Endosc. 2016;30(2):414–23.

37. Saik RP, Greenburg AG, Farris JM, Peskin GW. Spectrum of cholangitis. Am J Surg. 1975;130(2):143–50.

38. Kiriyama S, Takada T, Strasberg SM, Solomkin JS, Mayumi T, Pitt HA, Gouma DJ, Garden J, Buchler MW, Yokoe M, Kimura Y, Tsuyuguchi T, Itoi T, Yoshida M, Miura F, Yamashita Y, Okamoto K, Gabata T, Hata J, Higuchi R, Windsor JA, Bornnman PC, Fan ST, Singh H, de Santibanes E, Gomi H, Kusachi S, Murata A, Chen XP, Jagannath P, Lee SG, Padbury R, Chen MF, Dervenis C, Chan ACW, Supe AN, Liau KH, Kim MH, Kim SW. TG13 guidelines for diagnosis and severity grading of acute cholangitis. J Hepatobiliary Pancreat Sci. 2013;20:24–34.

39. Forsmark CE, Baillie J, AGA Institute Clinical Practice and Economics Committee, AGA Institute Governing Board. AGA Institute technical review on acute pancreatitis. Gastroenterology. 2007;132(5):2022–44.

40. Hernandez V, Pascual I, Almela P, Anon R, Herreros B, Sanchiz V, Minguez M, Benages A. Recurrence of acute gallstone pancreatitis and relationship with cholecystectomy or endoscopic sphincterotomy. Am J Gastroenterol. 2004;99(12):2417–23.

41. Mori T, Sugiyama M, Atomi Y. Gallstone disease: management of intrahepatic stones. Best Pract Res Clin Gastroenterol. 2006;20(6):1117–37.

42. Kim YT, Byun JS, Kim J, Jang YH, Lee WJ, Ryu JK, Kim SW, Yoon YB, Kim CY. Factors predicting concurrent cholangiocarcinomas associated with hepatolithiasis. Hepato-Gastroenterology. 2003;50(49):8–12.

Acute Cholangitis

12

Marko Bukur and Jaclyn Clark

Introduction

Acute cholangitis is an obstructive disease of the extrahepatic biliary tree that can be life-threatening without prompt intervention. Historically in a surgical disease, the methods toward achieving biliary decompression involve some of the most prolific surgical minds. In the late 1800s, several surgical techniques were set forth to deal with obstruction of the common bile duct (CBD). These included using forceps or fingers to crush or move stones externally, allowing for passage either through the ampulla or gallbladder [1]. Opening the common bile duct itself, known as a choledochotomy, was first successfully performed in 1889; however, this maneuver did not allow for retrieval of all CBD stones. Charles McBurney suggested opening the duodenum for large stones impacted at the ampulla [1]. Carrying a high surgical morbidity and mortality, techniques of open common bile duct exploration were honed over the next century. Adjuncts to open biliary surgery including intraoperative cholangiography were used to define CBD obstruction and anatomy [2]. The biggest advancement to the treatment of cholangitis, however, came in the 1970s and 1980s, when endoscopy emerged as a new interventional modality for CBD obstruction. Endoscopic retrograde cholangiopancreatography (ERCP) had the ability to establish biliary drainage not only by directly retrieving stones but by allowing continued drainage via sphincterotomy [3]. At first eligibility criteria for endoscopic management included those who had a previous cholecystectomy or those whose age or medical comorbidities were prohibitive for open surgery. ERCP has now become a mainstay in urgent biliary decompression. In addition to ERCP, laparoscopy has ushered in the new era of less invasive surgical management, with adaptations of all established open procedures, including transcystic and direct CBD exploration as well as transduodenal options. The purpose of this chapter is to review presentation, diagnosis, management, and outcomes of acute cholangitis.

Pathophysiology

Cholangitis results when two things happen: first biliary flow is obstructed and bile becomes secondarily infected. While the biggest risk factor for obstruction is cholelithiasis, secondary etiologies also include strictures, malignancy, postoperative/endoscopic instrumentation, and congenital anomalies [4]. Bile is usually sterile; however, 15–50% of those with cholelithiasis have positive bile cultures [5]. Several physiologic mechanisms are in place to prevent biliary stasis and infection, includ-

M. Bukur · J. Clark (✉)
Department of Surgery, NYU Langone Medical Center, New York, NY, USA
e-mail: Jaclyn.clark@nyumc.org

© Springer International Publishing AG, part of Springer Nature 2019
C. V. R. Brown et al. (eds.), *Emergency General Surgery*, https://doi.org/10.1007/978-3-319-96286-3_12

ing unhindered flow into the duodenum, phagocytosis of bacteria in the liver by Kupffer cells, as well as IgA and the bile salts in bile itself [6]. The source of bacterial contamination is not completely established. Postulated sources of bacteria in bile include portal venous seeding and ascent from the duodenum. Higher intrabiliary pressures can subsequently cause permeability and bacterial translocation, which could explain the bacteremia and systemic sepsis that can ensue [6]. The range of presentations of this disease are extremely variable, likely relating to the degree of obstruction, capacity for drainage, virulence of bacteria, and capacity of the host to withstand sepsis.

Clinical Presentation

The most common presenting symptom of cholangitis is fever (90%), followed by abdominal pain (70%) and jaundice (60%) [6]. Recognition of these most common clinical features of cholangitis can be first attributed to J.M. Charcot in 1877, who described a "hepatic fever" associated with right upper quadrant pain, fever, and jaundice [5]. The sensitivity and specificity of this triad have a wide range of values in the literature. While sensitivity ranged from 7.7% to 72%, specificity fell within a smaller range of 84–95%, suggesting those without these three elements are unlikely to have cholangitis [7]. In 1959, Benedict Reynolds published a series of cases of completely obstructing cholangitis with the aim of defining circumstances in which death was a certain outcome. He added altered mental status and hypotension to Charcot's triad to form the eponymous Reynolds' pentad [8]. While less than 15% of people present in this fashion, ability of cholangitis to cause sepsis and circulatory collapse should not be overlooked.

Diagnostic Studies

Laboratory values and imaging are essential components to the diagnosis of acute cholangitis. The most commonly ordered laboratory tests used in the evaluation of cholangitis are complete blood count (CBC), metabolic panel, aminotransferases, alkaline phosphatase, bilirubin, and coagulation panel. Each of these can provide clinically useful information but should not be relied upon exclusively to eliminate the diagnosis. Patients will classically have a leukocytosis, and liver panels will show elevated total and direct bilirubin levels as well as alkaline phosphatase, suggesting cholestasis. Abnormalities in the aminotransferases can also be seen and are often >500 IU/L depending on the degree of hepatocyte destruction. Biliary obstruction can cause elevation in the PT/INR due to malabsorption of vitamin K. This is important to consider when planning for interventions. It is important to draw blood cultures on those with suspicion of acute cholangitis, as bacteremia is common.

Ultrasound

No single imaging study exists to definitively diagnose cholangitis. In most other biliary diseases, imaging is performed to confirm a suspected diagnosis based on history, physical, and laboratory values; however, in cholangitis, diagnostic imaging is a supportive tool. While ultrasound has been the first modality to diagnose cholelithiasis and acute cholecystitis, it is less accurate for cholangitis. Due to its rapid availability and ability to be done at the bedside, its role is mostly confined to detecting dilatation of the biliary tree or observing a common bile duct (CBD) stone which can be difficult due to sonographer proficiency, body habitus, and bowel gas.

The extrahepatic common bile duct should be measured at the level of the right hepatic artery and not exceed 6 mm, while the intrahepatic bile ducts should not exceed 2 mm in size. With adequate sonographer experience, the level of biliary obstruction can be identified in 92% of patients, and overall sensitivity for choledocholithiasis can reach 75% [9]. It is important to emphasize that choledocholithiasis can also be present in the absence of biliary ductal dilation in 25–33% of cases [10]. Endoscopic ultrasonography (EUS) (Fig. 12.1) has considerably better sensitivity at detecting choledocholithiasis (96%) as opposed

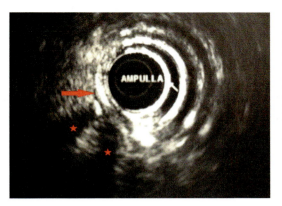

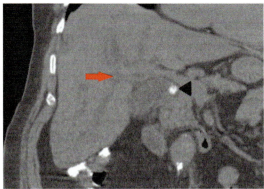

Fig. 12.1 Endoscopic ultrasound image taken at the level of the ampulla. Note the hyperechoic stones (arrow) and the hypoechoic posterior acoustic shadowing (stars inside)

Fig. 12.2 CAT scan of the abdomen showing a stone in a dilated common hepatic duct (black arrowhead) along with intrahepatic biliary dilation (red arrow)

to conventional sonography and may be considered in cases where this is equivocal as it avoids the associated risks of ERCP when used only for diagnostic purposes [11].

Computed Tomography

Computed tomography (CT) is not usually considered a preferred modality of choice in biliary disease. However, this is often the first study a patient will undergo when presenting to the emergency department with fever and abdominal pain. The sensitivity of CT to diagnose choledocholithiasis and biliary obstruction is variable, but reported to be around 80% [12]. Recently, several studies have examined subtle CT clues that support the diagnosis of acute cholangitis. These findings include dilation of the biliary tree, presence of stones, and transient hepatic attenuation differences, which essentially highlight nonstandard liver parenchymal enhancement due to alterations in blood flow [13] (Fig. 12.2). This pattern is primarily seen on the arterial phase of CT in patients with cholangitis, among other biliary pathologies [14]. One recent study found that CT had a sensitivity of 93% of CT for detecting acute cholangitis based on these patterns [15]. Peribiliary edema has also been used to support infection and therefore cholangitis on CT, with this pattern occurring over twice as frequently in patients with infected biliary obstruction [16].

CT comes with the advantages of being fast and readily available in most hospitals. Disadvantages include transport away from patient care areas, radiation, and intravenous contrast, which can contribute to acute kidney injury, especially in those patients with underlying renal dysfunction or end organ damage from sepsis.

Magnetic Resonance Imaging

Magnetic resonance imaging and magnetic resonance cholangiopancreatography (MRI, MRCP) has become a frequently used diagnostic tool to detect biliary obstruction due to its ability to highlight the biliary tract and suppress surrounding structures. It has a high sensitivity for identifying CBD obstruction between 80% and 100% with a specificity between 85% and 100% [17, 18]. MRCP creates a noninvasive cholangiogram by using signal difference between bile and the surrounding tissues as well as stones (Fig. 12.3). There are certain situations which are responsible for the variable sensitivity and specificity of MRCP for detecting biliary obstruction, including periampulary location due to the lack of bile and anatomy, motion artifact, and pneumobilia [19].

Like CT, MRCP can demonstrate CBD obstruction and be used in conjunction with other supporting elements of the patient presentation to support the diagnosis of cholangitis. In a pro-

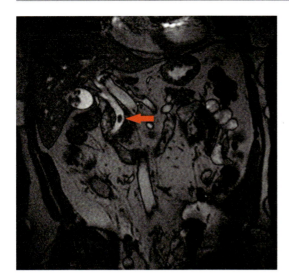

Fig. 12.3 T2-weighted MRCP showing a large stone in the common bile duct (red arrow)

spective study from 2012, Eun and colleagues have set forth some supplementary criteria on MRI that could suggest the diagnosis of cholangitis itself. These characteristics include increased periductal signal intensity, transient periductal signal difference, hepatic abscess, abscess, and a "ragged duct," which were frequent in patients with confirmed cholangitis [20].

MRI avoids radiation and is therefore the most useful study in the pregnant population. It cannot be used in patients with incompatible metal devices or implants and is difficult to tolerate for those with claustrophobia. Additionally, in some institutions MRI is not quickly and readily available, which can be imperative in severe cases. Though its diagnostic accuracy is the best of any noninvasive imaging study, its lack of therapeutic option after a diagnosis is established is its biggest drawback.

Cholangiography

Direct imaging of the biliary tree is the gold standard to locate the presence and level of CBD obstruction. This can be accomplished using either ERCP or the percutaneous transhepatic technique (PTC). While ERCP is widely accepted

as the premier treatment intervention for cholangitis, which will be discussed later, it also has diagnostic capability. Depending on clinical status, degree of suspicion of acute cholangitis, and ability to undergo less invasive diagnostic testing, ERCP can be used to diagnose biliary obstruction. The main advantage of this technique is the capability to immediately intervene and relieve the obstruction after the diagnosis is established (Fig. 12.4). While in mild cases the risks of the procedure outweigh the benefits, in patients with systemic manifestations, it presents an attractive option. There are several studies that have compared MRCP with ERCP as the gold standard for diagnosis of acute cholangitis, which have found that MRI has a similar diagnostic accuracy without the complications of an invasive procedure [21, 22]. ERCP is not without significant risks, notably including post-ERCP pancreatitis (2–10%) [23], hemorrhage, perforation, as well as the complications associated with procedural sedation. ERCP should be chosen carefully as the initial diagnostic study [24]. Predicting which asymptomatic patients will ultimately require ERCP is more difficult, but advanced age (>55), hyperbilirubinemia (>1.8 mg/dl), and common

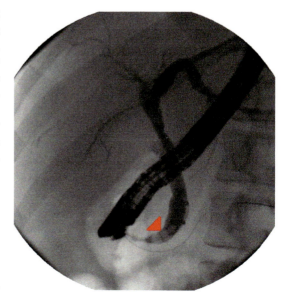

Fig. 12.4 An ERCP demonstrating a dilated common bile duct with multiple stones (red arrowhead)

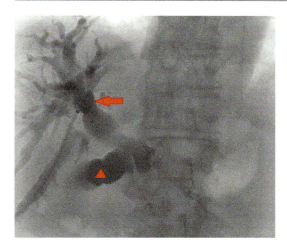

Fig. 12.5 A PTC demonstrating dilation of the intrahepatic biliary tree (red arrow) and tortuous common bile duct (red arrowhead)

duct dilation have all been shown to increase the likelihood of having a therapeutic ERCP [25].

PTC may be done at the patient's bedside under ultrasound guidance or in the fluoroscopy suite. After initial aspiration, a pigtail drainage catheter can be left in place for removal of further infected bile (Fig. 12.5). This temporizing measure can allow optimization of the patient's critical illness as well as any other underlying comorbidities. The drainage catheter should be left in place for 6 weeks to allow for establishment of a fibrous fistula tract prior to removal. In certain patients that are in a prohibitive surgical risk due to their underlying medical problems, conservative management with PTC cholangiography with stone extraction and catheter removal which can be accomplished successfully often without recurrence can be achieved [26]. Drawbacks to PTC include worsening sepsis from manipulation of the infected biliary tree and subsequent bacteremia, hemorrhage (including hemobilia), as well as biliary peritonitis.

Diagnostic Criteria and Severity Grading

A committee from Tokyo met to define standardized criteria for the diagnosis and management of cholangitis in 2007 and 2013. Because there are elements in a patient's history, physical exam, laboratory values, and imaging that contribute to the diagnosis of acute cholangitis, these criteria encompass elements from all of these categories. The guidelines include aspects based on (1) systemic inflammation, fever or chills, elevated white blood cell count, or C-reactive protein (CRP); (2) cholestasis, jaundice or abnormal liver function tests; and (3) imaging, biliary dilatation or evidence of a stricture, stone, or stent [27]. The diagnosis is suspected if a patient has evidence of systemic inflammation and cholestasis and considered definite if there is imaging evidence as defined above. Based on a retrospective study, the Tokyo Guidelines have increased sensitivity to 91% and specificity to 77% for diagnosis of acute cholangitis [28].

Taking this one step further, the Tokyo committee also aimed to develop a stratification based on clinical criteria to determine severity of illness that would identify patients who, if not intervened upon quickly, would have increased mortality. They retrospectively analyzed more than 1000 cases to determine these factors and came up with a grading system. Grade III (severe), patients presented with signs of organ system failure, grade II (moderate) patients had no improvement with antibiotics and resuscitation but no organ dysfunction, and grade I (mild) cases being those patients that responded to medical therapy alone [29].

Microbiology

In Western populations, bacterial pathogens are those most commonly responsible for acute cholangitis. Typical bacteria are those found in the gastrointestinal tract. Bile cultures are positive in 90% of cases of cholangitis [30]. Historically and currently, *Escherichia coli* is the most common organism isolated from bile cultures in patients with cholangitis (31–44%), followed by *Klebsiella* species (9–20%), and *Enterococcus* (3–34%) [31]. Anaerobes are not usually the predominant species isolated, but can coinfect bile in up to 50% of cases, with the most common organisms being *Bacteroides* sp., followed by *Clostridia* sp. [32]. Over the last several decades, there has been an increase in the number of procedures performed on the biliary tree and as such a rise in the number of healthcare-associated cholangitis infections. *Pseudomonas* species have become an important pathogen in these situations, and antibiotic therapy should be tailored accordingly.

Special Populations

Acute bacterial infection remains the most common cause of acute cholangitis in immunocompromised patients; however, it is worth mentioning other pathogens and populations that have special considerations. The immunocompromised host presents a challenge to both diagnose and treat, often with resistant and opportunistic pathogens. Acquired immunodeficiency syndrome (AIDS) patients have a propensity for biliary pathology including AIDS cholangiopathy. It can result from HIV itself, or a variety of opportunistic infections that cause ischemia and nerve damage to areas of the biliary tree, causing a secondary cholangitis. In only 50% of cases can a source be identified, which includes *Cytomegalovirus* (CMV), *Cryptosporidium parvum*, and *Mycobacterium avium complex*, among other organisms [33].

Liver transplant patients have a tendency toward cholangitis due to their immunocompromised state in addition to the presence of a biliary anastomosis, largely due to CMV [33]. This is treated with intravenous ganciclovir as well as stent placement for stricture-related disease.

Parasites

Though less of an issue in the Western population, parasites still account for episodes of cholangitis worldwide. Clonorchiasis is caused by small trematodes ingested with undercooked fish. They enter the biliary tree through the ampulla of Vater and migrate and lodge in medium- to small-sized ducts, causing obstruction and cholangitic

features. A significant burden of flukes can affect larger ducts and cause biliary obstruction and lead to bacterial cholangitis [34]. Therapy includes biliary decompression and an anti-helminthic agent, such as praziquantel [34]

Ascariasis is caused by a large round worm and is seen in tropical areas that can gain access to the biliary tree after being ingested. This worm causes cholangitis in several ways: their secretions cause sphincter of Oddi spasm and promote stone formation, cause necrosis and abscesses of the biliary tract, and can bring bacteria along to colonize bile [35]. A similar treatment strategy is employed, with biliary decompression, antibiotic therapy, and praziquantel.

Schistosomiasis is found in the Middle East, South America, Africa, China, and Japan and is characterized by trematode eggs that cause periportal inflammation and fibrosis [33]. It primarily affects the smaller peripheral ducts and can also be confused with acute bacterial cholangitis. It is also treated with biliary decompression and praziquantel.

Medical Management

The mainstays of treatment for acute cholangitis include resuscitation, antibiotic therapy, and decompression of the biliary obstruction. As discussed earlier, acute cholangitis is a diagnosis that encompasses a wide spectrum of clinical presentations, varying from mild to life-threatening organ dysfunction. Given its potentially devastating course, patients with high suspicion or diagnosis of acute cholangitis should be admitted to the hospital, administered antibiotics, and monitored for improvement. This is unlikely to succeed in those patients with complete biliary obstruction and will often progress to having moderate or severe disease.

Sepsis

Those with more severe disease-causing organ system dysfunction or signs of shock should be admitted to an intensive care unit (ICU) with central intravenous access, arterial blood pressure monitoring, and urinary catheter. Resuscitation in congruity with the 2016 guidelines set forth by the Surviving Sepsis Campaign should be undertaken [36]. Expedited volume administration with isotonic fluid should be empirically started and then targeted to hemodynamic parameters such as central venous and mean arterial pressure goals. Response to therapy can be assessed by monitoring continuous central venous gases, lactate measurements, and urine output. Should hemodynamic and resuscitative parameters be unobtainable, the first-line vasopressor of choice remains norepinephrine in most patients. After cultures are drawn, simultaneous early broad-spectrum antibiotic therapy is essential and should not be delayed. Any electrolyte abnormalities should be corrected. Medical management, while essential, is only a bridge toward patient optimization for definitive source control in the form of prompt biliary drainage.

Antibiotic Therapy

Early antibiotic therapy is imperative in treatment of cholangitis and should be guided toward the most common causative organisms. Selection of specific agents depends on each institution and its culture data, as well as host factors such as the severity of illness and likelihood of having a healthcare-associated infection.

Broadly, several categories of antibiotic are useful in treating community-acquired cholangitis of mild or moderate severity. These should be targeted toward *E. coli*, *Klebsiella*, and other enteric gram-negative pathogens. Penicillin derivatives such as second- and third-generation cephalosporins (cefoxitin and ceftriaxone, respectively) have broad gram-negative coverage. Ceftriaxone has been associated with biliary pseudolithiasis and had been avoided in biliary infections; however, this side effect is most prominent in children and is extremely rare [37]. The fluoroquinolone class (ciprofloxacin) has long been used for community-acquired intra-abdominal infections; however, there is a current trend of resistant organisms, and many institutions are avoiding this class of drug.

For a patient who presents with severe organ dysfunction and sepsis, it is important to target a wider spectrum of bacteria. The carbapenem class including imipenem and meropenem has activity against resistant gram-negative organisms, *Pseudomonas*, gram-positives including *enterococcus*, and anaerobes. The carbapenem class does not cover methicillin-resistant *Staphylococcus aureus* (MRSA). The ureidopenicillins include piperacillin with its beta-lactamase inhibitor tazobactam, which also have a wide spectrum of coverage including resistant gram-negatives, *Pseudomonas*, and anaerobes. Vancomycin can be added to cover enterococcus, which has largely become resistant to the aminoglycosides. The fourth-generation fluoroquinolone, moxifloxacin, can also be considered in this situation. It has activity against gram-negative organisms, anaerobes, and enterococcus. A randomized controlled trial showed it to be noninferior to piperacillin-tazobactam with amoxicillin-clavulanate, with just once daily dosing [38].

In a patient with the potential for a nosocomial infection (hospital or healthcare facility stay within 90 days), therapy should cover resistant gram negatives, *Pseudomonas*, enterococcus, MRSA, and anaerobes. One such regimen is vancomycin and piperacilin-tazobactam. If suspicion for vancomycin-resistant enterococcus is high, then linezolid should be added. While not routinely considered part of empiric coverage, antifungal coverage can be added if there is a history of malignant obstruction, pre-existing antibiotic or steroid use, immunocompromised state, or culture data showing yeast species [39].

In 2009 the Surgical Infection Society and the Infectious Disease Society of America penned guidelines to facilitate antibiotic choice for intra-abdominal infections [40]. The guidelines do not address cholangitis specifically, except in cases with a biliary-enteric anastomosis, in which case metronidazole should be added to the regimen to cover anaerobic bacteria. The Tokyo Guidelines from 2013 also address antibiotic management based on their own grading system for severity of disease [31]. They propose regimens that are penicillin, fluoroquinolone, and cephalosporin based, any of which can be applied depending on hospital resistance patterns and patient drug allergy. In all instances, antibiotics should be tailored to available culture data after empiric broad spectrum coverage is initiated and de-escalated when possible. In cases of mild cholangitis, generally only 2–3 days of antibiotics are recommended, while moderate to severe cases require 5–7 days assuming decompression has been accomplished [31].

Interventional Management

Ultimately, source control via biliary drainage is necessary for the successful treatment of acute cholangitis. Broadly, there are four categories of interventions to review: ERCP, percutaneous transhepatic biliary drainage (PTBD), laparoscopic surgical techniques, and their open counterparts.

ERCP

Endoscopic management has become the preferred treatment modality of acute cholangitis. It is 98% successful in clearing the CBD and providing biliary drainage [41]. ERCP can be used to image the common bile duct and biliary tree, clear the duct of stones and pus, and provide continued drainage via sphincterotomy or stenting. Patients with acute coagulopathy or that are on anticoagulation are not candidates for sphincterotomies due to increased bleeding risk, and can undergo balloon dilation, stent placement, or nasobiliary drainage instead.

An advanced endoscopist performs this procedure, which requires sedation and in some cases intubation when the patient is unstable. The endoscope is advanced through the mouth to the duodenum, and a catheter is fed through the ampulla of Vater. At this point pus or bile can be drained and sent for culture. Next, a sphincterotomy is performed, using electrocautery to incise the deep muscle layers of the sphincter of Oddi, allowing free drainage of stones and bile. If the

patient is unstable, decompression of the biliary tree with stenting should be the main objective to limit time under anesthesia, with delayed stone extraction or workup of stricture undertaken once the patient stabilizes. In stable patients with remaining stones, balloons and baskets are threaded past the stone to pull it toward and through the ampulla. Should a stone be too large to retrieve with this mechanism, mechanical lithotripsy can be performed to reduce the size of the stone to facilitate its removal. If the obstruction is caused by malignancy or stricture, a stent can be deployed to relieve the obstruction. Completion cholangiography can show the biliary tree without filling defects.

A large multicenter prospective study that set out to define rates and risk factors of complications related to ERCP showed that pancreatitis (5%), bleeding (2%), and perforation(0.003%) were the most frequently encountered [42]. Of those with pancreatitis, 0.4% had severe case, requiring over 10 days in the hospital. In certain patients with risk factors, peri-procedural indomethacin may reduce the rate of post ERCP pancreatitis [43]. Complication rates are lower for more experienced endoscopists. Post-procedure, patients should be monitored for pancreatitis using abdominal exam and lipase measurement.

Benefits of ERCP include its minimally invasive nature, wide availability, and remarkable success rate in treating CBD obstruction. ERCP has been compared to both percutaneous and surgical options. It has an equal success rate to open surgery; however, it has substantially less morbidity and mortality, especially in the elderly population [44].

Percutaneous Transhepatic Biliary Drainage

This technique involves percutaneous access to the biliary tract and is usually performed by interventional radiologist that uses fluoroscopy to correctly identify the biliary tract. Sedation and local anesthesia are required for analgesia. Puncture can be performed to target the right or left hepatic duct or the gallbladder, with the subcostal approach to the left duct being less painful [45]. Dilated peripheral ducts provide for more facile access to the biliary tract. External biliary drainage can be used to temporize the effects of sepsis, and a catheter is left in place to facilitate continued drainage. Through the catheter, many of the same interventions as ERCP can be performed, including balloon dilation and stenting [46, 47].

Where available ERCP with sphincterotomy and stenting is the first choice for biliary drainage in cholangitis due to its lower complications and higher success rate, however PTBD is a secondary option when ERCP fails [48]. PTBD can also be used for drainage in patients whose anatomy precludes ERCP, such as those with biliary-enteric anastomoses (i.e., Roux-en-Y).

Complications of this technique include catheter occlusion, dislocation, and recurrence of cholangitis with at least one complication noted in 40% of patients [49]. Hemobilia, occurring in 2.3%, can be a potentially life-threatening situation that requires angiographic intervention to remedy [50]. While not first line, PTBD remains an option in those patients for whom ERCP is unsuccessful and surgical intervention is too prohibitive.

Surgical Management

Principles of surgical biliary decompression have been honed over 100 years. Preoperative considerations include stability of the patient, comorbidities, and failure of endoscopic therapy.

Minimally Invasive Surgery

Laparoscopic common bile duct exploration has become an important option for surgical management of choledocholithiasis and cholangitis. The procedures described below are consistent with the current SAGES guidelines for laparoscopic biliary surgery [51] and are reflective of the authors preferences. This technique should only be considered in patients with mild to moderate disease on the Tokyo scale as those with severe disease are typically too unstable and would poorly tolerate the insufflation needed to perform this operation safely.

The patient is placed supine on the operating table arm tucking per surgeon preference. The patient is placed in the reverse Trendelenburg position with the right side up to clear small bowel and colon from the field. Abdominal access is achieved via open Hasson technique. Dissection begins as a laparoscopic cholecystectomy would, defining anatomic relationships and obtaining a critical view of safety prior to division of any structure. This entails identifying the hepatocystic triangle, a single duct, and a single artery entering the gallbladder and dissecting the lower third of the gallbladder off of the liver bed. This avoids harm to the CBD and portal structures. Once this is acquired, the CBD can be assessed for stones or inadvertent injury using intraoperative cholangiography to image the biliary tree. Additionally, intraoperatrive ultrasound can be used to detect stones in the CBD. Once IOC confirms obstruction or filling defects, the laparoscopic CBD exploration can begin.

Transcystic CBD Exploration

First, 1 mg of intravenous glucagon is given in conjunction with vigorous flushing of the CBD with saline through the cholangiogram catheter to relax the sphincter of Oddi. Fogarty balloons (3–5 French) can then be passed to try to retrieve stones via the cystic duct. This can be successful for smaller mobile stones (less than 8 mm). If this is not successful, a choledochoscope can be passed through an additional 5 mm laparoscopic port into the dilated cystic duct opening and attached to continuous irrigation. This can be used to confirm clearance or visualize stones. Retrieval baskets can be used and deployed to visualize the stone being pulled into the cystic duct. Cholangiography or repeat choledochoscopy can then be used to confirm stone clearance visually or by free flow of contrast into the duodenum.

Choledochotomy

If the CBD is dilated with impacted or large stones (>8 mm), a choledochotomy can be performed. This is generally done 1–2 cm distal from the junction of the cystic and common hepatic ducts (Fig. 12.6). We place two 4–0 PDS stay sutures at 10 and 2 o'clock positions to tent the CBD; this avoids the parallel 3 and 9 o'clock positions of the vasculature supplying the common bile duct. An anterior choledochotomy of 1 cm is made while placing the stay sutures under tension to prevent back wall injury. Through this, ductotomy Fogarty balloons (Fig. 12.7) or the choledochoscope can be placed, and retrieval (Fig. 12.8) can be attempted.

If there is an impacted stone that cannot be retrieved by any laparoscopic means, there are several options. Firstly, the stone can be left in place, and the CBD can be closed over a T-tube

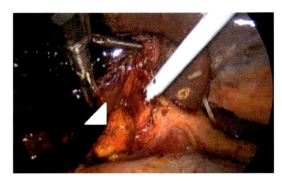

Fig. 12.8 Large common bile duct stone (white arrowhead) after being extracted using a biliary Fogarty

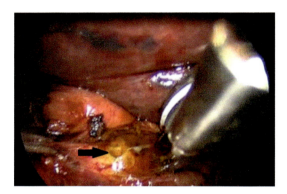

Fig. 12.6 Intraoperative photo of a laparoscopic common bile duct exploration. Anterior choledochocotomy is demonstrated (black arrow)

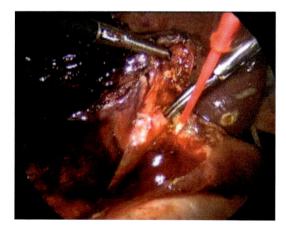

Fig. 12.7 A biliary Fogarty is used to clear the common bile duct via anterior choledochocotmy

providing drainage. Secondly, an intraoperative or postoperative ERCP can attempt removal with anterograde interventional assistance via the T-tube. In cases where this cannot be accomplished either intraoperatively or postoperatively, an open procedure involving a longitudinal duodenotomy and open sphincterotomy can be performed. This is not recommended in settings where interventional and advanced endoscopic expertise is readily available.

The CBD should be closed over a T-tube for all cases of acute cholangitis to allow for continued duct decompression. This should be placed to a gravity drainage bag, and the authors also prefer to utilize closed suction drainage in Morrison's pouch. Cholangiography can be performed through the T-tube, 2 or more weeks later after resolution of infection, and the drain can be removed if there are no signs of persistent obstruction. If there is low suspicion for biliary infection, the choledochotomy can be closed primarily with interrupted 4-0 PDS sutures. Alternatively, biliary drainage can be established via a transcystic catheter that is externalized.

Combined Procedures

Laparoscopy can be combined with ERCP if the surgeon does not feel comfortable performing a laparoscopic CBD exploration; however, this adds time and cost. It becomes especially useful, however, for direct access to the stomach in patients with Roux-en-Y anatomy. While laparoscopy generally has better morbidity and mortality for patients, there are several drawbacks including advanced laparoscopic techniques, readily available specialized instruments (i.e., choledochoscopes and stone extraction baskets), and suitable patient physiology to be performed safely.

Surgery Vs. Endoscopy

Biliary decompression is considered as the primary treatment of cholangitis. In less severe cases of acute cholangitis, elective biliary decompression may be planned by either endoscopy or laparoscopy. In severe cases, emergency endoscopic decompression should be performed as surgical treatment in these patients is associated with higher mortality [52, 53].

Open Surgery

Endoscopic and minimally invasive surgery have mostly obviated the need for an open surgery; however, open common bile duct exploration is always a fallback option for biliary drainage, particularly in unstable patients in which no endoscopic or interventional options exist. Open surgery carries risks of general anesthesia and the morbidity of a laparotomy. The technique, procedures, and adjuncts are analogous to those available laparoscopically. The most useful technique to employ in patients with severe cholangitis in situations such as these is open T-tube placement into the common bile duct. The authors prefer to use a right subcostal incision, but a midline incision is equally effective. The portal triad is exposed and structures dissected. Stay sutures are placed similarly to the laparoscopic procedure and an anterior ductotomy of 2 cm done longitudinally. A T-tube is then placed into the CBD and closed over horizontally placed 4-0 PDS sutures. Stone extraction should not be done at this time as the primary goal is to achieve biliary decompression and shorten the time the patient is under general anesthesia. The patient can then be further resuscitated, and once stabilized, transfer to a tertiary center that has ERCP/PTBD can be considered.

Post Intervention Care

Specific post-procedure considerations have been discussed above; however, there are some general tenets of care. After establishing adequate biliary drainage and antibiotic regimen appropriate for the patient, the patient should be admitted to a monitored setting. Resolution of leukocytosis and decreasing bilirubin should be expected if antibiotics and drainage are adequate. Any aberrant lab values associated with sepsis should also be checked regularly until normalization. Imaging should not be necessary, unless incomplete clearance of the CBD is suspected.

According to the IDSA and the Tokyo Guidelines, with complete drainage of biliary obstruction, antibiotic therapy for acute cholangitis should be continued for a total of 4–7 days, as longer durations were not associated with better outcomes [40]. In the event of bacteremia with enterococcus, 2 weeks of antibiotics are recommended [31]. If the CBD is not cleared completely, treatment should continue.

In those cases of acute cholangitis caused by gallstones, laparoscopic cholecystectomy is recommended. The NSQIP risk calculator [54] can be used to assess fitness for surgery and approximate operative risk. A discussion with the patient should review specific risks such as risk of recurrent cholangitis, biliary pancreatitis, or acute cholecystitis. The timing of elective cholecystectomy has been debated. In one retrospective review of 112 cases, patients who had surgery greater than 6 weeks after their bout of cholangitis had more intraoperative (28 vs 9%) and postoperative (42 vs 15%) complications compared to those who had surgery less than 6 weeks later [55]. Some studies have suggested that elective cholecystectomy reduces the risk of recurrent episodes of acute cholangitis [56, 57]. There are no data regarding cholecystectomy during the same admission vs. within 6 weeks.

Outcomes

Over the last 100 years, the mortality of acute cholangitis has greatly improved. Prior to 1980, the diagnosis carried greater than 50% mortality, but with modern interventions and management, this fell to 2–10% after 2000 [58]. Several studies have tried to investigate variables associated with worse outcome [59–61]. The highest mortality is seen in those patients who present with or develop signs of end-organ damage and sepsis related to cholangitis. The elderly also have worse outcomes after both mild and severe cholangitis vs. younger patients, with mortality rates of 10.8% vs 3.2%, respectively [44]. Delayed ERCP also has a negative effect on mortality, ICU stay, and organ failure [62, 63]. Those who present with malignant obstruction carry a higher mortality risk, related to the underlying disease process as well as patient comorbidities and chemotherapy [64]. For those who do not present with organ damage and sepsis, antibiotics and decompression have a mortality of less than 5% [59].

Conclusion

In summary, cholangitis compromises a wide clinical spectrum that has the potential to be life-threatening and systemic. If sepsis is present, emergent biliary decompression is necessary to achieve source control. Despite a historically high mortality, with early recognition and prompt intervention either endoscopic or surgical, outcomes are favorable.

References

1. McManus JE. The early history of surgery for common-duct stones; a brief review. N Engl J Med. 1956;254:17–20.
2. MacFadyen BV. Intraoperative cholangiography: past, present, and future. Surg Endosc. 2006;20(Suppl 2):S436–40.
3. Sivak MV Jr. Endoscopic management of bile duct stones. Am J Surg. 1989;158:228–40.
4. Kimura Y, Takada T, Kawarada Y, et al. Definitions, pathophysiology, and epidemiology of acute cholangitis and cholecystitis: Tokyo Guidelines. J Hepato-Biliary-Pancreat Surg. 2007;14:15–26.
5. Lipsett PA, Pitt HA. Acute cholangitis. Front Biosci. 2003;8:s1229–39.
6. Hanau LH, Steigbigel NH. Acute (ascending) cholangitis. Infect Dis Clin N Am. 2000;14:521–46.
7. Rumsey S, Winders J, MacCormick AD. Diagnostic accuracy of Charcot's triad: a systematic review. ANZ J Surg. 2017;87:232–8.
8. Reynolds BM, Dargan EL. Acute obstructive cholangitis; a distinct clinical syndrome. Ann Surg. 1959;150:299–303.
9. Laing FC. The gallbladder and bile ducts. In: Rumack C, Wilson S, Charbonneau J, editors. Diagnostic ultrasound. 2nd ed. Mosby-Year Book: St. Louis; 1998.
10. Millat B, Decker G, Fingerhut A. Imaging of cholelithiasis: what does the surgeon need? Abdom Imaging. 2001;26:3–6.
11. O'Neill DE, Saunders MD. Endoscopic ultrasonography in diseases of the gallbladder. Gastroenterol Clin N Am. 2010;39:289–305. ix.
12. Anderson SW, Lucey BC, Varghese JC, Soto JA. Accuracy of MDCT in the diagnosis of choledocholithiasis. AJR Am J Roentgenol. 2006;187:174–80.
13. Itai Y, Matsui O. Blood flow and liver imaging. Radiology. 1997;202:306–14.
14. Arai K, Kawai K, Kohda W, Tatsu H, Matsui O, Nakahama T. Dynamic CT of acute cholangitis: early inhomogeneous enhancement of the liver. AJR Am J Roentgenol. 2003;181:115–8.
15. Sugishita T, Higuchi R, Morita S, Ota T, Yamamoto M. Diagnostic accuracy of transient hepatic attenuation differences on computed tomography scans for acute cholangitis in patients with malignant disease. J Hepatobiliary Pancreat Sci. 2014;21:669–75.
16. Akaike G, Ishiyama M, Suzuki S, Fujita Y, Ohde S, Saida Y. Significance of peribiliary oedema on computed tomography in diagnosis and severity assessment of acute cholangitis. Eur J Radiol. 2013;82:e429–33.
17. Bilgin M, Toprak H, Burgazli M, et al. Diagnostic value of dynamic contrast-enhanced magnetic resonance imaging in the evaluation of the biliary obstruction. ScientificWorldJournal. 2012;2012:731089.
18. Pavone P, Laghi A, Catalano C, Panebianco V, Fabiano S, Passariello R. MRI of the biliary and pancreatic ducts. Eur Radiol. 1999;9:1513–22.
19. Irie H, Honda H, Kuroiwa T, et al. Pitfalls in MR cholangiopancreatographic interpretation. Radiographics. 2001;21:23–37.
20. Eun HW, Kim JH, Hong SS, Kim YJ. Assessment of acute cholangitis by MR imaging. Eur J Radiol. 2012;81:2476–80.
21. Lomas DJ, Bearcroft PW, Gimson AE. MR cholangiopancreatography: prospective comparison of a breath-hold 2D projection technique with diagnostic ERCP. Eur Radiol. 1999;9:1411–7.
22. Hekimoglu K, Ustundag Y, Dusak A, et al. MRCP vs. ERCP in the evaluation of biliary pathologies: review of current literature. J Dig Dis. 2008;9:162–9.
23. Thaker AM, Mosko JD, Berzin TM. Post-endoscopic retrograde cholangiopancreatography pancreatitis. Gastroenterol Rep (Oxf). 2015;3:32–40.
24. Freeman ML. Adverse outcomes of endoscopic retrograde cholangiopancreatography. Rev Gastroenterol Disord. 2002;2:147–68.
25. Williams EJ, Green J, Beckingham I, et al. Guidelines on the management of common bile duct stones (CBDS). Gut. 2008;57:1004–21.

26. Van Steenbergen W, Ponette E, Marchal G, et al. Percutaneous transhepatic cholecystostomy for acute complicated cholecystitis in elderly patients. Am J Gastroenterol. 1990;85:1363–9.

27. Kiriyama S, Takada T, Strasberg SM, et al. TG13 guidelines for diagnosis and severity grading of acute cholangitis (with videos). J Hepatobiliary Pancreat Sci. 2013;20:24–34.

28. Yokoe M, Takada T, Strasberg SM, et al. New diagnostic criteria and severity assessment of acute cholecystitis in revised Tokyo Guidelines. J Hepatobiliary Pancreat Sci. 2012;19:578–85.

29. Kiriyama S, Takada T, Strasberg SM, et al. New diagnostic criteria and severity assessment of acute cholangitis in revised Tokyo Guidelines. J Hepatobiliary Pancreat Sci. 2012;19:548–56.

30. van den Hazel SJ, Speelman P, Tytgat GN, Dankert J, van Leeuwen DJ. Role of antibiotics in the treatment and prevention of acute and recurrent cholangitis. Clin Infect Dis. 1994;19:279–86.

31. Gomi H, Solomkin JS, Takada T, et al. TG13 antimicrobial therapy for acute cholangitis and cholecystitis. J Hepatobiliary Pancreat Sci. 2013;20:60–70.

32. Marne C, Pallares R, Martin R, Sitges-Serra A. Gangrenous cholecystitis and acute cholangitis associated with anaerobic bacteria in bile. Eur J Clin Microbiol. 1986;5:35–9.

33. Catalano OA, Sahani DV, Forcione DG, et al. Biliary infections: spectrum of imaging findings and management. Radiographics. 2009;29:2059–80.

34. Lim JH, Mairiang E, Ahn GH. Biliary parasitic diseases including clonorchiasis, opisthorchiasis and fascioliasis. Abdom Imaging. 2008;33:157–65.

35. Shah OJ, Zargar SA, Robbani I. Biliary ascariasis: a review. World J Surg. 2006;30:1500–6.

36. Rhodes A, Evans LE, Alhazzani W, et al. Surviving sepsis campaign: international guidelines for management of sepsis and septic shock: 2016. Intensive Care Med. 2017;43:304–77.

37. de Moor RA, Egberts AC, Schroder CH. Ceftriaxone-associated nephrolithiasis and biliary pseudolithiasis. Eur J Pediatr. 1999;158:975–7.

38. Malangoni MA, Song J, Herrington J, Choudhri S, Pertel P. Randomized controlled trial of moxifloxacin compared with piperacillin-tazobactam and amoxicillin-clavulanate for the treatment of complicated intra-abdominal infections. Ann Surg. 2006;244:204–11.

39. Pappas PG, Kauffman CA, Andes DR, et al. Clinical practice guideline for the management of candidiasis: 2016 update by the Infectious Diseases Society of America. Clin Infect Dis. 2016;62:e1–50.

40. Solomkin JS, Mazuski JE, Bradley JS, et al. Diagnosis and management of complicated intra-abdominal infection in adults and children: guidelines by the Surgical Infection Society and the Infectious Diseases Society of America. Clin Infect Dis. 2010;50:133–64.

41. Tantau M, Mercea V, Crisan D, et al. ERCP on a cohort of 2,986 patients with cholelitiasis: a 10-year experience of a single center. J Gastrointestin Liver Dis. 2013;22:141–7.

42. Freeman ML, Nelson DB, Sherman S, et al. Complications of endoscopic biliary sphincterotomy. N Engl J Med. 1996;335:909–18.

43. Elmunzer BJ, Scheiman JM, Lehman GA, et al. A randomized trial of rectal indomethacin to prevent post-ERCP pancreatitis. N Engl J Med. 2012;366:1414–22.

44. Sugiyama M, Atomi Y. Treatment of acute cholangitis due to choledocholithiasis in elderly and younger patients. Arch Surg. 1997;132:1129–33.

45. Hayashi N, Sakai T, Kitagawa M, Kimoto T, Inagaki R, Ishii Y. US-guided left-sided biliary drainage: nine-year experience. Radiology. 1997;204:119–22.

46. Yee AC, Ho CS. Percutaneous transhepatic biliary drainage: a review. Crit Rev Diagn Imaging. 1990;30:247–79.

47. Lawson AJ, Beningfield SJ, Krige JE, Rischbieter P, Burmeister S. Percutaneous transhepatic self-expanding metal stents for palliation of malignant biliary obstruction. S Afr J Surg. 2012;50:54, 6, 8 passim.

48. Heedman PA, Astradsson E, Blomquist K, Sjodahl R. Palliation of malignant biliary obstruction: adverse events are common after percutaneous transhepatic biliary drainage. Scand J Surg. 2017;107(1):48–53. https://doi.org/10.1177/1457496917731192.

49. Nennstiel S, Weber A, Frick G, et al. Drainage-related complications in percutaneous transhepatic biliary drainage: an analysis over 10 years. J Clin Gastroenterol. 2015;49:764–70.

50. Rivera-Sanfeliz GM, Assar OS, LaBerge JM, et al. Incidence of important hemobilia following transhepatic biliary drainage: left-sided versus right-sided approaches. Cardiovasc Intervent Radiol. 2004;27:137–9.

51. Overby DW, Apelgren KN, Richardson W, Fanelli R, Society of American G, Endoscopic S. SAGES guidelines for the clinical application of laparoscopic biliary tract surgery. Surg Endosc. 2010;24:2368–86.

52. Jain MK, Jain R. Acute bacterial cholangitis. Curr Treat Options Gastroenterol. 2006;9:113–21.

53. Hui CK, Lai KC, Wong WM, Yuen MF, Lam SK, Lai CL. A randomised controlled trial of endoscopic sphincterotomy in acute cholangitis without common bile duct stones. Gut. 2002;51:245–7.

54. Risk calculator. 2017. At https://riskcalculator.facs.org/RiskCalculator/.

55. Li VK, Yum JL, Yeung YP. Optimal timing of elective laparoscopic cholecystectomy after acute cholangitis and subsequent clearance of choledocholithiasis. Am J Surg. 2010;200:483–8.

56. Targarona EM, Ayuso RM, Bordas JM, et al. Randomised trial of endoscopic sphincterotomy with gallbladder left in situ versus open surgery for common bileduct calculi in high-risk patients. Lancet. 1996;347:926–9.

57. Boerma D, Rauws EA, Keulemans YC, et al. Wait-and-see policy or laparoscopic cholecystectomy after endoscopic sphincterotomy for bile-duct stones: a randomised trial. Lancet. 2002;360:761–5.

58. Kimura Y, Takada T, Strasberg SM, et al. TG13 current terminology, etiology, and epidemiology of acute

cholangitis and cholecystitis. J Hepatobiliary Pancreat Sci. 2013;20:8–23.

59. Csendes A. Diaz JC, Burdiles P, Maluenda F, Morales E. Risk factors and classification of acute suppurative cholangitis. Br J Surg. 1992;79:655–8.

60. Tsujino T, Sugita R, Yoshida H, et al. Risk factors for acute suppurative cholangitis caused by bile duct stones. Eur J Gastroenterol Hepatol. 2007;19:585–8.

61. Gigot JF, Leese T, Dereme T, Coutinho J, Castaing D, Bismuth H. Acute cholangitis. Multivariate analysis of risk factors. Ann Surg. 1989;209:435–8.

62. Navaneethan U, Gutierrez NG, Jegadeesan R, et al. Factors predicting adverse short-term outcomes in patients with acute cholangitis undergoing ERCP: a single center experience. World J Gastrointest Endosc. 2014;6:74–81.

63. Khashab MA, Tariq A, Tariq U, et al. Delayed and unsuccessful endoscopic retrograde cholangiopancreatography are associated with worse outcomes in patients with acute cholangitis. Clin Gastroenterol Hepatol. 2012;10:1157–61.

64. Thompson J, Bennion RS, Pitt HA. An analysis of infectious failures in acute cholangitis. HPB Surg. 1994;8:139–44; discussion 45.

Gallstone Ileus

13

Chris Dodgion and Marc de Moya

Introduction

Gallstone ileus is a mechanical obstruction of the gastrointestinal tract caused by gallstones that enter the alimentary tract via a cholecystoenteric fistula. The etiology of the fistula often stems from episodes of cholecystitis or chronic inflammation of the gallbladder that forms adhesions to the surrounding bowel, usually the duodenum. The development of a large gallstone then causes pressure necrosis of the gallbladder wall resulting in bowel erosion and fistula formation. The subsequent passage of a gallstone (>2–2.5 cm) into the alimentary tract will tumble along until it reaches a point of narrowing causing a bowel obstruction that was historically mislabeled as an "ileus."

Eighty to 90% of all stones that enter the gastrointestinal tract are small and will pass spontaneously. The majority of stones (90%) that are responsible for the obstruction are >2.5 cm [1], and 60.5% of stones lodge just proximal to the ileocecal valve; other sites are less frequent: jejunum (16.5%), stomach (14.2%), sigmoid colon (4.1%), and duodenum (3.5%) [2, 3]. Obstruction is increasingly likely with smaller stones if patients have a history of inflammatory bowel disease, prior bowel obstructions, or diverticulitis, leading to decreased bowel intraluminal diameter though this is somewhat dependent on the location of the cholecystoenteric fistula. The second portion of the duodenum is the most common site of fistula formation (~68%) [4, 5] followed by gastric (5–13%), colonic (5–11%), and jejunal or ileal (2.5%) [6] (Fig. 13.1).

Epidemiology

The development of a gallstone ileus is a rare event, though first described in 1654 by Bartholin there were only 555 cases reported in the literature by 1954 [7]. Overall, only 0.3–0.5% of patients with choledocholithiasis will develop an obstruction related to a gallstone. Historically, 1–3% of all small bowel obstructions [8, 9] were thought to be secondary to gallstones, but a recent national evaluation using the National Inpatient Sample by Halabi et al. has shown rates as low as 0.095%. This represents an incidence of 500–600 patients per year [2].

However, both women and the elderly are disproportionately at risk for gallstone ileus. The mean age diagnosis is 74, and there is a 3:1 ratio

C. Dodgion (✉) · M. de Moya
Division of Trauma/Acute Care Surgery, Medical College of Wisconsin-Froedtert Trauma Center, Milwaukee, WI, USA
e-mail: cdodgion@mcw.edu

© Springer International Publishing AG, part of Springer Nature 2019
C. V. R. Brown et al. (eds.), *Emergency General Surgery*, https://doi.org/10.1007/978-3-319-96286-3_13

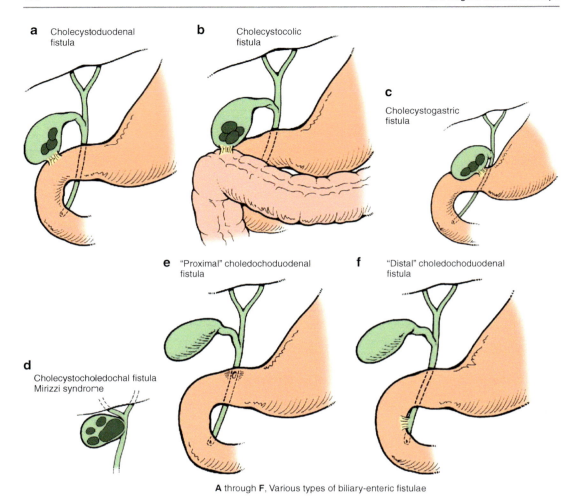

a Cholecystoduodenal fistula

b Cholecystocolic fistula

c Cholecystogastric fistula

d Cholecystocholedochal fistula Mirizzi syndrome

e "Proximal" choledochoduodenal fistula

f "Distal" choledochoduodenal fistula

A through **F**, Various types of biliary-enteric fistulae

Fig. 13.1 Types of biliary-enteric fistula [63]

of female predominance [2, 10]. In this select population of elderly female patients, gallstone ileus has been show to account for 22.5–25% of all nonischemic small bowel obstructions [3]. This lopsided distribution of patients is likely due in part to the increased rate of gallstone formation in women [11] and the relative pain tolerance of the elderly that decreases the rate of presentation with initial biliary symptoms.

Despite the low incidence of gallstone ileus, it has historically been associated with high morbidity and mortality. Early reported mortality rates were as high as 40–70% [7] but more recently have improved to 15–18% [3] or as low as 6% in recent national database studies [2, 10]. The high mortality rate is thought to be secondary to the advanced age, concomitant comorbidi-

ties, and delayed presentation. In a 6-year evaluation of NSQIP patients with gallstone ileus, Mallipeddi et al. found that 69% of patients had an ASA score of ≥3, frequently secondary to obesity (39%), diabetes (23%), hypertension (73%), coronary artery disease (10%) or COPD and tobacco use (12%). Most patients present 3–8 days after onset of symptoms and do not undergo a surgical intervention for another 3–4 days after presentation [4, 8, 9].

Signs and Symptoms

The symptoms associated with gallstone ileus are non-specific but often resemble that of a small bowel obstruction. Frequently, patients

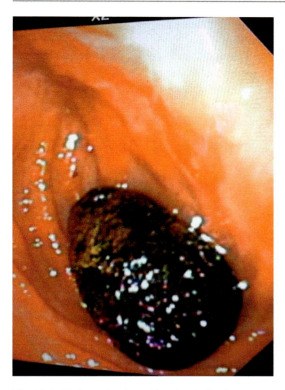

Fig. 13.2 Endoscopic view of intraluminal gallstone

describe episodic abdominal pain with intermittent-associated nausea and vomiting; often this is described as a "tumbling" type of obstruction from the passage of the stone along the gastrointestinal tract [12, 13] (Fig. 13.2). These obstructive symptoms with associated dehydration, electrolyte abnormalities, are much more common than signs or symptoms of biliary pathology – elevated LFTs (25%), jaundice (15%) [4], and RUQ pain (20%) [3, 14]. Though gallstone ileus is associated with chronic inflammation of the gallbladder and erosion of a stone into the gastrointestinal tract, only 50% of patients will have a prior history of biliary complaints [7, 8].

Historically only 20–50% of patients had the correct preoperative diagnosis [7, 15]. In part, this is secondary to the non-specific nature of the symptoms but also is a result of the insensitivity of abdominal X-rays. More contemporary series have increased the rate of preoperative diagnosis to approximately 77% with the use of CT scan and other imaging modalities.

Imaging

Abdominal X-ray

Given the non-specific nature of patients' presenting symptoms, abdominal imaging plays an important role in the diagnosis of gallstone ileus. The classic imaging findings on abdominal X-ray diagnostic of gallstone ileus are dilated bowel, pneumobilia, and a visualized gallstone often in the right lower quadrant. This is known as Rigler's triad, which was first described in 1941 when X-rays were the only available imaging study, and is pathognomonic for gallstone ileus [16, 17]. In Rigler's series of 14 cases, pneumobilia was present in 93% of cases [17]. However, less than 35% of patients display all three signs [18–20], and only 2/3 of Rigler's criteria are found in 50% of cases [21]. The overall sensitivity of abdominal X-ray for gallstone ileus is approximately 43% [22].

In part, the low sensitivity of abdominal X-ray is because only 15–30% of gallstones contain enough calcium to be radiopaque and even then they can be obscured by bowel gas [23]. Additionally, although pneumobilia is the most frequently seen sign on abdominal X-ray, there are a number of other conditions that can demonstrate this finding like emphysematous cholecystitis, suppurative cholangitis, and incompetent sphincter of Oddi (most common after ERCP or rarely blunt trauma) [3, 4, 22], and only 25% of all patients with pneumobilia have a cholecysto-enteric fistula [8].

Ultrasound

Abdominal ultrasound has been advocated to supplement X-ray findings as a low-cost alternative to CT scans, and adding ultrasound has improved the overall sensitivity of diagnosis to 73% [19, 22]. Specifically, ultrasound is more sensitive in identifying pneumobilia and ectopic gallstones [6]. Some additional advantages of ultrasound can be the identification of the site of the fistula [24], identification the site of obstruction in non-radiopaque stones [19], evaluation for additional stones within the biliary tree that might increase the risk of recurrence, and examination of the degree of biliary inflammation [4]. Finally, in those patients who undergo enterolithotomy alone, ultrasound can be useful to evaluate closure or persistence of a biliary enteric fistula [4].

Computed Tomography (CT)

More recently the high-resolution abdomen and pelvis CT scan with IV contrast has supplanted both ultrasound and abdominal X-rays in the diagnosis of gallstone ileus. CT has been shown to have a diagnostic sensitivity of 93% and a specificity of 100% [25] with Rigler's triad being identified in approximately 78% of patients [9, 15, 26–30] (Fig. 13.3). CT's improved diagnostic accuracy has assisted with decreasing the delay

in diagnosis and improving the historically high mortality rates [9, 15, 20, 30, 31]. Additionally, CT has an added advantage of inspection for other intra-abdominal pathology, assisting with localization of the site of obstruction and surgical planning and identification of concomitant stones that occur in 10–12% of patients and evaluating for associated intestinal ischemia.

Management

Resuscitation and relieving the obstruction in gallstone ileus are the primary goals of initial treatment. For most patients, this will require an urgent operation, but the exact method of intervention to relieve the obstruction and the need to address the fistula during the index operation is still being debated in the literature.

Enterolithotomy

The enterotomy for stone extraction is typically made >30 cm proximal to the site of obstruction to avoid any edema or inflammation around the site of the impaction. The enterotomy incision is made in a longitudinal fashion on the antimesenteric side of the bowel and closed in a transverse fashion, to avoid narrowing the lumen [5]. The exception to this is when the obstructed segment is ischemic or perforated which would require resection. Attempts should not be made to crush the gallstone in situ as this is more likely to damage the bowel wall than achieve meaningful results in relieving the obstruction or allowing distal passage of the stone [4]. During this operation, the entire small bowel should also be evaluated as there is a 5–10% rate of concomitant stones [32] (Fig. 13.4).

Fistula Closure

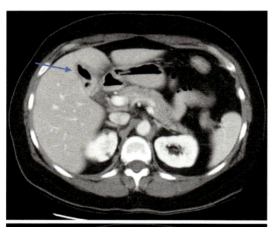
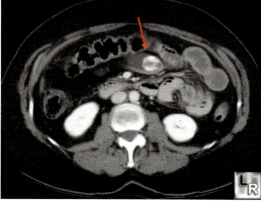

Fig. 13.3 *Pneumobilia (blue arrow), impacted gallstone (red arrow)

Fistula closure at the time of the index operation or as a second operation was historically controversial. Proponents for fistula closure cite less future biliary complications (cholecystitis and

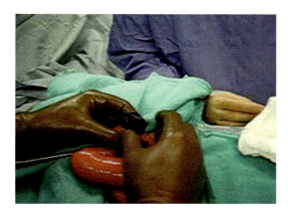

Fig. 13.4 Photo of enterolithotomy stone extraction

cholangitis), less recurrence, and concern for the presence or development of gallbladder carcinoma [33, 34]. Advocates against fistula closure cite that the gallbladder is typically shrunken down with significant pericholecystic inflammation, fibrosis, and distortion of biliary anatomy that increases the difficulty/complexity of both cholecystectomy and fistula repair and increases the chance of a common bile duct injury. Additionally, the inflamed tissue is at greater risk of postoperative leak after closure. Finally, enterolithotomy alone has a significantly shorter operative time which is essential in this typically debilitated infirmed patient who often presents with significant dehydration, possible shock, and multiple comorbidities.

A 40-year historical review (1953–1993) of 1001 patients by Reisner et al. showed a lower mortality rate with enterolithotomy alone (11.6%) vs 16.7% for those who underwent concomitant fistula closure [3]. Eighty percent of patients in the Reisner study were treated with enterolithotomy alone and 11% with enterolithotomy, cholecystectomy, and primary fistula closure. This mortality benefit for enterolithotomy alone was also supported by other smaller case series in those patients who are critically ill or elderly with significant comorbidities [35, 36]. Halabi et al. used the National Inpatient Sample in 2014 [2] to study 3268 cases of gallstone ileus from 2005 to 2009. In this cohort, 62% underwent enterolithotomy only, 19% underwent closure of the fistula tract, and 19%

underwent small bowel resection. The overall mortality rate was 6.7% with a significantly higher odds of mortality among those patients who underwent primary fistula closure (OR 2.86) and bowel resection (OR 2.96) after multivariate analysis.

In a 2013 NSQIP evaluation, Mallipeddi et al. evaluated 127 patients who were treated from 2005 to 2010. Seventy-four percent of patients underwent small bowel enterolithotomy, and 11% underwent an accompanying cholecystectomy with presumed fistula repair. They noted an overall morbidity of 35.4% and a mortality of 5.5% for all 127 patients and no significant difference in mortality with the addition of the cholecystectomy (5.3% vs 7.1%). The morbidity rate however was nearly double in those who underwent cholecystectomy (50% vs 25.7%, OR 3.52 $p = 0.04$).

Doko et al. evaluated a one-staged approach with primary fistula repair vs enterolithotomy alone in 30 patients over a 16-year period. They also found that mortality was comparable at 11% and 9%, respectively, but both operative duration was longer (40 min vs 140 min) and so were perioperative complication rates (61% vs 27%). Fistula closure remained associated with increased rate of postoperative complications even after multivariate adjustment for age, operative time, and duration of symptoms before hospitalization.

Recurrence

Overall 33–50% of patients who undergo enterolithotomy alone will have no further symptoms or recurrence, even without addressing the fistula [4, 5, 37]. Recurrence rates for gallstone ileus are 5–10% [3, 4, 8, 38, 39], 50% of which occur within the first 30 days postoperatively [40] with the majority of these being from secondary stones that were not identified at the time of the initial enterolithotomy [41]. Furthermore, of those with recurrence, only 10% require a subsequent operation [3]. Most (~80%) biliary fistulas shrink and close spontaneously without residual stones [3, 42].

Colonic Obstruction

Cases of colonic obstruction often occur in the sigmoid colon and is secondary to a cholecysto-colonic fistula or the rare passage of the stone past the ileocecal valve and an obstruction at the site of a diverticular, inflammatory, or malignant stricture [4, 43]. Often these patients will present with significant steatorrhea, weight loss, and fat-soluble vitamin deficiencies and have an increased rate of cholangitis. In these cases, sigmoid resection removing both the gallstone and the underlying stenosis and cholecystectomy with fistula repair is advocated [4]. In those patients without significant choleric enteropathy, only sigmoid resection is advocated.

Laparoscopic Intervention

Laparoscopic diagnosis and management of gallstone ileus has been described more recently in case reports and limited case series. Mongomery et al. first published his two cases of laparoscopic treatment of gallstone ileus in 1993 [44]. Both cases were in patients without a history of prior abdominal operations and were diagnosed laparoscopically. Only one of the patients had pneumobilia noted prior to surgery. Montgomery was able to successfully run the bowel and identify the point of obstruction at the terminal ileum. In both patients, a small laparotomy incision was made to externalize the small bowel to perform the enterolithotomy and primary closure extracorporeally. A cholecystectomy and fistula repair was not performed in either patient. No recurrence occurred in the subsequent 4-month follow-up period. Franklin et al. in 1994 described the first laparoscopic single-stage treatment of gallstone ileus with enterolithotomy and cholecystectomy with repair of the biliary fistula at the time of the initial operation [45]. However, given the higher rate of morbidity and mortality associated with addressing both the obstruction and the chole-cystoenteric fistula, most have not advocated for a laparoscopic single-stage approach.

Since those initial publications in the early 1990s, multiple other case reports and small case series have been published supporting either the more common laparoscopic-assisted enterolithotomy [46, 47] or a totally laparoscopic approach with intracorporeal stone extraction and enterotomy closure [48–50]. However, minimally invasive intervention for gallstone ileus remains infrequent with only about 10% of patients under laparoscopic treatment nationally, with a conversion to open rate of greater than 50% [2].

Advantages of the laparoscopic approach parallel those of other laparoscopic vs open procedure comparisons – shorter recovery period, decreased rate of wound infection, and decreased rate of incisional hernia. Challenges during laparoscopic intervention include concomitant comorbidities that may limit a patient's ability to tolerate pneumoperitoneum or a longer operation and a delayed presentation that can lead to dilated and edematous bowel that increases both the risk of laparoscopic entry and bowel manipulation. Furthermore, given the approximately 5% risk of additional stones [32], it is essential to complete a thorough evaluation of the remaining bowel which can be challenging without significant laparoscopic experience.

Thus, while laparoscopic management is technically feasible with lower rates of wound infection and earlier postoperative recovery, proper patient selection is key. In the cases reported, most of those undergoing laparoscopic intervention for gallstone ileus have less comorbidities, less bowel dilation, and no prior abdominal operations.

Endoscopic Therapy

Endoscopic extraction in gallstone ileus has also been described as a viable alternative to surgical intervention [51, 52]. Endoscopy has been used for either primary stone extraction or combined with different forms of lithotripsy with an overall success rate of approximately 10% [53–55]. The low overall success rate has been attributed to migration of the stone, failed lithotripsy, or secondary obstruction from large stone fragments after lithotripsy [55]. Endoscopic therapy has often reserved for those who are not operative candidates or those with proximal stones that cause gastric outlet (Bouveret Syndrome) or duodenal obstruction [53, 54, 56–58]. More distal stones have also been successfully treated using double balloon endoscopy [51], extracorporeal shockwave lithotripsy [52, 57] or colonic endoscopic mechanical lithotripsy [59]. Endoscopic intervention should be considered for those patients with an identified gallstone in an amenable location or in high-risk surgical candidates, but patients should be counseled that surgical intervention may still be necessary in the majority of cases.

Perioperative Complications

In recent studies, the rate of postoperative complications remains high in those patients undergoing surgery for gallstone ileus, ranging from 35% to 64% [2, 4, 10, 60]. Wound infection is the most common complication after surgery for gallstone ileus in most studies, occurring in 27–42% of patients in modern series [4, 10, 61] and 75% historically [1, 42]. Other common postoperative complications are acute renal failure, which has been seen in up to 30% of patients, followed by urinary tract infection (13%), ileus (13%), anastomotic leak, intra-abdominal abscess, enteric fistula (12%), and pneumonia (3%) [2]. Major complications (wound dehiscence, unplanned reintubation, myocardial infarction, stroke, septic shock) can occur in approximately 13% of patients [10]. While some series report no significant differences of postoperative complications between those patients treated by enterolithotomy or enterolithotomy, cholecystectomy, and fistula closure [32, 37, 62], both national evaluations by Halabi et al. Mallipeddi et al., have reported higher rates in those undergoing single-stage procedures with Mallipeddi et al. reporting rates of 27% vs 50% (Odds Ratio 3.58).

Recommendations

Only a handful of large studies have been done evaluating the management of gallstone ileus, and these are all retrospective in nature. The remaining studies are single institution limited case series. Thus, high-quality data is lacking; however, given the low incidence of gallstone ileus, this will likely continue to be a challenge. Surgical intervention remains the standard of care treatment for gallstone ileus. Based on the studies that have been done, we recommend that all patients with gallstone ileus undergo urgent enterolithotomy alone after adequate resuscitation, through a laparotomy for the majority of patients. We recommend against consideration of biliary fistula takedown at the primary operation or subsequently unless patients have gallbladder necrosis at the time of the initial operation, suffer from significant malabsorption issues and weight loss or develop recurrent obstruction, cholecystitis or cholangitis. Endoscopic lithotripsy can be considered for those with proximal obstruction or those who are nonoperative candidates. With careful patient selection and laparoscopic expertise, minimally invasive enterolithotomy alone may also be a treatment option.

References

1. Deitz DM, Standage BA, Pinson CW, McConnell DB, Krippaehne WW. Improving the outcome in gallstone ileus. Am J Surg. 1986;151(5):572–6.
2. Halabi WJ, Kang CY, Ketana N, Lafaro KJ, Nguyen VQ, Stamos MJ, Imagawa DK, Demirjian AN. Surgery for gallstone ileus: a nationwide comparison of trends and outcomes. Ann Surg. 2014;259(2):329–35.
3. Reisner RM, Cohen JR. Gallstone ileus: a review of 1001 reported cases. Am Surg. 1994;60(6):441–6.
4. Clavien PA, Richon J, Burgan S, Rohner A. Gallstone ileus. Br J Surg. 1990;77(7):737–42.
5. van Hillo M, van der Vliet JA, Wiggers T, Obertop H, Terpstra OT, Greep JM. Gallstone obstruction of the intestine: an analysis of ten patients and a review of the literature. Surgery. 1987;101(3):273–6.
6. Nuño-Guzmán CM. Gallstone ileus, clinical presentation, diagnostic and treatment approach. World J Gastrointest Surg. 2016;8(1):65–13.
7. Deckoff SL. Gallstone ileus; a report of 12 cases. Ann Surg. 1955;142(1):52–65.

8. Cooperman AM, Dickson ER, ReMine WH. Changing concepts in the surgical treatment of gallstone ileus: a review of 15 cases with emphasis on diagnosis and treatment. Ann Surg. 1968;167(3):377–83.

9. Ayantunde AA, Agrawal A. Gallstone ileus: diagnosis and management. World J Surg. 2007;31(6):1292–7.

10. Mallipeddi MK, Pappas TN, Shapiro ML, Scarborough JE. Gallstone ileus: revisiting surgical outcomes using National Surgical Quality Improvement Program data. J Surg Res. 2013;184(1):84–8.

11. Stinton LM, Shaffer EA. Epidemiology of gallbladder disease: cholelithiasis and cancer. Gut Liver. 2012;6(2):172–87.

12. Day EA, Marks C. Gallstone ileus. Review of the literature and presentation of thirty-four new cases. Am J Surg. 1975;129(5):552–8.

13. VanLandingham SB, Broders CW. Gallstone ileus. Surg Clin North Am. 1982;62(2):241–7.

14. Moss JF, Bloom AD, Mesleh GF, Deziel D, Hopkins WM. Gallstone ileus. Am Surg. 1987;53(8):424–8.

15. Chou J-W, Hsu C-H, Liao K-F, Lai H-C, Cheng K-S, Peng C-Y, Yang M-D, Chen Y-F. Gallstone ileus: report of two cases and review of the literature. World J Gastroenterol. 2007;13(8):1295–8.

16. Masannat Y, Masannat Y, Shatnawei A. Gallstone ileus: a review. Mt Sinai J Med. 2006;73(8):1132–4.

17. Rigler LG, Borman CN, Noble JF. Gallstone obstruction: pathogenesis and roentgen manifestations. J Am Med Assoc. 1941;117(21):1753–9.

18. Balthazar EJ, Schechter LS. Air in gallbladder: a frequent finding in gallstone ileus. AJR Am J Roentgenol. 1978;131(2):219–22.

19. Ripollés T, Miguel-Dasit A, Errando J, Morote V, Gómez-Abril SA, Richart J. Gallstone ileus: increased diagnostic sensitivity by combining plain film and ultrasound. Abdom Imaging. 2001;26(4):401–5.

20. Lassandro F, Gagliardi N, Scuderi M, Pinto A, Gatta G, Mazzeo R. Gallstone ileus analysis of radiological findings in 27 patients. Eur J Radiol. 2004;50(1):23–9.

21. Gaduputi V, Tariq H, Rahnemai-Azar AA, Dev A, Farkas DT. Gallstone ileus with multiple stones: where Rigler triad meets Bouveret's syndrome. World J Gastrointest Surg. 2015;7(12):394–7.

22. Wong CS, Crotty JM, Naqvi SA. Pneumobilia: a case report and literature review on its surgical approaches. J Surg Tech Case Rep. 2013;5(1):27–31.

23. Lasson A, Lorén I, Nilsson A, Nirhov N, Nilsson P. Ultrasonography in gallstone ileus: a diagnostic challenge. Eur J Surg. 1995;161(4):259–63.

24. Davies RJ, Sandrasagra FA, Joseph AE. Case report: ultrasound in the diagnosis of gallstone ileus. Clin Radiol. 1991;43(4):282–4.

25. Yu CY, Lin CC, Shyu RY, Hsieh CB, Wu HS, Tyan YS, Hwang JI, Liou CH, Chang WC, Chen CY. Value of CT in the diagnosis and management of gallstone ileus. World J Gastroenterol. 2005;11(14):2142–7.

26. Kirchmayr W, Mühlmann G, Zitt M, Bodner J, Weiss H, Klaus A. Gallstone ileus: rare and still controversial. ANZ J Surg. 2005;75(4):234–8.

27. Lassandro F, Romano S, Ragozzino A, Rossi G, Valente T, Ferrara I, Romano L, Grassi R. Role of helical CT in diagnosis of gallstone ileus and related conditions. AJR Am J Roentgenol. 2005;185(5):1159–65.

28. Lorén I, Lasson A, Nilsson A, Nilsson P, Nirhov N. Gallstone ileus demonstrated by CT. J Comput Assist Tomogr. 1994;18(2):262–5.

29. Swift SE, Spencer JA. Gallstone ileus: CT findings. Clin Radiol. 1998;53(6):451–4.

30. Reimann AJ, Yeh BM, Breiman RS, Joe BN, Qayyum A, Coakley FV. Atypical cases of gallstone ileus evaluated with multidetector computed tomography. J Comput Assist Tomogr. 2004;28(4):523–7.

31. Delabrousse E, Bartholomot B, Sohm O, Wallerand H, Kastler B. Gallstone ileus: CT findings. Eur Radiol. 2000;10(6):938–40.

32. Rodríguez-Sanjuán JC, Casado F, Fernández MJ, Morales DJ, Naranjo A. Cholecystectomy and fistula closure versus enterolithotomy alone in gallstone ileus. Br J Surg. 1997;84(5):634–7.

33. Berliner SD, Burson LC. One-stage repair for cholecyst-duodenal fistula and gallstone ileus. Arch Surg. 1965;90:313–6.

34. Warshaw AL, Bartlett MK. Choice of operation for gallstone intestinal obstruction. Ann Surg. 1966;164(6):1051–5.

35. Kasahara Y, Umemura H, Shiraha S, Kuyama T, Sakata K, Kubota H. Gallstone ileus. Review of 112 patients in the Japanese literature. Am J Surg. 1980;140(3):437–40.

36. Muthukumarasamy G, Venkata SP, Shaikh IA, Somani BK, Ravindran R. Gallstone ileus: surgical strategies and clinical outcome. J Dig Dis. 2008;9(3):156–61.

37. Tan YM, Wong WK, Ooi LLPJ. A comparison of two surgical strategies for the emergency treatment of gallstone ileus. Singap Med J. 2004;45(2):69–72.

38. Haq AU, Morris AH, Daintith H. Recurrent gall-stone ileus. Br J Radiol. 1981;54(647):1000–1.

39. Levin B, Shapiro RA. Recurrent enteric gallstone obstruction. Gastrointest Radiol. 1980;5(2):151–3.

40. Doogue MP, Choong CK, Frizelle FA. Recurrent gallstone ileus: underestimated. Aust N Z J Surg. 1998;68(11):755–6.

41. Mir SA, Hussain Z, Davey CA, Miller GV, Chintapatla S. Management and outcome of recurrent gallstone ileus: a systematic review. World J Gastrointest Surg. 2015;7(8):152–9.

42. Raiford TS. Intestinal obstruction caused by gallstones. Am J Surg. 1962;104:383–94.

43. Anseline P. Colonic gall-stone ileus. Postgrad Med J. 1981;57(663):62–5.

44. Montgomery A. Laparoscope-guided enterolithotomy for gallstone ileus. Surg Laparosc Endosc. 1993;3(4):310–4.

45. Franklin ME Jr, Dorman JP, Schuessler WW. Laparoscopic treatment of gallstone ileus: a case report and review of the literature. J Laparoendosc Surg. 1994;4(4):265–72.

46. Moberg AC, Montgomery A. Laparoscopically assisted or open enterolithotomy for gallstone ileus. Br J Surg. 2007;94(1):53–7.

47. Allen JW, McCurry T, Rivas H, Cacchione RN. Totally laparoscopic management of gallstone ileus. Surg Endosc. 2003;17(2):352.

48. Owera A, Low J, Ammori BJ. Laparoscopic enterolithotomy for gallstone ileus. Surg Laparosc Endosc Percutan Tech. 2008;18(5):450–2.

49. Sesti J, Okoro C, Parikh M. Laparoscopic enterolithotomy for gallstone ileus. J Am Coll Surg. 2013;217(2):e13–5.

50. Behrens C, Amson B. Laparoscopic management of multiple gallstone ileus. Surg Laparosc Endosc Percutan Tech. 2010;20(2):e64–5.

51. Kim YG, Byeon J-S, Lee SK, Yang D-H, Kim K-J, Ye BD, Myung S-J, Yang S-K, Kim J-H. Gallstone ileus successfully treated with endoscopic fragmentation by using double-balloon endoscopy (with video). Gastrointest Endosc. 2011;74(1):228–30.

52. Muratori R, Cennamo V, Menna M, Cecinato P, Eusebi LH, Mazzella G, Bazzoli F. Colonic gallstone ileus treated with radiologically guided extracorporeal shock wave lithotripsy followed by endoscopic extraction. Endoscopy. 2012;44(Suppl 2 UCTN (S 02)):E88–9.

53. Fujita N, Noda Y, Kobayashi G, Kimura K, Watanabe H, Shirane A, Hayasaka T, Mochizuki F, Yamazaki T. Gallstone ileus treated by electrohydraulic lithotripsy. Gastrointest Endosc. 1992;38(5):617–9.

54. Sackmann M, Holl J, Haerlin M, Sauerbruch T, Hoermann R, Heinkelein J, Paumgartner G. Gallstone ileus successfully treated by shock-wave lithotripsy. Dig Dis Sci. 1991;36(12):1794–5.

55. Lowe AS, Stephenson S, Kay CL, May J. Duodenal obstruction by gallstones (Bouveret's syndrome): a review of the literature. Endoscopy. 2005;37(1):82–7.

56. Bourke MJ, Schneider DM, Haber GB. Electrohydraulic lithotripsy of a gallstone causing gallstone ileus. Gastrointest Endosc. 1997;45(6):521–3.

57. Meyenberger C, Michel C, Metzger U, Koelz HR. Gallstone ileus treated by extracorporeal shockwave lithotripsy. Gastrointest Endosc. 1996;43(5):508–11.

58. Oakland DJ, Denn PG. Endoscopic diagnosis of gallstone ileus of the duodenum. Dig Dis Sci. 1986;31(1):98–9.

59. Zielinski MD, Ferreira LE, Baron TH. Successful endoscopic treatment of colonic gallstone ileus using electrohydraulic lithotripsy. World J Gastroenterol. 2010;16(12):1533–6.

60. Doko M, Zovak M, Kopljar M, Glavan E, Ljubicic N, Hochstädter H. Comparison of surgical treatments of gallstone ileus: preliminary report. World J Surg. 2003;27(4):400–4.

61. Rodríguez Hermosa JI, Codina Cazador A, Gironès Vilà J, Roig García J, Figa Francesch M, Acero Fernández D. Gallstone ileus: results of analysis of a series of 40 patients. Gastroenterol Hepatol. 2001;24(10):489–94.

62. Martinez Ramos D, Daroca Jose JM, Escrig Sos J, Paiva Coronel G, Alcalde Sanchez M, Salvador Sanchis JL. Gallstone ileus: management options and results on a series of 40 patients. Rev Esp Enferm Dig. 2009;101(2):117–20. 121-114.

63. Corvera CU, Reza JA. Chapter 42: Biliary fistulae and strictures A2. In: Jarnagin WR, editor. Blumgart's surgery of the liver, biliary tract and pancreas, 2-volume set. 6th ed. Philadelphia; 2017. p. 675–713.e679.

Acute Pancreatitis

14

Marc D. Trust, C. Yvonne Chung,
and Carlos V. R. Brown

Introduction

Acute pancreatitis is inflammation of the pancreas that may in turn lead to systemic inflammatory response and multi-organ dysfunction and failure. The spectrum of disease ranges from mild and self-limiting in the majority of patients to severe with multi-organ system failure and potential death. The disease accounts for 275,000 hospital admissions and $2.5 billion in healthcare costs yearly with increasing incidence in population-based studies [1, 2]. The rising incidence of acute pancreatitis is likely related to the growing obesity epidemic contributing to gallstone disease. Additionally, a nationwide database review also attributes the increase in acute pancreatitis hospital admissions to dramatic increase in chronic pancreatitis-related acute pancreatitis [3].

Despite increasing incidence of the disease, the associated mortality has decreased over time with the latest estimated overall mortality of 2%. Risk factors associated with increasing mortality are elderly age; presence of comorbidities, in particularly morbid obesity; hospital-acquired infections; and severe acute pancreatitis [1].

Etiology

The most common cause of acute pancreatitis is gallstone disease followed by alcohol [1, 2, 4]. Choledocholithiasis leads to obstruction of the pancreatic duct which results in blockage of pancreatic enzymes resulting in the acute inflammatory event. Alcohol, on the other hand, causes acute and chronic pancreatitis, and the mechanism involves both direct toxicity and an immunologic mechanism [5]. Diabetes and morbid obesity are both risk factors for acute pancreatitis [1]. A myriad of medications have also been implicated to cause acute pancreatitis, though the precise culprit drug is often impossible to identify. Genetic mutations and polymorphisms have also been linked with acute and chronic pancreatitis [1]. The exact cause of acute pancreatitis in some patients may be unknown, and the prevalence of idiopathic acute pancreatitis increases with patient age.

Epidemiologically, the risk of acute pancreatitis increases with age [6]. In men, acute pancreatitis is more likely to be related to alcohol, while in women it is more likely to be related to gallstones, endoscopic retrograde cholangiopancreatography (ERCP), autoimmune disorders, or idiopathic.

M. D. Trust (✉) · C. Y. Chung · C. V. R. Brown
Department of Surgery and Perioperative Care, Dell
Medical School at The University of Texas Austin,
Dell Seton Medical Center at The University of Texas,
Austin, TX, USA
e-mail: mdtrust@ascension.org

The incidence of acute pancreatitis in the pediatric patient population, though uncommon, is also found to be rising, though this may be related to the increasing use of serum tests in emergency department workups [7].

Diagnosis

The diagnosis of acute pancreatitis is made by meeting two of the three criteria: (1) clinical symptoms consistent with acute pancreatitis (e.g., acute epigastric abdominal pain), (2) serum lipase or amylase at least three times the normal limit, and (3) imaging findings characteristic of pancreatitis, most commonly on computer tomography [8]. It is important to note that roughly one in ten patients with acute pancreatitis can have normal serum amylase and lipase [9].

Initial evaluation of patients with acute pancreatitis should include detailed medical history, physical exam, routine laboratory serum tests, and abdominal imaging to evaluate for most common etiologies of pancreatitis. For patients with recurrent bouts of idiopathic pancreatitis, endoscopic ultrasound (EUS) may be reasonable to evaluate for biliary microlithiasis, neoplasm, and underlying chronic pancreatitis. The diagnostic yield of EUS as part of the evaluation for first or second admission for idiopathic acute pancreatitis was found to range from 32% to 88% in a systematic review [10].

By the most recent international consensus update on classifications and definitions related to acute pancreatitis, there are two types of acute pancreatitis: interstitial edematous pancreatitis and necrotizing pancreatitis [8]. The majority of patients with acute pancreatitis develop interstitial edematous pancreatitis, which is diffuse inflammatory edema involving the entire pancreas. Necrotizing pancreatitis develops in 5–10% of patients with necrosis of pancreatic parenchyma and/or peripancreatic tissue. Pancreatic and peripancreatic necrosis may remain sterile or become infected, which significantly increased morbidity and mortality, as prompt diagnosis and treatment are critical.

There are two phases of disease course – early and late – each with its corresponding mortality peaks [8]. The early phase lasts the 1–2 weeks and consists of the patient's systemic response – a constellation of symptoms and physiologic findings termed systemic inflammatory response syndrome (SIRS) – in reaction to pancreatic injury. Late phase of acute pancreatitis follows the acute phase and may last weeks to months. It is characterized by persistence of systemic inflammation and by the evolution of local complications [8]. Furthermore, the presence of necrosis or local complications may not yet be apparent on initial imaging, but their identification is not necessary during this phase. Repeat imaging is typically not necessary until approximately 1 week after admission, as local complications identified in this timeframe typically do not require treatment. In the late phase, systemic manifestations secondary to SIRS will continue, and local complications will also evolve.

Severity Classification

The original Atlanta classification of severity in 1992 [11] stratified severity into two categories, mild and severe, with severe pancreatitis characterized by organ failure and/or local complications. Over the next two decades, it was recognized that outcomes varied greatly depending on both the duration of organ failure and severity of local complications [12]. Because of these observations, the classification system was later amended into the 2012 revised Atlanta classification (Table 14.1) [8]. While mild disease was still characterized as lacking organ failure and any local or systemic complications, a new category of "moderately severe" was added. Moderately severe acute pancreatitis is characterized by local or systemic complications with transient (<48 h) organ failure. Severe acute pancreatitis is characterized by persistent organ failure, either single or multi-system, lasting more than 48 h [8]. Patients initially presenting with mild acute pancreatitis may worsen and thus should be evaluated daily as the disease course evolves and progresses.

Table 14.1 Severity of pancreatitis based on the revised Atlanta classification of 2012 [8] (transient < 48 h, persistent ≥ 48 h)

Severity	Organ failure	Local complications	Systemic complications
Mild	None	None	None
Moderately severe	Transient	+/−	+/−
Severe	Persistent	+/−	+/−

Table 14.2 Modified Marshall scoring system [8]

Organ system	0	1	2	3	4
Respiratory (PaO2/FiO2)	>400	301–400	201–300	101–200	≤100
Renal (serum creatinine, (mg/dl)	<1.4	1.4–1.8	1.9–3.6	3.6–4.9	>4.9
Cardiac (systolic blood pressure)	>90	<90, FR	<90, NFR	<90, pH <7.3	<90, pH <7.2

FR fluid responsive, *NFR* not fluid responsive

Both moderately severe and severe pancreatitis can manifest local and/or systemic complications. Local complications include pancreatic and peripancreatic fluid collections, gastric outlet dysfunctions, splenic and portal vein thrombosis, and colonic necrosis. Systemic complications are defined as the exacerbation of a pre-existing comorbidity secondary to the pancreatitis.

Published just prior to the revised Atlanta classification, the determinant-based classification system is slightly more extensive, including four categories of severity. Each category is also stratified based on the presence of local and/or systemic factors. Local determinants include the presence of pancreatic or peripancreatic necrosis, either sterile or infected, and systemic determinants include either transient or persistent organ failure. Mild pancreatitis lacks both local and systemic determinants while moderate pancreatitis is defined by the presence of either sterile necrosis and/or transient organ failure. Severe pancreatitis is defined by infected necrosis or persistent organ failure, while critical pancreatitis includes both infected necrosis and persistent organ failure [13]. Note that there is no incorporation of pre-existing comorbidities.

Despite the implications that local complications may have on treatment, it cannot be emphasized enough that organ failure is key determinant of severity. Furthermore, the extent of local complications does not correlate with the severity of pancreatitis. Organ systems of particular interest include the cardiac, respiratory, and renal system. Current guidelines recommend the use of the modified Marshal scoring system (Table 14.2) [8], in which each organ system is given a score based on varying degrees of dysfunction. A score of two or higher indicates organ failure for that particular system, and failure of at least two systems is considered multi-organ failure (MOF).

The American Association for the Surgery of Trauma (AAST) has expanded their scoring system of traumatic injuries to various organ systems to include emergency general surgery conditions. For acute pancreatitis, the scoring is graded from I to V, with each increasing grade signifying more severe disease. Grade I is limited to findings of mild edematous pancreatitis, while grade V involves findings such as extra-pancreatic involvement of necrosis such as colonic necrosis. This grading system defines clinical, imaging, operative, and pathologic criteria for each grade, allowing clinicians to appropriately grade the disease given various findings [14].

Severity Prognostication

Factors associated with increased mortality and complications include older age (>60 years), severe coexisting conditions, obesity, and chronic heavy alcohol use [1, 6]. Numerous scoring systems have been developed as models to predict the severity of disease progression, the earliest being Ranson's criteria introduced in 1974

(Table 14.3). However, these all are highly imperfect and subject to high false-positive rates, since the vast majority of patients do not develop severe acute pancreatitis.

In a single-institution comparison of Ranson's criteria, APACHE II, BISAP, Balthazar CTSI, and initial and 24-h C-reactive protein (CRP) using prospectively collective clinical data, the APACHE II was shown to have the highest accuracy in predicting severe pancreatitis. However, there was no statistical significance between paired comparisons between the APACHE II and the other scoring systems [21]. The BISAP was demonstrated to have similar accuracy of predicting development of severe acute pancreatitis to Ranson's,

APACHE II, and CTSI in a separate comparison [22]. Despite a myriad of severity scoring systems and painstaking comparisons, no one system has been demonstrated as clearly superior in predicting persistent organ failure in acute pancreatitis. The accuracy of scoring systems may improve when used in combination, but the cumbersome nature of most scoring system prohibits their widespread clinical use [23]. Despite these various models, current guidelines suggest that the best prognostication is highly reliant on clinician judgment and should include multi-dimensional approach to include baseline patient risk factors and comorbidities, risk stratification, and objective clinical response to initial therapy [24].

Table 14.3 Various acute pancreatitis severity prognostication scoring systems [15–20]

Scoring system, year	Components	Notes

Ranson criteria, 1974	On admission:
	  Age > 55
	  WBC > 16 K
	  Glucose >200 mg/dL
	  AST >250
	  LDH > 350
	At 48 h after admission:
	  Hct drop >10% from admit
	  BUN increase >5 mg/dL
	  Ca <8
	  Arterial pO2 < 60 mmHg
	  Base deficit >4
	  Fluid needs >6 L
		Requires 48 h for full score

Ranson criteria, modified for biliary pancreatitis, 1979	On admission:
	  Age > 70
	  WBC >18 K
	  Glucose >220
	  LDH > 400
	  AST >500
	At 48 h after admission:
	  Hct drop >10% from admit
	  BUN increase >2 mg/100 ml
	  Ca < 8
	  Base deficit >5
	  Fluid sequestration >4 L
		Requires 48 h for full score

Glasgow-Imrie, 1984	Age > 55 WBC >15 Blood glucose >10 mmol/L BUN >16 PaO2 < 60 mmHg Ca <2.0 mmol/L Albumin < 32 g/L LDH > 600 AST/ALT > 100	Requires 48 h of data for peak values

Table 14.3 (continued)

Scoring system, year	Components	Notes
APACHE II, 1989	History of severe organ failure or immunocompromised Acute renal failure Age Temperature Mean arterial pressure pH Heart rate Resp rate Na K Cr Hct WBC GCS	Estimates ICU mortality. Calculated within 24 h of ICU admission
CT severity index, 1990	Grading of pancreatitis (Balthazar score) 　A, normal pancreas: 0 　B, enlargement of pancreas: 1 　C, inflammatory changes in pancreas and 　　peripancreatic fat: 2 　D, ill-defined single peripancreatic fluid collection: 3 　E, two or more poorly defined peripancreatic fluid 　　collections: 4 Pancreatic necrosis 　None: 0 　≤30%: 2 　>30–50%: 4 　>50%: 6	Max score 10 0–3: mild AP 4–6: moderate AP 7–10: severe AP Does not account for systemic complications and organ failure Subject to inter-observer variability in interpretation
Modified CTSI, 2004	Pancreatic inflammation 　0: normal pancreas 　2: intrinsic pancreatic abnormalities with or without 　　inflammatory changes in peripancreatic fat 　4: pancreatic or peripancreatic fluid collection or 　　peripancreatic fat necrosis Pancreatic necrosis 　0: none 　2: 30% or less 　4: more than 30% Extrapancreatic complications 　2: one or more of pleural effusion, ascites, vascular 　　complications, parenchymal complications, and/or 　　gastrointestinal involvement	Max score 10 0–2: mild AP 4–6: moderate AP 8–10: severe AP
BISAP, 2008	BUN > 25 Impaired mental status 2 SIRS criteria or more Age > 60 Pleural effusion present	Calculated within 24 h of admission

Management

Management of acute pancreatitis should include accurate and timely diagnosis and triage, appropriate level of supportive care, monitoring and treatment of complications, and prevention of recurrence. For all forms of acute pancreatitis, supportive care is the mainstay of treatment. Patients with diagnosed or predicted moderately severe or severe acute pancreatitis should be admitted to an intensive care unit for appropriate monitoring and care. Adequate analgesia should be initiated. Parenteral opioid agents are often selected and, in a systematic database review, are found to decrease the need for supplemental analgesia [25]. Patients in respiratory failure should be managed with intubation and mechanical ventilation. Acute respiratory distress syndrome (ARDS) may be associated with the massive systemic inflammatory cascade brought by severe pancreatitis, and patients suspected to be in ARDS should be managed with lung-protective ventilation strategies with lower tidal volume, higher PEEP, and limiting inspiratory pressures [26].

Fluid Resuscitation

Because of the gastrointestinal fluid loss from emesis and poor oral intake as well as the severe inflammatory cascade and third spacing of fluids brought on by severe pancreatitis, these patients typically present in a hypovolemic state. They should be carefully assessed for signs of hypovolemia such as physical findings of dehydration, oliguria, hemoconcentration, and azotemia. While the data surrounding resuscitation is mixed, guidelines recommend that patients with these findings should be aggressively hydrated with intravenous fluids early on in their hospital course. A starting rate of infusion from 5 to 10 ml/kg/h is appropriate; however, the ideal duration of this rate of aggressive resuscitation is not yet known. There are, however, studies in the literature that have reported negative outcomes associated with aggressive hydration [27, 28], and because of these recent attention has been placed on goal-directed resuscitation using vital signs, laboratory values, and invasive cardiac parameters such as stroke volume variation to guide the need for continued aggressive resuscitation (Table 14.4) [24, 29, 30]. Regarding the choice of optimal resuscitation

Table 14.4 Goal-directed resuscitation end points [24, 29, 30]

Variable	Goal Value
Heart rate	<120 beats per minute
Mean arterial pressure	65–85 mmHg
Urine output	0.5–1.0 mL/kg/h
Hematocrit	35–44%, downtrending
Blood urea nitrogen	Downtrending
Stroke volume variation	<10–12%

fluid, crystalloid solution is preferred over colloids, with lactated ringers being the recommended crystalloid of choice.

Nutrition

In mild pancreatitis, oral feeding may be safely resumed upon improvement in abdominal pain, nausea, and laboratory markers. Randomized controlled trials have demonstrated safety in resuming a full diet, bypassing liquid or soft diets, as well as in initiating feeding without normalization of serum lipase level [31, 32]. In patients with severe pancreatitis, current guidelines based on moderate quality evidence recommend early (within 48 h of admission) enteral nutrition over delaying nutrition or initiation of parenteral nutrition [24]. This has been shown to decrease systemic infections, multi-organ failure, need for surgical interventions, and mortality. The mechanism behind this benefit is thought to be that early enteral nutrition prevents bacterial translocation. Administration of nutrition via the nasogastric route or orally is also safe, although patients may develop delayed emptying secondary to the pancreatitis and may not tolerate gastric nutrition. Parenteral nutrition (TPN) should only be used if enteral routes are not tolerated; however, current American Society for Parenteral and Enteral Nutrition (ASPEN) guidelines recommend waiting at last 7 days before initiation of TPN for patients at low risk of malnutrition [33].

Antibiotics

Previous literature suggested that the use of prophylactic antibiotics would prevent the onset of infection in necrotic tissue; however, the existing literature has not shown this to be true. A 2011 meta-analysis of 14 randomized controlled trials failed to show a reduction in mortality, pancreatic infection, or need for interventions with the use of prophylactic antibiotics [34]. Current guidelines recommend only using antibiotics for infected necrosis proven by FNA and culture or suspected infection based on imaging findings

[24]. According to the Infectious Disease Society of America guidelines on intra-abdominal infection, agents such as carbapenems or piparcillin-tazobactam that treat high-severity infections are the preferred agents [35].

Cholecystectomy

Patients with mild acute biliary pancreatitis should undergo laparoscopic cholecystectomy during the index admission. The safety and efficacy in preventing readmission for recurrent biliary pancreatitis of early cholecystectomy have been demonstrated in multiple systematic database reviews [36–38]. The timing of cholecystectomy for those with severe gallstone pancreatitis should be individualized based on clinical stability and possible local complication, such as the presence of peripancreatic fluid collections or necrosis.

Endoscopic Retrograde Cholangiopancreatography

Routine ERCP is not indicated in mild biliary pancreatitis in the absence of cholangitis or choledocholithiasis, as it does not significantly impact mortality and local or systemic complications [39]. In patients with cholangitis, ERCP is recommended within 24 h of admission: however, there is no strong evidence to support optimal timing of ERCP in patients without an urgent indication [24]. In those who do undergo ERCP with sphincterotomy, early cholecystectomy is still highly recommended as sphincterotomy prevents biliary pancreatitis but not other gallstone diseases such as cholecystitis or biliary colic.

Complications of Severe Pancreatitis

Infection

Infection in necrotic pancreatic tissue or the associated fluid collection is known to significantly increased morbidity and mortality. Typically, this

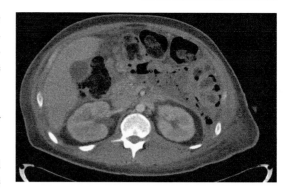

Fig. 14.1 Walled-off necrosis with gas in the fluid indicating infection

will manifest as a either an acute deterioration or failure to improve despite aggressive supportive care. Either of these two scenarios are an indication for repeat computed tomography imaging, as findings such as presence of gas within the pancreatic or peripancreatic tissue are sufficient to make the diagnosis of infection (Fig. 14.1). While routine image-guided percutaneous FNA of the necrotic tissue is not recommended, when infection is suspected although not clear based on imaging findings, sampling is then warranted to obtain gram stain and culture data to make a definitive diagnosis [8]. Once the diagnosis of infection is made, antibiotic therapy should be initiated, and interventions, either endoscopic or percutaneous, should be considered to obtain source control of the infected necrosis or fluid collections.

Fluid Collections

The revised 2012 Atlanta classification defines the various types of pancreatic fluid collections based on the morphological features of the parenchyma and the timing since the onset of pancreatitis (Table 14.5). Acute peripancreatic fluid collections are a complication of interstitial edematous pancreatitis, develop early, do not have a well-defined wall, and only contain fluid. In contrast, pancreatic pseudocysts (Fig. 14.2) have a well-defined wall and are present beyond 4 weeks after initial onset. They form as a result

Table 14.5 Pancreatic and peripancreatic fluid collections [8]

Morphology of pancreatitis	<4 weeks	>4 weeks
Interstitial edematous	Acute peripancreatic fluid collection	Pancreatic pseudocyst
Necrotizing	Acute necrotic collection	Walled-off necrosis

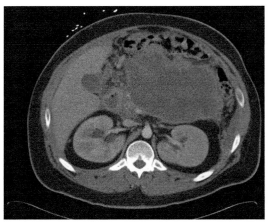

Fig. 14.3 Walled-off necrosis

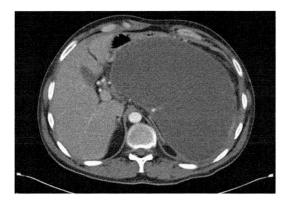

Fig. 14.2 Pancreatic pseudocyst

of leakage of pancreatic fluid from either main or branch ducts. Most importantly, to correctly be termed a pseudocyst, the collection should not contain any solid, necrotic material.

In the setting of necrotizing pancreatitis, acute necrotic collections arise early (<4 weeks) and contain both fluid and necrotic parenchyma or peripancreatic tissue and may be loculated. The presence of solid material is what differentiates this process from an acute peripancreatic fluid collection. Walled-off necrosis (Fig. 14.3) is a late phase (>4 weeks) entity with a well-defined wall. These too contain both fluid and solid contents consisting of necrotic pancreatic or peripancreatic tissue.

Abdominal Compartment Syndrome

Although many factors are associated with ACS, in patients with severe pancreatitis, the major pathophysiology results from inflammation and increased fluid within the peritoneal cavity secondary to this inflammation and massive fluid

administration. Intra-abdominal hypertension is defined as pressure greater than 12 mmHg, while abdominal compartment syndrome (ACS) is defined by persistent intra-abdominal pressure greater than 20 mmHg that is associated with new onset organ failure [24]. Typically, a firm, severely distended abdomen will be noted on physical exam, along with decreased urine output, hypotension, and/or difficultly with ventilation associated with elevated peak pressures if the patient is undergoing mechanical ventilation. Assessing bladder pressure provides an objective measurement of intra-abdominal pressure. Noninvasive management options include decompression of the intestines via nasogastric and rectal tube drainage, diuresis if volume overload is suspected, and measures to decrease abdominal wall tension such as adequate analgesia, sedation, and neuromuscular blockade. Decompressive laparotomy via a midline incision is the mainstay of invasive treatment, and although other options including percutaneous catheter drainage of ascites exist, laparotomy should be used in overt cases of ACS [40]. It cannot be stressed enough that in the acute setting, in the absence of infected pancreatic necrosis, no debridement should be attempted during surgical intervention for decompression. Doing so risks unnecessary complications such as inducing infection to sterile necrotic tissues, hemorrhage, and debridement of viable pancreatic tissue which may result in pancreatic insufficiency.

Hemorrhage

In the setting of acute pancreatitis, the release of pancreatic enzymes can have digestive effects on local tissue that result in hemorrhage from both pancreatic and peripancreatic tissue. Bleeding from small vessel can have local consequences; however, bleeding from major arterial complications such as a ruptured pseudoaneurysm may be fatal. Typically involving the splenic artery, pseudoaneurysms can also be seen in the gastroduodenal, pancreaticoduodenal, gastric, and hepatic arteries [41]. In the setting of acute hemorrhage, blood product resuscitation should be initiated and endovascular angioembolization should be attempted first in a stable patient. In an unstable patient not responsive to resuscitation, although open operations are associated with high morbidity and mortality in the setting of severe pancreatitis, surgical control of hemorrhage is required.

More commonly seen in chronic pancreatitis, mesenteric or portal vein thrombosis raise concern mostly for venous outflow obstruction causing mesenteric ischemia. Splenic vein thrombosis, however, can cause left-sided gastric varices that result in upper gastrointestinal hemorrhage. Endoscopic techniques typically can control acute hemorrhage, but a splenectomy is the treatment of choice to prevent recurrent bleeding episodes. Splenic artery angioembolization is also an option in a patient unfit for surgical intervention.

Interventions for Sterile Local Complications

Unlike infected necrosis and fluid collections, sterile processes do not require urgent intervention to mitigate the acute disease course. In fact, the vast majority of fluid collections will resolve spontaneously with conservative management. When these persist, however, they are associated with symptoms from gastric or biliary obstruction, bleeding, or may form pancreatic fistulae or ascites. While these issues indicate lack of resolution and warrant intervention, the most important factor in deciding to intervene is timing

from the initial episode. Interventions should not be attempted prior to 4–6 weeks. Traditionally managed with cystogastrostomy, endoscopic options have evolved to provide less invasive options for treatment of pseudocysts. One endoscopic option is transmural drainage, via either drainage or cystogastrostomy creation with an indwelling stent. Endoscopic ultrasound (EUS) is often used to verify cyst location and identify vascular structures to prevent hemorrhagic complications. Another option is transpapillary drainage which requires communication of the pseudocyst with the pancreatic duct. This relationship can be assessed with magnetic resonance cholangiopancreatography (MRCP) or ERCP, and, if present, a pancreatic duct stent will allow internal drainage and may negate the need for any further invasive intervention. If not amendable to endoscopic drainage or if these measures fail, surgical treatment with either a cystogastrostomy or cystojejunostomy is recommended. One randomized controlled trial of 40 patients showed similar success rates of endoscopic transmural drainage and surgical cystogastrostomy; however, surgical management was associated with longer hospital stay and higher cost [42]. This is promising for future treatment of pseudocysts; however, larger-scale data is needed to assess efficacy and, as this is an advanced endoscopic technique, may not be widely available.

Interventions for Infected Necrosis

Open pancreatic debridement or necrosectomy, once the standard of care, is associated with extremely high morbidity and mortality and has now widely been replaced by less invasive options. Indications for any intervention are limited to the presence of infection and need for source control to treat sepsis or failure to improve beyond approximately 4 weeks. This delay allows necrotic tissue to become a walled-off collection and also allows better visual differentiation of healthy pancreatic tissue. Unnecessary debridement of healthy pancreas helps avoid subsequent pancreatic insufficiency.

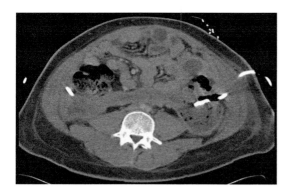

Fig. 14.4 Percutaneous drainage of infected fluid collection

Percutaneous Catheter Drainage

Image-guided percutaneous drainage of infected necrosis, acute necrotic collections, or walled-off necrosis should be the first step in management. These catheters are ideally placed via a retroperitoneal approach and in the subcostal position (Fig. 14.4). This will avoid peritoneal visceral complications, avoid violating the diaphragm and pleural space, and facilitate a step-up approach to debridement, which uses catheter guidance to locate collections needing debridement via less invasive approaches. These drains should be large bore to allow drainage of semisolid necrotic debris and prevent drain malfunction. If needed, drains can also be replaced for a larger caliber if patients fail to improve. Current guidelines are unable to recommend percutaneous drainage as a sole treatment modality as high-quality evidence comparing only drainage versus surgery is lacking [24, 43]. However, existing literature does show that a significant number of patients will improve with drainage alone and not require any further interventions. The best understood role of percutaneous drainage is allowing the delay of surgical intervention to a safer time in the course in the disease process, as well as facilitating less invasive debridement options when needed.

Endoscopic Debridement

With the growing range of endoscopic interventions, transmural endoscopic drainage and debridement of infected fluid collections and necrotic tissue became a possibility. This modality is useful when collections are immediately adjacent to the stomach or duodenum, however, may not be as successful when extensive peripancreatic and retroperitoneal debridement is required. Endoscopic ultrasound is an adjunct that can be used to help guide entry into the correct fluid collection as well identify major vascular structures to avoid hemorrhagic complications. In a low-powered randomized controlled study comparing endoscopic versus surgical debridement, either open or minimally invasive, patients who underwent endoscopic treatment had lower levels of inflammatory markers, post-procedural organ failure, and pancreatic fistulas and, however, did require more total procedures for adequate debridement [44]. This treatment option may be especially useful in patients with disconnected duct, allowing internal drainage of pancreatic fluid allowing fistulae to heal. Furthermore, endoscopic debridement can be combined with percutaneous drainage to further attempt to avoid unnecessary surgical intervention.

Minimally Invasive Necrosectomy

As mentioned previously, percutaneous and endoscopic interventions may not adequately treat the infection or control symptoms associated with extensive necrosis. When these options fail to achieve clinical improvement, more invasive measures debridement are indicated. Through a step-up approach, minimally invasive approaches such as video-assisted retroperitoneal debridement (VARD) are associated with better outcomes compared to open approaches. Most notably, a 2010 multicenter, randomized controlled trial showed a decrease in mortality or major complications from 69% to 40% in patients who were managed with a step-up and VARD approach [45]. Current guidelines further cite a three-fold reduction in organ failure and 50% reduction in mortality compared to open debridement [43].

Careful operative planning is key to prevention of iatrogenic complications. Imaging

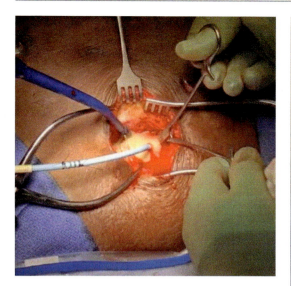

Fig. 14.5 Flank incision following percutaneous drain into the retroperitoneum

should be reviewed by the surgeon to identify the drain course in relation to necrotic collections requiring debridement, surrounding organs, and major vasculature. As drains are typically placed via the left, subcostal retroperitoneal approach, the patient is positioned in a right lateral decubitus position, although bilateral debridement may be necessary, in which case repositioning and repeat skin preparation may be necessary for debridement during a single operation. The supine position may also be used if bilateral debridement is required or if the patient's respiratory status will not tolerate lateral positioning. Using the previously placed percutaneous drains as a landmark, an approximately 5 cm skin incision is made in the flank and the drain is used to guide dissection into the retroperitoneum (Figs. 14.5, 14.6, 14.7, and 14.8). Any purulent fluid is evacuated and grossly necrotic tissues is gently debrided using ringed forceps. A laparoscopic port or camera directly through the incision are then inserted for deeper visualization of the retroperitoneal space and further debridement is done using forceps or a laparoscopic grasper. Care must be taken not to forcefully remove any tissue that is not easily debrided, as this may result in debridement

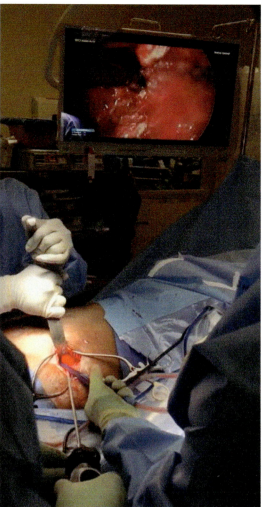

Fig. 14.6 Debridement of necrotic pancreatic parenchyma through flank incision

of viable pancreatic tissue or bleeding complications. If bleeding is encountered, control may be achieved with either packing or a laparoscopic clip applier. After copious irrigation of the cavity, the percutaneous drain is removed and replaced with large bore surgical drains. Post-operative lavage through these drains may be used. Given the contaminated nature, we opt to leave the skin incision open, managed with negative-pressure wound therapy, and allowed to close by secondary intention. Drains are left in place until the output volume is low and quality is serous [46, 47].

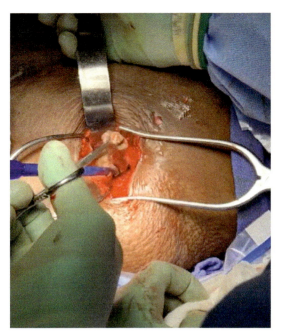

Fig. 14.7 Laparoscope inserted into the retroperitoneum through flank incision with visualization of the deep cavity

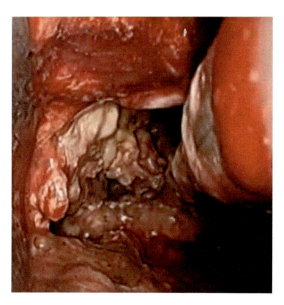

Fig. 14.8 Retroperitoneum surrounding necrotic parenchyma

Open Debridement

Options for open debridement include transperitoneal via a midline or chevron laparotomy incision or subcostal retroperitoneal approach. If the abdominal approach is chosen, the lesser sac is entered through the gastrocolic ligament. Fluid collections are evacuated and necrotic tissue or collections are gently debrided. Again, care is taken to gently debride and not forcefully remove tightly adherent tissue. Once adequate debridement has been completed and the lesser sac and retroperitoneum are irrigated, and if hemostasis is obtained, large bore drains are placed, and the abdomen is closed. These drains may also be used for postoperative lavage. If hemostasis is not obtained, we recommend packing the retroperitoneum and placing a temporary abdominal closure device with plans for a subsequent repeat laparotomy. As stated above, given the substantial morbidity and mortality associated with open debridement, this is no longer the recommended procedure of choice [43].

Conclusions

Acute pancreatitis is a problem that is commonly encountered by acute care surgeons that has a wide range of outcomes. Fortunately, most patients diagnosed with pancreatitis only suffer from the mild variant with excellent outcomes and little impact on their overall health. For patients who suffer from the most severe forms of pancreatitis, optimal treatment strategies have greatly evolved over the last 20 years with gradually improving outcomes. Excellent evidence-based guidelines currently exist that provide management strategies for all aspects of management, from diagnosis and initial supportive treatment, to the timing and the choice of appropriate intervention modalities when needed. Research is constantly ongoing to continue to optimize ways to manage this difficult disease process.

References

1. Forsmark CE, Vege SS, Wilcox CM. Acute pancreatitis. Campion EW, ed. N Engl J Med. 2016;375(20):1972–81.
2. Yadav D, Lowenfels AB. Trends in the epidemiology of the first attack of acute pancreatitis: a systematic review. Pancreas. 2006;33(4):323–30.
3. Krishna SG, Kamboj AK, Hart PA, Hinton A, Conwell DL. The changing epidemiology of acute pancreatitis hospitalizations: a decade of trends and the impact of chronic pancreatitis. Pancreas. 2017;46(4):482–8.
4. Johnson CD, Besselink MG, Carter R. Acute pancreatitis. BMJ. 2014;349:g4859.
5. Apte MV, Pirola RC, Wilson JS. Mechanisms of alcoholic pancreatitis. J Gastroenterol Hepatol. 2010;25(12):1816–26.
6. Yadav D, Lowenfels AB. The epidemiology of pancreatitis and pancreatic cancer. Gastroenterology. 2013;144(6):1252–61.
7. Morinville VD, Barmada MM, Lowe ME. Increasing incidence of acute pancreatitis at an American pediatric tertiary care center: is greater awareness among physicians responsible? Pancreas. 2010;39(1):5–8.
8. Banks PA, Bollen TL, Dervenis C, Gooszen HG, Johnson CD, Sarr MG, et al. Classification of acute pancreatitis – 2012: revision of the Atlanta classification and definitions by international consensus. Gut. 2013;62(1):102–11.
9. Rompianesi G, Hann A, Komolafe O, Pereira SP, Davidson BR, Gurusamy KS. Serum amylase and lipase and urinary trypsinogen and amylase for diagnosis of acute pancreatitis. Gurusamy KS, editor. Cochrane Database Syst Rev. Chichester: Wiley; 2017;4(4):CD012010.
10. Wilcox CM, Varadarajulu S, Eloubeidi M. Role of endoscopic evaluation in idiopathic pancreatitis: a systematic review. Gastrointest Endosc. 2006;63(7):1037–45.
11. Bradley EL. A clinically based classification system for acute pancreatitis. Summary of the International Symposium on Acute Pancreatitis, Atlanta, Ga, September 11 through 13, 1992. Arch Surg. 1993;128(5):586–90.
12. Banks PA. Acute pancreatitis: landmark studies, management decisions, and the future. Pancreas. 2016;45(5):633–40.
13. Dellinger EP, Forsmark CE, Layer P, Lévy P, Maraví-Poma E, Petrov MS, et al. Determinant-based classification of acute pancreatitis severity: an international multidisciplinary consultation. Ann Surg. 2012;256(6):875–80.
14. Data dictionaries for AAST grading system for EGS conditions [Internet]. Chicago: American Association for the Surgery of Trauma p12. Available from: http://www.aast.org/emergency-general-surgery-anatomic-grading-scales.
15. Ranson JH. The timing of biliary surgery in acute pancreatitis. Ann Surg. 1979;189(5):654–63.
16. Blamey SL, Imrie CW, O'Neill J, Gilmour WH, Carter DC. Prognostic factors in acute pancreatitis. Gut. 1984;25(12):1340–6.
17. Larvin M, McMahon MJ. APACHE-II score for assessment and monitoring of acute pancreatitis. Lancet. 1989;2(8656):201–5.
18. Balthazar EJ, Robinson DL, Megibow AJ, Ranson JH. Acute pancreatitis: value of CT in establishing prognosis. Radiology. 1990;174(2):331–6.
19. Mortelé KJ, Mergo PJ, Taylor HM, Wiesner W, Cantisani V, Ernst MD, et al. Peripancreatic vascular abnormalities complicating acute pancreatitis: contrast-enhanced helical CT findings. Eur J Radiol. 2004;52(1):67–72.
20. Wu BU, Johannes RS, Sun X, Tabak Y, Conwell DL, Banks PA. The early prediction of mortality in acute pancreatitis: a large population-based study. Gut. 2008;57(12):1698–703.
21. Cho JH, Kim TN, Chung HH, Kim KH. Comparison of scoring systems in predicting the severity of acute pancreatitis. World J Gastroenterol. 2015;21(8):2387–94.
22. Papachristou GI, Muddana V, Yadav D, O'Connell M, Sanders MK, Slivka A, et al. Comparison of BISAP, Ranson's, APACHE-II, and CTSI scores in predicting organ failure, complications, and mortality in acute pancreatitis. Am J Gastroenterol. 2010;105(2):435–41.
23. Mounzer R, Langmead CJ, Wu BU, Evans AC, Bishehsari F, Muddana V, et al. Comparison of existing clinical scoring systems to predict persistent organ failure in patients with acute pancreatitis. Gastroenterology. 2012;142(7):1476–82.
24. Working Group IAP/APA Acute Pancreatitis Guidelines. IAP/APA evidence-based guidelines for the management of acute pancreatitis. Pancreatology. 2013;13:e1–15.
25. Basurto Ona X, Rigau Comas D, Urrútia G. Opioids for acute pancreatitis pain. Basurto Ona X, editor. Cochrane Database Syst Rev. Chichester: Wiley; 2013;288(7):CD009179.
26. Fan E, Del Sorbo L, Goligher EC, Hodgson CL, Munshi L, Walkey AJ, et al. An official American Thoracic Society/European Society of Intensive Care Medicine/Society of Critical Care Medicine clinical practice guideline: mechanical ventilation in adult patients with acute respiratory distress syndrome. Am J Respir Crit Care Med. 2017;195(9):1253–63.
27. de-Madaria E, Martínez JF, Aparicio JR, Lluís F. Aggressive fluid resuscitation in acute pancreatitis: in aqua sanitas? Am J Gastroenterol. 2017;112(10):1617–8.

28. Mao E-Q, Fei J, Peng Y-B, Huang J, Tang Y-Q, Zhang S-D. Rapid hemodilution is associated with increased sepsis and mortality among patients with severe acute pancreatitis. Chin Med J. 2010;123(13):1639–44.

29. Aggarwal A, Manrai M, Kochhar R. Fluid resuscitation in acute pancreatitis. World J Gastroenterol. 2014;20(48):18092–103.

30. Trikudanathan G, Navaneethan U, Vege SS. Current controversies in fluid resuscitation in acute pancreatitis: a systematic review. Pancreas. 2012;41(6): 827–34.

31. Moraes JMM, Felga GEG, Chebli LA, Franco MB, Gomes CA, Gaburri PD, et al. A full solid diet as the initial meal in mild acute pancreatitis is safe and result in a shorter length of hospitalization: results from a prospective, randomized, controlled, double-blind clinical trial. J Clin Gastroenterol. 2010;44(7): 517–22.

32. Teich N, Aghdassi A, Fischer J, Walz B, Caca K, Wallochny T, et al. Optimal timing of oral refeeding in mild acute pancreatitis: results of an open randomized multicenter trial. Pancreas. 2010;39(7):1088–92.

33. McClave SA, Taylor BE, Martindale RG, Warren MM, Johnson DR, Braunschweig C, et al. Guidelines for the provision and assessment of nutrition support therapy in the adult critically ill patient: Society of Critical Care Medicine (SCCM) and American Society for Parenteral and Enteral Nutrition (A.S.P.E.N.). JPEN J Parenter Enteral Nutr. 2016;40(2):159–211.

34. Wittau M, Mayer B, Scheele J, Henne-Bruns D, Dellinger EP, Isenmann R. Systematic review and meta-analysis of antibiotic prophylaxis in severe acute pancreatitis. Scand J Gastroenterol. 2011;46(3):261–70.

35. Solomkin JS, Mazuski JE, Bradley JS, Rodvold KA, Goldstein EJC, Baron EJ, et al. Diagnosis and management of complicated intra-abdominal infection in adults and children: guidelines by the Surgical Infection Society and the Infectious Diseases Society of America. Clin Infect Dis. 2010;50(2):133–64.

36. Gurusamy KS, Nagendran M, Davidson BR. Early versus delayed laparoscopic cholecystectomy for acute gallstone pancreatitis. Gurusamy KS, editor. Cochrane Database Syst Rev. Chichester: Wiley; 2013;251(9):CD010326.

37. da Costa DW, Bouwense SA, Schepers NJ, Besselink MG, van Santvoort HC, van Brunschot S, et al. Same-admission versus interval cholecystectomy for mild gallstone pancreatitis (PONCHO):

a multicentre randomised controlled trial. Lancet. 2015;386(10000):1261–8.

38. van Baal MC, Besselink MG, Bakker OJ, van Santvoort HC, Schaapherder AF, Nieuwenhuijs VB, et al. Timing of cholecystectomy after mild biliary pancreatitis: a systematic review. Ann Surg. 2012;255(5):860–6.

39. Tse F, Yuan Y. Early routine endoscopic retrograde cholangiopancreatography strategy versus early conservative management strategy in acute gallstone pancreatitis. Tse F, editor. Cochrane Database Syst Rev. Chichester: Wiley; 2012;39(5):CD009779.

40. Kirkpatrick AW, Roberts DJ, De Waele J, Jaeschke R, Malbrain MLNG, De Keulenaer B, et al. Intra-abdominal hypertension and the abdominal compartment syndrome: updated consensus definitions and clinical practice guidelines from the World Society of the Abdominal Compartment Syndrome. Intensive Care Med. 2013;39(7):1190–206.

41. Mallick IH, Winslet MC. Vascular complications of pancreatitis. JOP. 2004;5(5):328–37.

42. Varadarajulu S, Bang JY, Sutton BS, Trevino JM, Christein JD, Wilcox CM. Equal efficacy of endoscopic and surgical cystogastrostomy for pancreatic pseudocyst drainage in a randomized trial. Gastroenterology. 2013;145(3):583–90.e1.

43. Mowery NT, Bruns BR, MacNew HG, Agarwal S, Enniss TM, Khan M, et al. Surgical management of pancreatic necrosis: a practice management guideline from the Eastern Association for the Surgery of trauma. J Trauma Acute Care Surg. 2017;83(2):316–27.

44. Bakker OJ, van Santvoort HC, van Brunschot S, Geskus RB, Besselink MG, Bollen TL, et al. Endoscopic transgastric vs surgical necrosectomy for infected necrotizing pancreatitis: a randomized trial. JAMA. 2012;307(10):1053–61.

45. van Santvoort HC, Besselink MG, Bakker OJ, Hofker HS, Boermeester MA, Dejong CH, et al. A step-up approach or open necrosectomy for necrotizing pancreatitis. N Engl J Med. 2010;362(16):1491–502.

46. Martin MJ, Brown CVR. Video-assisted retroperitoneal pancreatic debridement: a video-based guide to the technique. J Trauma Acute Care Surg. 2017;83(1):200–3.

47. van Santvoort HC, Besselink MGH, Horvath KD, Sinanan MN, Bollen TL, van Ramshorst B, et al. Videoscopic assisted retroperitoneal debridement in infected necrotizing pancreatitis. HPB. 2007;9(2):156–9.

Hepatic Abscess

15

Alexandra Brito and Leslie Kobayashi

Introduction

Hepatic abscesses are characterized by a suppurative fluid collection of invasive and multiplying microorganisms within the liver [1]. The primary organisms involved are bacteria accounting for approximately 80% of abscess, followed by parasites (amoebae), and rarely fungi [2]. Hepatic abscesses (HA) are rare, with an incidence ranging between 1/100000 to 86/100000 [3–6]. However, there is some indication in recent studies that the incidence of HA is increasing [5, 7]. Due to advances in diagnosis and management the mortality for HA is decreasing. The first review of pyogenic abscesses (PA) by Ochsner (1938) reported a mortality rate of 77% [8]. With the advent of percutaneous treatment in the 1980s, mortality rates fell to 24–50% [9–11]. Modern case series report mortality rates between 2.5% and 19%

[4, 6, 7, 12–16]. The population of patients affected by HA is shifting as well. The average age at diagnosis and number of comorbidities is increasing and the etiologies are shifting from primarily infectious to biliary and cryptogenic etiologies [7, 17].

Etiology

Amoebic Abscess

Amoebiasis is an infection caused by ingestion of mature cysts of *Entamoeba histolytica* which mature into trophozoites in the small intestine, migrate to the large intestine where they may invade the intestinal wall into the capillary system, and spread hematogenously to extra-intestinal sites [18]. HAs occur as a complication of gastrointestinal amoebic infections in fewer than 1% of cases [19, 20] and time between exposure and presentation can range from weeks to years [21]. In western countries amoebiasis is generally found in patients who have travelled to or migrated from endemic areas: mainly Mexico, Central and South America, India, and Africa [19–21]. For unclear reasons, amoebic HAs are ten times more common in males than females whereas amoebiasis is equally prevalent between the sexes [22]. This may be due to differences in predisposing factors or an intrinsic resistance to invasive disease such as relative iron deficiency anemia in women of

A. Brito
Department of Surgery,
UC San Diego Medical Center,
San Diego, CA, USA

L. Kobayashi (✉)
Department of Surgery, Division of Trauma,
Surgical Critical Care, Acute Care Surgery
and Burns, UC San Diego Medical Center,
San Diego, CA, USA
e-mail: lkobayashi@ucsd.edu

© Springer International Publishing AG, part of Springer Nature 2019
C. V. R. Brown et al. (eds.), *Emergency General Surgery*, https://doi.org/10.1007/978-3-319-96286-3_15

childbearing age [23]. Other risk factors include malnutrition, alcoholism, immunosuppression, and poor sanitation [21]. In addition, coinfection with bacteria can affect the invasiveness of *E. histolytica* by changing gene expression [24] or altering the oxygenation of the microenvironment to increase oxygen radicals [25, 26]. Rupture is a possible complication which most commonly occurs into the pleuropulmonary system rather than the peritoneum [17].

A second species of amoeba, *Entamoeba dispar*, has also been identified in amoebic HAs [27], but this strain is considered non-pathologic and coinfection is not thought to be of clinical significance [21]. Aspirate from amoebic HAs may show evidence of pathogenic and non-pathologic bacteria [27].

Pyogenic Abscess

Pyogenic hepatic abscesses are the most common etiology in western countries accounting for approximately 80% of cases [2]. Underlying causes are varied and include hematogenous spread, direct spread from adjacent organs, biliary disease, intrahepatic pathology, instrumentation of the liver or biliary tract, and cryptogenic causes. In most series, cryptogenic and biliary sources are the most common followed by cancer and other etiologies [12].

Hematogenous spread may be via the arterial or portal venous systems. In the earliest reviews of PAs, the most common identified trigger was pylephlebitis from appendicitis or less commonly diverticular disease [8]. Although appendicitis and diverticular disease still significantly increase the risk of PA [13, 28], improvements in treatment of these diseases have made this complication much less common. Similarly, arterial sources which are usually from distant disease have become less common with improved treatment of disseminated sepsis [29]. These infections are more likely to be monomicrobial and associated with underlying comorbidities [2]. Direct spread of infection may occur from infection of the hepatic flexure or rarely from migration of ingested foreign bodies [2, 30].

Biliary disease has become the most common identified etiology of PA in recent decades [17, 31]. Direct extension from cholecystitis is a rare complication often associated with gallbladder wall rupture and may resemble gallbladder malignancy on imaging [32]. Biliary obstruction due to stones, inflammation, ischemia (leading to bile duct necrosis), or congenital biliary abnormalities such as Caroli's disease may lead to bile stasis and ultimately ascending cholangitis. When this occurs, aspirate of the PA may be bilious providing an important clue to the underlying etiology [2]. In these cases the biliary obstruction must be relieved for PA treatment to be successful [33].

Intrahepatic pathology may also lead to bile stasis. Bile may pool in a congenital or hydatid cysts [2, 34] or necrotic tissue such as neoplasms which have outgrown their blood supply [35]; this stasis then predisposes to infection. It can be difficult to distinguish between neoplastic and nonneoplastic causes of HA by imaging and presentation, and a high degree of suspicion is necessary to avoid missing the diagnosis of underlying malignancy. If biopsy is not an option, repeat imaging after treatment of the abscess is recommended [2, 35]. Both long-term mortality and inhospital mortality from acute PA presentation are increased in the context of malignancy [16, 35, 36].

In addition to the structural changes that occur with malignancy which may predispose to necrosis and abscess formation, instrumentation as a part of treatment can also increase the risk of abscess formation. This may be from indwelling stents [37], stenosis of the hepatic artery or biliary drainage tract after pancreaticoduodenectomy [38, 39], or increased reflux of bile from choledo-cho-enterostomy [2, 39]. PA is also an infrequent but serious complication of chemoembolization (CE) and radiofrequency ablation (RFA) of intra-hepatic neoplasms [40]. Risk of developing PA after CE or RFA is increased in the presence of bilio-enterostomy [41], previous biliary drainage procedures [2], and hepatic metastases from neuroendocrine tumors [42], with larger areas of treatment [43] and with a history of diabetes or immunosuppression [40]. PA also appears to be more common with CE compared to RFA [44, 45]. Overall mortality from PA after CE has been reported as 15% [43].

Liver trauma may also introduce bacteria into the parenchyma causing PA. Usually the infection takes weeks to months to develop with the exception of *Clostridial* infection which can progress within hours [46]. The risk of PA formation is increased with operative management [47], more severe trauma with a larger area of necrosis, and following arterial embolization [48].

Liver transplantation (LT) is arguably the most invasive form of liver instrumentation. This combined with the mandatory aggressive immunosuppression creates an environment ideal for PA development. Incidence of bacterial infection after LT approach 70% in some series [49, 50]. Risk factors for PA after LT include age <20, biliary atresia, preoperative hypoalbuminemia, extended intensive care unit stay, need for hemodialysis, and biliary or vascular complications [46, 51]. Although method of biliary reconstruction has not been investigated in regard to PA risk specifically, bacteremia is 12 times more common in those with bilio-enterostomy compared to choledocho-choledochostomy [52].

Similarly to amoebic abscesses, there is an increased frequency of PAs in males compared to females, but the disparity is much less pronounced (~2:1) and is not consistent between studies [16, 31, 36, 53]. Older studies show a higher predominance in males compared to newer studies, which may be due to a shift in the most commonly identified etiology to biliary disease which is more frequent among females [8, 12].

Multiple comorbidities have been associated with increased risk of developing PA. These diseases include diabetes [36, 54], renal failure [55, 56], inflammatory bowel disease (IBD) [57], colorectal cancer [58], and splenectomy [56]. These causes share the feature of altered immune function, which is not surprising in the context of an infectious process. IBD and colorectal cancer additionally are associated with impairment of the

intestinal mucosa which is suspected to increase bacterial translocation into the portal circulation through the compromised mucosa [57]. With the average age of patients diagnosed with PA, increasing [5, 31, 59] comorbidities are increasingly important to take into consideration.

The microbiology of PA varies depending on region, underlying etiology, and the time period examined. In older studies, the most common bacteria isolated from PAs were *Escherichia coli* [60, 61]. In the past two decades, studies from several Asian countries [7, 28, 53, 62, 63] as well as North America [12, 53] have shown that *Klebsiella pneumonia* has become the most common isolate from PAs. Longitudinal studies have shown a trend of increasing prevalence of *Klebsiella* over several decades [7, 17]. This may be due to predominant etiologies shifting from intra-abdominal infections to biliary or cryptogenic sources, the increase in biliary instrumentation for hepatobiliary diseases, and changes in the local microbiome. The increase may also be partially artefactual due to advances in the ability to culture *Klebsiella* which has previously been difficult to isolate in artificial culture [64]. Important to note is the generally more favorable outcomes associated with *Klebsiella* PAs compared to other microbes [16, 65].

Key Points

1. Amoebic abscesses are more commonly found in younger patients, those from areas with endemic amoebiasis, and in males.
2. Pyogenic abscesses are much more common than amoebic abscesses.
3. Pyogenic abscesses are also more commonly found in males but with a less severe predominance than amoebic abscesses.
4. The most common causes of PA are cryptogenic and biliary infections.
5. Immunocompromised, biliary obstruction, manipulation and instrumentation, and RFA and CE increase the risk of PA.

Presentation and Diagnosis

The presentation of HA is varied and often non-specific. In the case of secondary infections, often the primary source will determine the patient's presenting symptoms. Aside from symptoms specific to a precipitating cause, most HA present with some combination of fever, chills, malaise, nausea, anorexia, vomiting, weight loss, diarrhea, and abdominal pain (Table 15.1). The most common symptoms are fevers, chills, and right upper quadrant abdominal pain [12, 36]. Clinical signs and symptoms are similar for both pyogenic and amoebic abscess, and history is a valuable tool in differentiating between the two. Younger age and a history of recent travel to areas with endemic amoebiasis should increase concern for amoebic etiology [21]. The patient may have had diarrhea preceding the onset of more systemic symptoms or right upper quadrant pain, but less than half of patients presenting with amoebic HA report diarrhea prior to diagnosis [21, 66]. In terms of timing, usually exposure to an endemic area is recent at the time of abscess diagnosis, but in some cases, the protozoa can be present and asymptomatic for months or even years [21].

Laboratory abnormalities which often accompany HA of any etiology include leukocytosis, transaminitis, hyperbilirubinemia, elevated C-reactive protein (CRP), and elevated alkaline phosphatase [21, 58]. It should also be kept in mind that tumor markers such as AFP, CEA, and CA 19-9 may be elevated even in the absence of malignancy [7]. Patterns of laboratory abnormalities do not reliably differentiate

Table 15.1 Signs and symptoms of hepatic abscess

Fever
Chills/rigors
Abdominal pain
Nausea/vomiting
Diarrhea
Weight loss
Jaundice/icterus
Leukocytosis
Transaminitis
Elevated alkaline phosphatase

between pyogenic and amoebic abscesses [21]. If there is any suspicion of amoebic abscess, blood antigen tests, which have sensitivity and specificity approaching 100% if any two antigen tests are used, should be done [27]. Blood cultures rarely identify protozoa, and stool studies are not sensitive nor specific for diagnosis of amoebic abscess [21]. Unlike other parasitic infections, eosinophilia is not generally present in amoebic HA [67].

With the non-specific presentation common to all HA regardless of source, a high index of suspicion is necessary and imaging the mainstay of diagnosis. Before the advent of advanced imaging studies, X-rays were primarily used to search for signs of HA including elevated right hemidiaphragm, right-sided pleural effusion, and air within the liver [12, 68]. The most commonly used modern imaging study for the diagnosis of HA is computed tomography (CT). Ultrasound (US) is a common alternative where resources are limited or when there is concern about exposing the patient to radiation or contrast. However, sensitivity and specificity for diagnosis of HA are better with CT than US, and CT has the added benefit of providing useful information on surrounding structures and possible etiologies such as biliary dilation and intra-abdominal infections [2, 69, 70]. The overall sensitivity of CT for HA is 97% [71].

CT findings indicating HA are extremely varied. Generally, they are seen as hypoattenuating areas in the liver which may have features of complex fluid including septations and heterogeneous enhancement with contrast or gas (Fig. 15.1a, b). They may also appear as dense masses indistinguishable from malignancy (even when underlying malignancy is not present) [71]. Abscesses which are early in development may appear as a cluster of microabscesses which later coalesce into a larger fluid collection [68] or a larger area which is hypodense and heterogeneous without clear borders which then develops a more obvious enhancing rim with or without a surrounding hypodense area of erythema creating a "target" appearance [2]. Distribution may vary with etiology; arterial etiology such as disseminated staphylococcal

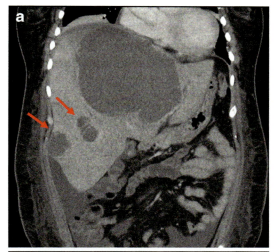

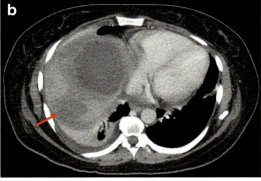

Fig. 15.1 Coronal (**a**) and axial (**b**) views of a large pyogenic hepatic abscess. Note there are also multiple satellite abscesses (arrows)

infection may form a military pattern, whereas portal venous sources such as appendicitis, diverticulitis, and amoebic infections tend to occur in the right lobe more than the left. This pattern has been attributed to portal streaming combined with the angulation of the left portal vein branch [12, 58, 72]. When a HA is identified, it is important to search for intra- or extra-hepatic pathology in the form of malignancy, infection, or structural abnormalities.

Amoebic abscesses are difficult to differentiate from PAs by imaging alone; however, they tend to have a more rounded appearance on CT scanning and are more likely to show the "target" pattern [68]. Ultrasound evaluation of amoebic abscesses generally reveal a round or oval, thick walled, hypoechoic fluid collection [70].

Rarely, a HA may perforate. Most commonly this results in a perihepatic fluid collection [73]. However, it is possible for the abscess to perforate through the diaphragm into the pleural space or into the abdominal cavity. Risks for perforation include cirrhosis, gas-forming abscesses, abscesses ≥6 cm, and other septic metastases [73]. Perforation increases the risk for protracted or complicated hospital course and may also increase mortality [73, 74].

Poor prognostic factors for PAs include APACHE II ≥15, increased urea, sepsis, shock, increased age, increased bilirubin, decreased albumin, concomitant malignancy, increased prothrombin time (PT), decreased hemoglobin, gas-forming abscesses, multidrug resistance, anaerobes, biliary origin, multiple abscesses, and increased abscess size [75].

Key Points

1. Symptoms of HA are generally non-specific, but the most common are fevers, chills, and right upper quadrant abdominal pain.
2. Imaging is the most sensitive and specific diagnostic modality to identify HA, with CT scan being the most commonly utilized and having the additional benefit of often identifying the underlying etiology of the abscess.
3. It is difficult to differentiate amoebic from PA by symptoms and imaging, history, and antigen testing are the most reliable means to differentiate the two types of HA.

Treatment

The treatment options for HA have evolved over the past decades. Classically the options were divided into medical and surgical. It is ideal to

Table 15.2 Outcomes for PA and amoebic abscess in appropriately selected cases

	Medical therapy	Percutaneous drain	Open surgery	Laparoscopic surgery
Pyogenic abscess				
Success rate	30–100	60–100	80–100	80–100
Morbidity	10–20	5–15	5–15	5–20
Mortality	0–100[a]	0–5	5–50	0–5
Amoebic abscess				
Success rate	70–90	90–100	90–100	100[b]
Morbidity	2–10	2–5	ID	0[b]
Mortality	<1	<1	ID	0[b]

Given changes in management, only data from the past 25 years was used in these estimates

ID insufficient data

[a]In the past 25 years when medical management is not successful, patients have been offered percutaneous drainage or surgery. The only recent cases found where deaths occurred with medical management only were those where patients refused further care

[b]Only one case of laparoscopic drainage of amoebic abscess was found

differentiate amoebic from pyogenic abscesses prior to intervention as amoebic abscesses very commonly respond to antibiotic treatment (metronidazole) only, whereas PA will commonly require percutaneous or surgical drainage (Table 15.2). Microbial diagnosis in PA generally requires aspiration and culture of the abscess as less than half of cases are associated with bacteremia on culture, and even in the presence of bacteremia, the culture results from abscesses and blood are only concordant in ~60% of cases [12, 61]. Blood cultures are more likely to be positive with *Klebsiella*-infected abscesses [53], which is consistent with its increased tendency to have metastatic complications such as meningitis and endophthalmitis.

Medical therapy for PA generally consists of broad spectrum antibiotics. In the case of severe sepsis, broad coverage with piperacillin-tazobactam and vancomycin is often used [2, 12]. Another common combination which covers the majority of responsible organisms is metronidazole and a third-generation cephalosporin such as ceftriaxone [7, 12, 16, 58]. This combination is used frequently in Asian countries and has the benefit of good central nervous system penetration with the rising frequency of metastatic lesions from K1 or magA mutant *Klebsiella* [76]. In western countries gentamycin is often added to the antimicrobial regimen [2, 31], but the risks of significant toxicities must be carefully weighed in a population with a high prevalence of comorbidi-

ties and renal dysfunction. Local resistance patterns should also be considered when choosing empiric antibiotics, and agents should be narrowed when species and susceptibilities become available. Although etiology of HA has been associated with increased frequency of specific pathogens, the patterns of association are not consistent, and frequency of pathogens has shifted over the past decade. As such narrowing antimicrobial treatment based on aspirate culture (or blood culture when aspirate is not available) is vital. Duration of antibiotic therapy is not clearly defined given the heterogeneity of presentation and etiology but generally varies between 2 and 6 weeks [2].

In the case of amoebic abscesses, the primary treatment of uncomplicated abscesses is metronidazole followed by a lumen-active agent such as iodoquinol to eliminate any remaining cysts in the colon [21, 77, 78]. This treatment is successful in up to 90% of patients with uncomplicated amoebic HA [79, 80]. Even in complex cases, medical treatment is successful in 70–80% of patients [81, 82].

Percutaneous Drainage

When medical management fails or the clinical situation requires a more aggressive approach, percutaneous drainage is the next option for treatment. Although percutaneous treatment was first described in 1953 [83], it took several decades to gain popularity. Since the late 1970s, percutaneous interventions have been increasingly used to spare patients the morbidity and mortality of open surgery [14, 17, 84]. There are many factors to consider when deciding between therapeutic approaches including abscess size, presence of loculations, and underlying cause. Although there is no official consensus on a size cutoff, there is good evidence in the literature to suggest that larger PAs (>3–5 cm) [75, 85, 86] have better outcomes with percutaneous drainage versus antibiotic treatment alone (Table 15.2). Percutaneous drainage includes both aspiration alone and catheter drainage. Outcomes of catheter drainage have been found to be superior in terms of success rate, clinical improvement, and days to reduce cavity size by 50% when compared to aspiration alone, even in studies where multiple aspirations were performed [36, 87]. Differences in hospitalization and procedure-related complications are similar.

Generally, the risk of failure of percutaneous drainage increases with size and number of abscesses [36, 88], presence of loculations [65, 89], as well as with underlying malignancy [88]. The effect of abscess loculations on failure rate differs greatly between studies, and as such this factor may be manageable with good interventional technique [36, 88]. While a daily output less than 30 mL is generally used for removal of surgical drains, waiting until daily output is less than 10–15 mL is associated with better outcomes [88, 90]. Other patient-specific factors that have been independently associated with failure of percutaneous therapy include ECOG performance status ≥ 2, hypertension, and raised serum total bilirubin [7, 75].

Percutaneous drainage of uncomplicated amoebic HA has not been shown to consistently improve outcomes compared to medical treatment in small, uncomplicated amoebic abscesses [23, 91, 92]. However, percutaneous drainage has been shown to be beneficial in select situations. In the case of treatment failure, very large abscesses (>8–10 cm), or those with high risk of rupture into the peritoneum or pericardium based on location, percutaneous drainage should be considered [65, 81, 82, 93, 94]. Similar to PAs, catheter drainage is more effective than aspiration alone with success rates of ~100% compared to less than 50%, respectively [81]. If secondary bacterial infection is suspected, the abscess should be treated as a PA.

In terms of technique, US or CT guidance is used to identify the cavity, a needle is used to enter the cavity, and the contents are aspirated and sent for culture. A drain (preferably large bore) catheter is then placed using the Seldinger technique. The imaging modality of choice should be used to identify loculations and place the drain in a manner such that of as many of the cavities as possible are drained.

Surgical

Before percutaneous drainage was well established, the alternative to medical therapy for both PAs and amoebic abscesses was open surgical drainage. This was associated with extremely high mortality rates [8, 95]. Although overall mortality rates continue to be higher in surgically treated versus percutaneous groups [84, 96], this is likely due to selection bias as only patients thought to have a high probability of failing percutaneous treatment have been treated primarily with surgery in recent decades [65]. In fact, more recent studies comparing percutaneous and surgical drainage for uncomplicated PAs larger than 5 cm showed similar complication rates between open surgical and percutaneous treatment groups (Table 15.2) [85].

Although percutaneous drainage is much less invasive, in terms of resolution of the abscess, surgery has a higher success rate overall [12, 63]. Both open and laparoscopic surgeries also have the benefit of addressing underlying etiology, particularly in the case of an underlying biliary pathology [97]. Both techniques also may use intraoperative ultrasound, although this is not always necessary if the abscess is visible on the surface of the liver [98]. Indications for surgical intervention include failure of percutaneous therapy, ruptures with peritonitis [73], and very large or multiple abscesses [99–101]. In the case that surgical intervention is not successful, repeat surgery or percutaneous drainage may be attempted [99, 102].

Open

Open surgical drainage procedures are generally performed through an upper midline or right subcostal incision. The area of the abscess is located often with the assistance of intraoperative ultrasound. The cavity is then opened and the aspirate sent for culture. The purulent material is evacuated using suction, and loculations broken up using blunt finger dissection. The abscess cavity should be irrigated thoroughly and hemostasis ensured before closure. A drain is generally left in place to provide further drainage for any remaining purulent material and any potential bile leak.

Although significant morbidity and mortality accompany open surgery including the effects of general anesthesia [84], it is a very effective means for evacuation of HA. One has complete and direct access to the liver, and adjunctive imaging such as intraoperative US is technically easier to use compared to laparoscopic approaches. There is the added benefit of access to the remainder of the abdomen as well, and a thorough washout decreases the risk of post-intervention peritonitis significantly compared to percutaneous drainage [85], Washout is also possible with laparoscopic therapy, although it is generally less thorough, and outcomes regarding peritonitis have not been directly examined [73],

When open surgery is compared directly with percutaneous drainage, success rate is higher and morbidity and mortality are similar [85], However, the majority of the reports of outcomes after open surgery for HA within the last 20 years refer to cases where the patient had either failed non-operative management or showed signs of peritonitis at presentation [99, 103]. The overall frequency of open surgical intervention has decreased [59, 103, 104] leading to a paucity of data on outcomes in modern series.

Laparoscopic

Laparoscopic surgery is an approach that has only recently begun to be used for treatment of HA. The abdomen is entered in a manner according to surgeon preference, and similar to open surgery, the abscess is located often with ultrasonic guidance, and the cavity is aspirated and then unroofed. Breaking up loculations can be more difficult to do with laparoscopic instruments without traumatizing the liver, so the success of this procedure is highly dependent on the skill and experience of the operating surgeon. Conversion rates are extremely low, generally reported as <1% [98, 108].

Laparoscopic drainage has been shown to have shorter operative times and faster recovery compared to open surgery [105]. However, this has only been examined retrospectively implying that patient selection may still affect outcomes. Laparoscopic drainage is most frequently used as a salvage treatment after failure of percutaneous drainage [99, 106]. In addition to ruling out contraindications to laparoscopy, the decision on whether laparoscopic surgery can be used instead of open depends on the location of the abscess/accessibility and surgeon comfort. Certain areas such as the caudate lobe may be safer to access through open surgery [107]. It is more difficult to obtain thorough drainage using a laparoscopic approach compared to open, but laparoscopic drainage has been shown to have acceptable results [65]. One study demonstrated an 11% primary treatment failure rate with laparoscopic drainage compared to 40% primary treatment failure with percutaneous drainage [65]. This study was not randomized as treatment modality was based on physician preference which ultimately resulted in patients with more severe disease being treated laparoscopically. Complication rates were similar (13% vs 17% percutaneous drain vs laparoscopic drain). Another study showed decreased length of hospital stay and earlier oral intake with laparoscopic vs open surgery, but again this study was not randomized, and open surgery patients were more likely to have more severe symptoms and greater deviation from normal lab values [97].

Mortality rates for HA have decreased with advances in therapy, with rates approaching 100% without treatment [109] reduced to 0% reported in many recent series where comprehensive treatment algorithms were used [59, 110]. The mortality rate also varies by region and underlying etiology.

Key Points

1. The majority of amoebic abscesses will resolve with medical management alone.
2. Drainage is recommend for most PA and very large amoebic abscesses and those amoebic abscesses at risk for rupture or failing medical treatment.
3. Percutaneous drainage is the least invasive manner of drainage and is frequently successful.
4. Surgical drainage is more successful than percutaneous, but has greater morbidity and possibly increased mortality.
5. When necessary surgical drainage can be performed via open or laparoscopic techniques.

References

1. Chiche L, Dargere S, Le Pennec V, Dufay C, Alkofer B. Pyogenic-liver abscess: diagnosis and management. Gastroenterol Clin Biol. 2008;32(12):1077–91.
2. Lardiere-Deguelte S, Ragot E, Amroun K, Piardi T, Dokmak S, Bruno O, et al. Hepatic abscess: diagnosis and management. J Visc Surg. 2015;152(4):231–43.
3. Jepsen P, Vilstrup H, Schonheyder HC, Sorensen HT. A nationwide study of the incidence and 30-day mortality rate of pyogenic liver abscess in Denmark, 1977-2002. Aliment Pharmacol Ther. 2005;21(10):1185–8.
4. Kaplan GG, Gregson DB, Laupland KB. Population-based study of the epidemiology of and the risk factors for pyogenic liver abscess. Clin Gastroenterol Hepatol. 2004;2(11):1032–8.
5. Meddings L, Myers RP, Hubbard J, Shaheen AA, Laupland KB, Dixon E, et al. A population-based study of pyogenic liver abscesses in the United States: incidence, mortality, and temporal trends. Am J Gastroenterol. 2010;105(1):117–24.
6. Tsai FC, Huang YT, Chang LY, Wang JT. Pyogenic liver abscess as endemic disease, Taiwan. Emerg Infect Dis. 2008;14(10):1592–600.
7. Lo JZ, Leow JJ, Ng PL, Lee HQ, Mohd Noor NA, Low JK, et al. Predictors of therapy failure in a series of 741 adult pyogenic liver abscesses. J Hepatobiliary Pancreat Sci. 2015;22(2):156–65.
8. Ochsner ADM, Murray S. Pyogenic abscess of the liver. Am J Surg. 1938;40:292–353.
9. Herbert DA, Fogel DA, Rothman J, Wilson S, Simmons F, Ruskin J. Pyogenic liver abscesses: successful non-surgical therapy. Lancet. 1982;1(8264):134–6.
10. Berger LA, Osborne DR. Treatment of pyogenic liver abscesses by percutaneous needle aspiration. Lancet. 1982;1(8264):132–4.
11. Bertel CK, van Heerden JA, Sheedy PF 2nd. Treatment of pyogenic hepatic abscesses. Surgical vs percutaneous drainage. Arch Surg. 1986;121(5):554–8.
12. Rahimian J, Wilson T, Oram V, Holzman RS. Pyogenic liver abscess: recent trends in etiology and mortality. Clin Infect Dis. 2004;39(11):1654–9.
13. Kuo SH, Lee YT, Li CR, Tseng CJ, Chao WN, Wang PH, et al. Mortality in Emergency Department Sepsis score as a prognostic indicator in patients with pyogenic liver abscess. Am J Emerg Med. 2013;31(6):916–21.
14. Mohsen AH, Green ST, Read RC, McKendrick MW. Liver abscess in adults: ten years experience in a UK centre. QJM. 2002;95(12):797–802.
15. Ruiz-Hernandez JJ, Leon-Mazorra M, Conde-Martel A, Marchena-Gomez J, Hemmersbach-Miller M, Betancor-Leon P. Pyogenic liver abscesses: mortality-related factors. Eur J Gastroenterol Hepatol. 2007;19(10):853–8.
16. Sohn SH, Kim KH, Park JH, Kim TN. Predictors of mortality in Korean patients with pyogenic liver abscess: a single center, retrospective study. Korean J Gastroenterol. 2016;67(5):238–44.
17. Huang CJ, Pitt HA, Lipsett PA, Osterman FA Jr, Lillemoe KD, Cameron JL, et al. Pyogenic hepatic abscess. Changing trends over 42 years. Ann Surg. 1996;223(5):600–7; discussion 607–9
18. CDC. Available from: https://www.cdc.gov/dpdx/amebiasis/index.html.
19. Haque R, Huston CD, Hughes M, Houpt E, Petri WA Jr. Amebiasis. N Engl J Med. 2003;348(16):1565–73.
20. Knobloch J, Mannweiler E. Development and persistence of antibodies to Entamoeba histolytica in patients with amebic liver abscess. Analysis of 216 cases. Am J Trop Med Hyg. 1983;32(4):727–32.
21. Wuerz T, Kane JB, Boggild AK, Krajden S, Keystone JS, Fuksa M, et al. A review of amoebic liver abscess for clinicians in a nonendemic setting. Can J Gastroenterol. 2012;26(10):729–33.
22. Maltz G, Knauer CM. Amebic liver abscess: a 15-year experience. Am J Gastroenterol. 1991;86(6):704–10.
23. Stanley SL Jr. Amoebiasis. Lancet. 2003;361(9362):1025–34.
24. Galvan-Moroyoqui JM, Del Carmen Dominguez-Robles M, Franco E, Meza I. The interplay between Entamoeba and enteropathogenic bacteria modulates epithelial cell damage. PLoS Negl Trop Dis. 2008;2(7):e266.
25. Bracha R, Mirelman D. Virulence of Entamoeba histolytica trophozoites. Effects of bacteria, microaerobic conditions, and metronidazole. J Exp Med. 1984;160(2):353–68.
26. Murray HW, Aley SB, Scott WA. Susceptibility of Entamoeba histolytica to oxygen intermediates. Mol Biochem Parasitol. 1981;3(6):381–91.

27. Reyna-Fabian ME, Zermeno V, Ximenez C, Flores J, Romero MF, Diaz D, et al. Analysis of the bacterial diversity in liver abscess: differences between pyogenic and amebic abscesses. Am J Trop Med Hyg. 2016;94(1):147–55.

28. Luo M, Yang XX, Tan B, Zhou XP, Xia HM, Xue J, et al. Distribution of common pathogens in patients with pyogenic liver abscess in China: a meta-analysis. Eur J Clin Microbiol Infect Dis. 2016;35(10):1557–65.

29. Dellinger RP, Levy MM, Carlet JM, Bion J, Parker MM, Jaeschke R, et al. Surviving Sepsis Campaign: international guidelines for management of severe sepsis and septic shock: 2008. Crit Care Med. 2008;36(1):296–327.

30. Matrella F, Lhuaire M, Piardi T, Dokmak S, Bruno O, Maestraggi Q, et al. Liver hilar abscesses secondary to gastrointestinal perforation by ingested fish bones: surgical management of two cases. Hepatobiliary Surg Nutr. 2014;3(3):156–62.

31. Chang AC. Ha NB, Satyadas T, Maddern G. Pyogenic liver abscess trends in South Australia. ANZ J Surg. 2015;85(3):179–82.

32. Stefanidis D, Sirinek KR, Bingener J. Gallbladder perforation: risk factors and outcome. J Surg Res. 2006;131(2):204–8.

33. Prost a la Denise J, Kianmanesh R, Castel B, Flamant Y, Msika S. Systemic sepsis after cholecystectomy. J Chir (Paris). 2008;145(3):278–83.

34. Reid-Lombardo KM, Khan S, Sclabas G. Hepatic cysts and liver abscess. Surg Clin North Am. 2010;90(4):679–97.

35. Law ST, Li KK. Is hepatic neoplasm-related pyogenic liver abscess a distinct clinical entity? World J Gastroenterol. 2012;18(10):1110–6.

36. Cai YL, Xiong XZ, Lu J, Cheng Y, Yang C, Lin YX, et al. Percutaneous needle aspiration versus catheter drainage in the management of liver abscess: a systematic review and meta-analysis. HPB (Oxford). 2015;17(3):195–201.

37. Pennington L, Kaufman S, Cameron JL. Intrahepatic abscess as a complication of long-term percutaneous internal biliary drainage. Surgery. 1982;91(6):642–5.

38. Gaujoux S, Sauvanet A, Vullierme MP, Cortes A, Dokmak S, Sibert A, et al. Ischemic complications after pancreaticoduodenectomy: incidence, prevention, and management. Ann Surg. 2009;249(1):111–7.

39. Yeo CJ, Cameron JL, Sohn TA, Lillemoe KD, Pitt HA, Talamini MA, et al. Six hundred fifty consecutive pancreaticoduodenectomies in the 1990s: pathology, complications, and outcomes. Ann Surg. 1997;226(3):248–57; discussion 257–60

40. Elias D, Di Pietroantonio D, Gachot B, Menegon P, Hakime A, De Baere T. Liver abscess after radiofrequency ablation of tumors in patients with a biliary tract procedure. Gastroenterol Clin Biol. 2006;30(6–7):823–7.

41. Woo S, Chung JW, Hur S, Joo SM, Kim HC, Jae HJ, et al. Liver abscess after transarterial chemoembolization in patients with bilioenteric anastomosis: frequency and risk factors. AJR Am J Roentgenol. 2013;200(6):1370–7.

42. Guiu B, Deschamps F, Aho S, Munck F, Dromain C, Boige V, et al. Liver/biliary injuries following chemoembolisation of endocrine tumours and hepatocellular carcinoma: lipiodol vs. drug-eluting beads. J Hepatol. 2012;56(3):609–17.

43. Shin JU, Kim KM, Shin SW, Min SY, Park SU, Sinn DH, et al. A prediction model for liver abscess developing after transarterial chemoembolization in patients with hepatocellular carcinoma. Dig Liver Dis. 2014;46(9):813–7.

44. Goldberg SN, Charboneau JW, Dodd GD 3rd, Dupuy DE, Gervais DA, Gillams AR, et al. Image-guided tumor ablation: proposal for standardization of terms and reporting criteria. Radiology. 2003;228(2):335–45.

45. Livraghi T, Solbiati L, Meloni MF, Gazelle GS, Halpern EF, Goldberg SN. Treatment of focal liver tumors with percutaneous radio-frequency ablation: complications encountered in a multicenter study. Radiology. 2003;226(2):441–51.

46. Oshima S, Takaishi K, Tani N, Hirano M, Ikeda K, Makari Y, et al. Two cases of liver abscess caused by Clostridium perfringens after transcatheter arterial chemoembolization. Gan To Kagaku Ryoho. 2013;40(12):1795–7.

47. Yoon W, Jeong YY, Kim JK, Seo JJ, Lim HS, Shin SS, et al. CT in blunt liver trauma. Radiographics. 2005;25(1):87–104.

48. Dabbs DN, Stein DM, Scalea TM. Major hepatic necrosis: a common complication after angioembolization for treatment of high-grade liver injuries. J Trauma. 2009;66(3):621–7; discussion 627–9

49. Kusne S, Fung J, Alessiani M, Martin M, Torre-Cisneros J, Irish W, et al. Infections during a randomized trial comparing cyclosporine to FK 506 immunosuppression in liver transplantation. Transplant Proc. 1992;24(1):429–30.

50. Kibbler CC. Infections in liver transplantation: risk factors and strategies for prevention. J Hosp Infect. 1995;30(Suppl):209–17.

51. Guckelberger O, Stange B, Glanemann M, Lopez-Hanninen E, Heidenhain C, Jonas S, et al. Hepatic resection in liver transplant recipients: single center experience and review of the literature. Am J Transplant. 2005;5(10):2403–9.

52. Nelson DB, Bosco JJ, Curtis WD, Faigel DO, Kelsey PB, Leung JW, et al. ASGE technology status evaluation report. Biliary stents. Update May 1999. American Society for Gastrointestinal Endoscopy. Gastrointest Endosc. 1999;50(6):938–42.

53. Lederman ER, Crum NF. Pyogenic liver abscess with a focus on Klebsiella pneumoniae as a primary pathogen: an emerging disease with unique clinical characteristics. Am J Gastroenterol. 2005;100(2):322–31.

54. Tsai MS, Lee HM, Hsin MC, Lin CL, Hsu CY, Liu YT, et al. Increased risk of pyogenic liver abscess

among patients with colonic diverticular diseases: a nationwide cohort study. Medicine (Baltimore). 2015;94(49):e2210.

55. Tsai LW, Chao PW, Ou SM, Chen YT, Shih CJ, Li SY, et al. Pyogenic liver abscess in end-stage renal disease patients: a nationwide longitudinal study. Hemodial Int. 2015;19(1):72–9.

56. Lai SW, Lai HC, Lin CL, Liao KF. Splenectomy correlates with increased risk of pyogenic liver abscess: a nationwide cohort study in Taiwan. J Epidemiol. 2015;25(9):561–6.

57. Lin JN, Lin CL, Lin MC, Lai CH, Lin HH, Kao CH. Pyogenic liver abscess in patients with inflammatory bowel disease: a nationwide cohort study. Liver Int. 2016;36(1):136–44.

58. Qu K, Liu C, Wang ZX, Tian F, Wei JC, Tai MH, et al. Pyogenic liver abscesses associated with nonmetastatic colorectal cancers: an increasing problem in eastern Asia. World J Gastroenterol. 2012;18(23):2948–55.

59. O'Farrell N, Collins CG, McEntee GP. Pyogenic liver abscesses: diminished role for operative treatment. Surgeon. 2010;8(4):192–6.

60. Alvarez Perez JA, Gonzalez JJ, Baldonedo RF, Sanz L, Carreno G, Junco A, et al. Clinical course, treatment, and multivariate analysis of risk factors for pyogenic liver abscess. Am J Surg. 2001;181(2):177–86.

61. Barnes PF, De Cock KM, Reynolds TN, Ralls PW. A comparison of amebic and pyogenic abscess of the liver. Medicine (Baltimore). 1987;66(6):472–83.

62. Pope JV, Teich DL, Clardy P, McGillicuddy DC. Klebsiella pneumoniae liver abscess: an emerging problem in North America. J Emerg Med. 2011;41(5):e103–5.

63. Cheng DL, Liu YC, Yen MY, Liu CY, Shi FW, Wang LS. Pyogenic liver abscess: clinical manifestations and value of percutaneous catheter drainage treatment. J Formos Med Assoc. 1990;89(7):571–6.

64. Advances in Klebsiella research and application: 2013 Edition. Atlanta: Scholarly Editions; 2013.

65. Tan L, Zhou HJ, Hartman M, Ganpathi IS, Madhavan K, Chang S. Laparoscopic drainage of cryptogenic liver abscess. Surg Endosc. 2013;27(9):3308–14.

66. Misra SP, Misra V, Dwivedi M, Singh PA, Barthwal R. Factors influencing colonic involvement in patients with amebic liver abscess. Gastrointest Endosc. 2004;59(4):512–6.

67. Reed SL. Amebiasis: an update. Clin Infect Dis. 1992;14(2):385–93.

68. Mortele KJ, Segatto E, Ros PR. The infected liver: radiologic-pathologic correlation. Radiographics. 2004;24(4):937–55.

69. Kimura K, Stoopen M, Reeder MM, Moncada R. Amebiasis: modern diagnostic imaging with pathological and clinical correlation. Semin Roentgenol. 1997;32(4):250–75.

70. Elzi L, Laifer G, Sendi P, Ledermann HP, Fluckiger U, Bassetti S. Low sensitivity of ultrasonography for the early diagnosis of amebic liver abscess. Am J Med. 2004;117(7):519–22.

71. Halvorsen RA, Korobkin M, Foster WL, Silverman PM, Thompson WM. The variable CT appearance of hepatic abscesses. AJR Am J Roentgenol. 1984;142(5):941–6.

72. Pathak S, Palkhi E, Dave R, White A, Pandanaboyana S, Prasad KR, et al. Relationship between primary colorectal tumour and location of colorectal liver metastases. ANZ J Surg. 2016;86(5):408–10.

73. Jun CH, Yoon JH, Wi JW, Park SY, Lee WS, Jung SI, et al. Risk factors and clinical outcomes for spontaneous rupture of pyogenic liver abscess. J Dig Dis. 2015;16(1):31–6.

74. Chou FF, Sheen-Chen SM, Lee TY. Rupture of pyogenic liver abscess. Am J Gastroenterol. 1995;90(5):767–70.

75. Chung YF. Pyogenic liver abscess – predicting failure to improve outcome. Neth J Med. 2008;66(5):183–4.

76. Fang CT, Chuang YP, Shun CT, Chang SC, Wang JT. A novel virulence gene in Klebsiella pneumoniae strains causing primary liver abscess and septic metastatic complications. J Exp Med. 2004;199(5):697–705.

77. Irusen EM, Jackson TF, Simjee AE. Asymptomatic intestinal colonization by pathogenic Entamoeba histolytica in amebic liver abscess: prevalence, response to therapy, and pathogenic potential. Clin Infect Dis. 1992;14(4):889–93.

78. Hughes MA, Petri WA Jr. Amebic liver abscess. Infect Dis Clin N Am. 2000;14(3):565–82, viii

79. Petri WA Jr, Singh U. Diagnosis and management of amebiasis. Clin Infect Dis. 1999;29(5):1117–25.

80. Ravdin JI. Amebiasis. Clin Infect Dis. 1995;20(6):1453–64; quiz 1465–6

81. Kale S, Nanavati AJ, Borle N, Nagral S. Outcomes of a conservative approach to management in amoebic liver abscess. J Postgrad Med. 2017;63(1):16–20.

82. Eastiak MF, Saifullah M, Islam MS, Hossain MJ, Mannan M, Mousumi MS, et al. Pigtail catheter in the management of liver abscess. Mymensingh Med J. 2015;24(4):770–5.

83. Mc FA, Chang KP, Wong CC. Solitary pyogenic abscess of the liver treated by closed aspiration and antibiotics; a report of 14 consecutive cases with recovery. Br J Surg. 1953;41(166):141–52.

84. Branum GD, Tyson GS, Branum MA, Meyers WC. Hepatic abscess. Changes in etiology, diagnosis, and management. Ann Surg. 1990;212(6):655–62.

85. Tan YM, Chung AY, Chow PK, Cheow PC, Wong WK, Ooi LL, et al. An appraisal of surgical and percutaneous drainage for pyogenic liver abscesses larger than 5 cm. Ann Surg. 2005;241(3):485–90.

86. Chung YF, Tan YM, Lui HF, Tay KH, Lo RH, Kurup A, et al. Management of pyogenic liver abscesses – percutaneous or open drainage. Singap Med J. 2007;48(12):1158–65; quiz 1165

87. Rajak CL, Gupta S, Jain S, Chawla Y, Gulati M, Suri S. Percutaneous treatment of liver abscesses: needle aspiration versus catheter drainage. AJR Am J Roentgenol. 1998;170(4):1035–9.

88. Haider SJ, Tarulli M, McNulty NJ, Hoffer EK. Liver abscesses: factors that influence outcome of percutaneous drainage. AJR Am J Roentgenol. 2017;209(1):205–13.

89. Hope WW, Vrochides DV, Newcomb WL, Mayo-Smith WW, Iannitti DA. Optimal treatment of hepatic abscess. Am Surg. 2008;74(2):178–82.

90. Ahmed S, Chia CL, Junnarkar SP, Woon W, Shelat VG. Percutaneous drainage for giant pyogenic liver abscess – is it safe and sufficient? Am J Surg. 2016;211(1):95–101.

91. Chavez-Tapia NC, Hernandez-Calleros J, Tellez-Avila FI, Torre A, Uribe M. Image-guided percutaneous procedure plus metronidazole versus metronidazole alone for uncomplicated amoebic liver abscess. Cochrane Database Syst Rev. 2009;(1):CD004886.

92. Van Allan RJ, Katz MD, Johnson MB, Laine LA, Liu Y, Ralls PW. Uncomplicated amebic liver abscess: prospective evaluation of percutaneous therapeutic aspiration. Radiology. 1992;183(3):827–30.

93. vanSonnenberg E, Mueller PR, Schiffman HR, Ferrucci JT Jr, Casola G, Simeone JF, et al. Intrahepatic amebic abscesses: indications for and results of percutaneous catheter drainage. Radiology. 1985;156(3):631–5.

94. Zafar A, Ahmed S. Amoebic liver abscess: a comparative study of needle aspiration versus conservative treatment. J Ayub Med Coll Abbottabad. 2002;14(1):10–2.

95. Jordan PH Jr. Treatment of amebic abscess of the liver by open surgical drainage. Ann Surg. 1955;141(1):70–6.

96. Mezhir JJ, Fong Y, Jacks LM, Getrajdman GI, Brody LA, Covey AM, et al. Current management of pyogenic liver abscess: surgery is now second-line treatment. J Am Coll Surg. 2010;210(6):975–83.

97. Tu JF, Huang XF, Hu RY, You HY, Zheng XF, Jiang FZ. Comparison of laparoscopic and open surgery for pyogenic liver abscess with biliary pathology. World J Gastroenterol. 2011;17(38):4339–43.

98. Aydin C, Piskin T, Sumer F, Barut B, Kayaalp C. Laparoscopic drainage of pyogenic liver abscess. JSLS. 2010;14(3):418–20.

99. Ng SS, Lee JF, Lai PB. Role and outcome of conventional surgery in the treatment of pyogenic liver abscess in the modern era of minimally invasive therapy. World J Gastroenterol. 2008;14(5):747–51.

100. Cioffi L, Belli A, Limongelli P, Russo G, Arnold M, D'Agostino A, et al. Laparoscopic drainage as first line treatment for complex pyogenic liver abscesses. Hepato-Gastroenterology. 2014;61(131):771–5.

101. Herman P, Pugliese V, Montagnini AL, Salem MZ, Machado MA, da Cunha JE, et al. Pyogenic liver abscess: the role of surgical treatment. Int Surg. 1997;82(1):98–101.

102. Tay KH, Ravintharan T, Hoe MN, See AC, Chng HC. Laparoscopic drainage of liver abscesses. Br J Surg. 1998;85(3):330–2.

103. Gallagher MC, Andrews MM. Postdischarge outcomes of pyogenic liver abscesses: single-center experience 2007-2012. Open Forum Infect Dis. 2017;4(3):ofx159.

104. Ferraioli G, Garlaschelli A, Zanaboni D, Gulizia R, Brunetti E, Tinozzi FP, et al. Percutaneous and surgical treatment of pyogenic liver abscesses: observation over a 21-year period in 148 patients. Dig Liver Dis. 2008;40(8):690–6.

105. Wang W, Lee WJ, Wei PL, Chen TC, Huang MT. Laparoscopic drainage of pyogenic liver abscesses. Surg Today. 2004;34(4):323–5.

106. Klink CD, Binnebosel M, Schmeding M, van Dam RM, Dejong CH, Junge K, et al. Video-assisted hepatic abscess debridement. HPB (Oxford). 2015;17(8):732–5.

107. Al Amer NA, Abd El Maksoud WM. Abscess of the caudate lobe of the liver, a rare disease with a challenging management: a case report. J Biomed Res. 2013;27(5):430–4.

108. Ekwunife CN, Okorie O, Nwobe O. Laparoscopy may have a role in the drainage of liver abscess: early experience at Owerri, Nigeria. Niger J Surg. 2015;21(1):35–7.

109. Lazarchick J, De Souza e Silva NA, Nichols DR, Washington JA 2nd. Pyogenic liver abscess. Mayo Clin Proc. 1973;48(5):349–55.

110. Zibari GB, Maguire S, Aultman DF, McMillan RW, McDonald JC. Pyogenic liver abscess. Surg Infect. 2000;1(1):15–21.

Small Bowel Obstruction

16

Amirreza T. Motameni and Jason W. Smith

Epidemiology

SBO is a condition leading to absence or abnormal progression and passage of intestinal content through the small bowel. SBO can be caused by mechanical or functional etiologies. The most common cause of SBO is adhesive disease, accounting for 65–75% of the cases [2]. The most common risk factor for development of small bowel obstruction is past surgical history of abdominal or pelvic operations. While the majority of patients who undergo transperitoneal surgery will develop postoperative adhesions, the risk of SBO can be as low as 1% after an appendectomy [1] and as high as 25% after restorative proctocolectomy via ileal pouch-anal anastomosis (IPAA) [18, 25]. Due to its commonality, SBO is of great socioeconomic significance, as a 10-year follow-up study reported 5.7% of all hospital readmissions to be due to adhesive SBO [17]. Estimated financial cost for patient care due to adhesion-related illnesses in the United States is reported at $1.3 billion [37].

Differential Diagnosis

SBO can be due to different underlying causes. Here we discuss common causes of SBO:

1. Adhesive small bowel obstruction: SBO caused by adhesions is the most common type of SBO, accounting for 65–75% of all cases (Fig. 16.1). The most important risk factor for the development of adhesive SBO is prior abdominal or pelvic operations. However, radiation, pelvic inflammatory disease (PID), and abscesses can also lead to adhesive SBO in patients with no prior abdominal surgeries.
2. Hernia: Hernias are the second leading cause of SBO in all patients and the most common cause of SBO in patients without history of prior abdominal surgical intervention. This emphasizes the importance of physical examination in all patients with SBO as hernias are often diagnosed with a thorough bedside examination. One caveat would be in patients with morbid obesity and prior complex ventral abdominal wall hernia repairs, where physical exam is often insensitive in identifying hernias and in these patients CT scans is instrumental. While the most common types of hernias leading to small bowel obstruction are incisional (Fig. 16.2), inguinal, or femoral hernias, one most always include internal hernias and paraesophageal hernias in the differential diagnosis.

A. T. Motameni · J. W. Smith (✉)
The Hiram C. Polk Jr. Department of Surgery,
University of Louisville School of Medicine,
Louisville, KY, USA
e-mail: j0smit19@louisville.edu

© Springer International Publishing AG, part of Springer Nature 2019
C. V. R. Brown et al. (eds.), *Emergency General Surgery*, https://doi.org/10.1007/978-3-319-96286-3_16

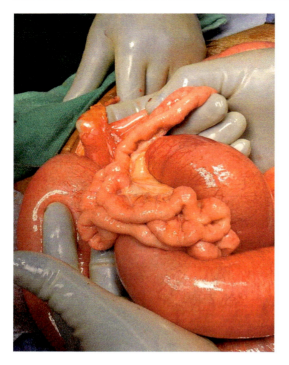

Fig. 16.1 57-year-old female with history of colonic resection presenting with small bowel obstruction. Single adhesive band found to be cause of obstruction

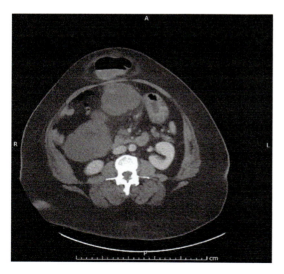

Fig. 16.2 58-year-old female presenting with an obstructing incisional hernia

3. Internal hernia: Roux-en-Y gastric bypass (RYGB) was a common surgical obesity procedure performed in the United States. One common complication inherent to this operation is the subsequent creation of potential spaces through which internal herniation can occur. Internal hernia must always be included in the differential diagnosis in the setting of prior RYGB and abdominal pain as 1–6% of patients experience SBO as a result of internal hernia [39]. The presence of "swirl sign" on CT scan is pathognomonic on CT scan [19]. With very few exceptions, internal hernia after RYGB is an indication for exploration as the consequences of missing the diagnosis results in potential for catastrophic bowel loss, morbidity, and mortality.

4. Neoplasm: Primary small bowel tumors are rare, accounting for 0.3% of all cancers. Of these rare cancers, adenocarcinoma and leiomyosarcoma are the most common, with carcinoid tumors and gastrointestinal stroma tumors (GIST) being much less common. Metastatic lesions to the small bowel are similarly rare, with lymphoma and melanoma being the most common of these etiologies. Diagnosis of small bowel neoplasm can be challenging, requiring appropriate imaging studies (see below) and clinical suspicion. Far more often, the small intestine is not the primary source of tumor or metastasis but becomes obstructed due to secondary tumor growth from an alternative intraperitoneal source of cancer [6].

5. Crohn's disease: An acute Crohn's disease exacerbation, intra-abdominal fluid collections, or strictures can serve as additional etiologies of SBO. The prevalence of small bowel strictures is common in this group of patients with a reported incidence of 7–15% [32, 48]. In the absence of absolute indications for exploration (pneumoperitoneum, peritonitis, etc.), the majority of patients with Crohn's disease who present with an acute Crohn's flare and stricture are successfully managed with medical management alone. The terminal ilium is often the most common anatomic location presenting with stricture in this patient population [5].

6. Intussusception: Intussusception is a rare diagnosis in adults as the cause of a small bowel obstruction. Defined as invagination of one segment of the bowel into an immediately

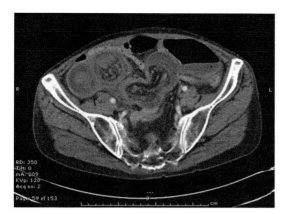

Fig. 16.3 32-year-old female presenting with 2 days history of nausea, vomiting, and bloody diarrhea. CT scan consistent with intussusception

adjacent segment, the incidence of adult intussusception leading to a SBO in adults is less than 0.3%. Pediatric patient more often present with this entity but, even in children, it is a rare occurrence. Most cases of intussusception are associated with a lead point causing the peristaltic movement of the bowel to intussuscept in that segment (Fig. 16.3). In adults, this is often associated with a malignancy, and the diagnosis is typically made in the operating room or on CT. Oncologic principles should be followed in all of these cases, which often require an oncologic resection including adequate margins and associated focal lymphadenectomy for best results [9, 29].

7. Foreign body (FB): Ingestion of FB is a common cause of small bowel obstruction. Risk factors for ingestion in the adult population are age, alcoholism, psychiatric disorders, and incarceration [45]. Symptoms associated with this pathology are diverse-acute respiratory failure, dyspepsia, GI bleeding, perforation, and GI obstruction. While most cases of FB ingestion can be managed either endoscopically or nonoperatively, 1–14% of patients ultimately require operative intervention [43]. Radiographic imaging can often identify the FB, and SBO due to FB ingestion is generally an indication for exploration.

8. Gallstone ileus: Gallstone ileus is a misnomer as the cause of the small bowel obstruction is not a functional ileus but rather a mechanical occlusion of the ileum. This often occurs at the ileocecal valve as a result of one or more large gallstones. Less than 1–3% of all cases of intestinal obstruction are due to gallstone ileus [22]. Gallstone ileus is more likely in the elderly patient population, and radiographic studies can be pathognomonic demonstrating pneumobilia, SBO, and FB at the ileocecal valve. SBO due to gallstone ileus is an indication for exploration as it will not resolve with nonoperative management.

Patient Presentation and Symptoms

Symptoms

The symptoms most commonly associated with acute small bowel obstruction include crampy abdominal pain accompanied by bloating and loss of appetite. A classic study of 300 patients suffering small bowel obstruction reported abdominal pain in 92% of patients and vomiting in 82% of patients [11]. The abdominal pain associated with small bowel obstruction is frequently described as periumbilical and colicky with spasms of pain occurring every few minutes in an intermittent, episodic fashion [36]. A progression from colicky to more focal and constant pain may indicate early focal peritonitis related to SBO complications such as ischemia, bowel necrosis, or focal perforation. With proximal small bowel obstruction (duodenum, proximal jejunum), nausea and vomiting can be severe, leading to significant electrolyte disturbances which must be managed and corrected prior to intervention. Obstipation (the lack of ability to pass flatus or stool) is often pathognomonic of the condition. The frequency of these symptoms is variable and depends upon both the cause and location of obstruction (proximal versus distal) within the GI tract.

Physical Examination

Overall, physical examination should focus on evaluating the patient for systemic sequelae of the bowel obstruction. The vomiting caused by the small bowel obstruction can often lead to severe dehydration. Systemic manifestations of dehydration include tachycardia, orthostatic hypotension, and reduced urine output. Dry mucus membranes, sunken periorbital areas, and poor skin turgor are physical exam signs that point toward severe dehydration. Fever is not generally associated with a bowel obstruction in the absence of complication but may be associated with infection (i.e., abscess) or other complications of obstruction (ischemia, necrosis, perforation). Hematemesis and hematochezia may be a sign of tumor, ischemia, inflammatory mucosal injury, or intussusception and are particularly concerning signs in the setting of a bowel obstruction.

Abdominal inspection will often identify abdominal distention in most patients with acute SBO. Abdominal inspection should also note surgical scars or evidence of abdominal wall hernia (including incisional hernia) or groin hernias. In numerous retrospective reviews, abdominal distension was the most frequent finding on physical examination, occurring in over 65% of patients. Although nausea and vomiting may be less severe in patients with distal small bowel obstruction compared with proximal obstruction, abdominal distention is greater because the more proximal bowel acts as a reservoir for gastrointestinal contents. Often, distention of the bowel results in tympany on percussion (hyperresonance) throughout the abdomen. Tenderness to light percussion suggests peritonitis. It is important to remember that in patients with a closed-loop obstruction, abdominal distention can be minimal.

Palpation of the abdomen is used to identify any abdominal wall or groin hernias, or abnormal masses, which, in the setting of small bowel obstruction, may indicate the source of obstruction. Digital rectal examination should be performed to identify fecal impaction or rectal mass as the source of obstruction even if a small bowel obstruction is presumed. Gross or occult blood may be related to intestinal tumor, ischemia, inflammatory mucosal injury, or intussusception and might help discern alternative etiologies of obstruction.

Laboratory and Imaging Evaluation of Small Bowel Obstruction

Laboratory Workup

CBC and BMP are helpful in management of patients with SBO. While laboratory values are nonspecific in the diagnosis of SBO, the presence or increasing leukocytosis can help in determining appropriate management of SBO as it can give insight into patient's pathology and the possibility of bowel ischemia. Margenthaler et al. reported patients undergoing exploration with adhesiolysis tend to have higher frequency of abnormal WBC count (> 11,000/mm^3) compared to patients requiring small bowel resection. However, patients who required small bowel resection tend to have significantly lower mean serum albumin levels compared with patients who required adhesiolysis [28]. Patient's with proximal SBO can have significant vomiting or have high nasogastric output that can result in a hypochloremic, hypokalemic metabolic alkalosis. An elevated creatinine and acute renal insufficiency or failure (ARF) can be seen in patients with dehydration and indicate need for more aggressive fluid resuscitation.

Imaging

Abdominal X-ray (AXR): X-ray is often the initial imaging study of choice as they can be obtained quickly, are relatively inexpensive, and can give general insight into the diagnosis of abdominal pain or obstruction. AXR can diagnose small bowel obstruction with a sensitivity and specificity of 79–83% and 67–83%, respectively, but can be normal in up 20% of patient with SBO [41]. Findings on plain radiography consistent with small bowel obstruction include the following:

• Dilated loops of bowel with air-fluid levels are pathognomonic for patients with SBO (Fig. 16.4) when present. However, it's important to keep in mind air-fluid levels are often absent in patients with proximal obstructions and other imaging findings such as dilated stomach can be helpful in diagnosis of proximal SBO [8].

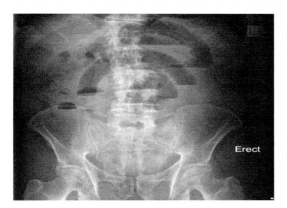

Fig. 16.4 Abdominal X-ray in a 42-year-old male with small bowel obstruction. Dilated loops of bowel and air-fluid levels can be seen in this image

- Proximal small bowel dilation with distal small bowel collapse – Small bowel obstruction can be diagnosed if the more proximal small bowel is dilated more than 2.5 cm (outer wall to outer wall), and the more distal small bowel is not dilated. The stomach may also be dilated prior to decompression.
- Loss of abdominal gas – A gasless abdomen may be due to complete filling of loops of bowel with sequestered fluid. A "string of pearls" sign may be seen in predominantly fluid-filled small bowel loops on upright or lateral films, as small amounts of intraluminal gas collect along the superior bowel wall separated by the valvulae conniventes.

Computed tomography (CT): Multidetector CT scanning is the most useful imaging study for the diagnosis and management of SBO. CT scan has a sensitivity of 95% and specificity of 96% for diagnosing SBO (Fig. 16.5) [26, 27]. In addition to diagnosing SBO, CT scans can be further helpful in diagnosing the underlying cause, such as identifying the specific location (i.e., transition point) and severity of SBO (partial versus complete); determining the etiology by identifying hernias, masses, or inflammatory changes; and identifying complications (ischemia, necrosis, perforation) [46]. Similar to the findings on plain abdominal radiography, a diagnosis of bowel obstruction on abdominal CT can be made by the findings of dilated proxi-

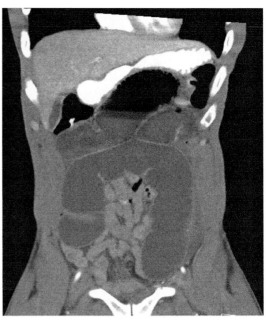

Fig. 16.5 21-year-old male with history of exploratory laparotomy after trauma presenting with small bowel obstruction. Collapsed and dilated loops of small bowel due to transition point in the pelvis can be seen in this image

mal bowel with distal collapsed bowel and air-fluid levels. Identifying the transition point between dilated and nondilated bowel, although not required to make the diagnosis of obstruction, may establish the location and cause of small bowel obstruction. However, the location of obstruction as identified on CT only correlates with the intraoperative locations in approximately 60–70% of patients [14]. In addition, the presence of a transition point on abdominal CT does not appear to accurately predict the need for immediate or delayed operative intervention and thus should not be used as a major initial criterion influencing a decision to operate [38]. Additional findings on abdominal CT scan consistent with a diagnosis of bowel obstruction include:

- Bowel wall thickening >3 mm (nonspecific)
- Mesenteric edema
- "Target sign"– Alternating hypo−/hyperdense layers, indicative of intussusception

- "Whirl sign" – Rotation of small bowel mesentery, suggesting a twist or a volvulus
- "Venous cutoff sign" – Venous flow to a loop of small bowel that is "cut off" suggests thrombosis

In general the administration of oral and intravenous contrast allows for the study to provide the best information. However, for those who cannot tolerate oral contrast, retained intraluminal fluid within dilated bowel loops usually provides adequate enhancement when evaluating patients for ischemic complications.

Magnetic resonance imaging (MRI) and abdominal ultrasonography (US): Abdominal MRI can be used to assess patients for a small bowel obstruction with sensitivity and specificity similar to CT scanning. However, the increased time for image acquisition and the need for repeated breath-holds to obtain high-quality images limit the general. Abdominal ultrasonography may be useful for the diagnosis of small bowel obstruction in selected patients though its specificity and sensitivity are less than CT and similar to AXR. Ultrasound is most useful in the emergency department to evaluate abdominal pain [20] and to assess for hernias that cannot be identified on patient exam and in patients with contraindications to CT, such as those with contrast allergies, pregnant patients, and critically ill patients for whom the study must be performed at the bedside [23].

Small bowel contrast studies: Therapeutic water-based hypertonic contrast administration for SBO (small bowel follow-through (SBFT) and enteroclysis) are of limited utility in the modern diagnosis of small bowel obstruction. Fluoroscopic findings consistent with small bowel obstruction are dilated loops of proximal small bowel opacification with contrast material and a change in the diameter of the small bowel at the transition zone (Fig. 16.6). The transition zone at the site of the SBO can be missed using small bowel follow-through because water-soluble contrast agents generally become diluted as they pass through dilated fluid-filled bowel loops. Thus, the degree of opacification may not be sufficient to identify the transition point at the site of obstruction. The transition zone, however,

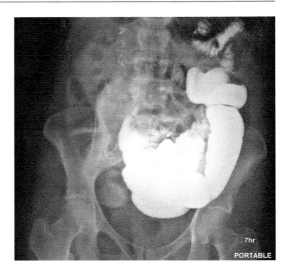

Fig. 16.6 Upper GI with small bowel follow-through (SBFT) in a 54-year-old female with multiple abdominal surgeries. Failure of contrast passing through small bowel after 7 h

can be readily identified with enteroclysis, particularly in patients with multiple obstructions and or chronic bowel obstructions. Enteroclysis is a procedure in which the duodenum is intubated with a tube, and a large volume of air and contrast (typically, barium and methylcellulose) is instilled directly into the small intestine while repeatedly imaging over time using fluoroscopy. Enteroclysis has some utility in the diagnosis and management of bowel obstruction related to inflammatory bowel disease and chronic obstructions as multiple areas of functional stenosis may need to be evaluated. However, in the acute setting, enteroclysis is not recommended as patients with acute small bowel obstruction tolerate the high volume of oral contrast material poorly. Also, it is preferable not to have large quantities of barium in the small bowel lumen if surgery or a perforation is a possibility.

Management

Initial Management

Patients who are diagnosed with acute small bowel obstruction generally require hospital admission for initial management that includes intravenous fluid therapy and electrolyte replacement. These patients should generally be admitted to a surgical service as studies have demonstrated shorter lengths of stay, fewer hospital charges, shorter times to surgery, and lower mortality rates than patients admitted to medical service [16, 33]. For patients who are admitted to a medical service, the use of clear-cut SBO treatment protocols have been shown to decrease time to surgical consultation and operative intervention and shorten hospital length of stay [30, 44].

In general, all patients with mechanical bowel obstruction should be made nil per os (NPO) to limit bowel distension and emesis. While surgical dogma teaches the need for early nasogastric tube (NGT) placement for decompression, there is currently little evidence to support this practice [21]. In patients with complete or high-grade small bowel obstruction, decompression of the distended stomach improves patient comfort and also minimizes the passage of swallowed air, which can worsen distension. Therefore, the need for NGT decompression in the setting of small bowel obstruction remains a matter of clinician judgment.

Patients with small bowel obstruction (particularly proximal obstructions) can have severe volume depletion, metabolic acidosis or alkalosis, and electrolyte abnormalities due to the nausea and vomiting resulting from the underlying pathophysiology of the disease. This is particularly true for patients seeking treatment later in the course of the disease progression with symptoms that have been present for several days prior to presentation. Upon admission, intravenous access in the form of two large-bore peripheral lines should be obtained for fluid resuscitation. Intravenous rehydration should be initiated using a balanced salt solution. Aggressive potassium repletion may be needed, but it is important to be certain the patient does not have acute kidney injury (acute renal failure) from severe dehydration, in which case potassium supplementation should be given cautiously until renal function is improved. Even in cases where signs and symptoms indicate urgent operative intervention, fluid resuscitation and repletion of electrolytes prior to surgery can significantly minimize complications

(i.e., hypotension) related to anesthesia induction agents.

In general, pain from mechanical bowel obstruction, which is crampy in nature, is often not amenable to treatment with analgesics, particularly opioids. Additionally, excessive administration of opiate pain medications in the setting of bowel obstruction may impede resolution of the obstruction. Pain management with opioids and other pharmacologic agents is reasonable in the setting of palliation.

Indication for Operative Management

Most patients suspected of having complicated bowel obstruction (complete obstruction, closed-loop obstruction, bowel ischemia, necrosis, or perforation) based upon clinical and radiologic examination should be taken to the operating room for abdominal exploration. Additionally, if malignancy is the suspected underlying cause of the small bowel obstruction, urgent or early intervention should be considered. Several studies have demonstrated that nonoperative management of malignant small bowel obstruction is associated with a high failure rate and high mortality [34]. However, it should be noted that palliative treatment of malignant bowel obstruction carries significant morbidity and mortality and setting realistic expectations with the patient is critical.

Overall, the incidence of need for operative intervention with adhesive obstruction is low. However, a significant change in clinical presentation and/or the development of a complicated obstruction (closed loop, perforation, and ischemia) during a trial of nonoperative management should prompt surgical exploration. Clinical signs and symptoms that are associated with worsening obstruction and possible bowel ischemia (Fig. 16.7) are nonspecific but include the following:

- Worsening leukocytosis
- Change in vital signs including tachycardia and hypotension

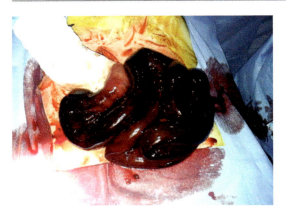

Fig. 16.7 75-year-old female presenting with small bowel obstruction and peritonitis. Necrotic bowel was found on exploration

- Metabolic acidosis
- Fever not present on admission
- Change in abdominal exam and/or the development of peritonitis.

These signs and symptoms correctly identify bowel ischemia in approximately 40–50% of cases [20, 40]. As always diligent monitoring of the patient's overall condition and following either the resolution or worsening of symptoms are imperative in the management of this condition.

Nonoperative Management

Patients without clinical or radiologic signs and symptoms of bowel ischemia or perforation can safely undergo initial nonoperative management. Progression to bowel ischemia in the setting of partial SBO is unlikely to occur with nonoperative management (3–6%), but patients need to be monitored with serial abdominal examinations and laboratory studies [24]. From a historical perspective, surgical dogma often recommended that patients with SBO (without indications for immediate surgical exploration) should be observed for no longer than 12–24 h after which time, if no improvement is seen, the patient should undergo exploration. Numerous studies have contradicted this approach, and in the absence of signs of complications of obstruction,

the patient may be observed for a longer period of time. Nonoperative management is overall successful in 65–80% of patients within 2–5 days of admission, especially in the setting of partial SBO and early postoperative SBO [7, 12].

Hypertonic Contrast in Partial SBO

In patients whose symptoms persist longer than 48 h following admission, the utilization of enteral water-soluble hypertonic contrast boluses may be beneficial [12, 13]. The water-soluble hypertonic contrast draws fluid into the lumen of the bowel due to its hypertonicity, thereby decreasing intestinal wall edema and stimulating intestinal peristalsis. After contrast administration, abdominal radiographs should be performed in order to follow the progression of the enteral contrast through the GI tract. In general, failure of the contrast to reach the colon within 24 h of administration suggests that surgical exploration is warranted.

A 2016 systematic review and meta-analysis demonstrated that water-soluble contrast predicted resolution of obstruction without surgery with a sensitivity of 92% and a specificity of 93%. Treatment with water-soluble hypertonic contrast also reduced the need for surgery, length of stay, and time to resolution of symptoms. There was no increased morbidity or mortality associated with water-soluble contrast [10]. Additionally, a multicenter prospective observational study compared patients treated at centers with and without a water-soluble contrast protocol, and those treated with protocols had a lower rate of operative exploration (21% vs 44%) and a reduced length of stay (4 days vs 5 days). In that study, multivariable regression demonstrated that the use of water-soluble hypertonic contrast in SBO was independently associated with successful nonoperative management [47]. It should be noted however that the Adhesive Small Bowel Obstruction Study (ASBOS) showed no difference in operative intervention or bowel resection between groups treated with water-soluble contrast and groups treated with normal saline. Additionally, contrary to prior studies, oral contrast administration did not shorten the length of hospital stay (3.5 days in both groups) [15, 42]. Overall, there is some evidence that the treatment of a bowel obstruction with an oral contrast challenge is helpful and very little evidence that it is harmful, thus it should be considered as a viable treatment modality in the management of small bowel obstruction.

Operative Techniques

Specific operative techniques needed to treat a bowel obstruction are primarily determined by the underlying etiology of the disease. However, the decision to transition to operative treatment for an uncomplicated bowel obstruction is primarily determined by the clinical status and progression of the patient and is often difficult. However, failure to regain bowel function after 5 days of nonoperative management suggests the need for operative management and delay beyond this time period has been associated with higher mortality and the need for longer hospitalization [4]. With regard to laparoscopic versus open surgical techniques for the treatment of this disease, a 2012 Eastern Association for the Surgery of Trauma (EAST) practice management guideline (PMG) determined: "Although previously reserved only for simple SBO, current literature supports the use of laparoscopy in complex SBO with dilated bowel and multiple previous abdominal operations. The appropriate setting not only depends on the patient but also on the surgeon's experience" [3]. Also noted within the EAST PMG for small bowel obstruction was the result of a 2012 meta-analysis of 29 studies and over 2000 patients that demonstrated a conversion rate of 29% and an enterotomy rate of less than 7% [31]. Patients with a single-band adhesive obstruction have a higher success rate but complex small bowel obstruction can be treated safely laparoscopically [35].

> ### Conclusion
> Small bowel obstruction is a common problem encountered by general surgeons and requires a thoughtful approach in order to

optimize outcomes. The most common etiology resulting in SBO is adhesive disease, accounting for 65–75% of all cases. CT scan is the imaging study of choice and allows for the diagnosis, localization, and characterization of the obstruction and is useful in providing information regarding complications of obstruction such as ischemia, perforation, and associated pathology. The majority (up to 75%) of patients are successfully managed with nasogastric decompression, fluid resuscitation, and bowel rest in the absence of indications for operative intervention. Indications for operative intervention include worsening leukocytosis, physiologic decompensation (change in vital signs including tachycardia and hypotension), metabolic acidosis, fever not present on admission, change in abdominal exam, and/or the development of peritonitis. In the event that operative management is required, both open and laparoscopic approaches are acceptable.

References

1. Ahlberg G, Bergdahl S, Rutqvist J, et al. Mechanical small-bowel obstruction after conventional appendectomy in children. Eur J Pediatr Surg. 1997;7:13–5.
2. Attard JA, Maclean AR. Adhesive small bowel obstruction: epidemiology, biology and prevention. Can J Surg. 2007;50:291–300.
3. Azagury D, Liu RC, Morgan A, et al. Small bowel obstruction: a practical step-by-step evidence-based approach to evaluation, decision making, and management. J Trauma Acute Care Surg. 2015;79:661–8.
4. Bauer J, Keeley B, Krieger B, et al. Adhesive small bowel obstruction: early operative versus observational management. Am Surg. 2015;81:614–20.
5. Boltin D, Levi Z, Halpern M, et al. Concurrent small bowel adenocarcinoma and carcinoid tumor in Crohn's disease – case report and literature review. J Crohns Colitis. 2011;5:461–4.
6. Catena F, Ansaloni L, Gazzotti F, et al. Small bowel tumours in emergency surgery: specificity of clinical presentation. ANZ J Surg. 2005;75:997–9.
7. Catena F, Di Saverio S, Coccolini F, et al. Adhesive small bowel adhesions obstruction: evolutions in diagnosis, management and prevention. World J Gastrointest Surg. 2016;8:222–31.
8. Catena F, Di Saverio S, Kelly MD, et al. Bologna guidelines for diagnosis and management of adhesive

small bowel obstruction (ASBO): 2010 evidence-based guidelines of the world society of emergency surgery. World J Emerg Surg. 2011;6:5.

9. Cera SM. Intestinal intussusception. Clin Colon Rectal Surg. 2008;21:106–13.

10. Ceresoli M. Coccolini F, Catena F, et al. Water-soluble contrast agent in adhesive small bowel obstruction: a systematic review and meta-analysis of diagnostic and therapeutic value. Am J Surg. 2016;211:1114–25.

11. Cheadle WG, Garr EE, Richardson JD. The importance of early diagnosis of small bowel obstruction. Am Surg. 1988;54:565–9.

12. Choi HK, Chu KW, Law WL. Therapeutic value of gastrografin in adhesive small bowel obstruction after unsuccessful conservative treatment: a prospective randomized trial. Ann Surg. 2002;236:1–6.

13. Choi HK, Law WL, Ho JW, et al. Value of gastrografin in adhesive small bowel obstruction after unsuccessful conservative treatment: a prospective evaluation. World J Gastroenterol. 2005;11:3742–5.

14. Colon MJ, Telem DA, Wong D, et al. The relevance of transition zones on computed tomography in the management of small bowel obstruction. Surgery. 2010;147:373–7.

15. Di Saverio S, Catena F, Ansaloni L, et al. Water-soluble contrast medium (gastrografin) value in adhesive small intestine obstruction (ASIO): a prospective, randomized, controlled, clinical trial. World J Surg. 2008;32:2293–304.

16. Diaz JJ Jr, Bokhari F, Mowery NT, et al. Guidelines for management of small bowel obstruction. J Trauma. 2008;64:1651–64.

17. Ellis H, Moran BJ, Thompson JN, et al. Adhesion-related hospital readmissions after abdominal and pelvic surgery: a retrospective cohort study. Lancet. 1999;353:1476–80.

18. Fazio VW, Ziv Y, Church JM, et al. Ileal pouch-anal anastomoses complications and function in 1005 patients. Ann Surg. 1995;222:120–7.

19. Fernandez-Moure J, Sherman V. Swirl sign – intestinal volvulus after roux-en-Y gastric bypass. N Engl J Med. 2017;376:e3.

20. Fevang BT, Jensen D, Svanes K, et al. Early operation or conservative management of patients with small bowel obstruction? Eur J Surg. 2002;168:475–81.

21. Fleshner PR, Siegman MG, Slater GI, et al. A prospective, randomized trial of short versus long tubes in adhesive small-bowel obstruction. Am J Surg. 1995;170:366–70.

22. Halabi WJ, Kang CY, Ketana N, et al. Surgery for gallstone ileus: a nationwide comparison of trends and outcomes. Ann Surg. 2014;259:329–35.

23. Jang TB, Schindler D, Kaji AH. Bedside ultrasonography for the detection of small bowel obstruction in the emergency department. Emerg Med J. 2011;28:676–8.

24. Jeong WK, Lim SB, Choi HS, et al. Conservative management of adhesive small bowel obstructions in patients previously operated on for primary colorectal cancer. J Gastrointest Surg. 2008;12:926–32.

25. Maclean AR, Cohen Z, Macrae HM, et al. Risk of small bowel obstruction after the ileal pouch-anal anastomosis. Ann Surg. 2002;235:200–6.

26. Maglinte DD, Reyes BL, Harmon BH, et al. Reliability and role of plain film radiography and CT in the diagnosis of small-bowel obstruction. AJR Am J Roentgenol. 1996;167:1451–5.

27. Mallo RD, Salem L, Lalani T, et al. Computed tomography diagnosis of ischemia and complete obstruction in small bowel obstruction: a systematic review. J Gastrointest Surg. 2005;9:690–4.

28. Margenthaler JA, Longo WE, Virgo KS, et al. Risk factors for adverse outcomes following surgery for small bowel obstruction. Ann Surg. 2006;243: 456–64.

29. Marsicovetere P, Ivatury SJ, White B, et al. Intestinal intussusception: etiology, diagnosis, and treatment. Clin Colon Rectal Surg. 2017;30:30–9.

30. Maung AA, Johnson DC, Piper GL, et al. Evaluation and management of small-bowel obstruction: an Eastern Association for the Surgery of Trauma practice management guideline. J Trauma Acute Care Surg. 2012;73:S362–9.

31. O'connor DB, Winter DC. The role of laparoscopy in the management of acute small-bowel obstruction: a review of over 2,000 cases. Surg Endosc. 2012;26:12–7.

32. Ohlsson B, Fork FT, Veress B, et al. Coexistent chronic idiopathic intestinal pseudo obstruction and inflammatory bowel disease. Gut. 2005;54:729–30.

33. Oyasiji T, Angelo S, Kyriakides TC, et al. Small bowel obstruction: outcome and cost implications of admitting service. Am Surg. 2010;76:687–91.

34. Paul Olson TJ, Pinkerton C, Brasel KJ, et al. Palliative surgery for malignant bowel obstruction from carcinomatosis: a systematic review. JAMA Surg. 2014;149:383–92.

35. Pearl JP, Marks JM, Hardacre JM, et al. Laparoscopic treatment of complex small bowel obstruction: is it safe? Surg Innov. 2008;15:110–3.

36. Rami Reddy SR, Cappell MS. A systematic review of the clinical presentation, diagnosis, and treatment of small bowel obstruction. Curr Gastroenterol Rep. 2017;19:28.

37. Ray NF, Denton WG, Thamer M, et al. Abdominal adhesiolysis: inpatient care and expenditures in the United States in 1994. J Am Coll Surg. 1998;186:1–9.

38. Scrima A, Lubner MG, King S, et al. Value of MDCT and clinical and laboratory data for predicting the need for surgical intervention in suspected small-bowel obstruction. AJR Am J Roentgenol. 2017;208:785–93.

39. Steele KE, Prokopowicz GP, Magnuson T, et al. Laparoscopic antecolic Roux-en-Y gastric bypass with closure of internal defects leads to fewer internal hernias than the retrocolic approach. Surg Endosc. 2008;22:2056–61.

40. Takeuchi K, Tsuzuki Y, Ando T, et al. Clinical studies of strangulating small bowel obstruction. Am Surg. 2004;70:40–4.

41. Van Oudheusden TR, Aerts BA, De Hingh IH, et al. Challenges in diagnosing adhesive small bowel obstruction. World J Gastroenterol. 2013;19: 7489–93.
42. Vather R, Josephson R, Jaung R, et al. Gastrografin in prolonged postoperative ileus: a double-blinded randomized controlled trial. Ann Surg. 2015;262:23–30.
43. Velitchkov NG, Grigorov GI, Losanoff JE, et al. Ingested foreign bodies of the gastrointestinal tract: retrospective analysis of 542 cases. World J Surg. 1996;20:1001–5.
44. Wahl WL, Wong SL, Sonnenday CJ, et al. Implementation of a small bowel obstruction guideline improves hospital efficiency. Surgery. 2012;152:626–32; discussion 632–4
45. Yamamoto H, Kita H, Sunada K, et al. Clinical outcomes of double-balloon endoscopy for the diagnosis and treatment of small-intestinal diseases. Clin Gastroenterol Hepatol. 2004;2:1010–6.
46. Zalcman M, Sy M, Donckier V, et al. Helical CT signs in the diagnosis of intestinal ischemia in small-bowel obstruction. AJR Am J Roentgenol. 2000;175:1601–7.
47. Zielinski MD, Haddad NN, Cullinane DC, et al. Multi-institutional, prospective, observational study comparing the Gastrografin challenge versus standard treatment in adhesive small bowel obstruction. J Trauma Acute Care Surg. 2017;83:47–54.
48. Zissin R, Hertz M, Paran H, et al. Small bowel obstruction secondary to Crohn disease: CT findings. Abdom Imaging. 2004;29:320–5.

Small Bowel Perforation

17

Eric M. Campion and Clay Cothren Burlew

Introduction

Non-traumatic perforation of the small bowel is a relatively rare occurrence. It requires prompt diagnosis and operative management to minimize morbidity and mortality. The etiology of small bowel perforations varies widely and can have a significant impact on management strategies. Clinicians that manage these patients should be aware of the diverse etiologies of small bowel perforation as they impact operative techniques, intraoperative care, postoperative management, and prognosis.

Clinical Presentation

Patients with small bowel perforation present along a spectrum of symptoms. Bowel perforation will result in some degree of contamination of the peritoneal cavity causing inflammation of the peritoneum and surrounding abdominal structures. This often leads to fever, abdominal pain, nausea, and vomiting. Physical examination reveals abdominal tenderness and frequently diffuse peritonitis. Peritonitis is identified on examination by rebound tenderness, guarding, and abdominal rigidity. The amount of peritoneal irritation will determine the severity of peritonitis and associated physical exam findings. If the perforation is being walled off by other abdominal structures, patients can present with mild pain and minimal signs of peritoneal irritation. Additionally, it is important to recognize that patients with conditions that cause an impaired inflammatory response, such as advanced AIDS, neutropenic patients, and patients taking high doses of immunomodulatory medications may not manifest peritonitis in the classic fashion. These patients may present with vague abdominal pain and sepsis without diffuse peritoneal signs.

The physiologic response to bowel perforation can vary widely, from a minor inflammatory response to severe septic shock. Prior to or concurrent with imaging studies, resuscitation of the patient should be the priority. This should include volume loading to correct adverse physiology and normalization of any reversible cardiomyopathy. Prompt administration of broad-spectrum antibiotics is warranted while the diagnositic workup proceeds [1]. This is imperative as severe physiologic compromise can result in cardiac arrest on induction of anesthesia. Markers of resuscitation such as lactate and arterial base deficit can help guide resuscitative efforts along with traditional endpoints such as blood pressure and urine output.

E. M. Campion · C. C. Burlew (✉)
Department of Surgery, Denver Health Medical Center/University of Colorado, Denver, CO, USA
e-mail: clay.cothren@dhha.org

© Springer International Publishing AG, part of Springer Nature 2019
C. V. R. Brown et al. (eds.), *Emergency General Surgery*, https://doi.org/10.1007/978-3-319-96286-3_17

Patients with abdominal pain and diffuse peritonitis should proceed to the operating room without delay. Plain abdominal radiographs will often demonstrate signs of hollow viscous perforation (such as free air). This combined with the physical exam is often enough information to proceed directly to the operating room.

Classically an abdominal series consists of three radiographs: a supine anteroposterior abdominal film, an upright abdominal film, and an upright chest film. Free air can be seen as a lucency under the diaphragm on upright abdominal or chest radiographs (Fig. 17.1). Other subtle findings can be identified on flat abdominal films suggesting the underlying etiology, such as bowel pneumatosis (ischemic bowel) or dilated bowel with air/fluid levels (bowel obstruction).

Computed tomography (CT) is being used with increasing frequency in the diagnosis of abdominal pain, often without plain abdominal films. CT imaging is very sensitive for intra-abdominal free air and will often localize the site of perforation with a high degree of specificity [2]. Specific findings concerning for bowel perforation on CT imaging are free air, extraluminal contrast extravasation, and visible transmural lesions of the intestinal wall [2]. This information can be useful to the operating surgeon but needs to be weighed against the time, expense, and radiation exposure when the diagnosis of a perforated viscous is obvious from clinical exam. When the clinical picture is less clear, CT imaging is often able to make the diagnosis of a perforated viscous and identify the etiology and any complications of the disease process.

Ultrasound is able to detect signs of bowel perforation but is limited by user dependence, poor patient cooperation due to pain, and obesity [3]. Signs of bowel perforation on ultrasound are strong reverberation above the liver, movement of reverberation with patient position, and probe pressure [2]. Ultrasound can also identify free fluid and decreased bowel activity which are non-specific but can be associated with bowel perforation.

Magnetic resonance imaging can be used in the diagnostic evaluation of patients with abdominal pain, including in cases of bowel perforation. This is often utilized in children and pregnant patients to limit radiation dosing to the patient. MRI is also being used with increasing frequency in patients with inflammatory bowel disease to limit lifetime radiation [4]. The utility of MRI as a first-line diagnostic tool has been limited due to its higher cost, lower availability, and limitations in patients with implanted devices and metallic foreign objects [3].

Etiology

Perforation of the small bowel can have a wide variety of causes. Many of these diverse etiologies can be suggested based on the patient's clinical presentation, making a thorough history and physical examination essential in identifying the correct diagnosis.

Small bowel obstruction is one of the leading causes of bowel perforation in the industrialized world. The majority of small bowel obstructions are related to adhesive disease from prior surgery or an incarcerated hernia. Small bowel obstruction leads to upstream bowel dilation. As the bowel dilates, it can cause venous outflow obstruction and ischemia leading to perforation. Patients generally present with abdominal pain, nausea, and vomiting prior to bowel perforation.

Most patients presenting with presumed adhesive disease-related small bowel obstruction can be treated with NG tube decompression, bowel rest, and increasingly modern protocols incorpo-

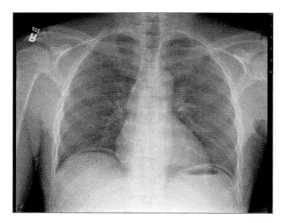

Fig. 17.1 Free air can be seen under both diaphragms in this upright chest radiograph

rating an oral contrast challenge that is diagnostic and often therapeutic [5]. However, evidence of bowel ischemia and/or perforation must be aggressively excluded at presentation and subsequently monitored for during the patient's hospital course (acidosis, increasing leukocytosis, increasing blood lactate, and worsening abdominal exam should prompt repeat investigation or operative intervention). Findings of ischemia on CT imaging or evidence of a "closed loop obstruction" where the intestine is obstructed in two places mandates urgent operative exploration. Patients presenting with a bowel perforation in the setting of bowel obstruction are not typically amenable to primary repair of the bowel, and segmental resection of the bowel is often required as the bowel may be dilated and/or ischemic.

Patients with an incarcerated hernia are typically identified on a thorough physical examination. When an incarcerated hernia is encountered, risk factors for bowel ischemia or perforation are assessed. These include significant erythema overlying the hernia, peritonitis on abdominal exam, elevated blood lactate levels or a metabolic acidosis, or imaging evidence consistent with bowel ischemia. In patients without clinical, laboratory, or imaging concerns for ischemia, urgent reduction of the hernia is warranted. Concern for bowel ischemia should lead to urgent operation with visualization of the bowel. Ischemic or perforated bowel from an incarcerated hernia requires resection. The hernia is then repaired to prevent recurrence of incarceration. One should avoid permanent mesh placement for herniorrhaphy in the setting of bowel perforation with contamination to prevent mesh infection [6].

Inflammatory Bowel Disease

Crohn's disease is a disorder that results in transmural inflammation of the intestinal wall. Acute perforation is uncommon, 2% of Crohn's patients in a recent study, but remains a significant indication for surgery [7]. The location of the perforation can be anywhere along the small bowel but most commonly occurs at the ileum. Patients on anti-inflammatory and biologic medications for Crohn's therapy can present in delayed fashion as these medications can mask the early signs and symptoms resulting in a benign physical exam and unremarkable laboratory values.

Operative management of small bowel perforation in Crohn's disease should be individualized. The segment including the perforation should be resected, rather than repaired. This should include the surrounding bowel that is clinically diseased, but there is no need to achieve microscopic margins or resect additional normal appearing bowel [8]. The chronicity of the perforation and the condition of the remaining intestine will determine operative management. Most patients will be amenable to a primary anastomosis of the bowel. In patients with delayed presentation and ileal perforation, occasional creation of a stoma is warranted. These patients are at increased risk for complications with one study showing a 20% rate of complications in patients with ileocecal resection for Crohn's disease [9]. Preoperative steroid therapy was a risk factor postoperative complications in this study. If Crohn's is suspected intraoperatively as a new diagnosis for the patient, postoperative colonoscopy should be performed to trigger appropriate treatment based on risk stratification. In addition, many centers perform postoperative endoscopic surveillance on all Crohn's patients to guide initiation of therapy post resection [10].

Acute Intestinal Ischemia

Acute intestinal ischemia can occur from obstructed arterial inflow, venous outflow, or a generalized low flow state. Bowel perforation in acute intestinal ischemia is a late complication of the disease process that results from the progression of bowel ischemia to infarction and then perforation. Risk factors for irreversible intestinal ischemia include elevated blood lactate, organ failure, and bowel loop dilation [11]. As free perforation is a late complication of this disease process, aggressive resuscitation is advocated to stabilize the patient for emergent surgery. Resection of the area of perforation with the

Fig. 17.2 An area of necrosis can be seen on the small bowel that was incarcerated in a femoral hernia

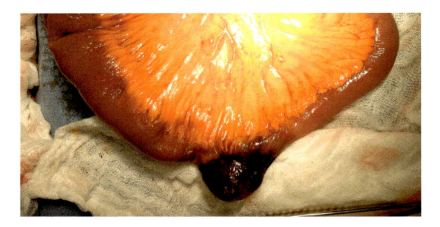

associated areas of ischemic and infarcted bowel is necessary. At initial operation, the viability of various areas of bowel may be questioned or unclear. A prudent strategy is to resect the areas of obvious necrosis and perforation, leave the bowel in discontinuity, and perform a second-look operation for repeat evaluations of the bowel (Fig. 17.2).

This permits physiologic restoration of the patient in the ICU, and often the segments of questionable bowel at the first exploration are found to be viable at repeat operation. The use of open abdomen techniques are often employed with this management approach. Anastomosis is performed after the viability of the bowel is assured. Conversely, ischemic segments that persist should be resected and the bowel anastomosis performed subsequently.

Meckel's Diverticulum

Meckel's diverticulum is the most common congenital abnormality of the intestinal tract and is thought to be a remnant of the omphalomesenteric duct. The overall incidence of complications of Meckel's diverticulum is between 4% and 16% [12]. The diverticulum is most commonly lined with intestinal type mucosa but not infrequently can have ectopic tissue. Obstruction of the lumen or erosion due to secretions of ectopic mucosa can cause perforation. Small bowel resection, including the diverticulum, is preferred over simple diverticulectomy in the setting of perforation [12].

Radiation Enteritis

Radiation enteritis is a clinical entity of acute and chronic changes of the small bowel in response to radiation injury. Acute radiation enteritis is due to the direct injury to the mucosa from radiation and can result in abdominal pain, diarrhea, and tenesmus. Chronic radiation enteritis is characterized by progressive obliterative endarteritis with exaggerated submucosal fibrosis [13] and can lead to perforation. Perforation in the background of radiation enteritis is complicated by the fact that the surrounding bowel is often abnormal with large segments of thickened fibrotic bowel. Given the radiation changes to the bowel, primary suture repair of the bowel is not typically feasible. Resection is typically performed and anastomosis can be attempted depending on the condition of the remaining bowel. Anastomotic leak occurs in 4–10% of patients [14, 15]. Alternatively, resection with ostomy creation is a safe strategy when there is not sufficient normal bowel for anastomosis.

Foreign Body

An ingested foreign body is an infrequent cause of perforation of the small intestine. Most foreign bodies that exit the stomach are able to pass through the small intestine without incident. Any number of foreign bodies can cause perforation with fish bones, chicken bones, and toothpicks being more commonly reported (Fig. 17.3).

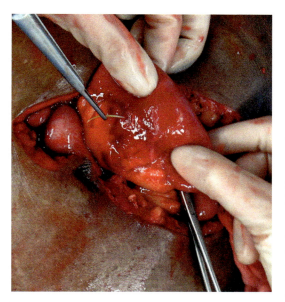

Fig. 17.3 A fish bone can be seen sticking through the bowel at a small perforation caused by the bone

Often, the small bowel can be repaired as the perforation is usually quite small. The acuity of the perforation and the condition of the bowel at the site will determine whether repair is feasible or resection with primary anastomosis will be necessary.

Infectious Causes

Bowel perforation can occur from a variety of infectious agents but is relatively rare in the developed world. However, it is important to be aware of these diagnoses given the incidence of international travel and immigration from countries where these diseases are endemic. Tuberculosis (TB) and salmonella typhi are the most common bacterial causes of intestinal perforation. Perforation due to tuberculosis is a rare complication of TB overall and a rare complication of intra-abdominal TB. Intestinal TB can for an ulcero-constrictive form which leads to strictures. Perforation is typically located just proximal to a stricture [16]. The perforation and associated stricture are typically resected [17]. As is true of Crohn's disease, the most difficult surgical conundrum is the state of the surrounding bowel at the area of perforation. Abdominal

TB is often associated with chronic abdominal infection with thickened, abnormal small bowel making anastomosis difficult. Purulent ascites is frequently present and should be sent for microbiologic analysis to confirm the diagnosis. Initiation of antimicrobial therapy for tuberculosis immediately postoperatively is critical. Antituberculous therapy selection is typically the same for pulmonary and abdominal TB.

Small bowel perforation associated with salmonella typhi is common in the developing world. Patients present with peritonitis after a typically long (weeks) febrile illness. The site of perforation is classically located at the ileum and is usually a solitary perforation [18]. As opposed to perforation with TB, these perforations can be amenable to primary repair if the patient presents early after perforation as the segment of bowel can be relatively normal. Mortality in the developing world remains high (15.4% overall) and is often associated with a delayed presentation of perforation [19]. In, itiation of broad-spectrum antibiotics with an agent sufficient to cover *S. typhi* should be started as soon as the diagnosis is made.

Neoplasms

Cancer of the small bowel is a relatively rare site for neoplasms accounting for only 1–3% of all gastrointestinal malignancies [20]. The overall prognosis of small bowel malignancy is poor but varies greatly based on type of neoplasm (GIST, adenocarcinoma, lymphoma, etc.). Perforation is a known complication of small bowel malignancy but remains uncommon. Management of perforation in the setting of suspected neoplasm remains resection and anastomosis in most instances. The only modification to the technique is the importance of taking a sufficient margin on either side of the lesion (10 cm) and resecting the mesentery supplying that segment for lymph node harvest.

Operative Considerations

Patients with perforated small bowel segment can present along a broad spectrum of physiologic perturbation. It is essential that adequate resuscitation precedes operative management. Volume resuscitation and broad-spectrum antibiotics are an essential part of the initial management of patients with small bowel perforation.

When the patient has been adequately resuscitated, as determined by improvement in patient physiology, base deficit and lactate, operative management can proceed. In rare cases, a patient must be taken to the operating room to achieve source control before being fully resuscitated. In this circumstance, the risks of cardiovascular collapse are weighed against the risk of delay to source control and aggressive resuscitation is continued during operation.

Laparotomy is the classic approach to small bowel perforation, but laparoscopic approaches are increasingly used with success. Many surgeons use a combined approach beginning with laparoscopy to identify the pathology along the gastrointestinal tract, and then a small laparotomy incision is able to be utilized to manage the identified perforation.

The vast majority of small bowel perforations can be managed with primary suture repair or resection and anastomosis. The choice of operative techniqe is most often influenced by the condition of the bowel at operation. Bowel that remains relatively normal in thickness, vascularity, and does not demonstrate significant pathology other than perforation is a candidate for primary repair (Fig. 17.4).

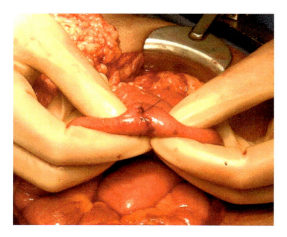

Fig. 17.4 A single layered running repair of the small bowel. 3-0 PDS suture is used

This can be performed in one or two layers based on the surgeon's preference. Abnormal bowel is often best managed by segmental resection and anastomosis. In rare cases, intestinal stomas can be created when bowel anastomosis is not practical or inflammation is too severe to resect a segment of distal bowel. This can occur when there is a long delay between perforation and presentation or when there is significant adhesion formation from prior operation or inflammation leading to a "frozen abdomen." When faced with this circumstance, the surgeon must make a risk/benefit decision regarding proceeding with further dissection and the risk of injuring the bowel versus bringing up a stoma. A distal small bowel stoma may be well tolerated but a proximal stoma can lead to nutritional deficiencies and significant volume problems. While placement of a stoma for small bowel perforation is rarely needed, it is an important tool for the emergency general surgeon. In the very rare case, where the bowel cannot be mobilized safely for resection or stoma, washout with drain placement and closure can be utilized.

The technique for bowel anastomosis in emergency surgery has come under significant debate with controversy surrounding the optimal choice between hand-sewn and stapled anastomosis. Several retrospective studies have shown a higher leak rate in stapled anastomosis in comparison to hand sewn during emergency surgery [21–23]. However, the most recent systematic review and a multicenter trial both did not find a difference in anastomotic leak rate between the two techniques [24, 25]. In the multicenter study, a prospective observational review of emergency general surgery patients, surgeons utilized hand-sewn anastomoses more often in sicker patients (lower hemoglobin levels, higher lactate, higher INR, lower albumin, worsened renal function, intraoperative vasopressors) [24]. These patients had a longer length of stay and a significant increase in mortality but no increase in anastomotic leaks. With more hand-sewn anastomoses being performed on patients with a higher acuity of illness and a presumed higher propensity to leak, it is distinctly possible that the hand-sewn technique may have a lower leak rate in this population. Based on the current literature, it is not possible to definitively suggest one technique over the other. However, it appears prudent to consider performing hand-sewn anastomoses in patients with abnormal bowel or significantly deranged physiology.

Another area of controversy in this patient population is the role of the "open abdomen." This technique involves leaving the abdominal wall fascia unapproximated at the initial operation with a planned reexploration within 24–48 h. The theoretical advantages of this strategy include the ability to reinspect the bowel to determine viability or to look for other pathology, repeated peritoneal irrigation, and restoration of deranged physiology prior to bowel anastomosis. The exact indications for utilizing this strategy are not well defined in the literature, but a recent World Society of Emergency Surgery position statement suggested that utilizing an open abdomen strategy should be considered in patients with a need for abbreviated laparotomy due to severe physiological derangement, need for delayed anastomosis, concern for ongoing bowel ischemia and ongoing contamination without source control and concern about severe bowel edema, and development of abdominal compartment syndrome [26]. This list of indications would seem to be a logical approach to utilizing the open abdomen in emergency general surgery. The multicenter study of suture technique also demonstrated a higher anastomotic leak rate in patients managed with the open abdomen, but this was felt to be more related to the severity of illness in this cohort as opposed to the technique itself [24]. When an open abdomen strategy is utilized, current recommendation is to use a negative pressure system on the abdomen in combination with a technique to maintain tension on the fascia. This will help ameliorate the retraction of the fascia and lead to a higher rate of primary fascial closure. The fascia should be closed as soon as the patient's physiology has improved and the indication for the open abdomen has been resolved. Every effort should be made to achieve fascial closure within 7 days [26].

Postoperative Considerations

After emergency surgery for bowel perforation, there is a lack of consensus surrounding the need for postoperative nasogastric decompression, timing of oral feeding, need for total parenteral nutrition, and the ideal methods for pain management. Studies have shown that early postoperative feeding in emergency general surgery patients is safe, but they have not been able to demonstrate significant improvement in patient outcomes [27]. As a matter of routine, the authors do not manage patients with small bowel perforation with a nasogastric tube unless there are signs of bowel obstruction at operation or in cases of significant intra-abdominal contamination and ileus. Nasogastric tubes are only inserted postoperatively in the minority of patients that develop significant nausea, vomiting, and ileus. Oral feeding is generally reinstituted as a patient's appetite returns and signs of gastrointestinal motility are noted.

Early postoperative mobilization is encouraged for all emergency general surgery patients. Pain control should be managed in a multimodality approach including the use of nonnarcotic medicines and local anesthetic techniques (epidural, TAP blocks, locoregional blocks, etc.) in addition to intravenous and oral narcotics.

Postoperative antibiotic duration is still an area of active study, but it is generally accepted that antibiotics should be discontinued within 24 h after operation unless evidence of preoperative abscess formation or other infection exists.

Complications

Patients with small bowel perforation are prone to any of the complications associated with abdominal operations. Intra-abdominal abscess formation is a frequent concern and can usually be managed successfully with percutaneous drain placement and antibiotics. Hernia formation can be seen as with any emergency laparotomy.

Anastomotic leak is a complication that can lead to significant morbidity in this population. Anastomotic leak has been noted to be 12.5% in a recent multicenter observational trial of emergency general surgery patients. This leak rate increased to 22% in patients managed with an open abdomen [24]. Anastomotic leaks that are recognized early after surgery are typically dealt with by repeat operation and either a second attempt at anastomosis (if a technical issue is suspected), further resection and anastomosis for ischemia or unhealthy bowel, or ostomy creation. Anastomotic leaks that present greater than 7–10 days after surgery present a more complex problem as adhesion formation and inflammation often leave the abdomen quite hostile. In this setting, draining the site of the leak either through interventional radiology techniques or through limited and careful operative exploration is often the best option. This controls sepsis and contamination with the goal of creating a controlled fistula. This fistula will often heal over 6–12 weeks with good nutritional support.

Conclusion

Small bowel perforation is a relatively rare event that can lead to significant morbidity and mortality. Appropriate resuscitation followed by timely and appropriate operative management can improve clinical outcomes. Operative technique should be tied to the etiology of the perforation and are often dependent on the condition of the surrounding small bowel. Knowledge of the diverse etiologies allows the clinician to determine operative techniques employed, postoperative adjunctive treatment, and risk of complications.

References

1. Rhodes A, Evans LE, Alhazzani W, Levy MM, Antonelli M, Ferrer R, et al. Surviving sepsis campaign: international guidelines for management of sepsis and septic shock: 2016. Crit Care Med. 2017;45(3):486–552.
2. Lo Re G, Mantia FL, Picone D, Salerno S, Vernuccio F, Midiri M. Small bowel perforations: what the radiologist needs to know. Semin Ultrasound CT MR. 2016;37(1):23–30.
3. Faggian A, Berritto D, Iacobellis F, Reginelli A, Cappabianca S, Grassi R. Imaging patients with ali-

mentary tract perforation: literature review. Semin Ultrasound CT MR. 2016;37(1):66–9.
4. Westerland O, Griffin N. Magnetic resonance enterography in crohns disease. Semin Ultrasound CT MR. 2016;37(4):282–91.
5. Loftus T, Moore F, VanZant E, Bala T, Brakenridge S, Croft C, et al. A protocol for the management of adhesive small bowel obstruction. J Trauma Acute Care Surg. 2015;78(1):13–9; discussion 19–21
6. Birindelli A, Sartelli M, Di Saverio S, Coccolini F, Ansaloni L, van Ramshorst GH, et al. 2017 update of the WSES guidelines for emergency repair of complicated abdominal wall hernias. World J Emerg Surg WJES. 2017;12:37.
7. Kim JW, Lee HS, Ye BD, Yang SK, Hwang SW, Park SH, et al. Incidence of and risk factors for free bowel perforation in patients with Crohn's disease. Dig Dis Sci. 2017;62(6):1607–14.
8. Yamamoto T, Watanabe T. Surgery for luminal Crohn's disease. World J Gastroenterol. 2014;20(1):78–90.
9. Fumery M, Seksik P, Auzolle C, Munoz-Bongrand N, Gornet JM, Boschetti G, et al. Postoperative complications after ileocecal resection in Crohn's disease: a prospective study from the REMIND group. Am J Gastroenterol. 2017;112(2):337–45.
10. Singh S, Nguyen GC. Management of Crohn's disease after surgical resection. Gastroenterol Clin N Am. 2017;46(3):563–75.
11. Nuzzo A, Maggiori L, Ronot M, Becq A, Plessier A, Gault N, et al. Predictive factors of intestinal necrosis in acute mesenteric ischemia: prospective study from an intestinal stroke center. Am J Gastroenterol. 2017;112(4):597–605.
12. Sagar J, Kumar V, Shah DK. Meckel's diverticulum: a systematic review. J R Soc Med. 2006;99(10):501–5.
13. Harb AH, Abou Fadel C, Sharara AI. Radiation enteritis. Curr Gastroenterol Rep. 2014;16(5):383.
14. Huang Y, Guo F, Yao D, Li Y, Li J. Surgery for chronic radiation enteritis: outcome and risk factors. J Surg Res. 2016;204(2):335–43.
15. Regimbeau JM, Panis Y, Gouzi JL, Fagniez PL, French University Association for Surgical Research. Operative and long term results after surgery for chronic radiation enteritis. Am J Surg. 2001;182(3):237–42.
16. Pattanayak S, Behuria S. Is abdominal tuberculosis a surgical problem. Ann R Coll Surg Engl. 2015;97(6):414–9.
17. Weledji EP, Pokam BT. Abdominal tuberculosis: is there a role for surgery? World J Gastrointest Surg. 2017;9(8):174–81.
18. Agu K, Nzegwu M, Obi E. Prevalence, morbidity, and mortality patterns of typhoid ileal perforation as seen at the University of Nigeria Teaching Hospital Enugu Nigeria: an 8-year review. World J Surg. 2014;38(10):2514–8.
19. Ugochukwu AI, Amu OC, Nzegwu MA. Ileal perforation due to typhoid fever – review of operative management and outcome in an urban centre in Nigeria. Int J Surg. 2013;11(3):218–22.

20. Rondonotti E, Koulaouzidis A, Yung DE, Reddy SN, Georgiou J, Pennazio M. Neoplastic diseases of the small bowel. Gastrointest Endosc Clin N Am. 2017;27(1):93–112.

21. Brundage SI, Jurkovich GJ, Grossman DC, Tong WC, Mack CD, Maier RV. Stapled versus sutured gastrointestinal anastomoses in the trauma patient. J Trauma. 1999;47(3):500–7; discussion 507–8

22. Brundage SI, Jurkovich GJ, Hoyt DB, Patel NY, Ross SE, Marburger R, et al. Stapled versus sutured gastrointestinal anastomoses in the trauma patient: a multicenter trial. J Trauma. 2001;51(6):1054–61.

23. Farrah JP, Lauer CW, Bray MS, McCartt JM, Chang MC, Meredith JW, et al. Stapled versus hand-sewn anastomoses in emergency general surgery: a retrospective review of outcomes in a unique patient population. J Trauma Acute Care Surg. 2013;74(5):1187–92; discussion 1192–4

24. Bruns BR, Morris DS, Zielinski M, Mowery NT, Miller PR, Arnold K, et al. Stapled versus hand-sewn: a prospective emergency surgery study. An American Association for the Surgery of Trauma multi-institutional study. J Trauma Acute Care Surg. 2017;82(3):435–43.

25. Naumann DN, Bhangu A, Kelly M, Bowley DM. Stapled versus handsewn intestinal anastomosis in emergency laparotomy: a systemic review and meta-analysis. Surgery. 2015;157(4):609–18.

26. Coccolini F, Montori G, Ceresoli M, Catena F, Moore EE, Ivatury R, et al. The role of open abdomen in non-trauma patient: WSES consensus paper. World J Emerg Surg WJES. 2017;12:39.

27. Klappenbach RF, Yazyi FJ, Alonso Quintas F, Horna ME, Alvarez Rodriguez J, Oria A. Early oral feeding versus traditional postoperative care after abdominal emergency surgery: a randomized controlled trial. World J Surg. 2013;37(10):2293–9.

Inflammatory Bowel Disease

18

Carey Wickham and Sang W. Lee

Inflammatory Bowel Disease Overview

Ulcerative colitis (UC) and Crohn's disease (CD) are idiopathic chronic inflammatory processes affecting the gastrointestinal tract. IBD is more common at northern latitudes with a high prevalence in North America and Europe. In the United States, a study looking at national insurance data found that both UC and Crohn's have an estimated prevalence of at least 200 per 100,000 adults [1]. The annual incidence of IBD has increased dramatically since the 1940s, with the steepest increases during the 1970s. There is also a gradient in the incidence of IBD in the United States, which increases from southern to northern latitudes. The incidence for both UC and CD ranges from approximately 0 to 20 per 100,000 [2]. There is also a genetic component of the pathogenesis of Crohn's and UC. Between 2% and 12% of patients with Crohn's and 8–14% of patients with UC have a family history of the disease. Twin studies have also demonstrated a concordance rate of 20–50% for Crohn's in monozygotic twins compared to 10% in dizy-

gotic twins and a concordance rate of 16% for UC in monozygotic twins compared to 4% in dizygotic twins. Multiple genetic loci are associated with IBD, with NOD2 on chromosome 6 being specifically associated with CD.

A number of other factors have been noted to have an association with IBD including the microbiome, adherent-invasive *Escherichia coli*, hygiene, medications, and diet. Smoking is thought to have a protective effect in UC, while it is associated with an increased primary risk of Crohn's as well as an increased risk of disease relapse. A recent study by Lunney et al. (2015) demonstrated that CD patients were more likely to smoke than UC patients (19.2% vs 10.2%, $p < 0.001$); however, smoking in CD was associated with an increased proportional surgery rate (45.8% vs 37.8%, $p = 0.045$), IBD-related hospitalization ($p = 0.009$), and incidence of peripheral arthritis (29.8% vs 22.0%, $p = 0.027$) [3]. Current smokers with UC demonstrated reduced corticosteroid utilization (24.1% vs 37.5%, $p = 0.045$), but no significant reduction in the rates of colectomy (3.4% vs 6.6%, $p = 0.34$) or hospital admission ($p = 0.25$) relative to nonsmokers. Former smokers with UC required proportionately greater immunosuppressive (36.2% vs 26.3%, $p = 0.041$) and corticosteroid (43.7% vs 34.5%, $p = 0.078$) therapies compared with current and never smokers. The deleterious effects of smoking, while less in UC than CD, support encouraging patient smoking cessation.

C. Wickham · S. W. Lee (✉)
Department of Colon & Rectal Surgery, University of Southern California, Keck School of Medicine, Los Angeles, CA, USA
e-mail: sangwl@med.usc.edu

© Springer International Publishing AG, part of Springer Nature 2019
C. V. R. Brown et al. (eds.), *Emergency General Surgery*, https://doi.org/10.1007/978-3-319-96286-3_18

Patients with both types of IBD can present with acute exacerbations potentially requiring operative intervention.

Ulcerative Colitis

Operative Indications

Emergent operative intervention for ulcerative colitis may be indicated in a number of different circumstances [4].

Acute fulminant colitis can occur in approximately 10% of patients with UC [5] and can present with sudden onset of bloody diarrhea, fecal urgency, abdominal pain, and anorexia. Patients can present with these symptoms at the time of diagnosis or later in the course of the disease. The additional findings of tachycardia, fever, leukocytosis, or hypoalbuminemia contribute to a more toxic picture. Patients may also have dehydration, anemia, hyponatremia, and hypokalemic alkalosis. Truelove and Witts first described the criteria for fulminant ulcerative colitis in 1955 (see Table 18.1) [6]. Up to 60% of patients fail to respond to intravenous steroids or cyclosporine [7, 8]. A slow or incomplete response to medical therapy leads to colectomy in two thirds of the patients within 1 year, and the majority of patients will have recurrent attacks [4].

Toxic megacolon may occur in patients with only left-sided colitis, as well as patients with extensive or pan-colitis. While the diagnosis is clinical, the hallmark feature is dilation of the colon, which can be segmental or pan-colonic. Toxic megacolon is differentiated from other causes of colonic dilation by systemic signs including fever, tachycardia, neutrophilic leukocytosis, anemia, dehydration, altered mental status, electrolyte derangements, and hypotension.

Table 18.1 Criteria for fulminant ulcerative colitis [6]

Criteria	Fulminant UC
Stool	>6 bloody BMs/day
Temperature	>37.5 °C
Heart rate	>90 bpm
Hemoglobin	<75% of normal
ESR	>30 mm/h
Transverse colon	>6 cm – Toxic megacolon

Rectal bleeding is common in UC and can vary from small amounts of blood per rectum to massive life-threatening hemorrhage. Even in the context of massive unremitting hemorrhage, not adequately responding to resuscitation with blood products, total colectomy with end ileostomy is typically effective for hemorrhage control. Total proctectomy is usually not necessary.

The risk of perforation is significantly increased for UC patients in the setting of acute colitis or toxic megacolon. Perforation results in 27–57% mortality. There are few hard signs of impending perforation as patients often do not exhibit classic signs of peritonitis due to immunosuppressive therapies. Persistent or increased dilation of the transverse colon, pneumatosis, and multiorgan failure are indications for emergent surgery [9]. A high level of suspicion should always be maintained when caring for these patients.

Initial management following inpatient admission should begin with laboratory tests including complete blood count, comprehensive metabolic panel, coagulation studies, type and screen, and blood cultures. Appropriate IV access should be obtained; large-bore peripheral IVs are preferred to central access if expedient large volume resuscitation is anticipated. Upright chest and abdominal radiographs should be obtained to evaluate for free air consistent with perforation and to evaluate colonic dilation. Stool studies should be sent to evaluate for infectious etiology, including *Clostridium difficile* PCR. Limited proctoscopy or flexible sigmoidoscopy with biopsy may be performed if patient does not have a prior tissue diagnosis; however, colonoscopy and barium enema are contraindicated in the setting of acute colitis. Resuscitation should be performed using isotonic fluids, with prompt correction of electrolyte abnormalities.

Medical management includes steroids and antibiotics. Fulminate colitis or toxic megacolon due to UC should be treated with steroids, most commonly hydrocortisone 100 mg every 6–8 h. Patients may already be taking cyclosporine, azathioprine, 6-mercaptopurine, or infliximab for induction or maintenance of symptom remission. Toxic megacolon or colitis with an infectious etiology, such as *C. difficile*, should not be treated with steroids. Empiric antibiotics with broad coverage of aerobic and anaerobic organisms such as a third- or fourth-generation cephalosporin and metronidazole may be used. Antibiotics should be narrowed or discontinued based on cultures, source control, and clinical improvement. Emergent surgical intervention should be pursued for peritonitis, free air, lack of improvement with medical management within 48–72 h, or clinical deterioration after admission [9].

Preoperative patient counseling is imperative and should always include discussion of stoma creation. Patients should be medically optimized with appropriate resuscitation, corrected electrolyte abnormalities, appropriate perioperative antibiotics, venous thromboembolism prophylaxis, and plans for postoperative steroid taper if applicable.

Surgical Strategies

The overarching surgical principle in patients who present with acute UC is to perform minimal surgery in maximally ill patients [4]. Patients are often malnourished, on chronic steroids, and immunosuppressed. The surgical procedure of choice in acute UC requiring emergent intervention is subtotal colectomy with end ileostomy. This allows for removal of the majority of the diseased colon, fecal diversion, and avoidance of pelvic dissection in an acutely ill patient, while preserving the option of future restoration of intestinal continuity on an elective basis. The major advantage of subtotal colectomy with end ileostomy as the index operation is that this is a minimal operation which can control disease symptoms and allow patients to recover until they are better able to tolerate a definitive surgery. Subtotal colectomy can adequately control acute hemorrhage and sepsis, while leaving virgin pelvic planes intact and being less likely to damage pelvic nerves.

The question of whether patients requiring emergent colectomy are best served by an open or a laparoscopic operation has been frequently investigated in the literature. Open procedures should be performed through a midline laparot-

omy, while laparoscopic port placement will vary depending upon the patient's exam and surgical history. Multiple studies have looked at performing laparoscopic versus open subtotal colectomy in the emergency setting [10–15]. Most of these show similar results for laparoscopic and open resections. Laparoscopic colectomy, including hand-assisted laparoscopy, results in similar to decreased postoperative morbidity, shorter time for return of bowel function, and decreased hospital length of stay. Not surprisingly, laparoscopic colectomy is associated with longer operative times. Toxic megacolon has a paucity of literature addressing possible laparoscopic intervention. Given the significant colonic distention decreasing available space for establishment of pneumoperitoneum, toxic megacolon should be approached with an open operation. Although it is safe and feasible to perform emergent laparoscopic colectomy in the appropriate setting, deciding between laparotomy or laparoscopy must be dependent on the patient's overall clinical condition and degree of abdominal distension [15]. Patients who are hemodynamically unstable should undergo an open operation (Table 18.2).

Surgical resection for UC can be performed as a single-stage, two-stage, or three-stage operation depending upon a number of factors reflecting the patient's overall health and current clinical condition. Determining the appropriate operative approach should also be impacted by perioperative steroid and other immunosuppressive medication use, the presence of intraoperative fecal spillage or free intestinal perforation, as well as surgeon preference. A single-stage operation should only be performed on an elective basis under ideal circumstances. It is not indicated under emergent circumstances for a number of reasons including the longer operative time, requirement of pelvic dissection for proctectomy, multiple anastomoses for the ileal pouch creation, and ileoanal anastomosis at high risk for leak.

Multiple-stage operations are more appropriate in the context of emergent colectomy in UC. Two-stage operations begin with proctectomy with creation of ileal pouch, ileal pouch anal anastomosis (IPAA), and diverting ileostomy,

Table 18.2 Staged operations for proctectomy with restoration of continuity

Operations	Single-stage	Two-stage (traditional)	Two-stage (modified)	Three-stage
1	Proctectomy; ileal pouch creation; ileal pouch anal anastomosis	Proctectomy; ileal pouch creation; ileal pouch anal anastomosis; diverting loop ileostomy	Subtotal colectomy; rectal stump or mucous fistula; end ileostomy	Subtotal colectomy; rectal stump or mucous fistula; end ileostomy
2		Loop ileostomy takedown	Completion proctectomy; ileal pouch creation; ileal pouch anal anastomosis	Completion proctectomy; ileal pouch creation; ileal pouch anal anastomosis; diverting loop ileostomy
3				Loop ileostomy takedown

followed by a second procedure to take down the ileostomy. Three-stage operations typically begin with a subtotal colectomy, end ileostomy, and creation of a rectal stump or a mucous fistula, with the goal of rapid resection of the diseased colon and avoiding the creation of an anastomosis in a toxic patient that could be complicated by leak.

The subsequent operations restore continuity with an IPAA or an ileorectal anastomosis with a diverting loop ileostomy, followed by a third operation for ileostomy takedown. In a study comparing laparoscopic two- and three-stage procedures in high-risk IBD patients, Mège et al. (2016) divided 185 patients into two groups, where the three-stage procedure group had a greater number of patients with Crohn's (16% vs 5%; $p < 0.04$) and a greater percentage of patients with emergent operation for acute colitis (37% vs 1%; $p < 0.0001$) [16]. Unsurprisingly, the cumulative operative time and length of stay were significantly longer with a three-stage operation (580 min, and 19 days vs 290 min and 10 days; $p < 0.0001$). They also found no significant difference between the two- and three-stage operations in terms of cumulative postoperative morbidity, anastomotic leak, wound infection, delay for stoma closure, delay for stoma function, and long-term morbidity. A retrospective study looking at two-stage compared to three-stage procedures found that the number of perioperative complications following two-stage operations was affected by surgeon experience ($p = 0.02$) but not by emergent status, use of

steroids, or use of antitumor necrosis factor agents. There was no increased risk of anastomotic leak with two-stage operations (odds ratio = 1.09; $p = 0.94$), and there was even a lower risk of anal stricture (odds ratio = 8.21; $p = 0.01$) with no differences in fistula or abscess formation or in pouch failure [17].

A modified two-stage operation for UC beginning with a subtotal colectomy with end-ileostomy, followed by ileal pouch creation and IPAA without ileostomy for fecal diversion, has recently been compared to the traditional two-stage operation for UC in the literature. Samples et al. (2017) found no significant difference in the 3-year cumulative incidence of pouch leaks between patients undergoing modified two-stage, compared with single or traditional two-stage, despite patients undergoing modified two-stage procedures being significantly more likely to receive an emergent operation (56.9% vs 0.0%; $p < 0.0001$), to have used a biologic within 2 weeks of surgery (32.1% vs 17.5%; $p = 0.003$), and to be taking high-dose steroids (60.4% vs 16.7%; $p \leq 0.0001$) [18]. A larger retrospective study published slightly earlier actually demonstrated a lower rate of anastomotic leak following IPAA (4.6% vs 15.7%, $p < 0.01$) despite significantly more preoperative enteral corticosteroid use (44.7% vs 33.2%, $p = 0.04$) and higher UC disease severity at presentation (86.9% patients with moderate/severe UC vs 73.1%, $p < 0.01$), in the modified two-stage group than the traditional two-stage group [19]. This suggests that diverting ileostomy may not reduce ileal pouch leak rates for IPAA in UC.

The decision to perform two- or three-stage operations for UC should be made based on the patient's clinical condition and the surgeon's experience.

Complications

Postoperative mortality is significantly higher after emergent surgery in UC (5.3%; 95% CI, 3.8–7.4%) compared to elective surgery (0.7%; 95% confidence interval [CI], 0.6–0.9%) [20]. Other potential postoperative concerns include infectious, thrombotic, and hemorrhagic complications.

Emergent surgery for UC carries a high risk of infectious complications. As with any colorectal operation, the postoperative complication most expected and feared is anastomotic leak from the ileal pouch, IPAA, or rectal stump. Surprisingly, a retrospective study by Hicks et al. (2014) demonstrated no significant difference in anastomotic leaks or abdominal sepsis in patients with severe UC undergoing emergent vs elective operations [21]. Short-term complications were increased with higher body mass index and urgency status ($p \leq 0.05$); however, surgeon inexperience and use of immunomodulators other than infliximab was associated with increased odds of long-term fistula/abscess (odds ratio, 5.56; $p = 0.05$) and pouch failure (odds ratio, 13.3; $p = 0.01$). These findings were similar to risk factors for anastomotic leak after nonemergent restorative proctectomy with IPAA for IBD [22]. Rectal stump leak after subtotal colectomy is another complication that can lead to pelvic sepsis. The incidence of rectal stump blowout ranges from 10% to 20%. Following subtotal colectomy, residual sigmoid colon can be fashioned into a low sigmoid mucous fistula, the transected rectosigmoid colon can be closed into the subcutaneous plane at the lower end of a midline wound, or the rectal stump can be closed at the level of the sacral promontory. Mucous fistulas are cumbersome for patients due to continuous drainage. Location of the rectal stump in the subcutaneous wound has a lower rate of pelvic sepsis but a higher rate of wound infections. Subcutaneous placement of the rectal stump, however, is associated with a lower total morbidity [23, 24]. Rectal stump tubes or drains may be placed to attempt to reduce the risk of rectal stump leak. Rectal

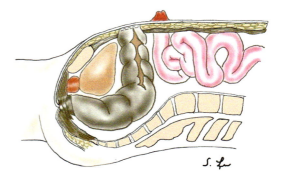

Fig. 18.1 Subcutaneous placement of rectal stump

stump lavage with iodine has also been proposed to avoid reoperation for rectal stump leak after emergent colectomy in UC [25] (Fig. 18.1).

Wound infection is a common complication after colorectal surgery [26]. Several studies looking at surgical site infections (SSI) in UC have shown that indicators of overall patient health are important risk factors. In emergent surgery for UC, diabetes, white blood cell count >15 cells/mm^3, intraoperative blood loss >200 mL, and intraoperative blood transfusion were all independent predictors of SSIs [27].

Patients with IBD are known to have a 1.5–3.5-fold increased risk for thrombotic complications, with a greater perioperative risk for patients with UC than Crohn's [28]. A review of NSQIP data demonstrated that venous thromboembolism (VTE) occurred with a higher frequency in patients with UC than in those with CD (3.3% vs 1.4%, $p < 0.001$). Deep vein thrombosis (DVT) and pulmonary embolism (PE) occurred a mean of 10.8 days postoperatively, and bleeding disorder, steroid use, anesthesia time, emergency surgery, hematocrit <37%, malnutrition, and functional status were all significantly associated ($p < 0.05$) with postoperative VTE in IBD [29]. While the mechanism for this increased risk of VTE is not well understood, PAI-1 antigen, active PAI-1, and intact thrombin activatable fibrinolysis inhibitor concentrations, as well as 50% clot lysis time and area under the curve on clot lysis profile, have been shown to be significantly associated with IBD (all $p < 0.05$) [30].

In patients who have had emergent colectomy for massive hemorrhage with a remaining rectum,

10–12% can have continued bleeding [31]. This can be managed non-operatively but may require another operation if severe. Significant bleeding is not otherwise a common complication of emergent surgery for UC.

Crohn's Disease

Operative Indications

Emergent operative intervention for Crohn's disease (CD) may be indicated in acute fulminant colitis, bowel obstruction, perforation, hemorrhage, or severe disease refractory to medical and non-operative management.

Acute fulminant colitis and toxic megacolon can occur in CD as well as in UC, with similar presenting signs and symptoms. Segmental colitis can also occur but typically lacks the severity of fulminant colitis or toxic megacolon. Perforation can also occur in CD and requires emergent operation [9]. High suspicion for perforation should be maintained in patients with a history of anti-TNF medications like infliximab or adalimumab, as there is some data supporting an association between anti-TNF medication and free perforation in CD [32].

Abscess formation is another common complication of CD, but it should be managed initially with percutaneous drainage. Operative intervention for abscesses should be avoided if possible. Failure to improve with adequate drainage and antibiotics may necessitate surgical intervention.

Rectal bleeding is less common in CD compared with UC, but patients with CD can still present with massive life-threatening hemorrhage. Given that Crohn's is segmental disease which can occur anywhere between the mouth and the anus, it is important to attempt to localize the bleeding during resuscitative efforts. If bleeding is localized but the patient does not respond appropriately to blood products, then targeted resection of the bleeding segment is indicated.

Bowel obstruction can be problematic in Crohn's. Intra-abdominal inflammation, masses, abscesses, and strictures can all cause intestinal obstruction. Operative management puts the patient at risk for development of more adhesive disease.

Initial management following inpatient admission should begin with laboratory tests including complete blood count, comprehensive metabolic panel, coagulation studies, type and screen, and blood cultures. Appropriate IV access should be obtained; large-bore peripheral IVs are preferred to central access if expedient large volume resuscitation is anticipated. Upright chest and abdominal radiographs should be obtained to evaluate for free air consistent with perforation and to evaluate colonic dilation. Limited proctoscopy or flexible sigmoidoscopy with biopsy may be performed if patient does not have a prior tissue diagnosis; however, colonoscopy and barium enema are contraindicated. Resuscitation should be performed using isotonic fluids, with prompt correction of electrolyte abnormalities.

Medical management includes steroids and antibiotics. Severe disease should be treated with steroids, typically hydrocortisone. Steroid therapy typically results in rapid suppression of disease. Immunosuppressant medications like azathioprine, 6-mercaptopurine, methotrexate, cyclosporine, tacrolimus, mycophenolate mofetil, or infliximab are used more for steroid-resistant disease or long-term maintenance of remission. Empiric antibiotics with broad coverage of aerobic and anaerobic organisms such as a third- or fourth-generation cephalosporin and metronidazole should be used, especially in the setting of abscesses or suppurative disease. Antibiotics should be narrowed or discontinued based on cultures, source control, and clinical improvement. Emergent surgical intervention should be pursued for peritonitis, free air, lack of improvement with medical management, or clinical deterioration after admission [9].

Preoperative patient counseling is imperative and should always include discussion of stoma creation. Patients should be medically optimized with appropriate resuscitation, corrected electrolyte abnormalities, appropriate perioperative antibiotics, venous thromboembolism prophylaxis, and plans for postoperative steroid taper if applicable.

Surgical Strategies

The overarching surgical consideration in patients with Crohn's is preserving functional small bowel length while adequately controlling the disease [4]. Surgical intervention should be geared toward minimizing resections and avoiding operative complications. Surgery is required in approximately 70% of patients with Crohn's disease, often requiring repeat interventions. These patients may benefit from minimally invasive approaches to reduce their risk of adhesive disease. Various bowel-sparing techniques, including strictureplasty, can be applied to reduce the risk of short-bowel syndrome.

Surgical intervention should be minimally invasive and laparoscopic whenever possible in Crohn's disease. Multiple studies have demonstrated longer operative duration with laparoscopic procedures; however, laparoscopy also resulted in significantly faster recovery of bowel function, with earlier oral intake tolerance, and shorter length of stay. Morbidity was lower for laparoscopic procedures compared with open procedures in CD (odds ratio, 0.57; 95% confidence interval, 0.37–0.87; $p = 0.01$). The rate of disease recurrence in CD was similar for both laparoscopic and open surgery [33]. Outcomes were also similar in laparoscopy performed for recurrent disease [34]. Minimally invasive approaches should be used whenever possible.

Segmental disease causing obstruction or perforation should be addressed with segmental resections. Laparoscopic ileocecectomy may often be indicated. Small bowel disease should be resected such that anastomoses are at areas of healthy tissue, and the overall small bowel length is conserved as much as possible. If obstruction is due to strictures, it may be tempting to perform strictureplasty to minimize resected small bowel; however, strictureplasty should not be performed in active Crohn's disease, phlegmon, and septic fistulas or in cases where the stricture site is at or close to a previous anastomosis site that has recurred within 12 months of the previous operation [35].

Complications

Postoperative complications with emergent operation for CD are similar to elective surgical complications and include leak, abscess, fistula, stricture, and bowel obstruction. Preoperative risk factors including low albumin level, preoperative steroids use, preoperative abscess, and history of prior surgeries may be associated with increased postoperative intraabdominal infectious complications, however, no association with anastomosis method, or therapy with biologics and immunomodulators has been demonstrated [36]. Risk of postoperative bowel obstruction is 12-fold higher in patients with CD undergoing colorectal surgery [37]. To a lesser extent than UC, Crohn's also has an increased risk of perioperative VTE [29].

One study also demonstrated a higher rate of catheter-associated blood stream infections in patients with CD receiving central venous catheters [38]. In patients with CD, postoperative mortality was significantly higher after emergent surgery (3.6%; 95% CI, 1.8–6.9%) compared to elective surgery (0.6%; 95% CI, 0.2–1.7%) [20]. Optimizing medical therapy, minimizing surgical interventions, and preserving small bowel length are important for reducing morbidity and mortality in CD.

References

1. Kappelman M, Rifas-Shiman S, Kleinman K, Ollendorf D, Bousvaros A, Grand R, Finkelstein J. The prevalence and geographic distribution of Crohn's disease and ulcerative colitis in the United States. Clin Gastroenterol Hepatol. 2007;5(12):1424–9.
2. Ananthakrishnan A. Epidemiology and risk factors for IBD. Nat Rev. 2015;12(4):205–17.
3. Lunney PC, Kariyawasam VC, Wang RR, Middleton KL, Huang T, Selinger CP, Andrews JM, Katelaris PH, Leong RW. Smoking prevalence and its influence on disease course and surgery in Crohn's disease and ulcerative colitis. Aliment Pharmacol Ther. 2015;42(1):61–70.
4. Michelassi F. Indications for surgical treatment in ulcerative colitis and crohn's disease. In: Michelassi F, Milsom JW, editors. Operative. strategies in inflammatory bowel disease. New York: Springer; 1999. p. 239.

5. Michelassi F, Finco C. Indications for surgery in inflammatory bowel disease: the surgeon's perspective. In: Kirsner JB, Shorter RG, editors. Inflammatory bowel disease. 4th ed. Baltimore: Williams & Wilkins; 1995. p. 771–83.

6. Truelove SC, Witts LF. Cortisone in ulcerative colitis. Final report on A therapeutic trial. Br Med J. 1955;29(4947):1041–8.

7. Kirsner JB, Palmer WL, Spencer JA, et al. Corticotropin (ACTH) and adrenal steroids in the management of ulcerative colitis: observations in 240 patients. Ann Int Med. 1959;50:89.

8. Edwards FC, Truelove SC. The course and prognosis of ulcerative colitis. Gut. 1963;4:299.

9. Tjandra JJ. Toxic colitis and perforation. In: Michelassi F, Milsom JW, editors. Operative strategies in inflammatory bowel disease, vol. 239. New York: Springer; 1999.

10. Ouaïssi M, Alves A, Bouhnik Y, Valleur P, Panis Y. Three-step ileal pouch-anal anastomosis under total laparoscopic approach for acute or severe colitis complicating inflammatory bowel disease. J Am Coll Surg. 2006;202:637–42.

11. Ouaïssi M, Lefevre JH, Bretagnol F, Alves A, Valleur P, Panis Y. Laparoscopic 3-step restorative proctocolectomy: comparative study with open approach in 45 patients. Surg Laparosc Endosc Percutan Tech. 2008;18:357–62.

12. Chung TP, Fleshman JW, Birnbaum EH, Hunt SR, Dietz DW, Read TE, Mutch MG. Laparoscopic vs. open total abdominal colectomy for severe colitis: impact on recovery and subsequent completion restorative proctectomy. Dis Colon Rectum. 2009;52: 4–10.

13. Marceau C, Alves A, Ouaissi M, Bouhnik Y, Valleur P, Panis Y. Laparoscopic subtotal colectomy for acute or severe colitis complicating inflammatory bowel disease: a case-matched study in 88 patients. Surgery. 2007;141:640–4.

14. Telem DA, Vine AJ, Swain G, Divino CM, Salky B, Greenstein AJ, Harris M, Katz LB. Laparoscopic subtotal colectomy for medically refractory ulcerative colitis: the time has come. Surg Endosc. 2010;24:1616–20.

15. Nash GM, Bleier J, Milsom JW, Trencheva K, Sonoda T, Lee SW. Minimally invasive surgery is safe and effective for urgent and emergent colectomy. Color Dis. 2010;12:480–4.

16. Mège D, Figueiredo MN, Manceau G, Maggiori L, Bouhnik Y, Panis Y. Three-stage laparoscopic Ileal pouch-anal anastomosis is the best approach for high-risk patients with inflammatory bowel disease: an analysis of 185 consecutive patients. J Crohn's Colitis. 2016;10(8):898–904.

17. Hicks CW, Hodin RA, Bordeianou L. Possible overuse of 3-stage procedures for active ulcerative colitis. JAMA Surg. 2013;148(7):658–64.

18. Samples J, Evans K, Chaumont N, Strassle P, Sadiq T, Koruda M. Variant two-stage Ileal pouch-anal anastomosis: an innovative and effective alternative to standard resection in ulcerative colitis. J Am Coll Surg. 2017;224(4):557–63.

19. Zittan E, Wong-Chong N, Ma GW, et al. Modified two-stage ileal pouch-anal anatomosis results in lower rate of anastomotic leak compared with traditional two-stage surgery for ulcerative colitis. J Crohns Colitis. 2016;10:766e772.

20. Singh S, Al-Darmaki A, Frolkis AD, Seow CH, Leung Y, Novak KL, Ghosh S, Eksteen B, Panaccione R, Kaplan GG. Pstoperative mortality among patients with inflammatory bowel diseases: a systematic review and meta-analysis of population-based studies. Gastroenterology. 2015;149(4):928–37.

21. Hicks CW, Hodin RA, Bordeianou L. Semi-urgent surgery in hospitalized patients with severe ulcerative colitis does not increase overall J-pouch complications. Am J Surg. 2014;207(2):281–7.

22. Sahami S, Bartels SA, D'Hoore A, Fadok TY, Tanis PJ, Lindeboom R, de Buck van Overstraeten A, Wolthuis AM, Bemelman WA, Buskens CJ. A multicentre evaluation of risk factors for anastomotic leakage after restorative proctocolectomy with Ileal pouch-anal anastomosis for inflammatory bowel disease. J Crohns Colitis. 2016;10(7):773–8.

23. Trickett JP, Tilney HS, Gudgeon AM, Mellor SG, Edwards DP. Management of the rectal stump after emergency sub-total colectomy: which surgical option is associated with the lowest morbidity? Color Dis. 2005;7(5):519–22.

24. Gu J, Stocchi L, Remzi F, Kiran RP. Intraperitoneal or subcutaneous: does location of the (colo)rectal stump influence outcomes after laparoscopic total abdominal colectomy for ulcerative colitis? Dis Colon Rectum. 2013;56(5):615–21.

25. Pellino G, Sciaudone G, Candilio G, Canonico S, Selvaggi F. Rectosigmoid stump washout as an alternative to permanent mucous fistula in patients undergoing subtotal colectomy for ulcerative colitis in emergency settings. BMC Surg. 2012;12(Suppl 1):S31.

26. Bhakta A, Tafen M, Glotzer O, Ata A, Chismark AD, Valerian BT, Stain SC, Lee EC. Increased incidence of surgical site infection in IBD patients. Dis Colon Rectum. 2016;59(4):316–22.

27. Coakley BA, Divino CM. Identifying factors predictive of surgical-site infections after colectomy for fulminant ulcerative colitis. Am Surg. 2012;78(4):481–4.

28. Wilson MZ, Connelly TM, Tinsley A, Hollenbeak CS, Koltun WA, Messaris E. Ulcerative colitis is associated with an increased risk of venous thromboembolism in the postoperative period: the results of a matched cohort analysis. Ann Surg. 2015;261(6):1160–6.

29. Wallaert JB, De Martino RR, Marsicovetere PS, Goodney PP, Finlayson SRG, Murray JJ, Holubar SD. Venous thromboembolism after surgery for inflammatory bowel disease: are there modifiable risk factors? Data from ACS NSQIP. Dis Colon Rectum. 2012;55(11):1138–44.

30. Bollen L, Vande Casteele N, Peeters M, Van Assche G, Ferrante M, Van Moerkercke W, Gils A. The

occurrence of thrombosis in inflammatory bowel disease is reflected in the clot lysis profile. Inflamm Bowel Dis. 2015;21(11):2540–8.

31. Robert JH, Sachar DB, Aufses AH Jr, Greenstein AJ. Management of severe hemorrhage in ulcerative colitis. Am J Surg. 1990;159(6):550–5.

32. Eshuis EJ, Griffioen GH, Stokkers PC, Ubbink DT, Bemelman WA. Anti tumour necrosis factor as risk factor for free perforations in Crohn's disease? A case-control study. Color Dis. 2012;14(5):578–84.

33. Tan JJ, Tjandra JJ. Laparoscopic surgery for Crohn's disease: a meta-analysis. Dis Colon Rectum. 2007;50(5):576–85.

34. Pinto RA, Shawki S, Narita K, Weiss EG, Wexner SD. Laparoscopy for recurrent Crohn's disease: how do the results compare with the results for primary Crohn's disease? Color Dis. 2011;13(3):302–7.

35. Jobanputra S, Weiss EG. Strictureplasty. Clin Colon Rectal Surg. 2007;20(4):294–302.

36. Huang W, Tang Y, Nong L, Sun Y. Risk factors for postoperative intra-abdominal septic complications after surgery in Crohn's disease: A meta-analysis of observational studies. J Crohn's Colitis. 2015;9(3):293–301.

37. Masoomi H, Kang CY, Chaudhry O, Pigazzi A, Mills S, Carmichael JC, Stamos MJ. Predictive factors of early bowel obstruction in colon and rectal surgery: data from the Nationwide inpatient sample, 2006-2008. J Am Coll Surg. 2012;214(5):831–7.

38. Uchino M, Ikeuchi H, Matsuoka H, Bando T, Ichiki K, Nakajima K, Takahashi Y, Tomita N, Takesue Y. Catheter-associated bloodstream infection after bowel surgery in patients with inflammatory bowel disease. Surg Today. 2014;44(4):677–84.

Small Bowel Sources of Gastrointestinal Bleeds

Shuyan Wei and Lillian S. Kao

Introduction

In adults, gastrointestinal (GI) bleeding from the small bowel is uncommon and accounts for 5–10% of all GI bleeds [1]. Historically, small bowel GI bleeds were also referred to as obscure GI bleeds, but with the advent of novel diagnostic strategies, the majority of small bowel GI bleeds can now be identified. They are usually suspected if persistent overt (presenting with melena or hematochezia) or occult (presenting with iron-deficiency anemia) bleeding occurs even though no source of bleeding has been discovered on routine esophagogastroduodenoscopy (EGD) and colonoscopy. This chapter will highlight the most common causes of small bowel GI bleeds, current diagnostic tools, diagnostic algorithms, and management recommendations for adults with suspected small bowel GI bleeds.

Sources of Small Bowel Gastrointestinal Bleeds in Adults

Small bowel GI bleeds usually refer to bleeding anywhere between the ligament of Treitz and the ileocecal valve. The most common causes of

small bowel GI bleeds in adults are vascular ectasias, neoplasms, ulcers caused by nonsteroidal anti-inflammatory drugs (NSAIDs), Crohn's disease, Dieulafoy's lesions, and Meckel's diverticula. Less common causes include small bowel varices, amyloidosis, vasculitis, infection, ischemia, intussusception, aortoenteric fistula, polyposis syndromes, Osler-Weber-Rendu syndrome, Plummer-Vinson syndrome, Ehlers-Danlos syndrome, and duplication cysts [1]. Additionally, any condition that leads to small bowel ulcerations has a potential to cause bleeding. These conditions include, but are not limited to, Zollinger-Ellison syndrome, radiation enteritis, lymphocytic enteritis, malnutrition, graft-versus-host disease, foreign body, and heavy metal poisoning.

Vascular Ectasias

Epidemiology Vascular ectasias (also called angiodysplasias or arteriovenous malformations) are the most common cause of small bowel GI bleeds in adults over 60 years of age and account for 30–40% of small bowel GI bleeds (Fig. 19.1 – *vascular ectasia*) [3]. Vascular ectasias are aberrant blood vessels that may be congenital but most often develop later in life. These aberrant blood vessels are thin-walled, dilated, and lined by the endothelium; they can occur in both the upper and lower GI tract. Endoscopically, these

S. Wei · L. S. Kao (✉)
Department of Surgery, McGovern Medical School at the University of Texas Health Science Center at Houston, Houston, TX, USA
e-mail: lillian.s.kao@uth.tmc.edu

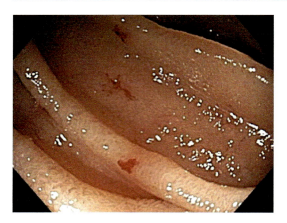

Fig. 19.1 Endoscopic view of small bowel vascular ectasia. (Reprinted with permission from Jackson and Strong [2])

lesions are red, flat, or slightly raised and range from 2 to 10 mm in size. The majority of people with vascular ectasias have synchronous lesions elsewhere in the GI tract. The cause of vascular ectasia formation is not well understood, although it has been suggested that chronic venous obstruction related to aging may contribute to their formation [4].

Risk factors Vascular ectasias are associated with other illnesses such as end-stage renal disease (ESRD), von Willebrand's disease, and aortic stenosis. In patients with ESRD, up to 30% of GI bleeds are attributable to vascular ectasias compared to 5% in those with normal kidney function [5]. The increased risk of GI bleeds due to vascular ectasia in ESRD patients may be in large due to uremia-induced platelet dysfunction and an overall higher tendency for bleeding in this patient population. GI vascular ectasias have been associated with inherited and acquired forms of von Willebrand's disease; 12% of individuals with acquired von Willebrand's disease are reported to also have GI vascular ectasias [6]. Bleeding from vascular ectasia in individuals with aortic stenosis is called Heyde's syndrome – first described by Edward Heyde in 1958. Heyde's syndrome is thought to be due to increased activation of von Willebrand factor-cleaving metalloprotease activity, whose activation is stimulated

by high shear stress induced by blood flow through a narrowed aortic valve. Bleeding from vascular ectasias would then occur secondary to this acquired coagulopathy [7]. A similar phenomenon is seen in people with left-ventricular assist devices [8].

Diagnosis and Treatment Bleeding from vascular ectasias is low grade in 85% of cases and painless. Endoscopy is the primary diagnostic tool for vascular ectasias. Incidentally discovered vascular ectasias during endoscopy that are not actively bleeding should not be treated. For actively bleeding vascular ectasias, endoscopic therapies are usually the first-line treatment option. Unfortunately, the evidence to support endoscopic treatment of vascular ectasia as superior to other therapies is weak, as there have been no randomized clinical trials evaluating treatment of vascular ectasias with endoscopic therapy compared with other treatment modalities [1]. Furthermore, studies show that up to 50% of endoscopically treated bleeding vascular ectasias will rebleed. Somatostatin analogs (e.g., octreotide) and thalidomide have been used in the medical management of vascular ectasias.

Prognosis Although bleeding stops spontaneously without intervention in 90% of cases, bleeding tends to recur [9].

Neoplasms

Epidemiology Small bowel neoplasms are rare and they are often diagnosed at later stages. They account for 3% of all GI tract tumors in the United States [10]. Their most common presenting symptoms are abdominal pain, nausea/vomiting, and weight loss; bleeding occurs in 23–41% of cases and intestinal obstruction in 22–26% of cases [11]. Small bowel tumors are a more frequent cause of small bowel GI bleeds in patients less than 40 years old. Primary small bowel neoplasms are less common than metastatic lesions from other sites of the body. Primary small bowel tumors can be benign (e.g., adenoma, lipoma, and leiomyoma) or malignant (e.g., carcinoid, adenocarcinoma, sarcoma, lymphoma). Specific tumor types tend to have a predilection for occurring in certain portions of the small bowel; for example, small bowel adenocarcinomas tend to occur in the duodenum (with the exception of in individuals with Crohn's disease), whereas carcinoid tumors tend to occur in the ileum. Benign tumors tend to increase in frequency from the duodenum to ileum [12].

Risk factors Risk factors associated with the development of primary small bowel neoplasms include hereditary cancer syndromes (e.g., hereditary nonpolyposis colorectal cancer or HNPCC, Peutz-Jeghers syndrome, and familial adenomatous polyposis or FAP), chronic inflammation (such as in Crohn's disease), smoking, a diet rich in saturated fats and refined sugars, and alcohol consumption [13, 14].

Diagnosis and Treatment Diagnosis of small bowel tumors varies depending on the type of tumor. Detailed diagnosis and treatment of each type of small bowel tumor is beyond the scope of this chapter. In brief, *carcinoid tumors* can be diagnosed by measuring 24-h urine 5-hydroxyindolacetic acid (5-HIAA) level or serum chromogranin A level. Somatostatin receptor scintigraphy (or octreotide scan) has a diagnostic sensitivity of up to 90% for detecting carcinoid tumors. Abdominal CT scans, magnetic resonance imaging (MRI), and positron emission tomography (PET) are also commonly used in the diagnostic workup of carcinoid tumors. Surgical resection is the only curative option for localized carcinoid tumor. Metastatic carcinoid disease is primarily managed by treatment of symptoms via octreotide and tumor debulking surgeries.

Small bowel adenocarcinomas are usually diagnosed at more advanced stages. Periampullary tumors tend to be diagnosed earlier (secondary to symptoms from biliary obstruction) by EGD, endoscopic ultrasound, or magnetic resonance cholangiopancreatography (MRCP). Barium contrast studies and CT scans can visualize more distal small bowel adenocarcinomas – with CT scans also having the advantage of evaluating for metastatic lesions. CT enterography (CTE) and MR enterography (MRE) are becoming more widely used for evaluation of small bowel pathology; these imaging modalities are discussed in further detail later in this chapter. Surgical resection is the only curative therapy for small bowel adenocarcinomas. Management of advanced or disseminated disease is targeted toward palliation of symptoms; chemotherapy has not been consistently shown to improve survival.

Gastrointestinal stromal tumors (GISTs) – the most common GI sarcoma – are usually diagnosed on upper endoscopy as a smooth, submucosal mass, or via abdominal CT scan. GISTs should not be routinely biopsied as there is an increased risk for rupture and recurrence. GISTs of the small bowel should be surgically resected. Neoadjuvant or adjuvant therapy with imatinib should be given to patients with marginally resectable GISTs or to those who undergo incomplete resection or have widespread disease.

Small bowel lymphomas encompass a variety of non-Hodgkin's lymphomas. Small bowel T-cell lymphomas are associated with celiac disease, and B-cell lymphomas should be considered in patients with immunodeficiency. CT scan is usually the diagnostic imaging of choice, and lesions suspicious for lymphomas should be biopsied and undergo immunohistochemical and cytogenetic testing. The mainstay of treatment for small bowel lymphomas is chemotherapy. Surgery is reserved for management of tumor complications, such as bleeding or bowel perforation.

Prognosis The 5-year survival rate for carcinoid tumor ranges from 54% to 65% for disseminated disease to well-differentiated localized disease. The 5-year survival for small bowel adenocarcinomas ranges from 10% to 65% for stage IV to stage I disease. Small bowel GISTs tend to have worse prognosis compared to gastric GISTs, and the 5-year survival for small bowel GISTs that undergo surgical resection is 40%. The 5-year survival for small bowel non-Hodgkin's lymphomas is 49% [15].

NSAID-Induced Ulcers

Epidemiology NSAIDs are well implicated in causing peptic ulcer disease. NSAIDs (such as ibuprofen, diclofenac, and celecoxib) are cyclooxygenase (COX) inhibitors and prevent the production of inflammatory prostaglandins to decrease pain and inflammation. NSAIDs and *Helicobacter pylori* infections can be attributed to 90% of duodenal ulcers. NSAIDs can also induce ulcer formation in the distal small bowel (and colon), especially in older adults and frequent NSAID users [16]. Ten percent of NSAID users have duodenal ulcers, and the prevalence of small bowel ulcers is difficult to estimate given the diagnostic challenge [17]. A Japanese study found that in 61 patients who used NSAIDs within 1 month prior to double-balloon endoscopy, approximately 50% of users had nonspecific small bowel mucosal breaks compared to only 5% observed in 600 control patients [18].

Pathogenesis NSAIDs induce small bowel ulcer formation via several mechanisms. First, NSAIDs inhibit the production of prostaglandins, which leads to decreased GI blood flow and mucus production resulting in small bowel damage. Second, enterohepatic circulation of NSAIDs absorbed in the small bowel is thought to induce small bowel damage through repeated exposure. This theory is supported by the finding that patients taking enteric-coated, sustained-release forms of NSAIDs develop small bowel ulcers more frequently than patients taking non-coated drug forms [19]. Third, it has been suggested that NSAIDs induce small bowel ulceration by directly damaging cell membranes of enterocytes and leads to enterocyte mitochondrial dysfunction, free radical release, and weakened integrity of the intestinal intercellular junctions, which ultimately exposes intestinal surfaces to caustic effects of intestinal contents [20]. Lastly, dysbiosis of the small intestine may facilitate NSAID-induced ulcer formation. Animal studies have shown an association between higher rates of small bowel ulcer formation and small bowel colonization by gram-negative bacteria in the setting of NSAID administration. Furthermore, studies have shown

that antibiotics against gram-negative bacteria reduce small bowel NSAID-induced ulcers [21]. The mechanism by which gram-negative bacteria augment NSAID-induced ulceration may be secondary to an inflammatory response triggered by their lipopolysaccharides [22].

Diagnosis and Treatment Endoscopy is the diagnostic modality of choice for NSAID-induced small bowel ulcers. On endoscopy, NSAID-induced small bowel ulcers are not macroscopically distinct from ulcers induced by other conditions, such as infection, ischemia, vasculitis, radiation, and inflammatory bowel conditions. Intestinal diaphragms – thin, concentric, weblike strictures with a small central lumen – are pathognomonic for NSAID-induced injury (Fig. 19.2 – *intestinal diaphragms*). NSAID-induced ulcers usually self-resolve once NSAIDs are discontinued, but intestinal diaphragms and strictures do not (Fig. 19.3 – *intestinal diaphragm dilation*). The latter may require treatment with endoscopic dilatation, needle-knife electroincision, surgical resection, or strictureplasty to resolve obstructive symptoms [25]. Patients who smoke tobacco should also undergo smoking cessation. Surgery is typically reserved for patients with perforated ulcers, refractory bleeding, and obstruction.

Crohn's Disease

Epidemiology The prevalence of Crohn's disease in North America is estimated to be 201 per 100,000 population [26]. Crohn's disease is a relapsing and remitting chronic inflammatory bowel disease of unclear etiology that predominantly affects the small intestines, and it can occur anywhere along the GI tract from the mouth to anus. Crohn's disease is characterized by transmural inflammation. The majority of patients (80%) have small bowel Crohn's disease, especially in the terminal ileum. Gastrointestinal symptoms include abdominal pain, diarrhea, bleeding, fistula formation between the bowel and adjacent structures, and malabsorption/weight loss. Individuals with Crohn's disease often have occult positive stools. Gross bleeding

Fig. 19.2 Gross specimen of intestinal diaphragms. (Reprinted with permission from Ullah et al. [23])

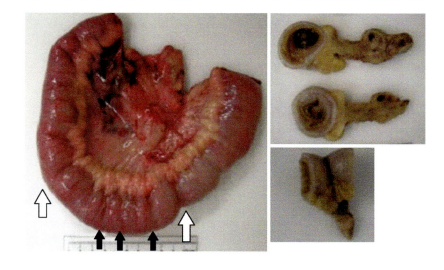

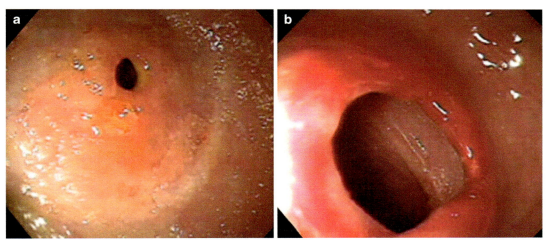

Fig. 19.3 Endoscopic view of intestinal diaphragm (**a**) pre-dilation and (**b**) post-dilation. (Reprinted with permission from Mehdizadeh and Lo [24])

may occur – especially with Crohn's colitis – although less common compared to patients with ulcerative colitis. When massive bleeding due to Crohn's disease does occur, the ileum is the most common source (66–83%), followed by the colon (13%) [27, 28].

Diagnosis and Treatment Computed tomographic angiography (CTA) is important in the preoperative assessment of brisk small bowel GI bleed prior to proceeding to the operating room. CTA allows for better identification of the bleeding source, especially in the presence of multiple

sites of small bowel Crohn's disease and if strictures are present that may limit the effectiveness of intraoperative enteroscopy [29]. Once the source of bleeding has been identified, hemostasis can be achieved through endoscopic interventions or surgical resection of the small bowel, depending on the clinical picture.

Meckel's Diverticulum

Epidemiology Meckel's diverticulum is a true diverticulum – meaning that it contains all layers of the small intestinal wall. It is the most common congenital GI abnormality. Meckel's diverticula in adult patients are often asymptomatic, and they are present in approximately 1–4% of the population. Clinically apparent Meckel's diverticulum can present with abdominal pain, bleeding, or obstruction. In cases of GI bleeds due to Meckel's diverticulum, there is usually adjacent ulceration of the small bowel secondary to the presence of acid-secreting ectopic gastric mucosa within the diverticulum. Ectopic gastric mucosa is the most commonly found ectopic tissue within a Meckel's diverticulum, followed by pancreatic and duodenal mucosa [30].

Diagnosis and Treatment If a symptomatic Meckel's diverticulum is suspected, Meckel's scintigraphy (or technetium-99 m pertechnetate) can be used to identify ectopic gastric mucosa within the diverticulum. This test has a higher sensitivity in children as compared to adults. Treatment for small bowel bleeding secondary to a Meckel's diverticulum involves surgical resection of the segment of intestine containing the Meckel's, because this removes the ulcerated small bowel that's usually located across the lumen from the diverticulum. In adults, incidentally discovered Meckel's diverticulum during surgery should not be resected.

Dieulafoy's Lesions

Epidemiology Dieulafoy's lesions are abnormal arteries in the submucosa that are exposed via small mucosal defects, with absence of inflammatory changes to suggest an overlying ulcer (Fig. 19.4 – *Dieulafoy's Lesions*). These vascular abnormalities can be up to 10 times greater in caliber compared to normal vasculature in their surroundings and are often described as "caliber-persistent." [32] The etiology and mechanism causing Dieulafoy's lesions to bleed is unclear. They are thought to be congenital lesions, and bleeding is hypothesized to result from a combination of mucosal atrophy secondary to pressure erosion of the overlying epithelium by the vessel and ischemic injury induced

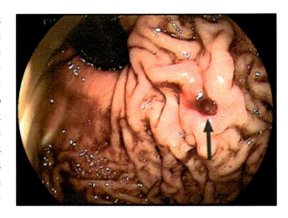

Fig. 19.4 Dieulafoy's lesion in the stomach. (Reprinted with permission from Close et al. [31])

by comorbid conditions, such as cardiovascular disease. Dieulafoy's lesions are more common in men (2 to 1 male to female predominance), older age (> 50 years), and people with comorbidities including cardiovascular disease, respiratory disease, and chronic renal failure. These lesions do not appear to be associated with peptic ulcer disease. Dieulafoy's lesions have been discovered in most parts of the GI tract; 74% are found in the stomach, 15% in the small bowel (predominantly in the duodenum), 5% at gastric anastomoses in people who have had prior surgery, and 6% in the colon and esophagus. GI bleeds secondary to Dieulafoy's lesions are self-limiting in 90% of cases.

Diagnosis and Treatment Dieulafoy's lesions are diagnosed on endoscopy. Endoscopic treatment with multimodal therapy (combination of injection therapy with thermal probe coagulation) or with endoscopic band ligation or clipping effectively treats bleeding up to 90% of the time, with low rates of reoccurrence [32].

Overview of Diagnostic Methods

Given the rarity of small bowel GI bleeds, small bowel sources are usually the last to be investigated during the workup of GI bleeds, unless initial imaging is concerning for small bowel malignancy. In the absence of small bowel malignancy, patients suspected to have a small bowel source of bleeding should have already undergone an upper endoscopy (EGD) and a lower endoscopy (colonoscopy) during which the source of bleeding had not been identified. The locations of small bowel GI bleeds lend to their diagnostic challenge as they are beyond the reach of the standard upper endoscope and colonoscope. Diagnostic tools to evaluate patients with suspected small bowel GI bleeds include video capsule endoscopy (VCE), computed tomographic enterography and magnetic resonance enterography (CTE and MRE), nuclear medicine scans, angiography, and enteroscopy. The 2015 American College of Gastroenterology guideline recommends performing a second-look endoscopy (particularly an upper endoscopy) prior to using another diagnostic tool, because a second-look endoscopy has been shown to detect previously missed sources in up to 60% of patients (Fig. 19.5 – Treatment algorithm [1]) [33]. The following section will highlight each diagnostic technique.

Video Capsule Endoscopy (VCE)

Video capsule endoscopy is the initial test of choice for non-massive GI bleeds suspected to be of small bowel origin after a repeat endoscopy fails to yield a bleeding source. Its advantages include being noninvasive with minimal patient discomfort and its ability to visualize the entire small bowel in up to 90% of patients. VCE's diagnostic yield for suspected small bowel GI bleeds is 83%, and it has a positive predictive value of 94–97% and a negative predictive value of 83–100% [34]. There are four different VCE devices available worldwide. They measure 26 × 11 mm^2 and are active over an 8–12 h period. Patients swallow the VCE device like they would a pill; the capsule takes pictures of the intestinal lumen during its transit and is eliminated in the feces. Studies suggest that VCE has the highest diagnostic yield if used within 2–3 days of overt suspected small bowel GI bleed [35].

An obvious limitation of the VCE is that it offers no therapeutic means. Furthermore, due to its quick transition through the duodenum, VCE

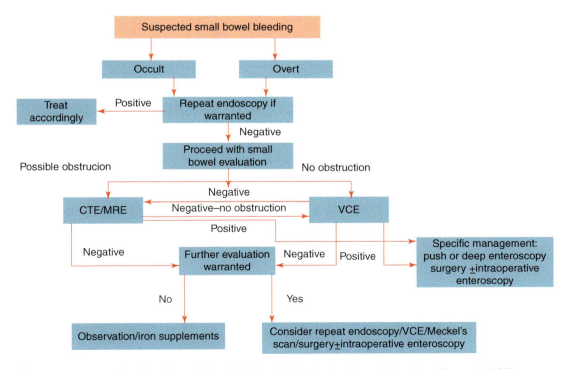

Fig. 19.5 Treatment algorithm for small bowel GI bleeds. (Reprinted with permission from Gerson et al. [1])

is poor at identifying duodenal lesions [36]. VCE should not be used if there is suspected bowel obstruction or bowel strictures because this increases the risk of capsule retention. Capsule retention – which is failure to pass the capsule 2 weeks after ingestion with radiographic confirmation on abdominal plain film – occurs in approximately 1.5% of patients who undergo this procedure for suspected small bowel GI bleeds. Capsule retention rate is much higher (up to 13%) in Crohn's patients [37]. Perforations due to VCE are extremely rare but have been reported. VCE should also be avoided in patients with gastrointestinal motility disorders or intestinal pseudo-obstruction. Patients with swallowing disorders should be carefully evaluated, and the capsule should be placed endoscopically to ensure proper entry into the alimentary tract. There is concern that VCE may interfere with cardiac pacemakers and implanted cardiac defibrillators, but its use in these patient populations is not contraindicated. Small case studies have shown no interference on these implantable devices in patients undergoing VCE [38, 39]. Patients should also not undergo magnetic resonance imaging (MRI) until they have passed the capsule.

Computed Tomographic or Magnetic Resonance Enterography (CTE or MRE)

CTE and MRE are cross-sectional imaging techniques used for diagnosis of possible small bowel GI bleeds in hemodynamically stable patients. Both require the ingestion of enteric contrast to aid in visualization of small bowel abnormalities. CTE is more often used than MRE due to its faster scan time and widespread availability. Diagnostic yield of CTE is only 40% in patients with suspected small bowel GI bleeds [40]. CTE appears to be superior to VCE in detecting intraluminal masses and inferior in detecting inflammatory or vascular small bowel lesions [41]. CTE and VCE are recommended as complementary diagnostic tools. CTE and MRE are excellent at delineating strictures in the small bowel that may

preclude VCE as a diagnostic option. MRE is less commonly performed, and there are few studies comparing its diagnostic ability to that of CTE. An advantage of MRE over CTE is that patients are exposed to less radiation with MRE.

Nuclear Medicine

Radionucleotide scans using technetium-99 (^{99m}Tc)-pertechnetate-labeled red blood cell (RBC) and ^{99m}Tc-pertechnetate offer additional diagnostic imaging options, especially in patients with slower rates of bleeding or suspected Meckel's diverticulum, respectively. ^{99m}Tc-pertechnetate-labeled red blood cell scintigraphy – commonly referred to as a tagged RBC scan – entails intravenous injection of ^{99m}Tc-pertechnetate-labeled autologous RBCs and obtaining abdominal imaging over the following 30–90 min. Additional imaging can be obtained every few hours for up to 1 day. The test is purely diagnostic, but its advantage lies in that delayed and intermittent bleeding may be more readily detected. Diagnostic yield is reported to be anywhere between 26% and 87%, and reported sensitivity and specificity are equally variable. ^{99m}Tc-pertechnetate scintigraphy – or Meckel's scan – can be used to detect the presence of ectopic gastric mucosa if a Meckel's diverticulum is suspected to be the cause of bleeding. ^{99m}Tc-pertechnetate is taken up and actively secreted by mucous cells within gastric mucosa, so a Meckel's scan does not detect bleeding but rather the presence of mucous-secreting gastric cells. Studies have shown that Meckel's scans are more sensitive in children than in adults. Specificity of a Meckel's scan is low (9%). False-positive scans could be due to bowel obstruction, ulcers, inflammation, neoplasms, duplication cysts, and arteriovenous malformations [42]. The 2015 American College of Gastroenterology guidelines strongly recommend that tagged RBC scintigraphy be used for diagnosis in patients with slower rates (0.1–0.2 mL/min) of overt suspected small bowel GI bleeds when VCE and deep enteroscopy cannot be performed [1].

Angiography

Conventional angiography and computed tomographic angiography (CTA) both have roles in the diagnosis and management of suspected small bowel GI bleeds. Conventional angiography should be the initial test of choice for acute, massive bleeding suspected to be from the small bowel in a hemodynamically unstable patient [1]. Conventional angiography allows for transarterial embolization to be performed at the time of diagnosis, and intraluminal blood or lack of bowel prep does not hinder its diagnostic ability. Conventional angiography has higher diagnostic yields in patients with brisk bleeding (0.5–1.0 mL/min) and is able to detect the source of small bowel GI bleeds, on average, in 50% of patients [43, 44]. Complications from conventional angiography with embolization include renal failure, thromboembolism, bowel infarction, and infection or bleeding from the arterial puncture site.

CTA is preferred over conventional angiography in hemodynamically stable patients with active bleeding from a suspected small bowel source [1]. CTA is able to detect bleeding occurring at slower rates (0.3 mL/min) compared to conventional angiography. CTA has a sensitivity of 89% and specificity of 85% in detecting the source of acute bleeding from the GI tract [45]. A major limitation of CTA is the inability to perform simultaneous intervention at the time of diagnosis. Similar to conventional angiography, patients must be actively bleeding at the time of CTA in order for contrast extravasation to be seen. A common concern for CTA is acute kidney injury from intravenous contrast administration.

Enteroscopy

There are several different types of enteroscopies that can be employed to examine the small bowel. These include push enteroscopy (PE), double-balloon enteroscopy (DBE), single-balloon enteroscopy (SBE), and intraoperative enteroscopy (IOE). *PE* is an extended upper endoscopy

performed with a longer PE scope or with a pediatric colonoscope. It reaches up to 90 cm past the ligament of Treitz. It is a good option for second-look endoscopy prior to undergoing VCE. Disadvantages of PE include patient discomfort and looping of the enteroscope in the stomach; the latter may be reduced by using an overtube to help stiffen the scope.

DBE and SBE use enteroscopes with balloons on the distal ends and both scopes use overtubes. DBE has a latex balloon on the end of the enteroscope and a second latex balloon on the overtube, whereas SBE has a silicone balloon on the end of the overtube only. DBE and SBE can be performed from an oral or anal approach. DBE is able to reach distances of 360 cm distal to the pylorus and 140 cm proximal to the ileocecal valve, with a diagnostic yield of DBE up to 80% in patients with small bowel GI bleeds [46]. DBE works by a series of pushing and pulling the enteroscope/overtube in coordination with alternately inflating and deflating the balloons on the overtube and the enteroscope. The overtube balloon anchors the overtube to the small bowel and allows for the scope (with balloon deflated) to be pushed forward. Subsequently, inflating the balloon on the advanced scope anchors the scope to the small bowel so the overtube (now with balloon deflated) can be advanced over the scope to catch up the distance gained (Fig. 19.6 – *DBE scope*). DBE is both diagnostic and therapeutic in

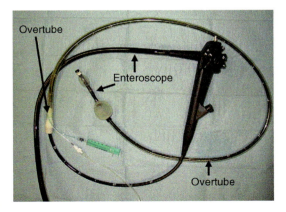

Fig. 19.6 Double-balloon enteroscope. (Reprinted with permission from May et al. [46])

the setting of small bowel GI bleeds. DBE scopes can perform tasks such as obtaining biopsies, coagulating bleeding sites, tattooing sites of interest, dilating strictures, and removing foreign bodies. Disadvantages to DBE include patient discomfort and long duration of the procedure. Overall complications after DBE are estimated to occur in 1.2% of patients, and these include perforation, bleeding, pancreatitis, and ileus [47].

SBE has a reported diagnostic yield of up to 74% in patients with suspected small bowel GI bleeds [48]. It works similarly to DBE, but instead of having a second balloon on the end of the enteroscope as an anchoring device, the endoscopist flexes the tip of the enteroscope against the bowel wall to anchor the scope as the overtube is advanced. Therapeutic options available with SBE are the same as those offered by DBE. Current data suggests that DBE and SBE are equivalent tools in the evaluation and treatment of suspected small bowel GI bleeds [49]. DBE and SBE may be unsuccessful in patients with extensive intraabdominal adhesions.

IOE is performed during laparotomy or laparoscopy. The enteroscope can be introduced orally, rectally, or through a surgical enterostomy in the small bowel. Any type of enteroscope can be used in this situation. In a two-center study comparing VCE with IOE, the latter was shown to have diagnostic yields of 100% in patients with overt bleeding and 50% in patients with occult bleeding [50]. Overall, diagnostic yield for IOE is up to 88%, but IOE has a high mortality rate of 2–17%. IOE should be reserved as a last resort for severe recurrent bleeding requiring transfusions not successfully diagnosed with other techniques (such as VCE and DBE/SBE) [51].

Overview of Treatment and Management

Treatment of small bowel GI bleeds varies depending on the source of bleeding, presence of ongoing blood loss, and the patient's hemodynamic status. As previously mentioned, conventional angiography is the best diagnostic and therapeutic option in hemodynamically unstable patients with acute, active bleeding suspected to be from a small bowel source. Angioembolization can be performed with permanent agents (such as microcoils or polyvinyl alcohol particles) or temporary agents (such as gelfoam) during conventional angiography to achieve hemostasis. Clinical success rates using permanent agents and temporary agents for angioembolization have been reported to be 98% and 71%, respectively. A 10-year retrospective study evaluating outcomes after super-selective angioembolization for GI bleeds reported a 2% incidence of post-embolization small bowel necrosis requiring surgical resection [52]. Angioembolization has also been used to treat postoperative small bowel GI bleeds. A small, retrospective study from Spain reported using angioembolization for treatment of postoperative GI bleeds in 21% of patients, and nearly half of these patients (45%) presented with anastomotic leak [53].

Surgical intervention may be necessary in some cases (such as bleeding due to Meckel's diverticulum or tumors) but generally needs diagnostic guidance from preoperative identification of the source and is often used as last resort. Patients with extensive bowel adhesions may require surgical lysis of adhesions for successful deep enteroscopy. A combination of conventional angiography and surgical therapy has also been described for small bowel GI bleeds. Patients undergo conventional angiography, and upon identification of the source, a catheter is left in place to intraoperatively inject methylene blue to highlight mesenteric vasculature feeding the bleeding source. This helps to localize the segment of bowel that requires surgical resection [54].

Endoscopy offers several treatment and diagnostic modalities for various sources of small bowel GI bleeds. Biopsies and polypectomies of suspicious ulcers and polyps can be obtained to diagnose cancers, vasculitis, infections, etc. Electrocautery, such as argon plasma coagulation, can be used to treat bleeding tissue, such as vascular ectasias. Sclerotherapy with epinephrine, alcohol, cyanoacrylate glue, and hypertonic glucose solution can be used, such as in the treatment of Dieulafoy's lesions. Band ligation and clips can be applied to visibly bleeding vessels.

Medical management of small bowel GI bleeds is an appropriate treatment in some settings. These management strategies are focused on treatment of anemia with oral or intravenous iron, and sometimes blood transfusions. Specific conditions, such as vascular ectasias, have been treated with somatostatin analogs such as octreotide and thalidomide. Somatostatin analogs are thought to reduce small bowel GI bleeds via decreasing splanchnic blood flow, decreasing angiogenesis, and improving platelet aggregation [55]. Somatostatin analogs have been shown to decrease transfusion requirements in multiple studies. Treatment protocols varied in their dosing (three times daily versus monthly depots) and duration (6–12 months) of treatment with somatostatin analogs, but outcomes between treatment and control groups show statistically significant improvement in those treated with somatostatin analogs [56]. Thalidomide is an antitumor necrosis factor immunomodulating agent with antiangiogenic properties. Studies have shown significant reduction in bleeding episodes in vascular ectasia patients treated with 4 months of thalidomide therapy [57]. However, adverse effects of thalidomide may not be tolerated by some patients; they include constipation, fatigue, and drowsiness. In the past, studies have investigated the use of estrogens in treatment of vascular ectasias, but this does not appear to be effective and is not recommended as an acceptable medical treatment option for this condition.

Conclusion

In conclusion, the 2015 American College of Gastroenterology guidelines strongly recommend that repeat endoscopic therapy (EGD and colonoscopy) should be the first-line diagnostic modality for suspected small bowel GI bleeds. If repeat EGD and/or colonoscopy fails to locate the source of bleeding, VCE or CTE/MRE should be performed next in the hemodynamically stable patient. If the source of bleeding is identified in the small bowel, deep enteroscopy or intraoperative enteroscopy should be performed to achieve hemostasis.

Persistent bleeding in stable patients with an unidentified source warrants repeat workup with second-look endoscopy, VCE, deep enteroscopy, etc. Active bleeding in a hemodynamically unstable patient is an indication for angiography. In cases where no source has been found despite thorough workup and evidence of bleeding persists, medical therapy with iron, somatostatin analogs, or antiangiogenic therapy is recommended.

References

1. Gerson LB, Fidler JL, Cave DR, et al. ACG clinical guideline: diagnosis and management of small bowel bleeding. Am J Gastroenterol. 2015;110(9):1265–87; quiz 1288
2. Jackson CS, Strong R. Gastrointestinal angiodysplasia: diagnosis and management. Gastrointest Endosc Clin N Am. 2017;27(1):51–62.
3. Clouse RE, Costigan DJ, Mills BA, et al. Angiodysplasia as a cause of upper gastrointestinal bleeding. Arch Intern Med. 1985;145(3):458–61.
4. Boley SJ, Sammartano R, Adams A, et al. On the nature and etiology of vascular ectasias of the colon. Degenerative lesions of aging. Gastroenterology. 1977;72(4 Pt 1):650–60.
5. Zajjari Y, Tamzaourte M, Montasser D, et al. Gastrointestinal bleeding due to angiodysplasia in patients on hemodialysis: a single-center study. Saudi J Kidney Dis Transpl. 2016;27(4):748–51.
6. Alhumood SA, Devine DV, Lawson L, et al. Idiopathic immune-mediated acquired von Willebrand's disease in a patient with angiodysplasia: demonstration of an unusual inhibitor causing a functional defect and rapid clearance of von Willebrand factor. Am J Hematol. 1999;60(2):151–7.
7. Hudzik B, Wilczek K, Gasior M. Heyde syndrome: gastrointestinal bleeding and aortic stenosis. CMAJ. 2016;188(2):135–8.
8. Singh G, Albeldawi M, Kalra SS, et al. Features of patients with gastrointestinal bleeding after implantation of ventricular assist devices. Clin Gastroenterol Hepatol. 2015;13(1):107–14.e101.
9. Poralla T. Angiodysplasia in the renal patient: how to diagnose and how to treat? Nephrol Dial Transplant. 1998;13(9):2188–91.
10. Siegel RL, Miller KD, Jemal A. Cancer statistics, 2017. CA Cancer J Clin. 2017;67(1):7–30.
11. Ciresi DL, Scholten DJ. The continuing clinical dilemma of primary tumors of the small intestine. Am Surg. 1995;61(8):698–702; discussion 702–3
12. Kemp CD, Russell RT, Sharp KW. Resection of benign duodenal neoplasms. Am Surg. 2007;73(11):1086–91.

13. Cross AJ, Leitzmann MF, Subar AF, et al. A prospective study of meat and fat intake in relation to small intestinal cancer. Cancer Res. 2008;68(22):9274–9.

14. Wu AH, Yu MC, Mack TM. Smoking, alcohol use, dietary factors and risk of small intestinal adenocarcinoma. Int J Cancer. 1997;70(5):512–7.

15. d'Amore F, Brincker H, Gronbaek K, et al. Non-Hodgkin's lymphoma of the gastrointestinal tract: a population-based analysis of incidence, geographic distribution, clinicopathologic presentation features, and prognosis. Danish Lymphoma Study Group. J Clin Oncol. 1994;12(8):1673–84.

16. Gibson GR, Whitacre EB, Ricotti CA. Colitis induced by nonsteroidal anti-inflammatory drugs. Report of four cases and review of the literature. Arch Intern Med. 1992;152(3):625–32.

17. Shin SJ, Noh CK, Lim SG, et al. Non-steroidal anti-inflammatory drug-induced enteropathy. Intest Res. 2017;15(4):446–55.

18. Matsumoto T, Kudo T, Esaki M, et al. Prevalence of non-steroidal anti-inflammatory drug-induced enteropathy determined by double-balloon endoscopy: a Japanese multicenter study. Scand J Gastroenterol. 2008;43(4):490–6.

19. Reuter BK, Davies NM, Wallace JL. Nonsteroidal anti-inflammatory drug enteropathy in rats: role of permeability, bacteria, and enterohepatic circulation. Gastroenterology. 1997;112(1):109–17.

20. Bjarnason I, Hayllar J, MacPherson AJ, et al. Side effects of nonsteroidal anti-inflammatory drugs on the small and large intestine in humans. Gastroenterology. 1993;104(6):1832–47.

21. Uejima M, Kinouchi T, Kataoka K, et al. Role of intestinal bacteria in ileal ulcer formation in rats treated with a nonsteroidal antiinflammatory drug. Microbiol Immunol. 1996;40(8):553–60.

22. Koga H, Aoyagi K, Matsumoto T, et al. Experimental enteropathy in athymic and euthymic rats: synergistic role of lipopolysaccharide and indomethacin. Am J Phys. 1999;276(3 Pt 1):G576–82.

23. Ullah S, Ajab S, Rao R, et al. Diaphragm disease of the small intestine: an interesting case report. Int J Surg Pathol. 2015;23(4):322–4.

24. Mehdizadeh S, Lo SK. Treatment of small-bowel diaphragm disease by using double-balloon enteroscopy. Gastrointest Endosc. 2006;64(6):1014–7.

25. Slesser AA, Wharton R, Smith GV, et al. Systematic review of small bowel diaphragm disease requiring surgery. Color Dis. 2012;14(7):804–13.

26. Gajendran M, Loganathan P, Catinella AP, et al. A comprehensive review and update on Crohn's disease. Dis Mon. 2018;64(2):20–57.

27. Matake H, Matsui T, Yao T. Inflammatory bowel disease – Crohn's diseaseNihon Rinsho. 1998;56(9):2349–53.

28. Cirocco WC, Reilly JC, Rusin LC. Life-threatening hemorrhage and exsanguination from Crohn's disease. Report of four cases. Dis Colon Rectum. 1995;38(1):85–95.

29. Michelassi F, Sultan S. Surgical treatment of complex small bowel Crohn disease. Ann Surg. 2014;260(2):230–5.

30. St-Vil D, Brandt ML, Panic S, et al. Meckel's diverticulum in children: a 20-year review. J Pediatr Surg. 1991;26(11):1289–92.

31. Close LN, Kumar NC, Glazer ES, Ong ES. A dieulafoy lesion as the cause of massive upper gastrointestinal bleeding after a distal pancreatectomy and splenectomy: case report and literature review. J Surg. 2013;1(2):3.

32. Lee YT, Walmsley RS, Leong RW, et al. Dieulafoy's lesion. Gastrointest Endosc. 2003;58(2):236–43.

33. Gerson LB. Small bowel bleeding: updated algorithm and outcomes. Gastrointest Endosc Clin N Am. 2017;27(1):171–80.

34. Delvaux M, Fassler I, Gay G. Clinical usefulness of the endoscopic video capsule as the initial intestinal investigation in patients with obscure digestive bleeding: validation of a diagnostic strategy based on the patient outcome after 12 months. Endoscopy. 2004;36(12):1067–73.

35. Yamada A, Watabe H, Kobayashi Y, et al. Timing of capsule endoscopy influences the diagnosis and outcome in obscure-overt gastrointestinal bleeding. Hepato-Gastroenterology. 2012;59(115):676–9.

36. Kong H, Kim YS, Hyun JJ, et al. Limited ability of capsule endoscopy to detect normally positioned duodenal papilla. Gastrointest Endosc. 2006;64(4):538–41.

37. Pennazio M. Capsule endoscopy: where are we after 6 years of clinical use? Dig Liver Dis. 2006;38(12):867–78.

38. Leighton JA, Sharma VK, Srivathsan K, et al. Safety of capsule endoscopy in patients with pacemakers. Gastrointest Endosc. 2004;59(4):567–9.

39. Leighton JA, Srivathsan K, Carey EJ, et al. Safety of wireless capsule endoscopy in patients with implantable cardiac defibrillators. Am J Gastroenterol. 2005;100(8):1728–31.

40. Wang Z, Chen JQ, Liu JL, et al. CT enterography in obscure gastrointestinal bleeding: a systematic review and meta-analysis. J Med Imaging Radiat Oncol. 2013;57(3):263–73.

41. Heo HM, Park CH, Lim JS, et al. The role of capsule endoscopy after negative CT enterography in patients with obscure gastrointestinal bleeding. Eur Radiol. 2012;22(6):1159–66.

42. Howarth DM. The role of nuclear medicine in the detection of acute gastrointestinal bleeding. Semin Nucl Med. 2006;36(2):133–46.

43. Rollins ES, Picus D, Hicks ME, et al. Angiography is useful in detecting the source of chronic gastrointestinal bleeding of obscure origin. AJR Am J Roentgenol. 1991;156(2):385–8.

44. Charbonnet P, Toman J, Buhler L, et al. Treatment of gastrointestinal hemorrhage. Abdom Imaging. 2005;30(6):719–26.

45. Wu LM, Xu JR, Yin Y, et al. Usefulness of CT angiography in diagnosing acute gastrointestinal bleeding: a meta-analysis. World J Gastroenterol. 2010;16(31):3957–63.

46. May A, Nachbar L, Ell C. Double-balloon enteroscopy (push-and-pull enteroscopy) of the small bowel: feasibility and diagnostic and therapeutic yield in patients with suspected small bowel disease. Gastrointest Endosc. 2005;62(1):62–70.

47. Mensink PB, Haringsma J, Kucharzik T, et al. Complications of double balloon enteroscopy: a multicenter survey. Endoscopy. 2007;39(7):613–5.

48. Manno M, Riccioni ME, Cannizzaro R, et al. Diagnostic and therapeutic yield of single balloon enteroscopy in patients with suspected small-bowel disease: results of the Italian multicentre study. Dig Liver Dis. 2013;45(3):211–5.

49. Domagk D, Mensink P, Aktas H, et al. Single- vs. double-balloon enteroscopy in small-bowel diagnostics: a randomized multicenter trial. Endoscopy. 2011;43(6):472–6.

50. Hartmann D, Schmidt H, Bolz G, et al. A prospective two-center study comparing wireless capsule endoscopy with intraoperative enteroscopy in patients with obscure GI bleeding. Gastrointest Endosc. 2005;61(7):826–32.

51. Leighton JA, Goldstein J, Hirota W, et al. Obscure gastrointestinal bleeding. Gastrointest Endosc. 2003;58(5):650–5.

52. Mejaddam AY, Cropano CM, Kalva S, et al. Outcomes following "rescue" superselective angioembolization for gastrointestinal hemorrhage in hemodynamically unstable patients. J Trauma Acute Care Surg. 2013;75(3):398–403.

53. Fernandez de Sevilla Gomez E, Vallribera Valls F, Espin Basany E, et al. Postoperative small bowel and colonic anastomotic bleeding. Therapeutic management and complications. Cir Esp. 2014;92(7):463–7.

54. Frydman J, Bahouth H, Leiderman M, et al. Methylene blue injection via superior mesenteric artery microcatheter for focused enterectomy in the treatment of a bleeding small intestinal arteriovenous malformation. World J Emerg Surg. 2014;9(1):17.

55. Szilagyi A, Ghali MP. Pharmacological therapy of vascular malformations of the gastrointestinal tract. Can J Gastroenterol. 2006;20(3):171–8.

56. Jackson CS, Gerson LB. Management of gastrointestinal angiodysplastic lesions (GIADs): a systematic review and meta-analysis. Am J Gastroenterol. 2014;109(4):474–83; quiz 484

57. Garrido A, Sayago M, Lopez J, et al. Thalidomide in refractory bleeding due to gastrointestinal angiodysplasias. Rev Esp Enferm Dig. 2012;104(2):69–71.

Mesenteric Ischemia

20

Meryl A. Simon and Joseph J. DuBose

Introduction

"Occlusion of the mesenteric vessels is apt to be regarded as one of those conditions of which the diagnosis is impossible, the prognosis hopeless and the treatment almost useless" [4].

Although the description of mesenteric ischemia by Cokkinis was written over 90 years ago, this vascular process remains a highly lethal but fortunately uncommon pathology. Given its rarity, the diagnosis is often delayed or missed, leading to high rates of associated morbidity and mortality. Early recognition and treatment remain paramount to success in treating this entity.

In this chapter, we will discuss mesenteric ischemia in terms of acute and chronic variants. We will also outline the pertinent epidemiology, etiology, diagnosis, and management of this clinically challenging pathology.

M. A. Simon
USAF, MC, David Grant USAF Medical Center;
University of California Davis Medical Center,
Division of Vascular and Endovascular Surgery,
Sacramento, CA, USA

J. J. DuBose (✉)
Department of Surgery, University of Maryland
School of Medicine, Baltimore, MD, USA

Acute Mesenteric Ischemia

Epidemiology Acute mesenteric ischemia (AMI) is a surgical emergency requiring prompt diagnosis and operative management. Although the prognosis differs based on etiology, the overall mortality ranges from 60% to over 80% [14, 17]. Despite imaging and therapeutic advancements, survival rates over time have failed to improve significantly.

AMI is fortunately rare, accounting for less than 1 in 1000 hospital admissions [18]. Women are more commonly affected, and the presenting age is typically 60–70 years. Comorbidities are common – including hypertension, peripheral arterial disease (PAD), coronary disease, atrial fibrillation, diabetes, renal disease, and chronic obstructive pulmonary disease (COPD) [24]. A patient's medical history will often guide the physician to the correct etiology of their AMI.

Etiology AMI can be classified as occlusive versus nonocclusive. Occlusive etiologies include embolic, thrombotic, or venous variants. Although the feared result of bowel ischemia can occur with each of these causes of occlusive ischemia, differentiating the cause is important in defining optimal treatment.

Arterial Embolization The most common cause of AMI is embolism – quoted at 40–50% of cases [14]. The culprit is usually a cardiac source, with

© Springer International Publishing AG, part of Springer Nature 2019
C. V. R. Brown et al. (eds.), *Emergency General Surgery*, https://doi.org/10.1007/978-3-319-96286-3_20

risk factors including arrhythmia, recent myocardial infarction, congestive heart failure, valve disorders, or a ventricular aneurysm. Any of these processes can lead to thrombus formation and subsequent embolization. One third of patients will have a history of a previous embolic event. A history of recent endovascular intervention should also be sought, as an alternate etiology can be due to atheroembolization. Other rare causes include embolization from an aortic aneurysm. The superior mesenteric artery (SMA) is the vessel most commonly affected due to its oblique angle of takeoff from the aorta. Most emboli will lodge distal to the first jejunal branches, once the vessel tapers in size. Approximately 50% will lodge distal to the middle colic artery – which results in a classic ischemic pattern seen, with the first portion of the small bowel along with the transverse colon spared [14] (Fig. 20.1).

Arterial Thrombosis Thrombosis is the second leading cause of AMI, comprising approximately 25% of cases [10]. This is often due to preexisting atherosclerotic disease, primarily at the origin of the visceral arteries. The SMA is often the cul-prit vessel. Upon questioning, the patient may provide a history of chronic mesenteric ischemic symptoms (postprandial abdominal pain and weight loss) and due to this will often have extensive visceral collateral development. This acute episode may also be the first presentation of a patients' mesenteric occlusive disease. In fact, autopsy results have shown that up to 10% of the population may harbor a >50% stenosis of one or more visceral vessels [21]. As will be discussed in the next section, patients with these chronic arterial narrowing pathologies will have underlying symptoms that present with a more gradual onset versus the acute symptomology observed with embolism. As occlusion occurs at the origin of the vessel, ischemia will encompass the entirety of the SMA territory, another distinguishing factor from embolization.

Nonocclusive Mesenteric Ischemia Nonocclusive mesenteric ischemia, or NOMI, accounts for 20% of AMI. Here, ischemia does not result from thrombosis or embolus but rather from a low flow state, which results in prolonged mesenteric vasospasm, leading to diminished intestinal perfusion. It is typically seen in critically ill patients

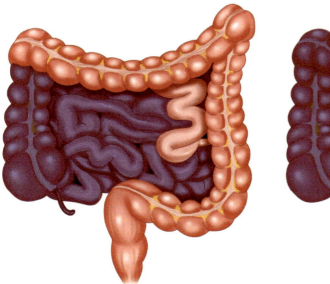
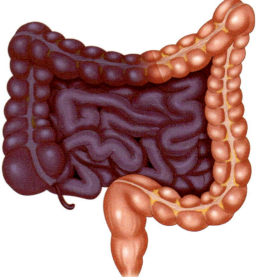

Fig. 20.1 Pattern of bowel ischemia seen in embolic (left) versus thrombotic (right) etiology. The left image shows sparring of the proximal jejunum and transverse colon

with failure of multiple organ systems and thus associated with a very high mortality rate. The mesenteric vessels undergo a prolonged period of vasoconstriction – often due to a combination of poor cardiac output from heart failure, hypovolemia, and the administration of vasoactive medications. NOMI can also be seen in illicit drug abuse, such as with cocaine, which also causes vasoconstriction.

Venous Thrombosis Mesenteric venous thrombosis (MVT) is thrombosis of the venous system of the intestines which include the superior mesenteric, inferior mesenteric, portal, and splenic veins. MVT can range in presentation from an asymptomatic incidental imaging finding to devastating bowel infarction. MVT is the least common cause of AMI, accounting for about 10% of cases, but carries a high mortality rate approaching 30% [14]. MVT can be classified as either primary (idiopathic) or secondary. Secondary is far more common, encompassing 90% of cases. Secondary causes have an underlying condition predisposing to thrombosis such as an inherited thrombophilia, malignancy, injury, or inflammatory states. Presentation and prognosis are related to extent and speed of venous involvement. Additionally, involvement of the superior mesenteric vein (SMV) incurs a higher risk of bowel infarction [1]. MVT is usually segmental. The outflow obstruction leads to focal edema, bowel distention, and finally hemorrhagic infarction [14].

Diagnosis

Presentation A high index of suspicion is paramount in making the diagnosis of acute mesenteric ischemia given its high morbidity, with a mortality that increases as diagnosis is delayed [14]. The classic symptom of AMI is abdominal pain which is out of proportion to physical exam findings. Until transmural bowel infarction occurs, there is minimal peritoneal irritation and thus little tenderness on exam. The presentation is often mistaken for other more common abdominal pathologies such as appendicitis, cholecysti-

tis, or diverticulitis, often leading to delays in the correct diagnosis.

For patients with AMI due to embolization, the abdominal pain is most commonly abrupt in onset. Yet, not all patients will present this way. Instead, patients may present with progression of pain over several hours to days. This is often the subgroup with preexisting chronic mesenteric disease, and due to collateral development, their symptoms may prove more insidious. Those with MVT are also likely to present with a more insidious course. Their pain can be highly variable and diffuse and present for days prior to presentation [9]. NOMI will also present as a prolonged course and often in a patient who cannot provide a history as they are usually critically ill. Regardless of the etiology, the abdominal exam can remain relatively benign until transmural necrosis takes place.

Laboratory There are no laboratory findings that are diagnostic for AMI. Additionally, compounding the difficulty in this diagnosis, patients may present with a normal set of laboratory values early in their clinical course. The most common abnormality seen is leukocytosis, which is nonspecific. Other common findings include hemoconcentration, along with elevated amylase, lactate dehydrogenase, and aspartate aminotransferase. Lactic acidosis can be seen, but unfortunately this is a late finding, often signifying bowel infarction has taken place [9].

D-dimer can be a useful test in cases of MVT. It is a sensitive marker for the early detection of AMI secondary to MVT, and some research even suggests its use as an indication of severity [23]. D-dimer is indeed sensitive, but it is not specific for MVT, as many other processes can lead its presence, but a negative test can likely exclude this diagnosis.

Testing for inherited hypercoagulable conditions such as antithrombin deficiency or Factor V Leiden can assist in identifying a secondary cause for MVT, but do not aid in the diagnosis of MVT.

Imaging Given the nonspecific presentation, a plain abdominal radiograph is often obtained, but findings may be normal in up to 25% of patients, especially early in the disease course [20]. The film may show signs of bowel edema or infarction – such as pneumatosis. Probably most useful is its ability to exclude other possible diagnoses.

Duplex ultrasound is typically an invaluable tool in the diagnosis and surveillance for chronic mesenteric ischemia, but has no significant role as an imaging modality in AMI for several reasons. Duplex is highly user dependent – experienced technologists are required and may not be available at many institutions nor at all hours. Additionally, abdominal studies are limited by the presence of bowel gas in the unprepped patient. Finally, the study requires constant abdominal compression to capture key images, which is not typically tolerated by the patient with acute ischemia.

Computed tomography angiography (CTA) has become the imaging modality of choice for the diagnosis of acute mesenteric ischemia. It has both a high sensitivity and specificity quoted at 93% and 95%, respectively, based on a 2010 meta-analysis [11]. The CTA is widely available, noninvasive, and expeditious. The vascular imaging quality obtained has continued to improve with the use of the multidetector CTA (MDCTA). The high-resolution images obtained have allowed the CTA to surpass traditional angiography as the first-line technique for diagnostic imaging (Fig. 20.2). Additionally, a variety of other intra-abdominal pathologies can be identified or excluded when the diagnosis is in question. It is important to mention that CTA studies are not without risk. The contrast utilized, which is often in the range of 100–125 ml, has the potential for both allergic reaction and contrast-induced nephropathy (CIN). CIN is not uncommon and is a leading cause of acute renal injury in the hospital setting and is associated with an increased overall mortality [6].

Angiography had previously been the "gold" standard study for AMI imaging prior to MDCTA technology. The benefits of this invasive study lie in its ability to provide both diagnostic information as well as a potentially therapeutic interven-

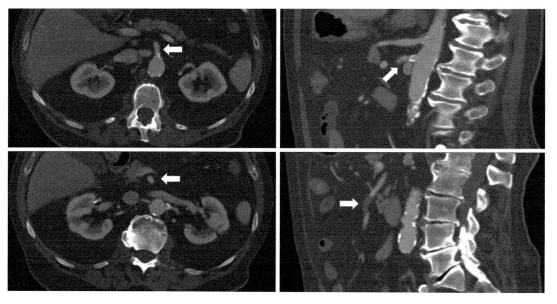

Fig. 20.2 This is a CT angiogram of a 70-year-old man who presented with several hours of acute abdominal pain. He was found to have an embolus to his SMA. The axial slice in the upper left shows the vessel origin. It does have atherosclerotic calcification but is patent. The lower left-hand image shows the SMA slightly distal to its take-off where it remains patent. The upper right-hand image is a sagittal view of the patent SMA origin. The right lower image is a sagittal view of the embolus shown by the white arrow. This patient underwent exploratory laparotomy with successful embolectomy without the need for bowel resection

tion (see section "Treatment" for more information). The risk of contrast-related renal injury, time to access an angiographic suite and to acquire the desired images, and invasive nature of the procedure have all made this traditional technique no longer the first step in imaging. Angiography is now often reserved for cases where the diagnosis remains in question, or when a thrombotic etiology is suspected, and the patient is seen early before bowel infarction has taken place. Additionally, angiography provides no information on the remainder of the abdominal organs, necessitating a laparotomy for bowel viability assessment.

Treatment

The initial management of a patient diagnosed with acute mesenteric ischemia begins with fluid resuscitation, electrolyte correction, hemodynamic monitoring, and placement of invasive lines in preparation for surgical exploration. Anticoagulation with heparin should be given as a bolus followed by a therapeutic drip if there are no contraindications. Heparin will prevent the propagation of further thrombosis. Additionally,

the administration of broad spectrum antibiotics should be strongly considered in order to mitigate the risk of intraluminal translocation of bacteria.

The basic surgical principles for AMI include revascularization before bowel resection (except for frank necrosis or bowel perforation) followed by a second-look laparotomy.

All patients with any concern for threatened bowel should be taken to the operating room. The best exposure for both bowel assessment and revascularization is through a midline vertical laparotomy. The patient is laid supine on the operating table, ideally one which can accommodate fluoroscopy if a completion angiogram is needed. The abdomen is widely prepared, and the anterior thighs are included in case the great saphenous vein must be harvested for a bypass. The bowel is assessed – and if there is neither frank transmural necrosis nor perforation with spillage, revascularization should take place first. Of note, if a large amount of bowel is nonviable, consideration should be given to aborting the procedure based on the patient's preoperative desires and a thoughtful discussion with the patient's family when they are not able to participate in these thought processes (Fig. 20.3). The

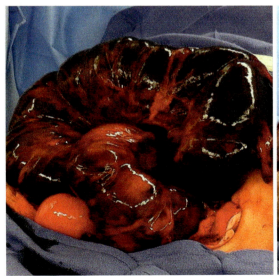 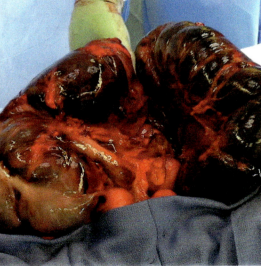

Fig. 20.3 An intraoperative photo of an exploratory laparotomy of a 40-year-old man who presented with 3 days of worsening abdominal pain. He was found to have thrombosis of the intra-abdominal aorta including the celiac axis and superior and inferior mesenteric arteries. Transmural necrosis was present throughout the entirety of the small bowel and colon

next steps will differ based on etiology. Embolectomy with either primary or patch closure is the technique of choice for embolism, while AMI due to thrombosis will require a bypass.

Embolism When AMI is due to an embolus to the SMA, the surgical treatment is embolectomy. There are multiple ways to access the superior mesenteric artery, and for embolectomy, the exposure of choice is identifying the vessel in its infra-pancreatic location. This is done by displacing the transverse colon and omentum cranially and retracting the small bowel to the patient's right. A horizontal incision is made in the peritoneum at the base of the transverse mesocolon. The SMA will lie to the left of the superior mesenteric vein. Often, the middle colic artery can be identified, and tracing this vessel proximally will identify the SMA. After circumferential dissection is completed, vessel loops can then be placed proximally and distally, as well as around all branches in the vicinity. Branches should be preserved if possible. Systemic heparin is administered. If the vessel is otherwise soft and healthy, a transverse arteriotomy is made. If a longitudinal arteriotomy is chosen, closure should be performed with a patch to avoid narrowing the vessel lumen. This may be a good option for a small vessel. Upon entering the vessel, thrombus can often be visualized and extracted. Additionally, manual "milking" of the vessel can express clot. Embolectomy catheters can be used, but care must be taken as the SMA is quite fragile. A 2 or 3 French balloon is used distally, while a 3 or 4 French balloon is employed proximally. Embolectomy proceeds until brisk blood flow is encountered. If not, there is likely missed thrombus. Once the embolectomy is complete, the arteriotomy is closed with interrupted suture (or with a vein patch) and flow is restored. The SMA should now be pulsatile. Branches should also be assessed for pulsation or Doppler signal. If there is lack of signal or concern for retained embolus, an angiogram can be helpful.

Once perfusion is restored, the bowel is reassessed. Necrotic segments are resected, and the bowel is left in discontinuity. A temporary abdominal closure of choice is placed, with planned second look in 24–48 h.

Thrombosis For thrombotic disease, the surgical management is typically visceral artery bypass. Consideration can also be given to stenting. As the disease is located at the vessels origin off the aorta, the exposure differs from that described above, and there are multiple bypass options available.

The SMA can be exposed in its sub-pancreatic location but from a lateral rather than anterior approach, as was seen for embolectomy. The first steps are similar – the transverse colon is reflected up, and the small bowel is retracted to the right. The additional step is to mobilize the fourth portion of the duodenum by dividing the ligament of Treitz. The SMA will be identified in the peritoneal tissue cranial to the duodenum. Remember to open the peritoneum longitudinally to maximize exposure. For further exposure, the pancreas can be retracted superiorly to the level where the left renal vein crosses anterior to the aorta. This exposed the SMA distal to the atherosclerotic disease found at its origin and will be the site for the distal bypass anastomosis.

The inflow of the bypass can originate in either an antegrade or retrograde fashion. Antegrade inflow is typically the supraceliac aorta. Retrograde inflow can come from the infrarenal aorta, the right common iliac or left common iliac arteries. Prosthetic conduits are often preferred, such as an externally supported polytetrafluoroethylene (PTFE) graft because they avoid the need for vein harvest, provide an appropriate size match, and are more resistant to kinking. If gross peritoneal contamination is present, then utilization of a vein conduit is preferred.

The preferred technique by most is a retrograde "C" loop from the right common iliac artery (Fig. 20.4). The retrograde approach avoids the need for supraceliac dissection and aortic clamping. The right side is preferred as the sympathetic nerve plexuses run along the left common iliac artery. The bypass is created in an end-to-side fashion off the iliac and either end-to-end or end-to-side onto the SMA. End-to-side

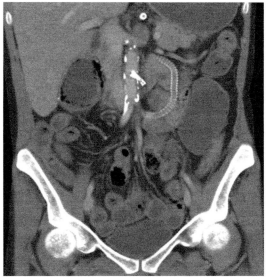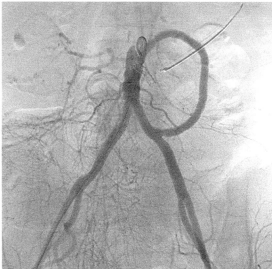

Fig. 20.4 This patient presented with acute-on-chronic mesenteric ischemia due to occlusion of a previously placed graft. She had a left common iliac to SMA loop graft with PTFE. The CTA on the left shows the occluded bypass. The angiogram on the right was taken after successful graft thrombectomy

has the additional benefit of preserving flow to any proximal branches which may remain patent.

A short bypass from the infrarenal aorta to the SMA from the same exposure can also be created. This bypass also uses a prosthetic conduit and requires minimal additional dissection. The limiting factor though is often the existence of atherosclerotic disease in this segment of the aorta.

An alternative option to bypass is endovascular stenting. A short lesion at the origin of the vessel is ideal for this technique, so the CTA should be reviewed prior to this decision. The SMA can be exposed as above and accessed with a needle. This technique is known as retrograde open mesenteric stenting (ROMS) as described by the Dartmouth group [22]. A hydrophilic wire should be used to traverse the lesion. Care is taken to not injure the vessel and cause a dissection or perforation. A self-expanding stent (covered or bare metal) is used, with projection into the aorta to not miss the proximal extent of the lesion. This technique can also be performed from a transfemoral or transbrachial approach, but the physician would need to be certain no bowel is at risk as this does not allow for intestinal viability evaluation. Endovascular approaches are most appropriate for the rare patient caught very early in presentation.

Venous thrombosis All patients with symptomatic mesenteric venous thrombosis should be systemically anticoagulated as soon as able. In patients with incidentally detected splanchnic thrombosis, no anticoagulation is the recommendation by the American College of Chest Physicians guidelines [8]. Conservative management can be safely instituted in patients without peritoneal findings. Anticoagulation alone will often lead to recanalization and can avoid the resection of bowel which has not progressed to transmural infarction. In patients caught early before transmural necrosis, nonoperative management has shown similar rates of morbidity, mortality, and survival [2].

Patients with MVT and peritonitis should be taken to the operating room for exploration. If frank bowel necrosis is encountered, resection and anastomosis should take place. If bowel viability is questionable, the abdomen should be temporarily closed for a planned second look in 24–48 h as done for embolism or thrombosis.

Seldom, open thrombectomy or endovascular thrombolysis can be considered. Thrombectomy works best in situations of recent thrombosis isolated to the superior mesenteric vein. These procedures are performed so rarely, that most of the available literature is from case reports or case series. Endovascular techniques described include thrombolysis, either by way of a transhepatic or superior mesenteric artery route, suction thrombectomy, or direct open approach. These procedures have been shown to improve symptoms and limit bowel resection, but they come with high complication rates, such as life-threatening gastrointestinal hemorrhage [7]. These procedures should be reserved for patients with severe disease or who fail anticoagulation alone.

Once the patients clinical picture improves and no further invasive procedures are likely, the transition to an oral anticoagulant should take place. For patients who present with a clear temporary cause, anticoagulation can be limited to 3–6 months. For most patients, the etiology is idiopathic, and therapy should be indefinite given its high rate of recurrence [5].

Nonocclusive Ischemia The principal treatment for NOMI is medical therapy. This involves improving intestinal perfusion with intravenous fluids and stopping offending agents such as vasoactive medications. Surgical exploration is reserved for cases of suspected peritonitis. Arteriography can be performed as both a diagnostic and potentially therapeutic modality but is often limited by the acutely ill nature of these patients, who may not be stable for transport to an endovascular suite.

If performed, the angiogram findings suggestive of NOMI include diffuse mesenteric vessel narrowing, a pattern of "string of sausages" – where areas of dilatation and narrowing alternate in the intestinal branches, spasm of the mesenteric arcades, and impaired filling of the intramural vessels [19]. Many have advocated for the infusion of vasodilator agents at the time of diagnostic angiogram to relieve the spasm. The most common medications used include nitroglycerine, papaverine, and prosta-

glandin E_1 (PGE_1). Some series have shown good success with continuous infusions, such as Mitsuyoshi et al. who showed an 8/9 patient survival in those treated with PGE_1 versus a 69% (9/13) mortality rate in those not treated [13]. Although the groups differed based on time to diagnosis (the untreated group all occurred before the incorporation of MDCTA in diagnostic workup), it does show a potential role for vasodilator therapy. This therapy is not without risk. Nitroglycerin and papaverine cannot be given systemically without the untoward effect of hypotension, so intra-catheter administration is required. PGE_1 inhibits platelet aggregation which can increase the risk of hemorrhage.

Chronic Mesenteric Ischemia

Epidemiology Chronic mesenteric ischemia (CMI) is an uncommon cause of abdominal pain, yet the presence of atherosclerotic involvement in the visceral vasculature approaches 20% in the over 65 years of age population [16]. Despite this, most patients will remain asymptomatic. CMI accounts for less than 1 in 100,000 hospital admissions and less than 2% of gastrointestinal admissions [12]. Like acute mesenteric ischemia, CMI is a rare disease process which requires a high index of suspicion to diagnosis. This often leads to a delay in diagnosis, which is often reached only after an extensive workup has been completed.

Etiology Atherosclerosis of the visceral vessels is the most common cause of CMI, accounting for over 90% of cases. The atherosclerotic lesions are seen at the origins of the visceral arteries, most commonly the celiac axis and superior mesenteric artery (SMA). This is often referred to as "aortic spill over," and patients may be found to have calcifications of the origins of multiple vessels, including the renal arteries as well [3].

Other less common causes of CMI include fibromuscular dysplasia, vasculitides such as Takayasu's arteritis or polyarteritis nodosa, median arcuate ligament syndrome, chronic dissections, or radiation arteritis. Processes involving the supraceliac aorta may also manifest with CMI symptoms such as aortic coarctation.

This section will focus on CMI due to atherosclerosis.

Diagnosis

Presentation The classic presentation is that of a patient in their sixth decade of life, more commonly a woman, who complains of postprandial abdominal pain. The onset of pain is typically within 15–30 min of a meal and can last for hours thereafter. The pain is described as dull and crampy. The presence of this pain after each meal leads to the development of "food fear" which then leads to the other classic finding of weight loss.

On physical examination, the CMI patient can appear cachectic. The abdominal exam is often unremarkable, but a bruit may be appreciated. Other vascular beds should be assessed, as patients with atherosclerosis in the territory will have disease elsewhere.

Laboratory There is no laboratory test that is diagnostic for CMI, but nutrition labs should be checked (such as albumin and prealbumin) and will usually show evidence of malnutrition.

Imaging Diagnosis of CMI is made through imaging. Similar to the studies used for AMI, computed tomography angiography (CTA) and angiography have key roles.

Additionally, mesenteric duplex ultrasonography is now the screening test of choice given its noninvasive nature and ability to provide a high sensitivity for the presence of visceral artery stenosis. Additionally, duplex can be used for surveillance after revascularization. Although each vascular lab will use its own criteria for diagnosis, all diagnoses are based on peak systolic velocity (PSV) measurements. Most commonly, a significant stenosis of the SMA is diagnosed by a PSV > 275 cm/s, while a PSV > 200 cm/s signifies a significant celiac stenosis [12].

Once the diagnosis is made by duplex, further imaging with CTA or conventional angiography is obtained for interventional planning.

Treatment

Although the technical aspects of CMI treatment are beyond the scope of this chapter, there are a few key points to take away. Revascularization should be pursued for all symptomatic patients. For asymptomatic disease, there are no guidelines to suggest operative intervention.

As technology continues to evolve, more patients with CMI are now undergoing endovascular intervention (angioplasty and stenting), with open traditional mesenteric bypass being reserved for endovascular failure, stent occlusion, or non-atherosclerotic etiologies.

The debate about whether to revascularize just the SMA or both the SMA and celiac arteries is ongoing, but there is no data to suggest that two vessels are better than one. What the literature does show is that open operations for CMI is successful, with good long-term symptom relief and low operative mortality [15].

Conclusion

Acute and chronic mesenteric ischemia are rare but potentially devastating disease processes. Given their infrequent nature, delays in diagnosis are common. Mesenteric pathology requires a high index of suspicion, and once identified, a rapid workup and management strategy must be implemented.

References

1. Amitrano L, Guardascione MA, Scaglione M, Pezzullo L, Sangiuliano N, Armellino MF, Manguso F, Margaglione M, Ames PR, Iannaccone L. Prognostic factors in noncirrhotic patients with splanchnic vein thromboses. Am J Gastroenterol. 2007;102:2464.
2. Brunaud L, Antunes L, Collinet-Adler S, Marchal F, Ayav A, Bresler L, Boissel P. Acute mesenteric venous thrombosis: case for nonoperative management. J Vasc Surg. 2001;34:673–9.

3. Chandra A, Quinones-Baldrich WJ. Chronic mesenteric ischemia: how to select patients for invasive treatment. Semin Vasc Surg. 2010;23:21–8.
4. Cokkinis A. Mesenteric vascular occlusion. South Med J. 1926;19:655.
5. Dentali F, Ageno W, Witt D, Malato A, Clark N, Garcia D, Mccool K, Siragusa S, Dyke S, Crowther M. Natural history of mesenteric venous thrombosis in patients treated with vitamin K antagonists: a multi-centre, retrospective cohort study. Thromb Haemost. 2009;102:501–4.
6. From AM, Bartholmai BJ, Williams AW, Cha SS, Mcdonald FS. Mortality associated with nephropathy after radiographic contrast exposure. Mayo Clin Proc. 2008;83:1095–100.
7. Hollingshead M, Burke CT, Mauro MA, Weeks SM, Dixon RG, Jaques PF. Transcatheter thrombolytic therapy for acute mesenteric and portal vein thrombosis. J Vasc Interv Radiol. 2005;16:651–61.
8. Kearon C, Akl EA, Comerota AJ, Prandoni P, Bounameaux H, Goldhaber SZ, Nelson ME, Wells PS, Gould MK, Dentali F, Crowther M, Kahn SR. Antithrombotic therapy for VTE disease: antithrombotic therapy and prevention of thrombosis, 9th ed: American College of Chest Physicians Evidence-Based Clinical Practice Guidelines. Chest. 2012;141:e419S–96S.
9. Kumar S, Sarr MG, Kamath PS. Mesenteric venous thrombosis. N Engl J Med. 2001;345:1683–8.
10. Lock G. Acute intestinal ischaemia. Best Pract Res Clin Gastroenterol. 2001;15:83–98.
11. Menke J. Diagnostic accuracy of multidetector CT in acute mesenteric ischemia: systematic review and meta-analysis. Radiology. 2010;256:93–101.
12. Mitchell EL, Moneta GL. Mesenteric duplex scanning. Perspect Vasc Surg Endovasc Ther. 2006;18:175–83.
13. Mitsuyoshi A, Obama K, Shinkura N, Ito T, Zaima M. Survival in nonocclusive mesenteric ischemia: early diagnosis by multidetector row computed tomography and early treatment with continuous intravenous high-dose prostaglandin E(1). Ann Surg. 2007;246:229–35.
14. Oldenburg WA, Lau LL, Rodenberg TJ, Edmonds HJ, Burger CD. Acute mesenteric ischemia: a clinical review. Arch Intern Med. 2004;164:1054–62.
15. Park WM, Cherry KJ, Chua HK, Clark RC, Jenkins G, Harmsen WS, Noel AA, Panneton JM, Bower TC, Hallett JW, Gloviczki P. Current results of open revascularization for chronic mesenteric ischemia: a standard for comparison. J Vasc Surg. 2002;35:853–9.
16. Roobottom C, Dubbins P. Significant disease of the celiac and superior mesenteric arteries in asymptomatic patients: predictive value of Doppler sonography. AJR Am J Roentgenol. 1993;161:985–8.
17. Schoots I, Koffeman G, Legemate D, Levi M, Van Gulik T. Systematic review of survival after acute mesenteric ischaemia according to disease aetiology. Br J Surg. 2004;91:17–27.
18. Schoots IG, Levi MM, Reekers JA, Lameris JS, Van Gulik TM. Thrombolytic therapy for acute superior mesenteric artery occlusion. J Vasc Interv Radiol. 2005;16:317–29.
19. Siegelman SS, Sprayregen S, Boley SJ. Angiographic diagnosis of mesenteric arterial vasoconstriction. Radiology. 1974;112:533–42.
20. Smerud MJ, Johnson CD, Stephens DH. Diagnosis of bowel infarction: a comparison of plain films and CT scans in 23 cases. Am J Roentgenol. 1990;154:99–103.
21. Walker TG. Mesenteric ischemia. Seminars in interventional radiology: © Thieme Medical Publishers; USA. 2009. p. 175–83.
22. Wyers MC, Powell RJ, Nolan BW, Cronenwett JL. Retrograde mesenteric stenting during laparotomy for acute occlusive mesenteric ischemia. J Vasc Surg. 2007;45:269–75.
23. Yang S, Fan X, Ding W, Liu B, Meng J, Wang K, Wu X, LI J. D-dimer as an early marker of severity in patients with acute superior mesenteric venous thrombosis. Medicine. 2014;93:e270.
24. Zettervall SL, Lo RC, Soden PA, Deery SE, Ultee KH, Pinto DS, Wyers MC, Schermerhorn ML. Trends in treatment and mortality for mesenteric ischemia in the United States from 2000 to 2012. Ann Vasc Surg. 2017;42:111–9.

Acute Appendicitis

21

Brittany Bankhead-Kendall
and Pedro G. R. Teixeira

Background

Acute appendicitis is one of the most common acute surgical conditions in the United States. In 1886, Dr. Reginald Fitz first used the term acute appendicitis to describe an inflammatory condition of the right lower quadrant that was starting to be treated surgically with success [1]. In the nineteenth century, Dr. Charles McBurney went on to author a series of papers describing appendicitis definitively as a surgical disease. According to his observation, this condition was commonly associated with focal pain and tenderness at one specific location in the right lower quadrant later became widely known as "McBurney's point" [2, 3].

As progressive advances in surgical technique, antiseptic principles, and antibiotic therapy occurred, the mortality associated with this condition began a steady decline and reached single-digit rates in the early 1940s, a remarkable treatment success for a disease that had previously touted 50% mortality rates [4]. Currently, approximately 11 per 10,000 patients a year present with clinical evidence of appendicitis, leading to 300,000 appendectomies performed each year across the United States. Lifetime risk of acute appendicitis for males is 8.6% and 6.7% for females [5].

Diagnosis

Clinical presentation of acute appendicitis is characterized by the acute onset of nausea, vomiting, abdominal pain, anorexia, and fever. In many cases, history and physical exam alone are enough for a clinical diagnosis and to warrant surgical exploration. Dr. Alfredo Alvarado sought to create a scoring system to combine subjective complaints with objective physical exam and laboratory findings to establish the diagnosis and identify patients who needed to be observed and those who needed an operation [6]. The components of the Alvarado score include symptoms, signs, and laboratory work (Table 21.1).

This score, which was initially proposed to discriminate between patients that should be observed (scores 5 or 6) and those who should be operated on (score 7 or higher), later became a tool to identify patients with intermediate risk for appendicitis who would need imaging investigation. A systematic review performed to investigate the value of the Alvarado score for predicting acute appendicitis found that a score less than 5 can accurately rule out appendicitis, but a score of 7 or higher lack specificity to identify those patients requiring surgical exploration. This

B. Bankhead-Kendall · P. G. R. Teixeira (✉)
Department of Surgery and Perioperative Care,
University of Texas at Austin, Dell Medical School,
Austin, TX, USA
e-mail: pgteixeira@austin.utexas.edu

© Springer International Publishing AG, part of Springer Nature 2019
C. V. R. Brown et al. (eds.), *Emergency General Surgery*, https://doi.org/10.1007/978-3-319-96286-3_21

Table 21.1 Alvarado score

	Points
Symptoms	
Migration	1
Anorexia	1
Nausea-vomiting	1
Signs	
Tenderness in the right lower quadrant	2
Rebound pain	1
Fever	1
Laboratory	
Leukocytosis	2
Shift to the left	1
Total score	10

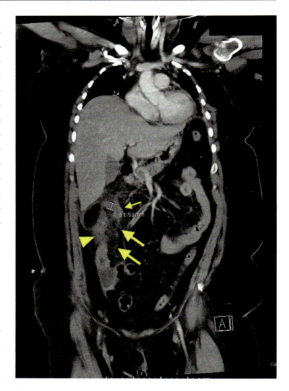

Fig. 21.1 CT scan image (coronal section) demonstrating dilated appendix (small arrow), with adjacent fat stranding (large arrows), and periappendicular free fluid (arrowhead), suggestive of acute appendicitis

finding suggests that additional imaging is warranted even for patients with a high score [7].

Negative appendectomy is not without its own significant morbidity risk from the operation. Diagnostic imaging outperforms the Alvarado score [8], and its utilization has led to a decrease in negative appendectomies, without an impact in decreasing incidence of perforation [9]. Options for imaging include ultrasound, computerized tomography (CT) scan, and magnetic resonance imaging (MRI). Ultrasound as an initial imaging modality as part of a diagnostic algorithm has been shown to be a useful tool [10]. Ultrasound for the evaluation of acute appendicitis yields a high positive predictive value, but negative or inconclusive findings cannot be used to rule out appendicitis, and these patients warrant further imaging, which is often a CT scan.

A normal appendix on ultrasound is a blind-ending tubular structure arising from the cecum with normal diameter (≤6–7 mm) and normal wall thickness (≤2 mm). An inflamed appendix will be dilated, non-compressible, and often immobile with a thickened wall. The presence of adjacent free fluid or fecalith can also be suggestive of acute appendicitis. Quality of evaluation of the appendix via ultrasound is often highly dependent on the operator performing the exam.

CT scan findings of acute appendicitis are closely related to those described for the ultrasound but less operator-dependent. These findings include dilated appendix, periappendicular fluid, adjacent fat stranding, presence of a fecalith (Figs. 21.1, 21.2, and 21.3), and absence of luminal contrast or gas in the appendix. CT scan can also suggest alternative diagnoses and also identify complications such as rupture, phlegmon, and abscess that may necessitate alternative nonoperative management (Fig. 21.4).

MRI is available, but less frequently used, in the diagnoses of acute appendicitis. Its utility lies more heavily in the pregnant and pediatric populations where the lack of ionizing radiation justifies the increased costs compared to CT scans.

Sensitivity for each imaging modality is quite good for ultrasound, CT scan, and MRI (75–90%, 90–100%, and 97–100%, respectively), as well as their positive predictive value (91–94%, 92–98%, and 98%). Overall, CT scan provides higher sensitivity and specificity compared to

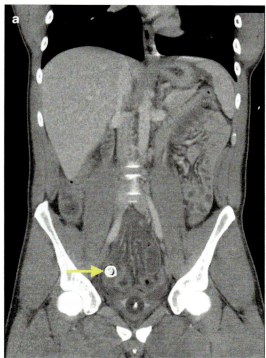

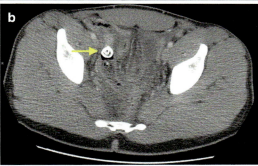

Fig. 21.2 (**a**, **b**) CT scan images (axial and coronal sections) demonstrating a large fecalith (arrows)

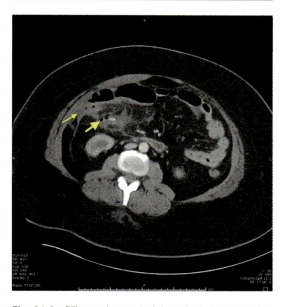

Fig. 21.3 CT scan image (axial section) demonstrating presence of extraluminal air adjacent to the appendix (large arrow), with adjacent free fluid (small arrow), suggestive of acute perforated appendicitis

ultrasound [11–13] (Table 21.2) and leads to decreased indicidence of negative appendectomies, without the associated cost increase of the MRI. In children, however, graded-compression ultrasound has sensitivity and specificity comparable to those from CT scan without the potential harm of ionizing radiation [14]. Likewise, MRI is a reasonable alternative when ultrasound is inconclusive and the radiation exposure associated with CT scan modality is contraindicated, as in the pregnant women population.

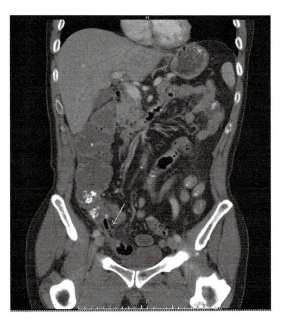

Fig. 21.4 CT scan image (coronal section) demonstrating presence of extraluminal air adjacent to the appendix (arrow), suggestive of acute perforated appendicitis

Table 21.2 Comparison of imaging modalities used for the diagnosis of acute appendicitis

	Sensitivity	Specificity	Accuracy	PPV	NPV
Ultrasound	75–90%	86–100%	87–96%	91–94%	89–97%
CT Scan	90–100%	91–99%	94–98%	92–98%	95–100%
MRI	97–100%	92–98%	92–99%	98%	100%

Nonoperative Management

Nonoperative Management for Uncomplicated Appendicitis

Challenging the dogma of operative treatment as the primary approach to uncomplicated appendicitis – defined as acute appendicitis without abscess, phlegmon, or other loculated adjacent fluid collections – multiple studies, including several randomized controlled trials, have investigated the role of nonoperative treatment with antibiotics as the primary treatment for this condition [15–22]. These studies suggest that nonoperative treatment with antibiotics is a safe initial treatment modality for patients with uncomplicated appendicitis but is associated with significant failure rates. As the number of patients now being treated nonoperatively increases, significant controversy still exists regarding this treatment pathway. A meta-analysis summarizing the findings of studies investigating the nonoperative management of uncomplicated appendicitis found a 20% chance of recurrence after conservative treatment within 1 year [15]. Of those recurrences, 20% presented with perforated or gangrenous appendicitis, thereby raising the question whether a failure rate of 20% within 1 year, with a quarter of those presenting worse than their initial presentation, is acceptable or not. Supporters of the nonoperative strategy emphasize that appendectomy may be avoided in a large proportion of these patients, thereby reducing operative rate and surgical risks, as well as overall costs.

Critics of the nonoperative strategy stress that a significant number of patients in these studies were treated without imaging confirmation of appendicitis, which may falsely increase the success rate of the nonsurgical cohorts. In 2015, Salminen et al. conducted a randomized, multicenter clinical trial including 530 adult patients who had uncomplicated acute appendicitis confirmed by CT scan. Patients were randomized to early open appendectomy or antibiotics (3 days IV ertapenem followed by 7 days oral levofloxacin and metronidazole) with 1-year follow-up. In the nonoperative group, 27% of patients required appendectomy within 1 year of presentation, which led to the conclusion that "among patients with CT-proven, uncomplicated appendicitis, antibiotic treatment did NOT meet the pre-specified criterion for noninferiority compared with appendectomy" [23]. Despite failing to demonstrate that antibiotics alone were not inferior to appendectomy, this study was accompanied by an editorial stating that "the time has come to consider abandoning routine appendectomy for patients with uncomplicated appendicitis" as diagnostic capabilities become more precise and broad-spectrum antibiotics more effective [24]. That same year, an article in the New England Journal of Medicine recommended that "…pending more information regarding the effectiveness of an antibiotics-first approach and the longer-term outcomes of this strategy, patients interested in considering an antibiotics first approach should be encouraged to participate in clinical trials" [25]. Although most agree that more research is required to fully support the use of antibiotics alone as the primary treatment modality for uncomplicated appendicitis, the evidence so far strongly suggests that albeit associated with significant failure rates, this strategy is a safe alternative to appendectomy. Therefore, the ideal patient-centered treatment plan for those presenting with this condition should include a detailed discussion about the current treatment options aiming at a well-informed shared decision.

Nonoperative Management for Complicated Appendicitis

Patients presenting with a right lower quadrant phlegmon or abscess are better treated with nonoperative management, as immediate surgical treatment is associated with a threefold increase in morbidity, including unnecessary ileocecal resection or right hemicolectomy [26]. Nonoperative treatment in this setting has a success rate of 93%; however percutaneous drainage (Fig. 21.5) is necessary in 20%. The risk of recurrence was less than 10% and often associated with the presence of an appendicolith.

Operative Management

After the first laparoscopic appendectomy was described by Semm [27], the use of this technique increases and has now become the most frequently performed appendectomy technique (Fig. 21.6) [28–31]. Theoretical advantages to laparoscopy are congruent with any laparoscopic or minimally invasive procedure: Less pain, shorter recovery time, faster return to work, decreased inflammatory response, decreased formation of adhesions, and better cosmetic results. Differently to what has been demonstrated in other surgical procedures, the benefits for the laparoscopic appendectomy compared to the open approach have been difficult to prove. Multiple trials have been performed to evaluate the role of laparoscopy for patients undergoing appendectomy, with most of them demonstrating benefits that were marginal or of questionable clinical relevance [31–41]. A Cochrane review of laparoscopic versus open surgery concluded with a recommendation in favor of the laparoscopic approach but with the caveat that the benefits of laparoscopy compared to open are small and of questionable clinical significance [42]. According to this pooled data review, laparoscopic appendectomy, which is currently the most common technique being used, was found to be associated with less postoperative pain, shorter hospital stay, and faster return to work; however significant heterogeneity among the studies included in that review weakens the significance of its findings. Regarding to surgical site infection, open appendectomy has been repeatedly demonstrated to be associated with higher rates of wound infection, while laparoscopic appendectomy is associated with increased rates of intra-abdominal abscess [31, 36, 43]. Overall, open and laparoscopic appendectomies provide clinically similar results.

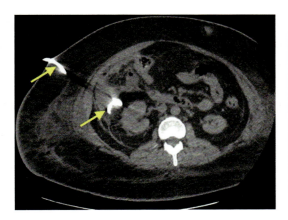

Fig. 21.5 CT scan axial images demonstrating perforated appendicitis with abscess treated with percutaneous CT-guided drainage (pigtail drain highlighted with arrows)

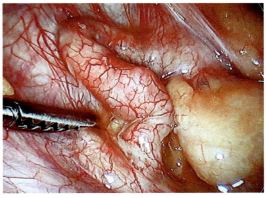

Fig. 21.6 Laparoscopic view of an inflamed appendix, demonstrating a dilated organ with serosal vascular congestion and the presence of periappendicular fluid

Appendectomy Timing

Immediate appendectomy to prevent perforation has been challenged by recent studies supporting a semielective approach to acute appendicitis [30, 44–47]. However, increased morbidity associated with appendectomy delay has been reported [48–50]. Because of this potential morbidity risk associated with surgical delay, prompt surgical intervention remains the safest approach for patients with the diagnosis of acute appendicitis. In our own review of over 4000 patients undergoing appendectomy for acute appendicitis at an urban academic tertiary center, 64% of patients underwent appendectomy more than 6 h after admission (overall average time 11 h and 50 min). After adjusting for age, gender, leukocytosis, perforation, and laparoscopy, a delay greater than 6 h from surgical admission to appendectomy was independently associated with increased rates of surgical site infection. For the subgroup of patients without perforation, patients who underwent appendectomy within 6 h had a 42% relative risk reduction in surgical site infection rates. Those who developed an infection remained an additional 5 days in the hospital and the incurred costs associated with it [51].

Duration of Postoperative Antibiotic Treatment

For those undergoing operative treatment of appendicitis, and without evidence of perforation, abscess, or local peritonitis, only prophylactic administration of narrow-spectrum antibiotics should be given, and these should then be discontinued within 24 h (Class I-A evidence) [52]. For patients with perforated appendicitis, fixed short courses of postoperative antibiotic treatment have been demonstrated to be safe and effective, with evidence to suggest that a 3-day course is equally effective to a 5-day course [53, 54].

Appendicitis During Pregnancy

Appendicitis is the most common non-obstetrical condition requiring emergent surgery during pregnancy [55]. Half of these cases occur during the second trimester [56]. Appendicitis in pregnancy is associated with low birth weight, preterm birth, babies who are small for gestational age, low APGAR scores, and preeclampsia/eclampsia [56–58]. Increased fetal mortality from 7–10% to 24% has been reported in association with ruptured appendicitis [59, 60].

Diagnostic challenges in pregnancy are secondary to limiting exposure of the patient and fetus to ionizing radiation with imaging, as well as the anatomic and physiologic changes of pregnancy. Gestational symptoms can often mimic those of acute appendicitis, specifically nausea/vomiting, and lower abdominal pain. Immunologically, pregnant patients will often not develop a fever. Physiologically, tachycardia is not uncommon, and the leukocytosis frequently seen in pregnant patients can be difficult to discern from a new infectious process.

These diagnostic challenges and fear of perforation (and subsequent increased fetal mortality) often lead to increased negative explorations, with some studies showing 25–50% rate of negative appendectomies in pregnant women [58, 61, 62]. The risk of these negative appendectomies is that a negative surgical exploration is not inconsequential and comes with its own overall fetal loss of 4% after negative exploration. Most importantly, among pregnant women who sustained fetal loss or early delivery after undergoing appendectomy, almost 1 in 3 had a negative appendectomy [63]. This boasts the need for accurate diagnosis often supported by appropriate imaging modalities in pregnancy.

Optimal ultrasound has sensitivity of 100%, specificity of 96%, and accuracy of 98%. Unfortunately, an enlarged uterus can limit graded compression used during ultrasound; additionally, while CT carries 99% negative predictive value, its potential detrimental effects of radiation limit its ideal use in pregnant patients [64]. In a survey study, radiologists from 183 departments in the

United States chose to use CT over MRI when presented with a scenario of a pregnant patient with appendicitis during the second and third trimester. The same radiologist however switched to MRI instead of CT scan if the patients were in their first trimester [65]. According to a statement by the American College of Radiology, MRI is acceptable for patients in any stage of pregnancy after a risk/benefit assessment is performed [66].

Regarding the choice of surgical technique for appendectomy, the use of laparoscopy should have special considerations during pregnancy. In addition to the anatomic changes of the gravid uterus and the challenges it could invoke on a laparoscopic approach, fetal physiologic effects should be considered as well. Fetal acidemia occurs during pneumoperitoneum with CO_2 in animal models [67]. A systematic review and meta-analysis of laparoscopic versus open approach in pregnancy summarized the available studies investigating this issue [68]. While ten of the studies showed a similar relative risk in either approach, a study by McGory et al. [63] favored the open approach, ultimately skewing the overall relative risk toward favoring an open approach.

With the increasing literature demonstrating the safety of nonoperative treatment of appendicitis with antibiotics and considering the risks of fetal loss and preterm delivery associated with surgical exploration, it is natural to cogitate the nonoperative treatment modality for patients who present with appendicitis while pregnant. The application of a nonoperative approach for this patient population however must be considered with much caution as pregnant patients have not been included in studies investigating safety and efficacy of nonoperative strategy.

Incidental Appendectomy

Performance of an incidental appendectomy during elective or emergency abdominal surgery would only make sense if no significant morbidity increase could be attributable to the incidental appendectomy. When appropriate risk adjustment statistical techniques were used to investigate this issue, the added risk of the incidental appendectomy became apparent [69]. This added risk probably outweighs the benefit of avoiding a future operation for appendicitis. From a cost analysis perspective, incidental appendectomy as a preventive measure has not been found to be effective either [70, 71]. The potential increase in morbidity and cost inefficacy suggest that routine incidental appendectomy should not be performed.

Interval Appendectomy

The risk of recurrent appendicitis in patients successfully treated nonoperatively ranges from 8% to 21% [72, 73]. Interval appendectomy is not an innocuous procedure, with complication rates ranging from 3% to 18% [73–78]. The case against interval appendectomy has been presented [13], and consideration to appendectomy after successful nonoperative treatment of acute appendicitis should be reserved for those cases that recur.

However, the concern for a malignancy in the adult population treated nonoperatively for an episode of acute appendicitis cannot be ignored [75]. Approximately 2% of patients older than 40 years old treated nonoperatively for an appendiceal mass or abscess will have a diagnosis other than appendicitis, including Crohn's disease or a malignancy. They should therefore undergo a colonoscopy during follow-up to rule out other causes for the appendiceal mass or abscess [26].

In summary, interval appendectomy is not always indicated because of considerable risks of complications and lack of clinical benefit.

Summary

- Liberal imaging is warranted in the diagnostic evaluation of appendicitis. Negative or inconclusive ultrasound findings cannot rule out appendicitis and should be followed by CT scan or MRI.
- Nonoperative treatment with antibiotics is a safe initial treatment for uncomplicated

appendicitis and associated with significant decrease in complications but a high failure rate.

- Routine incidental appendectomy is not warranted due to increased risk of complications.
- Interval appendectomy is not warranted because of significant complication risks and no demonstrated clinical benefit.
- Open and laparoscopic appendectomies provide clinically similar results overall.
- Antibiotic duration after appendectomy for non-perforated cases are considered prophylactic (<24 h) and for perforated cases are equally effective at a 3-day regimen versus 5 days.
- Increased morbidity of surgical site infections associated with appendectomy delay suggests that prompt surgical intervention remains the safest approach.
- Optimal management during pregnancy requires essential diagnostic accuracy preoperatively, as negative appendectomy is associated with significant incidence of fetal loss. MRI is a reasonable alternative to CT scan in this population.

References

1. Fitz RH. Perforating inflammation of the vermiform appendix. Am J Med Sci 1886;92:321–346.
2. McBurney C. II. The indications for early laparotomy in appendicitis. Ann Surg 1891;13(4):233–254.
3. McBurney C. IV. The incision made in the Abdominal Wall in cases of appendicitis, with a description of a new method of operating. Ann Surg 1894;20(1):38–43.
4. Cantrell JR, Stafford ES. The diminishing mortality from appendicitis. Ann Surg 1955;141(6):749–758.
5. Addiss DG, Shaffer N, Fowler BS, Tauxe RV. The epidemiology of appendicitis and appendectomy in the United States. Am J Epidemiol 1990;132(5):910–925.
6. Alvarado A. A practical score for the early diagnosis of acute appendicitis. Ann Emerg Med 1986;15(5):557–564.
7. Ohle R, O'Reilly F, O'Brien KK, Fahey T, Dimitrov BD. The Alvarado score for predicting acute appendicitis: a systematic review. BMC Med 2011;9:139.
8. Sun JS, Noh HW, Min YG, Lee JH, Kim JK, Park KJ, et al. Receiver operating characteristic analysis of the diagnostic performance of a computed tomographic examination and the Alvarado score

for diagnosing acute appendicitis: emphasis on age and sex of the patients. J Comput Assist Tomogr 2008;32(3):386–391.
9. SCOAP Collaborative, Cuschieri J, Florence M, Flum DR, Jurkovich GJ, Lin P, et al. Negative appendectomy and imaging accuracy in the Washington state surgical care and outcomes assessment program. Ann Surg 2008;248(4):557–563.
10. Poortman P, Oostvogel HJM, Bosma E, Lohle PNM, Cuesta MA, de Lange-de Klerk ESM, et al. Improving diagnosis of acute appendicitis: results of a diagnostic pathway with standard use of ultrasonography followed by selective use of CT. J Am Coll Surg 2009;208(3):434–441.
11. Cobben L, Groot I, Kingma L, Coerkamp E, Puylaert J, Blickman J. A simple MRI protocol in patients with clinically suspected appendicitis: results in 138 patients and effect on outcome of appendectomy. Eur Radiol 2009;19(5):1175–1183.
12. Singh A, Danrad R, Hahn PF, Blake MA, Mueller PR, Novelline RA. MR imaging of the acute abdomen and pelvis: acute appendicitis and beyond. Radiographics 2007;27(5):1419–1431.
13. Tekin A, Kurtoğlu HC, Can I, Öztan S. Routine interval appendectomy is unnecessary after conservative treatment of appendiceal mass. Color Dis 2008;10(5):465–8.
14. Rosen MP, Ding A, Blake MA, Baker ME, Cash BD, Fidler JL, et al. ACR appropriateness criteria® right lower quadrant pain—suspected appendicitis. J Am Coll Radiol 2011;8(11):749–755.
15. Varadhan KK, Neal KR, Lobo DN. Safety and efficacy of antibiotics compared with appendicectomy for treatment of uncomplicated acute appendicitis: meta-analysis of randomised controlled trials. BMJ 2012;344:e2156.
16. Vons C, Barry C, Maitre S, Pautrat K, Leconte M, Costaglioli B, et al. Amoxicillin plus clavulanic acid versus appendicectomy for treatment of acute uncomplicated appendicitis: an open-label, non-inferiority, randomised controlled trial. Lancet 2011;377(9777):1573–1579.
17. Styrud J, Eriksson S, Nilsson I, Ahlberg G, Haapaniemi S, Neovius G, et al. Appendectomy versus antibiotic treatment in acute appendicitis. A prospective multicenter randomized controlled trial. World J Surg 2006;30(6):1033–1037.
18. Hansson J, Körner U, Ludwigs K, Johnsson E, Jönsson C, Lundholm K. Antibiotics as first-line therapy for acute appendicitis: evidence for a change in clinical practice. World J Surg 2012;36(9):2037–2038.
19. Eriksson S, Granström L. Randomized controlled trial of appendicectomy versus antibiotic therapy for acute appendicitis. Br J Surg 1995;82(2):166–169.
20. Farahnak M, Talaei-Khoei M, Gorouhi F, Jalali A, Gorouhi F. The Alvarado score and antibiotics therapy as a corporate protocol versus conventional clinical management: randomized controlled pilot study of approach to acute appendicitis. Am J Emerg Med 2007;25(7):3–3.

21. Mason RJ, Moazzez A, Sohn H, Katkhouda N. Meta-analysis of randomized trials comparing antibiotic therapy with appendectomy for acute uncomplicated (no abscess or phlegmon) appendicitis. Surg Infect 2012;13(2):74–84.

22. Di Saverio S, Sibilio A, Giorgini E, Biscardi A, Villani S, Coccolini F, et al. The NOTA study (non operative treatment for acute appendicitis): prospective study on the efficacy and safety of antibiotics (amoxicillin and clavulanic acid) for treating patients with right lower quadrant abdominal pain and long-term follow-up of conservatively treated suspected appendicitis. Ann Surg 2014;260(1):109–117.

23. Salminen P, Paajanen H, Rautio T, Nordström P, Aarnio M, Rantanen T, et al. Antibiotic therapy vs appendectomy for treatment of uncomplicated acute appendicitis: the APPAC randomized clinical trial. JAMA 2015;313(23):2340–2348.

24. Livingston E, Vons C. Treating appendicitis without surgery. JAMA 2015;313(23):2327–2328.

25. Flum DR. Clinical practice. Acute appendicitis--appendectomy or the "antibiotics first" strategy. N Engl J Med 2015;372(20):1937–1943.

26. Andersson RE, Petzold MG. Nonsurgical treatment of appendiceal abscess or phlegmon: a systematic review and meta-analysis. Ann Surg 2007;246(5):741–748.

27. Semm K. Endoscopic appendectomy. Endoscopy 1983;15(2):59–64.

28. Anderson JE, Bickler SW, Chang DC, Talamini MA. Examining a common disease with unknown etiology: trends in epidemiology and surgical Management of Appendicitis in California, 1995-2009. World J Surg 2012, 36, 2787.

29. Bulian DR, Knuth J, Sauerwald A, Ströhlein MA, Lefering R, Ansorg J, et al. Appendectomy in Germany-an analysis of a nationwide survey 2011/2012. Int J Color Dis 2012;28(1):127–138.

30. Ingraham AM, Cohen ME, Bilimoria KY, Ko CY, Hall BL, Russell TR, et al. Effect of delay to operation on outcomes in adults with acute appendicitis. Arch Surg 2010;145(9):886–892.

31. Ingraham AM, Cohen ME, Bilimoria KY, Pritts TA, Ko CY, Esposito TJ. Comparison of outcomes after laparoscopic versus open appendectomy for acute appendicitis at 222 ACS NSQIP hospitals. Surgery 2010;148(4):625–35–discussion635–7..

32. Kim MJ, Fleming FJ, Gunzler DD, Messing S, Salloum RM, Monson JRT. Laparoscopic appendectomy is safe and efficacious for the elderly: an analysis using the National Surgical Quality Improvement Project database. Surg Endosc 2011;25(6):1802–1807.

33. Page AJ, Pollock JD, Perez S, Davis SS, Lin E, Sweeney JF. Laparoscopic versus open appendectomy: an analysis of outcomes in 17,199 patients using ACS/NSQIP. J Gastrointest Surg 2010;14(12):1955–1962.

34. Martin LC, Puente I, Sosa JL, Bassin A, Breslaw R, McKenney MG, et al. Open versus laparoscopic appendectomy. A prospective randomized comparison. Ann Surg 1995;222(3):256–61–discussion261–2..

35. Tan-Tam C, Yorke E, Wasdell M, Barcan C, Konkin D, Blair P. The benefits of laparoscopic appendectomies in obese patients. Am J Surg 2012;203(5):609–612.

36. Tuggle KR-M, Ortega G, Bolorunduro OB, Oyetunji TA, Alexander R, Turner PL, et al. Laparoscopic versus open appendectomy in complicated appendicitis: a review of the NSQIP database. J Surg Res 2010;163(2):225–228.

37. Katkhouda N, Mason RJ, Towfigh S, Gevorgyan A, Essani R. Laparoscopic versus open appendectomy: a prospective randomized double-blind study. Ann Surg 2005;242(3):439.

38. Mason RJ, Moazzez A, Moroney JR, Katkhouda N. Laparoscopic vs open appendectomy in obese patients: outcomes using the American College of Surgeons National Surgical Quality Improvement Program database. J Am Coll Surg 2012;215(1):88–99–discussion99–100..

39. Tzovaras G, Baloyiannis I, Kouritas V, Symeonidis D, Spyridakis M, Poultsidi A, et al. Laparoscopic versus open appendectomy in men: a prospective randomized trial. Surg Endosc 2010;24(12):2987–2992.

40. Li X, Zhang J, Sang L, Zhang W, Chu Z, Li X, et al. Laparoscopic versus conventional appendectomy--a meta-analysis of randomized controlled trials. BMC Gastroenterol 2010;10:129.

41. Guller U, Hervey S, Purves H, Muhlbaier LH, Peterson ED, Eubanks S, et al. Laparoscopic versus open appendectomy: outcomes comparison based on a large administrative database. Ann Surg 2004;239(1):43–52.

42. Sauerland S, Jaschinski T, Neugebauer EA. Laparoscopic versus open surgery for suspected appendicitis. Cochrane Database Syst Rev 2010;(10):CD001546.

43. Fleming FJ, Kim MJ, Messing S, Gunzler D, Salloum R, Monson JR. Balancing the risk of postoperative surgical infections: a multivariate analysis of factors associated with laparoscopic appendectomy from the NSQIP database. Ann Surg 2010;252(6):895–900.

44. Yardeni D, Hirschl RB, Drongowski RA, Teitelbaum DH, Geiger JD, Coran AG. Delayed versus immediate surgery in acute appendicitis: do we need to operate during the night? J Pediatr Surg 2004;39(3):464–469.

45. Abou-Nukta FF, Bakhos CC, Arroyo KK, Koo YY, Martin JJ, Reinhold RR, et al. Effects of delaying appendectomy for acute appendicitis for 12 to 24 hours. Arch Surg 2006;141(5):504–507.

46. Kearney D, Cahill RA, O'Brien E, Kirwan WO, Redmond HP. Influence of delays on perforation risk in adults with acute appendicitis. Dis Colon Rectum 2008;51(12):1823–1827.

47. Stahlfeld K, Hower J, Homitsky S, Madden J. Is acute appendicitis a surgical emergency? Am Surg 2007 73(6):626–9–discussion629–30..

48. Busch M, Gutzwiller FS, Aellig S, Kuettel R, Metzger U, Zingg U. In-hospital delay increases the risk of perforation in adults with appendicitis. World J Surg 2011;35(7):1626–1633.

49. Ditillo MFM, Dziura JDJ, Rabinovici RR. Is it safe to delay appendectomy in adults with acute appendicitis? Ann Surg 2006;244(5):656–660.

50. Omundsen M, Dennett E. Delay to appendicectomy and associated morbidity: a retrospective review. ANZ J Surg 2006;76(3):153–155.

51. Teixeira PGR, Sivrikoz E, Inaba K, Talving P, Lam L, Demetriades D. Appendectomy timing: waiting until the next morning increases the risk of surgical site infections. Ann Surg 2012;256(3):538–543.

52. Solomkin JS, Mazuski JE, Bradley JS, Rodvold KA, Goldstein EJC, Baron EJ, et al. Diagnosis and management of complicated intra-abdominal infection in adults and children: guidelines by the surgical infection society and the Infectious Diseases Society of America. Surg Infect 2010;11(1):79–109.

53. van Rossem CC, Schreinemacher MHF, Treskes K, van Hogezand RM, van Geloven AAW. Duration of antibiotic treatment after appendicectomy for acute complicated appendicitis. Br J Surg 2014;101(6):715–719.

54. van Rossem CC, Schreinemacher MHF, van Geloven AAW, Bemelman WA, Snapshot appendicitis collaborative study group. Antibiotic duration after laparoscopic appendectomy for acute complicated appendicitis. JAMA Surg 2016;151(4):323–329.

55. Tamir IL, Bongard FS, Klein SR. Acute appendicitis in the pregnant patient. Am J Surg 1990;160(6):571–5–discussion575–6..

56. Mazze RI, Källén B. Appendectomy during pregnancy: a Swedish registry study of 778 cases. Obstet Gynecol 1991;77(6):835–840.

57. Wei P-L, Keller JJ, Liang H-H, Lin H-C. Acute appendicitis and adverse pregnancy outcomes: a nationwide population-based study. J Gastrointest Surg 2012;16(6):1204–1211.

58. Andersen B, Nielsen TF. Appendicitis in pregnancy: diagnosis, management and complications. Acta Obstet Gynecol Scand 1999;78(9):758–762.

59. Yilmaz HG, Akgun Y, Bac B, Celik Y. Acute appendicitis in pregnancy--risk factors associated with principal outcomes: a case control study. Int J Surg 2007;5(3):192–7.

60. Ueberrueck T, Koch A, Meyer L, Hinkel M, Gastinger I. Ninety-four appendectomies for suspected acute appendicitis during pregnancy. World J Surg 2004;28(5):508–511.

61. Hale DA, Molloy M, Pearl RH, Schutt DC, Jaques DP. Appendectomy: a contemporary appraisal. Ann Surg 1997;225(3):252–261.

62. Hée P, Viktrup L. The diagnosis of appendicitis during pregnancy and maternal and fetal outcome after appendectomy. Int J Gynaecol Obstet 1999;65(2):129–135.

63. McGory ML, Zingmond DS, Tillou A, Hiatt JR, Ko CY, Cryer HM. Negative appendectomy in pregnant women is associated with a substantial risk of fetal loss. J Am Coll Surg 2007;205(4):534–540.

64. Lim HK, Bae SH, Seo GS. Diagnosis of acute appendicitis in pregnant women: value of sonography. AJR Am J Roentgenol 1992;159(3):539–542.

65. Jaffe TA, Miller CM, Merkle EM. Practice patterns in imaging of the pregnant patient with abdominal pain: a survey of academic centers. AJR Am J Roentgenol 2007;189(5):1128–1134.

66. Kanal EE, Borgstede JPJ, Barkovich AJA, Bell CC, Bradley WGW, Felmlee JPJ, et al. 2002 American College of Radiology White Paper on MR safety. AJR. 178, 1335–1347.

67. Hunter JG, Swanstrom L, Thornburg K. Carbon dioxide pneumoperitoneum induces fetal acidosis in a pregnant ewe model. Surg Endosc 1995;9(3):272–7–discussion277–9..

68. Wilasrusmee C, Sukrat B, McEvoy M, Attia J, Thakkinstian A. Systematic review and meta-analysis of safety of laparoscopic versus open appendicectomy for suspected appendicitis in pregnancy. Br J Surg 2012;99(11):1470–1478.

69. Wen SW, Hernandez R, Naylor CD. Pitfalls in non-randomized outcomes studies. The case of incidental appendectomy with open cholecystectomy. JAMA 1995;274(21):1687–1691.

70. Sugimoto T, Edwards D. Incidence and costs of incidental appendectomy as a preventive measure. Am J Public Health 1987;77(4):471–475.

71. Wang HT, Sax HC. Incidental appendectomy in the era of managed care and laparoscopy. J Am Coll Surg 2001;192(2):182–188.

72. Puapong D, Lee SL, Haigh PI, Kaminski A, Liu I-LA, Applebaum H. Routine interval appendectomy in children is not indicated. J Pediatr Surg 2007;42(9):1500–1503.

73. Hall NJ, Jones CE, Eaton S, Stanton MP, Burge DM. Is interval appendicectomy justified after successful nonoperative treatment of an appendix mass in children? A systematic review. J Pediatr Surg 2011;46(4):767–771.

74. Oliak D, Yamini D, Udani VM, Lewis RJ, Arnell T, Vargas H, et al. Initial nonoperative management for periappendiceal abscess. Dis Colon Rectum 2001;44(7):936–941.

75. Willemsen PJ, Hoorntje LE, Eddes E-H, Ploeg RJ. The need for interval appendectomy after resolution of an Appendiceal mass questioned. Dig Surg 2002;19(3):216–222.

76. Lugo JZ, Avgerinos DV, Lefkowitz AJ, Seigerman ME, Zahir IS, Lo AY, et al. Can interval appendectomy be justified following conservative treatment of perforated acute appendicitis? J Surg Res 2010;164(1):91–94.

77. Eriksson S, Styrud J. Interval appendicectomy: a retrospective study. Eur J Surg 2003;164(10):771–774.

78. Iqbal CW, Knott EM, Mortellaro VE, Fitzgerald KM, Sharp SW, St Peter SD. Interval appendectomy after perforated appendicitis: what are the operative risks and luminal patency rates? J Surg Res 2012;177(1):127–130.

Diverticulitis

22

Anuradha R. Bhama, Anna Yegiants,
and Scott R. Steele

Introduction

The prevalence of diverticulosis in the United
States has increased in recent years, affecting
approximately 70% of people over the age of 80,
with the incidence increasing with age [1–3]. In
Western countries, diverticular disease usually
involves the left colon, with as many as 99% of
patients having some amount of disease in the
sigmoid colon [1]. Approximately 20% of
patients with diverticulosis will develop diverticulitis in their lifetime [1, 4]. Diverticulitis results
in over 300,000 hospitalizations, 1.5 million days
of inpatient hospital care, and costs $2.4 billion
per year [2–5].

A majority of colonic diverticula are located
in the sigmoid colon. Diverticulosis is thought to
develop from a combination of increased intraluminal colonic pressure in the sigmoid colon and
age-related erosion of the mucosal wall. This

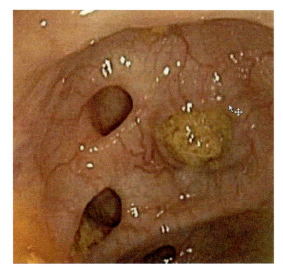

Fig. 22.1 Appearance of diverticulosis on endoscopy

results in points of weakness at the insertion of
the vasa recta, resulting in outpouchings of the
colonic wall (Fig. 22.1) [6]. The diverticula in are
not true diverticula, which are full thickness; they
are only comprised of mucosa, submucosa, and
serosa and are, therefore, false diverticula.
Diverticulitis is thought to be caused obstruction
by fecaliths or small food particles causing localized trauma, inflammation, and microperforation.
Diverticulitis can present along a spectrum of
severity, from mild inflammation to microperforation, to free perforation. A perforation can be
walled off by omentum, mesentery, pericolonic

A. R. Bhama
Department of Colorectal Surgery, Cleveland Clinic
Foundation, Cleveland, OH, USA

A. Yegiants
Case Western Reserve University School of
Medicine, Cleveland, OH, USA

S. R. Steele (✉)
Department of Colorectal Surgery, Cleveland Clinic,
Cleveland, OH, USA
e-mail: steeles3@ccf.org

fat, or adjacent organs such as the bladder, which may lead to development of an abscess or fistulizing disease. In severe cases, patients can present with life-threatening free perforation and peritonitis. For patients presenting with an episode of acute diverticulitis, identifying disease severity and subsequent treatment strategy is the first step.

Initial Presentation and Work-Up

A majority of patients evaluated in the emergency room with diverticulitis present with a chief complaint of abdominal pain. When evaluating a patient with diverticulitis, it is imperative to first identify hemodynamic stability. Even in the setting of tachycardia, most patients are relatively stable, and outside of free perforation and sepsis, often allowing time for evaluation. Delineating between a stable patient and an unstable patient will identify the patients that potentially require emergent operative intervention. This classification of stable versus unstable can be made swiftly by assessing the patient's vital signs and physical exam. Once this delineation is made, the work-up can continue in an algorithmic fashion (Fig. 22.2).

In the stable patient, the work-up should begin with a thorough history and physical examination. History should focus on a detailed description of

abdominal pain and any associated symptoms. Based on typical presentation, often patients have already been seen by the referring physician, and the consult comes complete with labs, a CT scan demonstrating the classical appearance, and a "diagnosis." However, this is not always the cases; and even when presented like this, it is imperative as the surgeon to work through the finer points. Typically, the abdominal pain is focused in the left lower quadrant, but given the potential redundancy of the sigmoid colon, pain may also be experienced in the midportion of the lower abdomen and right lower quadrant. Patients often will complain of nausea, decreased appetite, and even vomiting. Typically during early stages of the disease process, obstructing symptoms are uncommon, and most patients continue to pass flatus and may continue to have bowel movements. Blood in the stool is typically not associated with diverticulitis and should prompt consideration of alternative diagnoses such as malignancy or ischemic colitis. It is important to elicit any signs and symptoms of complicated disease, such as pneumaturia or fecaluria, which are signs of fistulizing disease to the bladder (Fig. 22.3). Similarly, the passage of flatus per vagina is also concerning of fistulizing disease to the uterus or vagina. A full medical and surgical history should be taken, as well as a review of all medications and allergies.

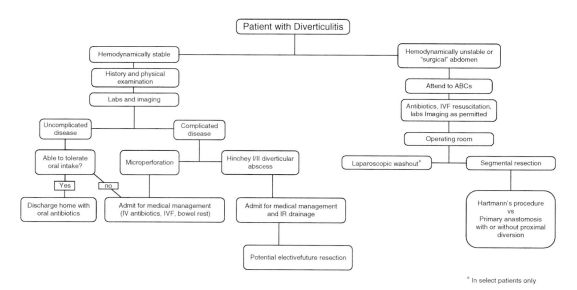

Fig. 22.2 Algorithm for the treatment of acute sigmoid diverticulitis

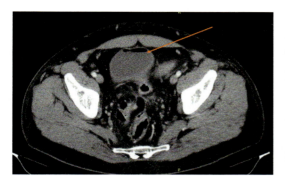

Fig. 22.3 Appearance of colovesical fistula on CT scan. Arrow demonstrates air in the bladder from the colovesical fistula

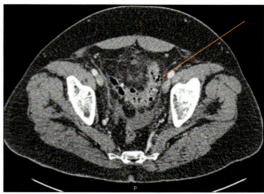

Fig. 22.4 Appearance of diverticulitis on CT scan

It is important to note the number and frequency of any prior episodes of diverticulitis and how they were treated. These factors may not influence immediate management, but will help counsel the patient regarding future elective surgery. All patients should be asked about their most recent colonoscopy and if there is any personal history of colon polyps or cancer. If there is a history of malignancy, noting the surgical and adjuvant treatments and surveillance will help distinguish between diagnoses of primary diverticulitis versus a recurrent colon cancer. Family history of colon cancer should also be noted. Malignancy of the sigmoid colon can share symptoms of diverticulitis; therefore it is imperative to evaluate patients accordingly. Similarly, several other pathologies besides cancer may lead to symptoms similar to diverticulitis, such as irritable bowel syndrome, inflammatory bowel disease, gynecologic pathologies, appendicitis, or ischemic colitis. A thorough history and physical examination should help delineate between these diagnoses.

A physical examination should take note of fevers and any variations in vital signs. The abdomen should be examined with attention paid to any peritoneal signs. Patients with mild disease typically experience pain in the left lower quadrant with deep palpation. Typically, rebound tenderness is not present, though voluntary guarding is common. In more severe disease, focal peritonitis may be present, but may not necessarily warrant urgent surgical exploration. Distension of the abdomen may be a sign of development of possible obstruction. A rectal examination should

be performed to evaluate for any anorectal pathologies as well as assess for sphincter tone. Any worrisome comorbid conditions should be identified that may require attention and possible intervention. Any patient who presents with uncomplicated diverticular disease may develop a smoldering clinical course and require operative intervention; management of comorbid conditions should be handled in a fashion that prepares the patient for surgery if needed. For example, medications such as clopidogrel and warfarin should be held and replaced with easily reversible medication substitutions, such as heparin, if indicated. Blood work should include a complete blood count, comprehensive metabolic panel, urinalysis, and coagulation parameters in patients on anticoagulants. In stable patients, CT scan of the abdomen and pelvis with oral and intravenous contrast should be obtained as the initial imaging study [7–9]. CT will typically demonstrate thickening of the sigmoid colon wall with associated fat stranding (Fig. 22.4) but may also demonstrate other findings that may influence decision-making (see below).

Uncomplicated Diverticulitis

The treatment plan of patients with diverticulitis depends upon the clinical severity of the disease. Select patients with mild diverticulitis, who are tolerating oral intake, may be discharged home from the emergency department with oral antibiotics [10]. In order to safely treat diverticulitis on an outpatient basis, it is imperative that the patients are able to maintain hydration and nutrition. Ciprofloxacin (500 mg twice daily) and metronidazole (250 mg three times daily) or amoxicillin/clavulanic acid (500/250 mg twice daily) are typical outpatient antibiotic regimens for diverticulitis. Patients should be cautioned regarding signs and symptoms that warrant reevaluation by a physician, such as worsening abdominal pain, worsening fevers, inability to tolerate medications, or inability to tolerate an oral diet. A recent review demonstrated that 12.5% of patients discharged from the emergency room will return or be readmitted within 30 days, but only 1% will require emergency surgery [11]. Women and patients with free fluid are at risk for failure of outpatient therapy [12]. Any patient with diverticulitis who is unable to tolerate oral intake should be admitted to the hospital for hydration, bowel rest, and pain control [13]. Antibiotics are also given intravenously, though there is limited data in their efficacy. A recent randomized control trial comparing medical treatment with and without antibiotics of first episode of diverticulitis demonstrated no difference in mortality, ongoing/complicated/recurrent diverticulitis, sigmoid resection, readmission, or adverse events [14]. In fact, length of stay was significantly shorter in the observation group without antibiotics. Several other studies have suggested that antibiotics may be omitted in the treatment of uncomplicated diverticulitis, but further research is necessary to confidently conclude that antibiotic treatment may be abandoned [15, 16]. Until further studies elucidate the safety of omitting antibiotics, it remains standard practice to treat diverticulitis with antibiotics. Common regimens include ceftriaxone/metronidazole, ampicillin/sulbactam, piperacillin/tazobactam, and ciprofloxacin/metronidazole. Individual hospital antibiograms are helpful in guiding choice of antibiotics. Non-operative management of simple diverticulitis is successful in as many as 93% of patients [17]. These patients should be seen in follow-up to ensure resolution of their symptoms. If patients have had several episodes of diverticulitis, a discussion regarding possible outpatient surgery may be warranted.

Complicated Diverticulitis

Complicated diverticulitis includes any patient who is found to have a perforation, abscess, pneumoperitoneum, obstruction, or fistula. These patients should be admitted to the hospital for conservative management including bowel rest, IV fluid hydration, and IV antibiotics and possible abscess drainage. Microperforated diverticulitis is considered diverticulitis in which a small perforation has occurred, small amounts of gas escaped the lumen, and then sealed off. This results in pneumoperitoneum that is either pericolic or free air. There has been a recent evolution in considerations for patients with pneumoperitoneum. Traditionally, any signs of pneumoperitoneum warranted operative exploration. Frequently, these patients underwent emergent sigmoid resection with creation of an end colostomy. However, in patients who are hemodynamically stable without signs of systemic sepsis and/or a surgical abdomen, frequently a small amount of pneumoperitoneum may be observed and treated conservatively [18]. On CT scan, these patients may have a small amount of extraluminal air or a sliver of air just above the liver, though on exam these patients often do not have a "surgical" abdomen (Fig. 22.5). Without concern for active ongoing leakage of air through the perforation, these patients may be admitted for conservative treatment and closely observed. This includes bowel rest, IV hydration, IV antibiotics, and serial abdominal exams. These patients should be monitored closely; patients with deterioration should be considered for emergent surgery. A vast majority of these patients typically improve with this treatment plan and are able to be evaluated as an outpatient for elective resection.

Another common clinical scenario is that of a diverticular abscess seen on CT imaging (Fig. 22.6). The Hinchey classification is typically used to describe these abscesses, with type I being a pericolic abscess and type II being a pelvic abscess. These patients should be admitted to the hospital for IV hydration, IV antibiotics, pain control and bowel rest. Any coagulopathy should be corrected prior to invasive interven-

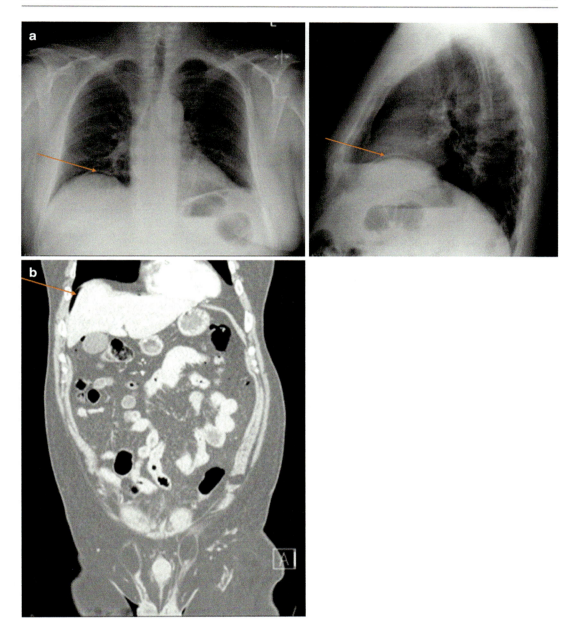

Fig. 22.5 Small sliver of free air above the liver – visible on chest X-ray and CT scan. (**a**) Arrows demonstrate sliver of free air under the diaphragm. (**b**) Arrows demonstrate sliver of free air under the diaphragm

tions. Abscesses occur in up to 20% of patients who present with diverticulitis, and these abscesses should be drained by interventional radiology if possible. No official size criteria for abscess drainage exist though several studies have examined the necessary abscess size for drainage. In general abscesses smaller than 3 cm typically resolve with intravenous antibiotics, fluid hydration, and bowel rest, while larger abscesses require interventional draiage [17, 19]. Abscesses larger than 5 cm typically fail treatment with antibiotics alone and eventually require drainage [20, 21]. Several studies have demonstrated that abscess drainage helps to avoid

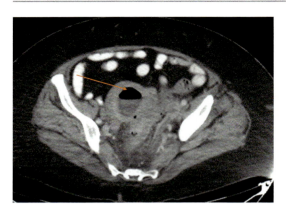

Fig. 22.6 Diverticular abscess on CT. Arrow demonstrates a pericolic diverticular abscess

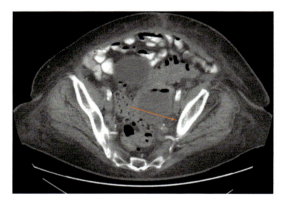

Fig. 22.7 Abscess due to diverticulitis not amenable to CT drainage. Arrow demonstrates an abscess that is not drainable by interventional radiology techniques. Note the abscess is obstructed by the bowel located anterior to the abscess, the bony pelvis lateral, and the blood vessels located posteriorly

urgent colectomy in these patients [19, 20, 22–24]. In patients with small abscesses without clinical improvement, the abscess may be aspirated, as the abscess cavity may be too small to accommodate the tip of a typical pigtail drainage catheter. There must be a clear path from the skin to the abscess, unobstructed by bowel, bone, vessels, etc. In some situations, an abscess may not be amenable to radiologic-guided drainage due to location (Fig. 22.7). In these scenarios, patients may be treated with antibiotics; if no improvement has occurred in several days, repeat CT scan may demonstrate progression of the abscess in size and location making it amenable to radiologic drainage. In situations where the abscess is

not amenable to drainage and the patient does not improve with antibiotic therapy, segmental colectomy is indicated. Patients with diverticular abscesses who are successfully treated without surgical intervention should later be evaluated in the outpatient setting and counselled regarding the potential need for elective surgical resection.

Patients presenting in with frank peritonitis or systemic sepsis must be managed in an expeditious fashion. Up to 25% of patients presenting with diverticulitis require urgent operation [13]. Airway protection and IV access should be assessed and secured immediately. Aggressive fluid resuscitation should begin immediately and IV antibiotics should be administered. Blood work should include complete blood count, comprehensive metabolic panel, lactate, coagulation parameters, urinalysis, and arterial blood gas as needed. Simultaneously, a focused history and physical examination should be performed. A plain X-ray may be obtained to evaluate for pneumoperitoneum. Aggressive resuscitation and administration of broad-spectrum IV antibiotics should occur in the emergency department during the initial evaluation. A CT scan may be obtained in patients who are not in extremis at the discretion of the surgeon. This may help localize the source of pneumoperitoneum to the upper or lower GI tract. It is not uncommon for a patient with pneumoperitoneum from an upper GI source to also have incidental diverticulosis; lack of inflammation of the sigmoid colon points toward an upper GI source. The transverse colon may be secondarily inflamed in the setting of upper GI perforation, but transverse colon diverticulitis and perforation are exceedingly rare [25, 26]. A CT scan that demonstrates inflammation of the sigmoid colon with a copious amount of pneumoperitoneum and free fluid should be classified as Hinchey III (purulent peritonitis) or Hinchey IV (feculent peritonitis). These patients should undergo immediate operative intervention. There are several surgical options available, including resection with colostomy (i.e., Hartmann's procedure), resection with primary anastomosis, resection with primary anastomosis and proximal diversion, laparoscopic peritoneal lavage and drainage, proximal drainage, and damage control surgery.

The gold standard operation for perforated diverticulitis is a Hartmann's procedure consisting of sigmoid resection with creation of an end colostomy. Ideally, the patient is marked preoperatively by an enterostomal therapist for ideal stoma placement. This operation is performed with the patient in modified lithotomy position. A generous lower midline incision is made and the abdomen is explored and the purulent contamination is irrigated. The sigmoid colon is mobilized off of the retroperitoneum by mobilizing along the white line of Toldt. The extent of the resection should include the entire sigmoid colon down to soft, pliable, healthy rectum distally. Proximally, the descending colon should be mobilized only to the extent to which an end colostomy can be brought to the skin level to create a colostomy; full mobilization of the splenic flexure is typically not necessary. Complete mobilization of the splenic flexure during this operation may increase the risk of colostomy prolapse. Additionally, during eventual colostomy reversal, keeping the splenic flexure tissue planes untouched will ease in mobilization of the colon during colostomy reversal. Care should be taken to avoid injury to the ureter, which may be secondarily inflamed. If necessary, a ureteral stent may be placed; though this will aid in identification of ureteral injury, placement of ureteral stents has never been shown to prevent ureteral injury. It is not necessary to perform a high ligation of the inferior mesenteric artery unless there is high suspicion for an underlying malignancy. Transection should occur at the top of the rectum, distal to where the tinea coalesce and where the rectum is soft and pliable. The rectal stump is managed by oversewing the staple line with polypropylene suture and leaving long tails in order to aid in identification of the rectal stump during future stoma reversal operations. The abdomen should be irrigated copiously, and the placement of drains (both transabdominal and transanal) is left to the discretion of the surgeon. A Foley catheter or mushroom drain may be used as a transanal drain. The abdominal wound should be copiously irrigated and may be closed with staples and intervening wicks.

Hartmann's procedure and reversal carry an aggregate morbidity of 20%, with a stoma complication rate of 10% and wound complication rate of 29% [27]. Colostomies remain permanent in over 30% of patients. Risk factors for nonreversal include age, ASA score, pulmonary comorbidities, preoperative blood transfusion, perforation, and anticoagulation [28]. Based upon patient hemodynamics and comfort level of the surgeon, Hartmann's procedure is always a safe option for perforated diverticulitis [29]. Recently, there has been increasing interest in alternatives to Hartmann's procedure. Depending on the stability of the patient and safety assessment by the surgeon, primary anastomosis with or without proximal diversion is an option. Several studies have compared the safety and cost of performing a primary anastomosis (PA) or primary anastomosis with proximal diversion (PAPD) with Hartmann's procedure (HP). PAPD has been reported to have a mortality of 9% and morbidity of 75%, with a stoma reversal rate of 90%, shorter hospital stay, and decreased costs [2, 4]. A large National Surgical Quality Improvement Program study comparing HP, PA, and PAPD demonstrated no significant difference in mortality or postoperative surgical site infections for these three procedures [30]. A recent randomized control trial comparing patients undergoing HP and PAPD demonstrated no difference in mortality or morbidity but did demonstrate that, at 18 months, 96% of PAPD patients and 65% of HP patients had a stoma reversal [31]. In certain situations, primary anastomosis may be performed without proximal diversion, with significantly improved outcomes compared to Hartmann's procedure [32]. The patient's condition should drive the decision whether or not to perform an anastomosis. Factors to consider include history of immunosuppression or malnutrition, higher ASA score, current hemodynamic status, and large volume blood loss. It is necessary that the descending colon proximally and the distal rectum are healthy and uninflamed with adequate blood supply. If there is question as to the quality of these tissues, an anastomosis should not be performed. It is to the surgeon's discretion as to which procedure to elect, and if the patient is unstable, it is wise to perform the procedure with which the surgeon is most comfortable and familiar with.

Recent attention has been drawn to another alternative to Hartmann's procedure – laparoscopic peritoneal lavage with drainage. This procedure purports benefits of decreased morbidity and mortality, avoidance of a stoma, and avoidance of anastomotic complications. First described in 1996 by O'Sullivan, this procedure typically involves laparoscopic evaluation of the abdomen to differentiate between purulent and feculent peritonitis [33]. A 12 mm trocar is placed at the umbilicus and two additional 5 mm trocars are placed. The abdomen is then irrigated with 3–9 L of warm saline solution. Adhesions to the sigmoid colon are not taken down as they may be sealing the initial perforation. Several large drains are left in the pelvis and near the sigmoid colon. These patients are maintained on antibiotics for 7–10 days. Several studies have evaluated laparoscopic lavage and have demonstrated mixed results regarding morbidity, mortality, and colostomy formation. The DILALA trial randomized patients with Hinchey grade III to laparoscopic lavage or Hartmann's procedure. Significant differences were identified between the two groups including increased operative time and increased postoperative length of stay for Hartmann's procedure [34]. A meta-analysis of recent studies demonstrated that laparoscopic lavage had an increased rate of reoperation and need for IR drainage compared to colon resection but had a decreased rate of stoma formation. There was no difference in mortality [35]. The Ladies trial was a multicenter parallel group, randomized trial comparing laparoscopic lavage to Hartmann's procedure in patients with feculent peritonitis. This trial was terminated early due to high rates of short-term morbidity and reinervention in the laparoscopic lavage group [36]. A recent multicenter trial from several European centers conducted the Ladies trial which consisted to two arms - one comparing laparoscopic lavage with sigmoidectomy, and the other comparing the Hartmannn's procedure with the resection and primary anastomosis with diverting ostomy. Unfortunately, the lavage portion of the trial had to be prematurely terminated secondary to higher morbidity and mortality in the lavage group after only 90 patients (odds ratio 1.28, 95% CI 0.54–3.03, p = 0.58), as lavage was determined not be be superior to sigmoid resection. Ongoing trials are underway to evaluate the long-term efficacy of this approach.

Given the limitations of the available current literature, this operative strategy should be adopted with extreme caution and an understanding that routine utilization of laparoscopic lavage is not yet standard of care.

Conclusion

Several elements should influence the decision for management of acute diverticulitis in the emergent setting. Severity of illness will determine if the patient may be treated as an outpatient or requires hospitalization, and CT imaging is the best imaging modality to help determine therapy. All patients who require admission to the hospital, regardless of severity, should be treated with antibiotics, bowel rest, hydration, and pain control. The patient's hemodynamic state and physical exam findings should drive the decision for emergent operation. In patients requiring an operation, there is controversy regarding the operation of choice. Hospital factors (availability of ICU, IR availability, etc.), surgeon comfort level, and patient comorbidities should influence the decision of which operation to perform.

References

1. Heise CP. Epidemiology and pathogenesis of diverticular disease. J Gastrointest Surg. 2008;12(8):1309–11. https://doi.org/10.1007/s11605-008-0492-0.
2. Shaheen NJ, Hansen RA, Morgan DR, et al. The burden of gastrointestinal and liver diseases, 2006. Am J Gastroenterol. 2006;101(9):2128–38. https://doi.org/10.1111/j.1572-0241.2006.00723.x.
3. Everhart JE, Ruhl CE. Burden of digestive diseases in the United States part III: liver, biliary tract, and pancreas. Gastroenterology. 2009;136(4):1134–44. https://doi.org/10.1053/j.gastro.2009.02.038.
4. D a E, Mack TM, Beart RW, Kaiser AM. Diverticulitis in the United States: 1998-2005: changing patterns of disease and treatment. Ann Surg. 2009;249(2):210–7. https://doi.org/10.1097/SLA.0b013e3181952888.
5. DeFrances CJ, Cullen K A, Kozak LJ. National hospital discharge survey: 2005 annual summary with detailed diagnosis and procedure data; 2007.
6. Strate LL, Modi R, Cohen E, Spiegel BMR. Diverticular disease as a chronic illness: evolving epidemiologic and clinical insights. Am J

Gastroenterol. 2012;107(10):1486–93. https://doi.org/10.1038/ajg.2012.194.

7. Baker ME. Imaging and interventional techniques in acute left-sided diverticulitis. J Gastrointest Surg. 2008;12(8):1314–7. https://doi.org/10.1007/s11605-008-0490-2.

8. Sarma D, Longo WE. Diagnostic imaging for diverticulitis. J Clin Gastroenterol. 2008;42(10):1139–41. https://doi.org/10.1097/MCG.0b013e3181886ed4.

9. Destigter KK, Keating DP. Imaging update: acute colonic diverticulitis. Clin Colon Rectal Surg. 2009;22(3):147–55. https://doi.org/10.1055/s-0029-1236158.

10. Biondo S, Golda T, Kreisler E, et al. Outpatient versus hospitalization Management for Uncomplicated Diverticulitis. Ann Surg. 2014;259(1):38–44. https://doi.org/10.1097/SLA.0b013e3182965a11.

11. Sirany AME, Gaertner WB, Madoff RD, Kwaan MR. Diverticulitis diagnosed in the emergency room: is it safe to discharge home? J Am Coll Surg. 2017;225:21.

12. Etzioni DA, Chiu VY, Cannom RR, Burchette RJ, Haigh PI, Abbas MA. Outpatient treatment of acute diverticulitis: rates and predictors of failure. Dis Colon Rectum. 2010;53(6):861–5. https://doi.org/10.1007/DCR.0b013e3181cdb243.

13. Beckham H, Whitlow CB. The medical and nonoperative treatment of diverticulitis. Clin Colon Rectal Surg. 2009;22(3):156–60. https://doi.org/10.1055/s-0029-1236159.

14. Daniels L, Ünlü Ç, de Korte N, et al. Randomized clinical trial of observational versus antibiotic treatment for a first episode of CT-proven uncomplicated acute diverticulitis. Br J Surg. 2017;104(1):52–61. https://doi.org/10.1002/bjs.10309.

15. Shabanzadeh DM, Wille-Jørgensen P. Antibiotics for uncomplicated diverticulitis. Cochrane Database Syst Rev. 2012;11:CD009092. https://doi.org/10.1002/14651858.CD009092.pub2.

16. Chabok A, Påhlman L, Hjern F, Haapaniemi S, Smedh K. Randomized clinical trial of antibiotics in acute uncomplicated diverticulitis. Br J Surg. 2012;99(4):532–9. https://doi.org/10.1002/bjs.8688.

17. Dharmarajan S, Hunt SR, Birnbaum EH, Fleshman JW, Mutch MG. The efficacy of nonoperative management of acute complicated diverticulitis. Dis Colon Rectum. 2011;54(6):663–71. https://doi.org/10.1007/DCR.0b013e31820ef759.

18. Costi R, Cauchy F, Le Bian A, Honart JF, Creuze N, Smadja C. Challenging a classic myth: pneumoperitoneum associated with acute diverticulitis is not an indication for open or laparoscopic emergency surgery in hemodynamically stable patients. A 10-year experience with a nonoperative treatment. Surg Endosc. 2012;26(7):2061–71. https://doi.org/10.1007/s00464-012-2157-z.

19. Siewert B, Tye G, Kruskal J, Sosna J, Opelka F. Impact of CT-guided drainage in the treatment of diverticular abscesses: size matters. Am J Roentgenol.

2006;186(3):680–6. https://doi.org/10.2214/AJR.04.1708.

20. Ambrosetti P, Chautems R, Soravia C, Peiris-Waser N, Terrier F. Long-term outcome of mesocolic and pelvic diverticular abscesses of the left colon: a prospective study of 73 cases. Dis Colon Rectum. 2005;48(4):787–91. https://doi.org/10.1007/s10350-004-0853-z.

21. Kumar RR, Kim JT, Haukoos JS, et al. Factors affecting the successful management of intra-abdominal abscesses with antibiotics and the need for percutaneous drainage. Dis Colon Rectum. 2006;49(2):183–9. https://doi.org/10.1007/s10350-005-0274-7.

22. Durmishi Y, Gervaz P, Brandt D, et al. Results from percutaneous drainage of Hinchey stage II diverticulitis guided by computed tomography scan. Surg Endosc. 2006;20(7):1129–33. https://doi.org/10.1007/s00464-005-0574-y.

23. Brandt D, Gervaz P, Durmishi Y, Platon A, Morel P, Poletti PA. Percutaneous CT scan-guided drainage vs. antibiotherapy alone for Hinchey II diverticulitis: a case-control study. Dis Colon Rectum. 2006;49(10):1533–8. https://doi.org/10.1007/s10350-006-0613-3.

24. Kaiser AM, Jiang J-K, Lake JP, et al. The Management of Complicated Diverticulitis and the role of computed tomography. Am J Gastroenterol. 2005;100(4):910–7. https://doi.org/10.1111/j.1572-0241.2005.41154.x.

25. Chughtai SQ, Ackerman NB. Perforated diverticulum of the transverse colon. Am J Surg. 1974;127(5):508–10. https://doi.org/10.1016/0002-9610(74)90306-7.

26. Shperber Y, Halevy A, Oland J, Orda R. Perforated diverticulitis of the transverse colon. Dis Colon Rectum. 1986;29(7):466–8. https://doi.org/10.1007/BF02561589.

27. Salem L, Anaya DA, Roberts KE, Flum DR. Hartmann's colectomy and reversal in diverticulitis: a population-level assessment. Dis Colon Rectum. 2005;48(5):988–95. https://doi.org/10.1007/s10350-004-0871-x.

28. Riansuwan W, Hull TL, Millan MM, Hammel JP. Nonreversal of hartmann's procedure for diverticulitis: derivation of a scoring system to predict nonreversal. Dis Colon Rectum. 2009;52(8):1400–8. https://doi.org/10.1007/DCR.0b013e3181a79575.

29. Oberkofler CE, Rickenbacher A, Raptis DA, et al. A multicenter randomized clinical trial of primary anastomosis or Hartmann's procedure for perforated left colonic diverticulitis with purulent or fecal peritonitis. Ann Surg. 2012;256(5):819–26.7. https://doi.org/10.1097/SLA.0b013e31827324ba.

30. Tadlock MD, Karamanos E, Skiada D, et al. Emergency surgery for acute diverticulitis: which operation? A National Surgical Quality Improvement Program study. J Trauma Acute Care Surg. 2013;74(6):1385–91.; quiz 1610. https://doi.org/10.1097/TA.0b013e3182924a82.

31. Bridoux V, Regimbeau JM, Ouaissi M, Mathonnet M, Mauvais F, Houivet E, Schwartz L, Mege D, Sielezneff I, Sabbagh CTJ. No Hartmann's procedure or primary anastomosis for generalized peritonitis due to perforated diverticulitis: a prospective multicenter randomized trial (DIVERTI). J Am Coll Surg. 2017;225:798.

32. Constantinides VA, Tekkis PP, Senapati A. Prospective multicentre evaluation of adverse outcomes following treatment for complicated diverticular disease. Br J Surg. 2006;93(12):1503–13. https://doi.org/10.1002/bjs.5402.

33. O'Sullivan GC, Murphy D, O'Brien MG, Ireland A. Laparoscopic management of generalized peritonitis due to perforated colonic diverticula. Am J Surg. 1996;171(4):432–4. https://doi.org/10.1016/S0002-9610(97)89625-0.

34. Angenete E, Thornell A, Burcharth J, et al. Laparoscopic lavage is feasible and safe for the treatment of perforated diverticulitis with purulent peritonitis. Ann Surg. 2016;263(1):117–22. https://doi.org/10.1097/SLA.0000000000001061.

35. Galbraith N, Carter JV, Netz U, et al. Laparoscopic lavage in the Management of Perforated Diverticulitis: a contemporary meta-analysis. J Gastrointest Surg. 2017;21(9):1491–9. https://doi.org/10.1007/s11605-017-3462-6.

36. Vennix S, Musters GD, Mulder IM, et al. Laparoscopic peritoneal lavage or sigmoidectomy for perforated diverticulitis with purulent peritonitis: a multicentre, parallel-group, randomised, open-label trial. Lancet. 2015;386(10000):1269–77. https://doi.org/10.1016/S0140-6736(15)61168-0.

Clostridium difficile Infection

23

Aela P. Vely and Paula Ferrada

Introduction

Clostridium difficile infection (CDI) has been recognized since the1970s. The past two decades have seen an increase in frequency and severity of cases, leading to a steady rise in mortality [1–3]. In 2011 in the United States, there were 29,000 deaths within 30 days of diagnosis from CDI and almost 500,000 cases reported [3]. CDI is now the most common hospital-acquired infection, requiring increased mobilization of health-care resources and costs [2]. Those changes have been attributed to the rise of more virulent strains in North America and Europe.

Clostridium difficile (C. diff) is a gram-positive anaerobic bacteria, naturally present in the colon, that either produce toxins (TcdA and/or TcdB) or not. These toxins can cause a chronic or acute infection in the colon through inflammation and injury of the intestinal barrier [4]. The infection usually occurs after a change in the balance of the intestinal flora, where *C. diff* is able to proliferate unchecked. Oftentime, this imbalance is attributed to the intake of antimicrobials (a single dose

can be sufficient) or a weakened immune system in hospitalized patients exposed to spore in the environment. Both toxins translocate into cells, causing disruption in the cell morphology and subsequent death. They also stimulate inflammatory reactions causing increased permeability of the intestinal membrane and release of pro-inflammatory agents that when combined lead to pseudomembranous colitis, malabsorption, and diarrhea [5]. It remains unclear how the toxins affect the severity of the strains of *C. difficile*. Clinical presentation can vary from simple diarrhea to fulminant disease requiring ICU admission and emergent surgery. Risk factors identified for CDI include advanced age (over 60), exposure to antimicrobials, previous hospitalizations, colon surgery, inflammatory bowel disease, and decreased gastric acid [6, 7]. However, in more recent years, patients otherwise healthy have been noted to present with more severe cases.

Initial Presentation and Evaluation

The patient with CDI will often present with diarrhea that can be associated with or without abdominal pain. As mentioned prior, the typical patient would have been an elderly patient over 60, from a long-term care facility. But younger patients, living in the community, suffer more and more from symptomatic CDI. The diagnosis is often suspected but not always confirmed. It is imperative to

A. P. Vely
Division of Acute Care Surgical Services, Virginia Commonwealth University, Richmond, VA, USA

P. Ferrada (✉)
VCU Surgery Trauma, Critical Care and Emergency Surgery, Richmond, VA, USA
e-mail: paula.ferrada@vcuhealth.org

© Springer International Publishing AG, part of Springer Nature 2019
C. V. R. Brown et al. (eds.), *Emergency General Surgery*, https://doi.org/10.1007/978-3-319-96286-3_23

establish whether the patient has recently had exposure to antibiotics, a recent hospitalization, or an exposure to an individual with CDI. A differential diagnosis including other infectious/noninfectious etiologies for diarrhea should be kept in mind. Hence determining the duration and severity of the symptoms is essential. Possible triggers such as recent meals, sick relatives, or recent travels should be investigated. Durations of more than 1–2 weeks suggest a more indolent course and possibly another etiology, and patterns of alternating diarrhea and constipation should also be established. Patients should also be asked about the consistency, color, or smell of the stool, which can be—although not always—liquid, mucous-like, and foul smelling. In addition, patients who have been hospitalized and have a persistent or rising leukocytosis or fever associated with diarrhea should be tested for C. diff, especially if they received antibiotics during the course of their admission or are on longer-term PPI [8–16].

On examination it is not uncommon to find patients to have soft, non-tender but distended abdomen and severe complicated disease. Peritonitis is an absolute indication for surgery, but patients that require surgery might present without this ominous sign. Leukocytosis, elevated creatinine from baseline, and signs of metabolic acidosis are concerning signs for severe infections.

There are several tests used to evaluate for the presence of active CDI, but the most popular is a combination of C. difficile antigen test (GDH), used as an initial test for the presence of the bacteria, and PCR assays that confirm the presence of the toxin. Those tests can take several hours to several days.

Initial Management

CDI may have a wide and varied presentation. In order to help the clinician better treat their patients, attempts have been made to establish a stratification and classification of the patients into mild, moderate, and severe disease. There are different criteria to establish the level of

severity. For simplicity, we will use the criteria used by IDSA and SHEA. Patients with WBC less than 15,000 and serum creatinine less than 1.5 the baseline with or without diarrhea or fevers have mild to moderate disease. Patients with values higher than the above associated with hypotension or shock are considered severe/complicated disease.

Mild to Moderate Disease

For patients with mild to moderate disease, a C. diff toxin test should be sent to confirm CDI while the patient is placed on contact precautions to avoid further dissemination of disease. It is of critical importance starting treatment as soon as possible with IV or PO metronidazole at a dose of 500 mg q8h. If the patient is on antibiotics, every attempt to terminate those antibiotics as early as clinically feasible should be made.

Supportive care to these patients should be provided with intravenous fluids, electrolyte replacement, and be kept NPO with serial abdominal exams. Although in some mild cases a diet can be considered, it should be kept in mind that CDI can have both diarrhea and ileus pictures intermixed and a propensity to escalate to a more severe picture quickly. Hence, keeping the patient NPO in the first couple of days of treatment allows some time to gauge the response to the treatment.

If the patient's clinical picture does not improve or worsens—without meeting criteria for severe disease—it is reasonable to escalate treatment from metronidazole to oral vancomycin. In most cases, with stable clinical pictures but no response to treatment, an escalation will happen after 5–7 days. Oral vancomycin should also be considered as a first-line drug for pregnant or nursing patients. The dose of vancomycin is 125 mg PO (or PR) q6h. The antibiotic course should be 10–14 days.

More recently, a newer drug, fidaxomicin, has been used to treat CDI with high success rate, low recurrences, and overall better outcomes than vancomycin. It is, similarly to vancomycin, poorly absorbed orally and has limited systemic side effects. It also appears to not completely deplete the gut's natural flora, which is likely one of the causes for its low recurrence rates. The dose of fidaxomycin is 200 mg PO q12h for 10–14 days. At this time, it is used mostly in cases of failure to respond to metronidazole and/ or vancomycin, but it may soon become more prominently used.

At any point during the course of treatment, the patient, initially deemed to have mild to moderate disease, can evolve to a more severe picture, and regularly reassessing one's patient is important.

Severe/Complicated Disease

Patients with WBC over 15,000 and creatinine 1.5 times higher than baseline (keep in mind that in patient with low baseline, that number can still appear as "normal") are considered severe CDI. Again, it can be associated, or not, with diarrhea or fever. A high index of suspicion should be used, to send test to confirm suspicion, and supportive fluid resuscitation should be initiated. Again, patient should be placed NPO, other antibiotics discontinued as soon as clinically indicated, and empiric treatment with antibiotics should be initiated.

In severe cases, metronidazole 500 mg IV q8h should be given concomitantly with vancomycin 500 mg PO q6h (if able) and 500 mg PR q6h. The duration of the treatment should be 10–14 days as well. Serial abdominal exams are crucial, and frequent clinical re-evaluation is key to determining the timing or need for surgical intervention. If the patient develops signs of shock with hypotension, fever, altered mental status, or peritoneal signs, this patient needs emergent surgery. If the patient shows signs of deterioration or no response to treatment, it is pivotal to make the decision for early surgical intervention.

Surgical Intervention

Subtotal Colectomy

The standard of care for severe or complicated CDI remains subtotal colectomy (or total abdominal colectomy). One pitfall in the surgical management of CDI is underappreciating the severity of disease during surgery. As CDI is a mucosal process, the colon may look relatively normal or only mildly edematous at the time of operation. However, if the operation is being performed for the treatment of CDI, only a subtotal colectomy should be performed, as partial colectomy is associated with an unacceptably high rate of mortality [17]. After subtotal colectomy and depending on the hemodynamic stability of the patient, once the colon is removed, an end ileostomy can be matured or the patient can be left in discontinuity with the placement of a temporary abdominal closure. In the latter, the patient will return to the operating room within 24–48 h for end ileostomy after resuscitation in the ICU.

Loop Ileostomy and Colonic Lavage

A subtotal colectomy is a morbid procedure and less morbid surgical approaches have been considered. Loop ileostomy and colonic lavage is one such that has gained some traction for the treatment of severe, complicated CDI. Since it is less extensive, this can be performed laparoscopically or open, depending on the surgeon's skill and the hemodynamic state of the patient.

A loop of distal ileum should be brought up to create a loop ileostomy. A tube should be inserted in the efferent limb, past the ileocecal valve. An intraoperative antegrade lavage of the colon should be performed with 8 L of warmed GoLytely solution. The tube should be kept in place to allow for antegrade vancomycin enema administration, 500 mg every 8 h for 10–14 days [18, 19].

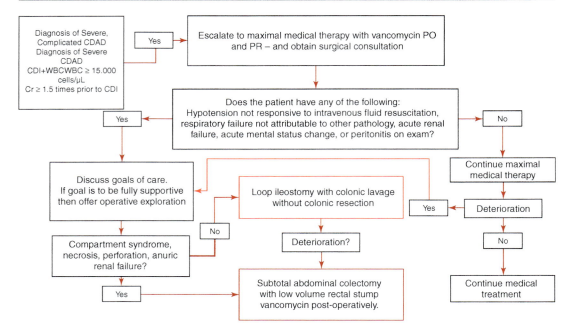

Fig. 23.1 Protocol for treatment of C diff

Absolute contraindications for this procedure are ischemia or necrosis of the colon, distal obstruction, or intra-abdominal compartment syndrome. Additionally, if clinical improvement is not noted shortly after the procedure, the patient will require a prompt return to the operating room for a subtotal colectomy.

At our institution we have a protocol for the surgical treatment of *C. diff*—see Fig. 23.1.

Postoperative Management

The patient with a rectal stump should undergo continued administration of rectal vancomycin, very gently, to prevent a blowout as well as IV metronidazole, in the same doses as mentioned above, to complete a 10-day course from the day of surgery. In patients with a diverting loop ileostomy, vancomycin antegrade enema will need to be administrated to the tune of 500 mg every 8 h, as well as metronida-

zole 500 mg IV every 8 h, for 10 days after surgery. This patient who underwent surgery will be returning to the ICU for supportive care, NPO, NGT decompression, and vasopressors as needed.

Prevention

As the frequency and severity of CDI continue to increase, it is the responsibility of all, patients, family members, and members of the healthcare team, to prevent the spreading of CDI to others. We should continue to educate the importance of contact precautions, systematic hand washing with soap and water (alcohol-based hand sanitizers are not effective against *C. diff* spores), and minimizing the use of computers, stethoscopes, and other adjuncts from one room to the next without thorough washing. The staff should educate patients suffering from CDI and their loved ones in the proper techniques of preventions.

Signs on the doors should be placed systematically to alert the providers of the reason for contact isolation. Stethoscopes should be designated for every room/patient. Computers and machines should be wiped down entirely when entering and leaving the room.

References

1. Vindigni SM, Surawicz CM. C. Difficile infection: changing epidemiology and management paradigms. Clin Transl Gastroenterol. 2015;6(7):e99. https://doi.org/10.1038/ctg.2015.24.
2. Khanna S, et al. The growing incidence and severity of Clostridium difficile infection in inpatient and outpatient settings. Expert Rev Gastroenterol Hepatol. 2010;4:409–16.
3. Lessa FC, et al. Burden of Clostridium difficile Infection in the United States. N Engl J Med. 2015;372:825–34. https://doi.org/10.1056/NEJMoa1408913.
4. Sun X, et al. The Enterotoxicity of Clostridium difficile Toxins. Toxins (Basel). 2010;2(7):1848–80.
5. Voth DE, Ballard JD. Clostridium difficile Toxins: Mechanism of Action and Role in Disease. Clin Microbiol Rev. 2005;18(2):247–63. https://doi.org/10.1128/CMR.18.2.247-263.2005.
6. Vestcinsdottir I, et al. Risk factors for Clostridium difficile toxin-positive diarrhea: a population-based rospective case-control study. Eur J Clin Microbiol Infect Dis. 2012;31(10):2601–10. Epub 2012 Mar 23.
7. Rodemann JF, et al. Incidence of Clostridium difficile infection in inflammatory bowel disease. Clin Gastroenterol Hepatol. 2007;5(3):339–44.
8. Halabi WJ, et al. Clostridium difficile colitis in the United States: a decade of trends, outcomes, risk factors for colectomy, and mortality after colectomy. J Am Coll Surg. 2013;217(5):802–12. https://doi.org/10.1016/j.jamcollsurg.2013.05.028. Epub 2013 Sep 4.
9. Surawicz CM, et al. Guidelines for diagnosis, treatment, and prevention of Clostridium difficile infections. Am J Gastroenterol. 2013;108(4):478–98.; quiz 499. https://doi.org/10.1038/ajg.2013.4.
10. Cohen SH, et al. Clinical practice guidelines for Clostridium difficile infection in adults: 2010 update by the society for healthcare epidemiology of America (SHEA) and the infectious diseases society of America (IDSA). Infect Control Hosp Epidemiol. 2010;31(5):431–55. https://doi.org/10.1086/651706.
11. van der Wilden GM, et al. Fulminant Clostridium difficile colitis: prospective development of a risk scoring system. J Trauma Acute Care Surg. 2014;76(2):424–30. https://doi.org/10.1097/TA.0000000000000105.
12. Zar FA, et al. A comparison of vancomycin and metronidazole for the treatment of Clostridium difficile-associated diarrhea, stratified by disease severity. Clin Infect Dis. 2007;45(3):302–7. Epub 2007 Jun 19.
13. Louie TJ, et al. Fidaxomicin versus vancomycin for Clostridium difficile infection. N Engl J Med. 2011;364(5):422–31. https://doi.org/10.1056/NEJMoa0910812.
14. Ofosu A. Clostridium difficile infection: a review of current and emerging therapies. Ann Gastroenterol. 2016;29(2):147–54.https://doi.org/10.20524/aog.2016.0006.
15. Dallal RM, et al. Fulminant Clostridium difficile: An Underappreciated and Increasing Cause of Death and Complications. Ann Surg. 2002;235(3):363–72.
16. Lamontagne F, et al. Impact of emergency colectomy on survival of patients with fulminant Clostridium difficile colitis during an epidemic caused by a hypervirulent strain. Ann Surg. 2007;245(2):267–72.
17. Ferrada P, et al. Timing and type of surgical treatment of Clostridium difficile-associated disease: a practice management guideline from the Eastern Association for the Surgery of Trauma. J Trauma Acute Care Surg. 2014;76(6):1484–93. https://doi.org/10.1097/TA.0000000000000232.
18. Neal MD, et al. Diverting loop ileostomy and colonic lavage: an alternative to total abdominal colectomy for the treatment of severe, complicated Clostridium difficile associated disease. Ann Surg. 2011;254(3):423–7 discussion 427–9. https://doi.org/10.1097/SLA.0b013e31822ade48.
19. Ferrada P, Callcut R, Zielinski MD, et al, EAST Multi-Institutional Trials Committee. Loop ileostomy versus total colectomy as surgical treatment for Clostridium difficile-associated disease: an Eastern Association for the Surgery of Trauma multicenter trial. J Trauma Acute Care Surg. 2017;83(1):36–40.

Large Bowel Obstruction: Current Techniques and Trends in Management

Andrew T. Schlussel and Erik Q. Roedel

Introduction

The management of an acute large bowel obstruction (LBO) remains one of the most complex surgical diseases presenting in the emergency setting. Historically, operative treatment was the standard of care, extirpating the pathology and oftentimes creating a permanent stoma [1]. The acute blockage of fecal flow often results in an overt need for laparotomy; nevertheless, having a systematic and algorithmic approach to the management of a LBO will significantly influence the patient's quality of life (Fig. 24.1). It is imperative that the surgeon not only treat the obstructing process but also consider the underlying etiology. Many LBOs are mechanical in origin; however, nonmechanical causes such as pseudo-obstructions have also been described. Both benign and malignant diseases, with either intrinsic or extrinsic compression, may result in obstruction, and the underlying disease and patient's physiology will often dictate the treatment required. As experience and technology has advanced in the management of acute colonic emergencies, several treatment options are available, and all should be in the armamentarium of the acute care surgeon.

Etiology

The pathophysiology of a LBO most commonly occurs due to the progressive narrowing of the colon lumen due to an intrinsic process. Colorectal cancer is the third most common malignancy and is the third leading cause of cancer-related death in the United States [2]. An obstruction will be the initial presentation in 10–33% of these cases, accounting for over 50% of all LBOs [3–5]. A diverticular stricture is reported to be the second most common cause of intrinsic obstruction with a prevalence ranging between 10% and 20%. Additionally, acute diverticulitis may also result in a LBO due to an inflammatory process or abscess formation. Volvulus, which accounts for 10–17% of LBOs, typically develops in the sigmoid colon and cecum [5]. Diseases such as ischemic colitis, radiation enteritis, Crohn's disease (CD), and endometriosis may also present as an obstructive process; however, these are much less common.

Malignant obstructions are most likely to form in the descending colon and rectosigmoid junction. Often it may be difficult to differentiate between benign and malignant pathology, and this will further add to the complex decision-

A. T. Schlussel (✉)
Department of Surgery, Madigan Army Medical Center, Tacoma, WA, USA

E. Q. Roedel
Department of Surgery, Tripler Army Medical Center, Honolulu, HI, USA

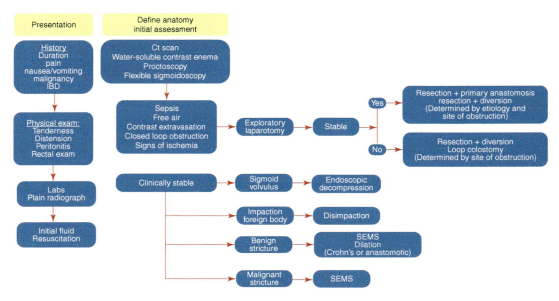

Fig. 24.1 Evaluation and treatment algorithm for the management of an acute large bowel obstruction

making process. Extrinsic compression either from carcinomatosis or extra colonic malignancies may result in an acute obstruction, and rarely postoperative adhesions may significantly occlude the colon. It is critical that a thorough history and physical is performed as this will guide the subsequent steps in determining the diagnosis and treatment.

Pathophysiology

The nature of the obstruction will often dictate the patient's clinical status, as well as the urgency in which an intervention must be rendered. The colon is a resilient organ, with great compliance, and patients can often tolerate an obstructive process for several days before an emergent situation arises. When the ileocecal valve is not competent, large bowel contents may decompress proximally, and this prevents the development of a closed-loop obstruction and subsequent perforation. The effects of colonic distention on perfusion have been evaluated in a dog model by Boley and colleagues. Findings demonstrated that once an intraluminal pressure has reached above 30 mmHg, there is an immediate fall in intestinal

blood flow, a decrease in the oxygen extraction by the intestine, and ultimately intestinal ischemia, hypoxia, and perforation [6]. The timing in which this develops is dependent on the severity and duration of the obstruction.

The mechanical effects inflicted on each portion of the colon are dependent on wall tension. The degree of tensile force on the wall is proportional to the pressure generated in the colon and the diameter of the at-risk segment as dictated by the law of Laplace [7]. Therefore, the cecum, which has the largest diameter, will have the greatest degree of tension distributed in this segment. This incremental rise of intraluminal pressure will result in a hypoxic environment generated at the level of the mucosa and submucosa, and subsequent perforation will ensue [6, 8].

Presentation

The initial presentation of an acute LBO may be variable based on the degree, timing, and etiology of the disease (Table 24.1). Typically, an obstruction secondary to a colonic volvulus will present in a rapid fashion, versus a diverticular stricture or malignant process which may be more chronic.

Table 24.1 Etiology of large bowel obstruction

Malignant disease	Benign disease
Colon cancer	Diverticular disease
Rectal cancer	Volvulus: cecal or sigmoid
Carcinoid	Fecal impaction
Lymphoma	Foreign body
Gastrointestinal stromal tumor	Ischemic colitis
Extrinsic compression from metastatic carcinoma	Inflammatory bowel disease
	Colonic pseudo-obstruction
	Anastomotic stricture
	Adhesions
	Hernia

Some signs and symptoms may be subtle, compared to others who present with a profound physiologic derangement. Patients may develop a prodrome of symptoms to include bloating, obstipation or constipation, thinning of the stool caliber, and colicky or cramping abdominal pain. Emesis is often a late sign of disease progression if decompression through the ileocecal valve has occurred. As previously discussed, when the ileocecal valve is competent, a closed-loop obstruction will result, and patients experience progressive dilation, pain, and eventual perforation [8].

Physical exam may demonstrate a distended tympanic abdomen, with an associated dominant mass. Signs of focal abdominal tenderness and peritonitis warrant urgent operative intervention, as one must be concerned for associated ischemia or perforation. A digital rectal exam should be performed in all patients to identify a distal rectal or anal cancer, stricture from a prior low colorectal anastomosis, foreign body, or fecal impaction. When feasible, proctoscopy may be performed at the bedside to evaluate the rectum and distal sigmoid colon; however, care must be made not to over distend the colon as this may worsen the patient's condition.

Colonic dilation may result in severe volume depletion and electrolyte disturbances due to fluid shifts in the intestinal luminal, bacterial overgrowth, and concomitant emesis. Overt septic shock may be present with more advanced disease. Following an initial assessment, complete blood work should be performed to include a complete blood count, chemistry, and lactic acid levels. Acid-base abnormalities should be noted to guide the initial resuscitation, and a serum creatinine should be evaluated prior to administering intravenous contrast. When the suspicion for a malignancy is high, a carcinoembryonic antigen (CEA) level should be obtained, and complete imaging of the chest abdomen and pelvis to identify metastatic disease must be performed.

The initial management as well as a thorough workup of the acute obstruction should occur simultaneously. The patient's volume status must be addressed and fluid resuscitation should commence in the emergency room. In addition to closely monitoring the patient's vital signs and laboratory results, a Foley catheter should be placed for an accurate measurement of urine output. Nasogastric tube decompression should be performed in patients with active nausea, ongoing emesis, or if small bowel dilatation is recognized on imaging. If the patient does not mandate immediate operative exploration, then observation in a monitored setting is critical.

Although often overlooked due to the ease of obtaining advanced imaging, a flat and upright abdominal and chest plain film should be performed to evaluate for free perforation which would warrant operative exploration. These films can provide insight to the location of the obstruction, size of the cecum, as well as subtle findings associated ischemia. Although there is no exact correlation between cecal diameter and ischemia or perforation, 12 cm is generally a cutoff that warrants concern; however, perforations have occurred with a smaller luminal dilation [9–12]. Furthermore, these images are diagnostic for either a sigmoid or cecal volvulus, with the colon mesentery of the volvulized segment oriented toward the quadrant of concern. Swenson and colleagues demonstrated that plain radiographs were unable to determine the diagnosis of a cecal and sigmoid volvulus in 85% and 49% of patients, respectively. Therefore, additional imaging is required when clinical suspicion is high [13]. The inability to interpret a plain film should not delay identifying the correct diagnosis.

Advanced Imaging

Once the stability of the patient has been determined, and there is no urgent surgical intervention required, a more thorough radiographic evaluation of the patient is performed. Computed tomography (CT) of the abdomen and pelvis has become the diagnostic modality of choice in the setting of a LBO due to its near-ubiquitous availability, technical easy to obtain, and it provides rapid access to high-quality images (Fig. 24.2). This imaging modality has largely replaced contrast enemas (CE) and endoscopy as an initial test. CT is a critical tool in the event of any diagnostic dilemma. When performed correctly, this study provides quality information regarding intra-abdominal pathology and can help differentiate between intrinsic and extrinsic compression of the colon. CT has a reported sensitivity and specificity of over 90%, with an accuracy of 94% in correctly identifying the level of obstruction and 81% in determining the correct diagnosis

[14]. In a study by Frager and colleagues, a CT scan was found to have a significantly greater sensitivity, accuracy, and negative predictive value in the evaluation of a LBO when compared to a contrast enema [14]. Intravenous, oral, and rectal contrast may be administered to further increase the accuracy and quality of the study. In addition, these adjuncts have resulted in the overall improvement of both false-negative and false-positive rates [14]. Based on these advantages, a CT scan should be strongly considered as the initial diagnostic test of choice in the evaluation of an acute LBO.

Contrast enemas have historically been the gold standard in the diagnosis of a LBO. It is recommended to instill water-soluble contrast for this study rather than barium, as there is a risk of peritonitis secondary to barium if a perforation occurs (Fig. 24.3). Contrast enemas are beneficial as they may further elucidate details about the obstructing lesion anatomy. This includes size, tortuosity, or whether the lumen has a benign smooth appearance versus a malignant one. These characteristics provide important insight if endoluminal stenting is to be considered. This

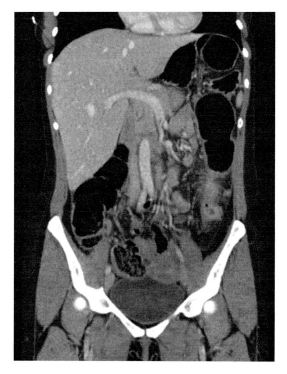

Fig. 24.2 Computed tomography demonstrating sigmoid stricture with proximal dilation

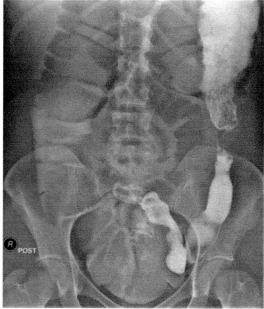

Fig. 24.3 Water-soluble contrast enema of sigmoid stricture

modality has a sensitivity of 96% and specificity of 98% in identifying the level of obstruction. These findings are similar to CT scan but significantly greater compared to plain radiographs [15]. In a patient with volvulus a "bird's beak" or tapering of the lumen can be observed [13, 16]. Due to the decreased accessibility, increased variability of administration, risk of perforation, and associated patient discomfort, water-soluble CE should be considered as a radiographic adjunct to CT, or for preprocedural planning for colonic stent placement, as will be discussed below [5].

Endoscopy

Flexible sigmoidoscopy should also be considered while evaluating the stable patient with a LBO. This procedure imparts minimal risk to the patient and is often readily available and requires no sedation. The risk of perforation is rare; however, carbon dioxide insufflation should be used as this has been found to have a lower risk of perforation when compared to air. Carbon dioxide is absorbed 250 times faster than air and this will minimize the degree of distention proximal to the disease [17]. This diagnostic and therapeutic tool will identify a rectal or sigmoid mass, allow for biopsies to be obtained, and provide information for consideration of stent placement simultaneously. In addition, if a sigmoid volvulus is encountered detorsion can be performed, and an emergent condition can now be mitigated to a semi-elective one.

Management

Traditionally all patients with a large bowel obstruction required operative exploration. In the setting of a patient with a closed-loop obstruction, evidence of ischemia, or findings of a perforation with a subsequent physiologic insult, the decision for surgical intervention is relatively straightforward. Volume resuscitation should be ongoing as the operating room is prepared, adequate vascular access should be confirmed, and

the patient should receive appropriate parenteral antibiotic coverage against anaerobic and gram-negative bacteria. A stoma marking both for a colostomy and an ileostomy should be placed on the patient while awake. When possible, this should be performed in the supine, sitting, and standing positions. However, this may be challenging in patients who are in acute distress. Maturing a stoma in an emergency setting has been associated with poor outcomes, and every effort to obtain a preoperative enteric stomal therapist site marking should be made [18]. A thorough discussion with the anesthesia service should be performed to ensure appropriate ongoing volume repletion. The patient and family should be fully informed on the gravity of the situation which includes a significantly elevated rate of stoma creation. In the stable patient, without signs of impending abdominal sepsis, a nonoperative and potentially endoscopic approach can be considered. This process may be as straightforward as fecal disimpaction or as complex as the placement of a self-expanding metallic stent (SEMS) to temporarily alleviate the obstructive process. Presently, this strategy has become more accepted, and in the appropriately selected patient, this is a viable option to avoid a technically challenging and potentially morbid operation.

Operative Management

Right-Sided Obstruction

Proximal or right-sided obstructions have traditionally been treated with right colectomy and ileocolic anastomosis and can be safely performed in most patients [19]. The decision to perform a primary anastomosis requires the surgeon to assess the patient's overall clinical status, their physiology during surgery, and bowel viability at the proximal and distal resection margins. The incidence of an anastomotic leak was not significantly different when primary anastomosis was performed in the setting of obstruction (10%) compared to no obstruction (6%) [20]. When clinical factors are questionable, a proximal protective loop ileostomy may be performed to mitigate the effects of an anastomotic leak if one subsequently occurs. Furthermore, in the unstable patient presenting with generalized peritonitis, as in the setting of cecal perforation, this may require resection of the obstructed segment with an end ileostomy and consideration of a distal mucous fistula [4]. If the distal colon is unable to be brought to the skin surface, it may be secured in the subcutaneous tissue at the stoma site or midline incision.

Greater than one half of LBOs are caused by a malignant process; therefore, an oncologic resection should be pursued when approaching these lesions. Current recommendations are that a segmental resection be performed which includes the lymphatic and vascular drainage of the tumor [21]. For lesions in the cecum or ascending colon, resection should include the distal terminal ileum through the transverse colon, with proximal ligation of the ileocolic vascular pedicle and division of the right branch of the middle colic artery. Tumor spread occurs through a submucosal plane; consequently, a minimum margin of 5–7 cm proximal and distal to the mass should be obtained [21]. Obstructing masses at the hepatic flexure and transverse colon should be managed with an extended right colectomy including a high ligation of the middle colic artery.

A laparoscopic resection may be considered by a surgeon with appropriate training and experience. There are multiple factors which will add to the complexity of this operation. The presence of an obstruction will diminish the working space available in the intra-abdominal cavity; additionally, the distended colon will have a significant stool burden and may be friable and compromised due to ischemia. This may result in a higher degree of iatrogenic injury when the colon and small intestine are handled by laparoscopic instruments. Complete laparoscopic or hand-assisted laparoscopic colectomy has been shown to be safe and effective when performed by those proficient in this technique; however, one should have a low threshold to convert to an open approach [22, 23]. Furthermore, if proceeding with a laparoscopic approach, a sound oncologic operation must be performed.

In the elective setting, a colectomy performed through a minimally invasive approach has been shown to decrease hospital length of stay and risk of postoperative adverse events [24–28]. Due to the significant differences in outcomes reported for emergent open colectomy when compared to elective minimally invasive colectomy, it is naturally appealing to explore stenting as a bridge to elective surgery in right-sided LBO. There have been several retrospective studies showing that in centers with appropriate support and experienced providers, stenting can be safe and effective [29–31]. Evidence for this practice is limited, and due to technical challenges, it should only be attempted by an experienced endoscopist. Procedural details and clinical outcomes following endoscopic stenting will be discussed below.

Left-Sided Obstruction

While right-sided obstructions are predominantly treated by primary resection and anastomosis, the management of a left-sided obstruction is far more complicated and controversial. Due to a high risk of anastomotic leak, these patients have been generally treated with either diversion alone for decompression or resection and end colostomy [20]. In a less ideal surgical candidate, those with compromised bowel, intraoperative instability, or evidence of perforation at the site of obstruction, a Hartmann's procedure (resection and end colostomy) may still be necessary.

More recently, it is recommended that the surgical treatment of left-sided obstructions be individualized to the patient. Postoperative outcomes appear to be similar and potentially better following primary resection for left-sided lesions [32, 33]. The operative approach should be based on location of the lesion, completeness and chronicity of the obstruction, benign or malignant pathology, nutritional status, and history of radiation or an immunocompromised state. In patients who remain stable, with low operative risk factors and a proximal colon that is not severely distended or ischemic, segmental resection with primary anastomosis can be considered [34, 35]. A side-to-end or side-to-side anastomosis can be utilized to correct for a size mismatch in the setting of chronically dilated but healthy proximal colon. Decompression of a severely dilated colon can often be advantageous to allow for better manipulation of the colon to perform a resection; the addition of colonic irrigation may also be done simultaneously in selected cases [36, 37].

The utilization of intraoperative on-table colonic lavage is preferred by some surgeons in the management of left-sided obstruction. This procedure is performed in an attempt to relieve the stool burden, allow for an intraoperative colonoscopy when indicated, and aid in creating a primary anastomosis with efforts to minimize the risk of an anastomotic leak [38]. Recent data, including a randomized trial, has demonstrated equivalent outcomes between colonic lavage versus those who only received manual evacuation of the colon [39–41]. Multiple techniques for this procedure have been described. Regardless of the methods used for irrigation, the colon is first fully mobilized and vascular ligation is performed. Following mobilization Otsuka et al. recommend inserting an irrigation catheter through the appendix or cecum, a non-crushing bowel clamp is placed on the terminal ileum to prevent proximal flow of stool, and the colon is then fully irrigated. Once the fecal residue is softened by the warm irrigation, it is drained out the catheter into a collection bag, the resection and anastomosis is then performed [39]. Lim and colleagues advise dividing the colon proximal to the site of obstruction and placing that end into a basin. After manual decompression of any hard-bulky stool from the colon, an appendicostomy is created in the mid-appendix and a 16 French Foley catheter is placed into the cecum and secured in place. The terminal ileum is occluded with a bowel clamp, and the colon is irrigated with 4–8 liters of saline. Once completed an appendectomy is performed. Interestingly, in this cohort of patient, there was no significant difference in the time to recovery of bowel function, hospital length of stay, risk of wound infection, and rate of anastomotic leak [40]. Due to the variability in outcomes when on-table lavage is implemented, this operative step should only be considered when technically necessary to create an anastomosis.

Subtotal Colectomy

An alternative effort to avoid stoma creation is performing a subtotal or total abdominal colectomy with ileorectal or ileosigmoid anastomosis. Although this may be an appealing operation to perform in the acute setting, with a similar risk of morbidity and mortality, this procedure will result in a significant alteration in bowel function as well as a decrease in quality of life compared to those undergoing a segmental resection [42, 43]. It is important to ascertain the patient's defecatory function preoperatively, as someone with incontinence at baseline will have significant difficulties postoperatively. Indications to perform this operation include a synchronous neoplasm proximally or a known hereditary colorectal cancer syndrome, ischemia of the cecum, or a perforation proximal to the obstructing lesion [44]. Determining when to perform a subtotal colectomy should be based on the patient's clinical status, comorbid conditions, degree of fecal continence, and intraoperative findings.

Rectal Obstruction

Obstruction secondary to a rectal cancer is a clear sign of locally advanced disease and careful evaluation, and staging is critical to determining the best initial treatment of the patient. While proximal rectal cancers causing obstruction may be bridged with an endoluminal stent, mid and distal rectal masses have a higher rate of failure [45]. In patients with complete obstruction, loop colostomy provides both proximal and distal decompression and allows for the timely resumption of a diet. Patients who present in the emergency care setting will most likely demonstrate abdominal symptoms. However, if an endoscopically obstructed rectal cancer is identified, the patient should be referred for immediate neoadjuvant chemoradiotherapy. This cohort can safely be managed without proximal diversion or stenting, with only a 4.3% risk of progressing to a complete and clinically significant obstruction [46].

Nonoperative Therapies

Disimpaction

A colonic obstruction may occur as a result of significant fecal impaction or a retained foreign body. Although not often considered a surgical emergency, fecal impaction is associated with 1.3% of LBOs. This develops at a greater rate in patients with spinal cord injuries, leading to a reported risk of mortality as high as 16% [47]. Oftentimes disimpaction can occur manually or with the aid of enemas and sedation. When stool is inspissated proximally, or in the setting of a large calcified fecalith, an endoscopic approach may be required to alleviate the impaction. Under colonoscopic guidance, stool can be broken up with a water irrigator, or large calcified stool can be extracted with a Roth Net® retriever.

When approaching a retained foreign body endoscopically, there are multiple tools that may be utilized. Depending on the object inserted, this may be removed in the emergency bay; however, this oftentimes requires moderate sedation. Simple insufflation may disrupt the vacuum effect of the rectum and allow for decent of the object. An endoscopic balloon or Foley catheter can be placed proximally to aid in bringing the foreign body down into the anal canal. Additionally, a large snare or long wire folded into snare tubing can be utilized to lasso the object and extract it. In cases where endoscopic retrieval is unsuccessful, general anesthesia should be induced. When transanal extraction fails, despite complete relaxation and paralysis, milking of the object distally either laparoscopically or through an open laparotomy incision is necessary. Furthermore, creation of a proximal longitudinal colotomy with transabdominal extraction may be required. This defect should then be closed in a transverse fashion. If a perforation of the colon or rectum is discovered, this may be repaired primarily based on the size of the defect and viability of surrounding tissue. It is critical that following successful removal of any object, the mucosa should be evaluated endoscopically for any significant damage.

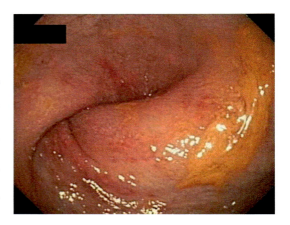

Fig. 24.4 Pinwheel sign of colonic mucosa from sigmoid volvulus

Decompression

Endoscopic decompression is the first-line treatment of choice in the management of acute sigmoid volvulus in the stable patient without evidence of perforation. This procedure functions as both a diagnostic and therapeutic intervention. The colonoscope should be inserted and passed carefully to the level of obstruction. A classic pinwheel sign of the colonic mucosa can be identified at the volvulus site (Fig. 24.4). Gentle insufflation and pressure result in detorsion of the colon and its mesentery, relieving ischemia and decreasing intraluminal pressure. This maneuver is successful in 85–95% of patients with a sigmoid volvulus [48]. The scope may then be advanced proximal to the volvulized point to assess mucosal integrity and to suction any additional fluid or air from the lumen (Fig. 24.5). A long colonic decompression tube should be placed to minimize the risk of recurrent volvulus (Fig. 24.6). These patients should be observed for recurrence, and sigmoid colectomy is recommended during the index hospital admission as there is a 60% risk of recurrence [49]. Decompression is not advised in the setting of cecal volvulus unless the patient is of prohibitive surgical risk. Endoscopic management has a high failure rate, and patients have a greater risk of ischemia, necessitating a more urgent operation

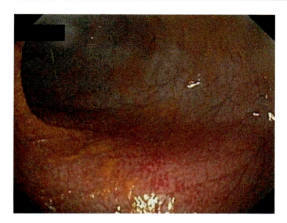

Fig. 24.5 Assessment of colonic mucosa and decompression of a sigmoid volvulus

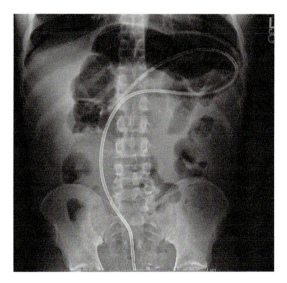

Fig. 24.6 Placement of long colonic decompression tube

[50]. These patients should be appropriately resuscitated and ileocolectomy is recommended. A primary anastomosis may be performed in the majority of patients unless clinically unstable [5].

Dilation

Endoscopic balloon dilation is a suitable treatment option for select cases of LBO in the stable patient. The circumferential radial expansion balloon system utilized in this procedure distributes pressure evenly around the bowel wall. The mechanical effects of this balloon result in a decreased the risk of perforation and prevent slippage above or below the stricture during dilation. This technique should be considered in the management of benign disease to include inflammatory bowel disease (IBD) and anastomotic strictures. Dilation alone has a greater success rate, and lower risk of complications, when alleviating an obstruction secondary to a short fibrotic stricture.

Crohn's disease is a transmural inflammatory process that has an associated risk of either inflammatory or fibrotic stricture formation in up to 30% of patients [51]. Dilation in the setting of CD has a risk of perforation as high as 10%. Risk factors for this complication include hospitalized patients with active mucosal inflammation, malnutrition, and chronic steroid use [52]. The etiology of an anastomotic stricture may be multifactorial. This complication may be secondary to the suture or stapling technique, mucosal ischemia, suture or staple line ischemia, or the effects of prior radiation therapy [53]. These risks factors must be considered when determining the appropriate intervention for these patients. In general, an anastomotic stricture is defined as a luminal diameter that an endoscopist cannot pass a standard 13-mm-diameter adult colonoscope through. Dilation may be performed with either an over-the-wire (OTW) balloon or through-the-scope (TTS) balloon dilation system (Fig. 24.7). The risk of perforation is low, and Di Giorgio and colleagues found no significant difference in either technique. However, the majority of patients required more than one dilation [53]. Creating a radial cut in the stricture with a precut sphincterotome may aid in successful dilation. This technique has also been reported as an independent procedure by creating radial cuts in four quadrants of the stricture with no additional balloon dilation [54]. If there is any concern for perforation following the procedure, a water-soluble contrast enema may be obtained. If a perforation is discovered, this may require antibiotics or an urgent exploration depending on the severity of injury. Caution must be taken to ensure there is

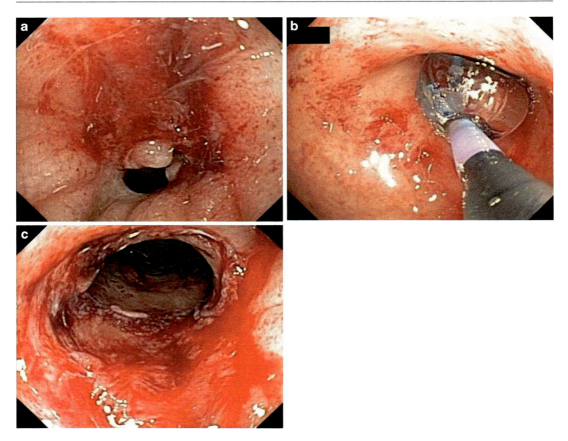

Fig. 24.7 Anastomotic stricture and dilation. (**a**) Anastomotic stricture prior to dilation, (**b**) dilation of stricture with a through-the-scope balloon system, (**c**) successful dilation of anastomotic stricture

no evidence of recurrent cancer prior to pursuing anastomotic dilation. Biopsies should be obtained, and an alternative treatment option should be considered in this situation [55]. Although there is a paucity of data in the utilization of endoscopic balloon dilation in the setting of an acute LBO, this is an effective option in the appropriately selected patient and may avoid a laparotomy and stoma creation.

Self-Expanding Metallic Stent Placement

The utilization of SEMS in the setting of LBO has become popularized over the past few decades since its inception in 1991 by Dohmoto who reported on the efficacy of this procedure in

the palliative treatment of a metastatic LBO [56]. Shortly thereafter Tejero and colleagues applied this technique as a temporary measure in the setting of a malignant LBO, in order to decompress the colon, to allow for a bowel preparation, and to bridge these patients to an elective operation [57]. Since the introduction of this procedure, the deployment of a SEMS has been used as a strategy in the treatment of malignant obstructions or as palliative measure in those with incurable disease. There have been more recent reports in the placement of colonic stents for benign disease. This procedure temporizes an emergent situation and may act as a "bridge to surgery," in patients with curable malignant or benign disease. The ability to provided prolonged endoscopic decompression for a period of days to weeks can provide time for a full bowel preparation, await a histologic diagnosis, perform a proximal endoscopic evaluation for synchronous lesions, and allow for a laparoscopic resection and primary anastomosis in a semi-elective fashion. Ultimately the goal is to transition an emergent operation into an elective one, reducing the risk of postoperative mortality, morbidity, and stoma creation. Furthermore, the placement of SEMS has been associated with an overall improvement in quality of life for these patients [58].

Technical Aspects

Prior to SEMS placement, it is critical that all appropriate material and equipment for the procedure are available. The current Food and Drug Administration-approved stents are composed of either nitinol, cobalt-chromium-nickel, or stainless steel. Similar to dilators, these are designed as either TTS or OTW devices (Table 24.2) [59]. An uncovered stent is utilized to prevent SEMS migration; therefore, removal may only be performed at the time of surgical resection (Fig. 24.8). Due to the diameter of the TTS system and the friction generated in the working channel when looping occurs, an adult or therapeutic colonoscope with a 3.7–4.2 mm diameter instrument channel is required to accommodate the device. By placing the SEMS through the scope, the device can be deployed as far proximally as the scope can reach, including the right colon and ileum if required [59, 60]. However, when managing a LBO secondary to an obstructing rectal process, it is imperative that the distal aspect of the stent be positioned at least 6 centimeters from the anal verge to prevent severe tenesmus and anal pain from the device [61].

Preoperative imaging to include a CT scan or water-soluble contrast enema is helpful in determining if there is a complete obstruction. If present, this may prevent passage of a guidewire, which is the first critical step of SEMS insertion. However, Small and colleagues have demonstrated that the lack of luminal flow of contrast on

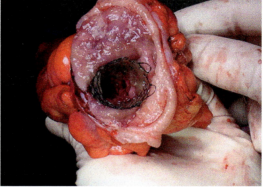
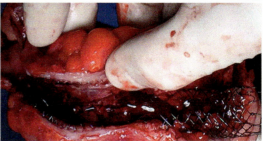

Fig. 24.8 Self-expanding metallic stent removed at time of surgical resection

Table 24.2 Food and Drug Administration-approved colonic stents [59]

Industry name	Composition	Diameter	Type of device
Boston Scientific			
Ultraflex Precision Colonic	Nitinol	25 mm + 30 mm proximal flare	OTW Nonreconstrainable
Wallstent Enteral	Elgiloy (cobalt-chromium-nickel)	20 mm and 22 mm	TTS Reconstrainable
Wallflex Enteral Colonic	Nitinol	(a) 25 mm body + 30 mm proximal flare (b) 22 mm body + 27 mm proximal flare	TTS Reconstrainable
Cook Endoscopy			
Colonic Z-stent	Stainless steel	25 mm	OTW

OTW Over the wire, *TTS* Through the scope

a water-soluble enema is not a contraindication to stent placement [62]. These imaging techniques provide anatomic information regarding the stricture. Factors that may influence the complexity of stent placement and aid in preprocedural planning include the length of the stricture and the degree of angulation. Previous studies have reported that shorter strictures with a median length of 40 mm and those with a wider colonic angulation at the distal extent of the stricture (median 121°) had a greater rate of successful stent deployment and decompression [63]. Identifying any signs of perforation is important prior to proceeding with stent placement, as this could rapidly change an urgent situation into an emergent one. It is recommended to perform the procedure under fluoroscopic guidance when possible [61]. Once the endoscope is passed to the level of the stricture, a 0.035-inch hydrophilic guidewire can be inserted through the working channel of the scope, and this should be positioned as far proximal to the stricture as possible (Fig. 24.9). Care should be made to ensure adequate control of the guidewire once inserted. A biopsy of the lesion should not be performed at the time of the SEMS placement as this may lead to a greater risk of perforation during deployment. An endoscopic retrograde cholangiopancreatography (ERCP) catheter may then be

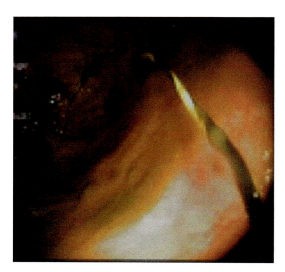

Fig. 24.9 Guidewire placed through obstructing colonic stricture

passed over the guidewire and contrast injected to opacify the lumen and confirm appropriate positioning. The catheter is then removed, and the TTS system is passed over the guidewire and deployed inside the stricture under fluoroscopic guidance. The proximal landing zone of the stent is observed radiographically and the distal aspect is visualized endoscopically. It is critical to maintain the device within the stricture during the entire deployment to avoid incorrect placement. Some devices may be reconstrained to allow for small adjustments during placement; however, this must be known prior to stent selection (Figs. 24.10 and 24.11). Once the SEMS is fully deployed, an abdominal radiograph is obtained to confirm appropriate positioning (Fig. 24.12). The stricture should be fully traversed, and the stent displays an hourglass-like configuration with both ends open on either side of the lesion. Balloon dilation is not required to augment decompression [61]. Due to the technical complexity of this procedure, Lee and colleagues recommend at least 30 SEMS insertions to achieve proficiency [64].

Outcomes of Colonic Stenting

The advent of SEMS in the management of an acute LBO has played an integral role in both benign and malignant diseases. Emergent colonic resection in the setting of a LBO is associated with a significantly worse outcome and a greater rate of stoma creation when compared to elective colorectal surgery. Mortality rates range as high as 15% at 30 days and 12% at 90 days for emergent colectomy, versus an elective colorectal resection having a 2.1% risk of mortality at 90 days [65, 66]. Furthermore, operative morbidity has been reported as high as 50% following emergent colectomy [67]. In addition, endoscopic decompression may allow for a completion colonoscopy to evaluate for synchronous tumors. This not only provides the best oncologic procedure but allows for a well-informed decision of the operative plan [5, 68]. Unfortunately, upward of 60% of patients who require a colostomy under urgent or emergent circumstances

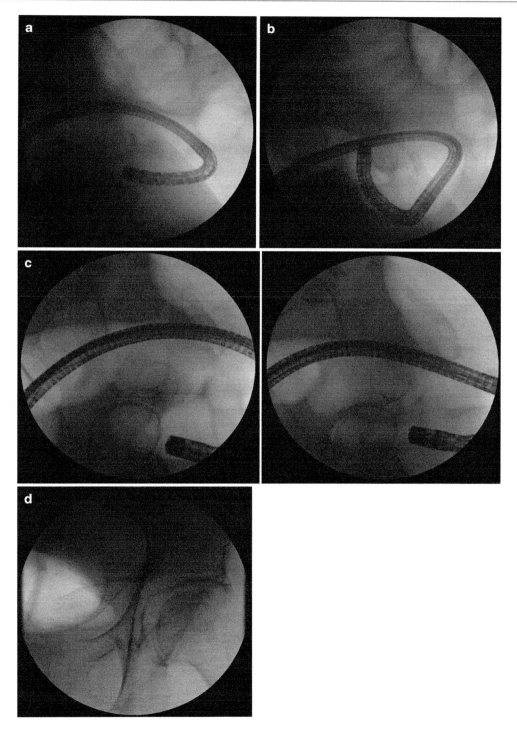

Fig. 24.10 Fluoroscopic guidance for self-expanding metallic stent deployment. (**a**) Colonoscope passed to level of obstruction, (**b**) guidewire passed through the lesion, (**c**) stent partially deployed, (**d**) stent deployed with hourglass shape across the lesion

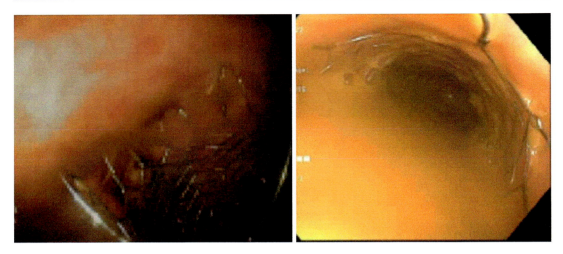

Fig. 24.11 Endoscopic visualization of the distal landing zone following stent deployment with successful decompression

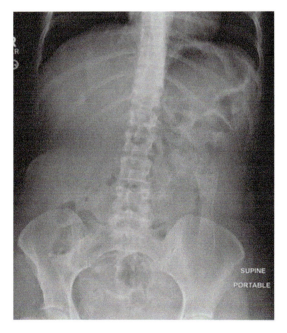

Fig. 24.12 Abdominal radiograph following colonic stent placement

will never be reversed [69, 70]. Additionally, colostomy reversal is fraught with multiple complications to include anastomotic leak, with an overall morbidity rate of 16%. These findings support an effort to avoid an emergent colonic resection when possible [71]. Cumulative rates of stoma creation following an acute LBO second-

ary to metastatic colorectal cancer were found to be significantly less following SEMS (15%) compared to primary colectomy (29%) at 1 year [67]. Although Kavanagh and colleagues have questioned the benefit of SEMS as a bridge to surgery, they recognized this intervention is associated with a significantly lower risk of requiring a total abdominal colectomy in the emergency setting (4% vs. 23%; $p = 0.03$) [72].

Clinical and technical success rates of SEMS deployment range from 73% to 95% [58, 63, 73–75]. The utilization of endoscopic colonic stenting as a bridge to surgery has now become a strong recommendation in the most recent update of the American College of Colon and Rectal Surgery (ASCRS) Clinical Practice Guidelines for the management of obstructing left-sided colon cancer with potentially curable disease [21]. Furthermore, these guidelines, in addition to two retrospective studies, have demonstrated the efficacy of SEMS and interval colectomy in the setting of right-sided and transverse colon cancer. Therefore, this approach should be considered to provide decompression and an opportunity to perform a minimally invasive operation [21, 31, 76]. A decision analysis review by Targownik et al. reported not only a reduction in stoma formation and mortality but a significant decrease in cost for those requiring SEMS vs. emergent resection [77].

Malignant Disease

Despite advances in colorectal cancer screening, greater than one third of patients may present with a malignant LBO. The majority of current literature focuses on the utilization of this technique in cancer patients as either a palliative measure or a bridge to surgery [78, 79]. A Cochrane library review on the use of colorectal stents in the management of malignant bowel obstructions from 2011 concluded that stenting had no advantage over emergency surgery. This systematic review of five randomized trials identified a greater clinical success rate with primary resection; however, a longer hospital length of stay and a significantly greater risk of blood loss were reported in the surgical arm compared to endoluminal stenting [80]. Subsequently, Jimenez-Perez and colleagues, in a multicenter international randomized trial, demonstrated the efficacy of SEMS as a bridge to elective resection, with a 90% clinical success rate and only a 6% risk of stoma formation [81]. A randomized trial of 48 patients identified SEMS to be safe and provided a means to perform a laparoscopic resection and create a primary anastomosis. This approach resulted in improved perioperative complications to include a decrease in blood loss, postoperative pain control, anastomotic leak, wound infection, and rate of permanent stoma formation. From an oncologic standpoint, stenting as a bridge to surgery resulted in a greater median lymph node harvest (23 nodes) compared to an open emergent intervention, with only 11 nodes obtained. These findings may significantly affect the patient's prognosis [82].

The median survival of stage IV colorectal cancer has significantly improved from 9 to 12 months to greater than 24 months with advancements in chemotherapy; however, a cure from chemotherapy alone is rare [83] [84]. The long-term effects of endoscopic stenting when placed as a palliative measure may be questioned as the life expectancy increases with advanced disease. Stent patency rates at 12 months are approximately 50%. SEMS placement is associated with an increased frequency of subsequent operations or repeat stent placement at 1 year,

and this may result in significant morbidity [85, 86]. In a retrospective risk-adjusted analysis of 345 patients from the New York State Department of Health Statewide Planning and Research Cooperative System, patients undergoing stent placement were associated with a significantly decreased hospital length of stay, blood transfusion requirement, use of total parenteral nutrition, hospital charges, and death when compared to stoma creation as a palliative procedure. Furthermore, in this analysis, there was no significant difference in hospital readmission at 90 days and 1 year or the need for operative intervention at 90 days between these cohorts [86]. The long-term clinical success of SEMS is debatable; therefore, future surgical resection may be warranted based on the patient's clinical status and response to systemic chemotherapy [85].

Benign Disease

As experience and technology has grown with the use of SEMS for malignant disease, its success has now been applied in the setting of benign pathology. Technical placement is often more challenging as these strictures tend to be longer with a more torturous colonic wall. The majority of supporting evidence to date includes small case series, with a paucity of large retrospective data. Endoscopic stenting has been reported in the treatment of LBO secondary to anastomotic stricture, CD, diverticular stricture, radiation induced, and ischemic colitis. Technical success in stent placement is high (85–100%), and colonic decompression is achieved between 71% and 86% of the time [87, 88]. Diverticular strictures have been evaluated to the greatest extent. Cautious and careful SEMS placement is required as the risk of complications is reported as high as 38–71%. This includes the risk of stent migration, perforation, reobstruction, fistula formation, and stent fracture [73, 88, 89]. Small and colleagues evaluated 23 cases of an acute LBO secondary to benign disease and demonstrated that the majority (87%) of complications were identified 7 days following stent insertion. These patients were successfully bridged from an urgent to an elective operation, and over half were able to avoid a colostomy [73]. Levine et al. reported on the long-term follow-up of endoscopic stenting for five anastomotic strictures in the setting of CD. Mean patency length was over 30 months, with one complication. There is even a greater paucity of data in the management of de novo strictures in fibrostenotic CD, and the risk of malignancy must be strongly considered in these circumstances [90]. There is certainly a role for SEMS in a benign acute LBO; however, stent placement should be performed by an experienced endoscopist. Long-term stent placement appears to influence the risk of perforation; therefore, it is recommended this intervention be a means to convert an emergent operation to a semi-elective one with goals to minimize surgical complications and stoma creation.

Complications

Regardless of the indication for endoluminal stenting, this procedure has associated risks and potential complications. Small and colleagues demonstrated an overall complication rate of 24%, with the majority of adverse outcomes identified greater than 7 days following stent insertion. Minor complications to include hematochezia, fevers/bacteremia, and tenesmus all occurred <5% of the time. The overall rate of perforation was 8%, with a risk of stent occlusion and migration being 8% and 7%, respectively. Complications were significantly greater following palliative stenting, with a mean time to perforation of 27 days [62]. At a median time of 116 days post-stent placement, Gianotti and colleagues identified a 43% risk of complications. The rate of hospital readmission secondary to SEMS complications has been reported at 34% [91]. In a prospective multicenter trial of 182 patients by Jimenez-Perez et al., the risk of procedurally related major complications was 3.3%. The risk of perforation requiring surgical intervention was 1.7%. In addition, persistent obstruction occurred in 1.1% of cases, and transient bleeding occurred in one patient. Delayed postprocedural complications occurred in 4.2% of

patients, with one colonic perforation presenting 6 days after stent insertion. This is one of the largest reviews to date evaluating SEMS as a bridge to surgery, and this data supports the safety of this intervention [81]. Although stent-related perforation rates are low, there is a trend toward an increase in cancer recurrence and a potential decrease in disease-free survival following SEMS if complicated by a perforation. Furthermore, subclinical perforation is of concern as this may also impact overall survival [92]. There is limited data regarding the oncologic safety of SEMS. Despite these findings, previous studies have identified similar rates of both overall and cancer-specific survival [72, 93]. Reports on the outcomes following endoscopic colonic stenting are variable; nevertheless, multiple studies support the safety and efficacy of this approach. Patients should be well-informed, and the surgeon should be vigilant in detecting any complications when proceeding with this intervention.

Conclusion

Despite advances in the management of acute colorectal conditions, the treatment of a large bowel obstruction remains a complex surgical decision-making process. The presentation of this condition is quite variable, ranging from subtle findings to overt physiologic decompensation. The patient's presentation and clinical status will often dictate which intervention is required. However, in the era of advanced flexible endoscopy and minimally invasive surgery, patients now have an opportunity to potentially bridge an urgent or emergent operation to one that is semi-elective. This may avoid the significant morbidity associated with a laparotomy, as well as the risks of a permanent colostomy. Presently, there are multiple strategies to treat these patients, and the acute care surgeon should be well-versed in these techniques. Regardless of all the technology available, some patients may still require the creation of a stoma, and this should never be viewed as an unsuccessful operation. Each case should be individualized based on clinical status, comorbidities, location, as well as etiology of the obstruction. The patient should be well-informed on the risks, both operatively and oncologically, prior to any intervention. Nevertheless, maintaining a thoughtful algorithmic approach in the treatment of this condition will ultimately result in better outcomes and quality of life for these patients.

References

1. Byrne JJ. Large bowel obstruction. Am J Surg. 1960;99:168–78.
2. Siegel R, Desantis C, Jemal A. Colorectal cancer statistics, 2014. CA Cancer J Clin. 2014;64(2):104–17.
3. Athreya S, et al. Colorectal stenting for colonic obstruction: the indications, complications, effectiveness and outcome--5 year review. Eur J Radiol. 2006;60(1):91–4.
4. Lopez-Kostner F, Hool GR, Lavery IC. Management and causes of acute large-bowel obstruction. Surg Clin North Am. 1997;77(6):1265–90.
5. Yeo HL, Lee SW. Colorectal emergencies: review and controversies in the management of large bowel obstruction. J Gastrointest Surg. 2013;17(11):2007–12.
6. Boley SJ, et al. Pathophysiologic effects of bowel distention on intestinal blood flow. Am J Surg. 1969;117(2):228–34.
7. Stillwell GK. The law of Laplace. Some clinical applications. Mayo Clin Proc. 1973;48(12):863–9.
8. Saegesser F, et al. Intestinal distension and colonic ischemia: occlusive complications and perforations of colo-rectal cancers. A clinical application of Laplace's law. Chirurgie. 1974;100(7):502–16.
9. Vanek VW, Al-Salti M. Acute pseudo-obstruction of the colon (Ogilvie's syndrome). An analysis of 400 cases. Dis Colon Rectum. 1986;29(3):203–10.
10. Sawai RS. Management of colonic obstruction: a review. Clin Colon Rectal Surg. 2012;25(4):200–3.
11. Saunders MD. Acute colonic pseudo-obstruction. Gastrointest Endosc Clin N Am. 2007;17(2):341–60. vi-vii.
12. Melzig EP, Terz JJ. Pseudo-obstruction of the colon. Arch Surg. 1978;113(10):1186–90.
13. Swenson BR, et al. Colonic volvulus: presentation and management in metropolitan Minnesota, United States. Dis Colon Rectum. 2012;55(4):444–9.
14. Frager D, et al. Prospective evaluation of colonic obstruction with computed tomography. Abdom Imaging. 1998;23(2):141–6.
15. Chapman AH, McNamara M, Porter G. The acute contrast enema in suspected large bowel obstruction: value and technique. Clin Radiol. 1992;46(4):273–8.
16. Vandendries C, et al. Diagnosis of colonic volvulus: findings on multidetector CT with three-dimensional reconstructions. Br J Radiol. 2010;83(995):983–90.
17. Luning TH, et al. Colonoscopic perforations: a review of 30,366 patients. Surg Endosc. 2007;21(6):994–7.
18. Park JJ, et al. Stoma complications: the Cook County Hospital experience. Dis Colon Rectum. 1999;42(12):1575–80.
19. Morita S, et al. Outcomes in colorectal surgeon-driven Management of Obstructing Colorectal Cancers. Dis Colon Rectum. 2016;59(11):1028–33.
20. Phillips RK, et al. Malignant large bowel obstruction. Br J Surg. 1985;72(4):296–302.
21. Vogel JD, et al. The American Society of Colon and Rectal Surgeons clinical practice guidelines for the treatment of Colon Cancer. Dis Colon Rectum. 2017;60(10):999–1017.
22. Di Saverio S, et al. Intracorporeal anastomoses in emergency laparoscopic colorectal surgery from a series of 59 cases: where and how to do it - a technical note and video. Color Dis. 2017;19(4):O103–o107.
23. Li Z, et al. Comparative study on therapeutic efficacy between hand-assisted laparoscopic surgery and conventional laparotomy for acute obstructive right-sided Colon Cancer. J Laparoendosc Adv Surg Tech A. 2015;25(7):548–54.
24. Mistrangelo M, et al. Laparoscopic versus open resection for transverse colon cancer. Surg Endosc. 2015;29(8):2196–202.
25. Fernandez-Cebrian JM, et al. Laparoscopic colectomy for transverse colon carcinoma: a surgical challenge but oncologically feasible. Color Dis. 2013;15(2):e79–83.
26. Zeng WG, et al. Outcome of laparoscopic versus open resection for transverse Colon Cancer. J Gastrointest Surg. 2015;19(10):1869–74.
27. Wu Q, et al. Laparoscopic colectomy versus open colectomy for treatment of transverse Colon Cancer: a systematic review and meta-analysis. J Laparoendosc Adv Surg Tech A. 2017;27(10):1038–50.
28. Zhao L, et al. Long-term outcomes of laparoscopic surgery for advanced transverse colon cancer. J Gastrointest Surg. 2014;18(5):1003–9.
29. Amelung FJ, et al. Emergency resection versus bridge to surgery with stenting in patients with acute right-sided colonic obstruction: a systematic review focusing on mortality and morbidity rates. Int J Color Dis. 2015;30(9):1147–55.
30. Arai T, et al. Efficacy of self-expanding metallic stent for right-sided colonic obstruction due to carcinoma before 1-stage laparoscopic surgery. Surg Laparosc Endosc Percutan Tech. 2014;24(6):537–41.
31. Ji WB, et al. Clinical benefits and oncologic equivalence of self-expandable metallic stent insertion for right-sided malignant colonic obstruction. Surg Endosc. 2017;31(1):153–8.
32. Faucheron JL, et al. Emergency surgery for obstructing colonic cancer: a comparison between right-sided and left-sided lesions. Eur J Trauma Emerg Surg. 2017;44:71.

33. Lee YM, et al. Emergency surgery for obstructing colorectal cancers: a comparison between right-sided and left-sided lesions. J Am Coll Surg. 2001;192(6):719–25.
34. Goyal A, Schein M. Current practices in left-sided colonic emergencies: a survey of US gastrointestinal surgeons. Dig Surg. 2001;18(5):399–402.
35. Kozman DR, et al. Treatment of left-sided colonic emergencies: a comparison of US, UK and Australian surgeons. Tech Coloproctol. 2009;13(2):127–33.
36. Khoo RE, et al. Tube decompression of the dilated colon. Am J Surg. 1988;156(3 Pt 1):214–6.
37. Chiappa A, et al. One-stage resection and primary anastomosis following acute obstruction of the left colon for cancer. Am Surg. 2000;66(7):619–22.
38. Sasaki K, et al. One-stage segmental colectomy and primary anastomosis after intraoperative colonic irrigation and total colonoscopy for patients with obstruction due to left-sided colorectal cancer. Dis Colon Rectum. 2012;55(1):72–8.
39. Otsuka S, et al. One-stage colectomy with intraoperative colonic irrigation for acute left-sided malignant colonic obstruction. World J Surg. 2015;39(9):2336–42.
40. Lim JF, et al. Prospective, randomized trial comparing intraoperative colonic irrigation with manual decompression only for obstructed left-sided colorectal cancer. Dis Colon Rectum. 2005;48(2):205–9.
41. Kam MH, et al. Systematic review of intraoperative colonic irrigation vs. manual decompression in obstructed left-sided colorectal emergencies. Int J Color Dis. 2009;24(9):1031–7.
42. You YN, et al. Segmental vs. extended colectomy: measurable differences in morbidity, function, and quality of life. Dis Colon Rectum. 2008;51(7):1036–43.
43. Ghazal AH, et al. Colonic endolumenal stenting devices and elective surgery versus emergency subtotal/total colectomy in the management of malignant obstructed left colon carcinoma. J Gastrointest Surg. 2013;17(6):1123–9.
44. Danis J. Single-stage treatment for malignant left-sided colonic obstruction: a prospective randomized clinical trial comparing subtotal colectomy with segmental resection following intraoperative irrigation. Br J Surg. 1996;83(9):1303.
45. Hunerbein M, et al. Palliation of malignant rectal obstruction with self-expanding metal stents. Surgery. 2005;137(1):42–7.
46. Patel JA, et al. Is an elective diverting colostomy warranted in patients with an endoscopically obstructing rectal cancer before neoadjuvant chemotherapy? Dis Colon Rectum. 2012;55(3):249–55.
47. Wrenn K. Fecal impaction. N Engl J Med. 1989;321(10):658–62.
48. Mangiante EC, et al. Sigmoid volvulus. A four-decade experience. Am Surg. 1989;55(1):41–4.
49. Baker DM, et al. The management of acute sigmoid volvulus in Nottingham. J R Coll Surg Edinb. 1994;39(5):304–6.
50. Rabinovici R, et al. Cecal volvulus. Dis Colon Rectum. 1990;33(9):765–9.
51. Cosnes J, et al. Long-term evolution of disease behavior of Crohn's disease. Inflamm Bowel Dis. 2002;8(4):244–50.
52. Chen M, Shen B. Endoscopic therapy in Crohn's disease: principle, preparation, and technique. Inflamm Bowel Dis. 2015;21(9):2222–40.
53. Di Giorgio P, et al. Endoscopic dilation of benign colorectal anastomotic stricture after low anterior resection: a prospective comparison study of two balloon types. Gastrointest Endosc. 2004;60(3):347–50.
54. Bravi I, et al. Endoscopic electrocautery dilation of benign anastomotic colonic strictures: a single-center experience. Surg Endosc. 2016;30(1):229–32.
55. Pietropaolo V, et al. Endoscopic dilation of colonic postoperative strictures. Surg Endosc. 1990;4(1):26–30.
56. Dohmoto M. New method: endoscopic implantation of rectal stent in palliative treatment of malignant stenosis. Endosc Dig. 1991;3:1507–12.
57. Tejero E, et al. New procedure for the treatment of colorectal neoplastic obstructions. Dis Colon Rectum. 1994;37(11):1158–9.
58. Young CJ, et al. Improving quality of life for people with incurable large-bowel obstruction: randomized control trial of colonic stent insertion. Dis Colon Rectum. 2015;58(9):838–49.
59. Baron TH. Expandable gastrointestinal stents. Gastroenterology. 2007;133(5):1407–11.
60. Repici A, et al. Stenting of the proximal colon in patients with malignant large bowel obstruction: techniques and outcomes. Gastrointest Endosc. 2007;66(5):940–4.
61. Garcia-Cano J. Colorectal stenting as first-line treatment in acute colonic obstruction. World J Gastrointest Endosc. 2013;5(10):495–501.
62. Small AJ, Coelho-Prabhu N, Baron TH. Endoscopic placement of self-expandable metal stents for malignant colonic obstruction: long-term outcomes and complication factors. Gastrointest Endosc. 2010;71(3):560–72.
63. Boyle DJ, et al. Predictive factors for successful colonic stenting in acute large-bowel obstruction: a 15-year cohort analysis. Dis Colon Rectum. 2015;58(3):358–62.
64. Lee JH, et al. The learning curve for colorectal stent insertion for the treatment of malignant colorectal obstruction. Gut Liver. 2012;6(3):328–33.
65. Morris EJ, et al. Thirty-day postoperative mortality after colorectal cancer surgery in England. Gut. 2011;60(6):806–13.
66. Allievi N, et al. Endoscopic stenting as bridge to surgery versus emergency resection for left-sided malignant colorectal obstruction: an updated meta-analysis. Int J Surg Oncol. 2017;2017:2863272.
67. Lee HJ, et al. The role of primary colectomy after successful endoscopic stenting in patients with obstructive metastatic colorectal cancer. Dis Colon Rectum. 2014;57(6):694–9.

68. Vitale MA, et al. Preoperative colonoscopy after self-expandable metallic stent placement in patients with acute neoplastic colon obstruction. Gastrointest Endosc. 2006;63(6):814–9.
69. Zarnescu Vasiliu EC, et al. Morbidity after reversal of Hartmann operation: retrospective analysis of 56 patients. J Med Life. 2015;8(4):488–91.
70. Pearce NW, Scott SD, Karran SJ. Timing and method of reversal of Hartmann's procedure. Br J Surg. 1992;79(8):839–41.
71. Vermeulen J, et al. Avoiding or reversing Hartmann's procedure provides improved quality of life after perforated diverticulitis. J Gastrointest Surg. 2010;14(4):651–7.
72. Kavanagh DO, et al. A comparative study of short- and medium-term outcomes comparing emergent surgery and stenting as a bridge to surgery in patients with acute malignant colonic obstruction. Dis Colon Rectum. 2013;56(4):433–40.
73. Small AJ, Young-Fadok TM, Baron TH. Expandable metal stent placement for benign colorectal obstruction: outcomes for 23 cases. Surg Endosc. 2008;22(2):454–62.
74. Tierney W, et al. Enteral stents. Gastrointest Endosc. 2006;63(7):920–6.
75. Watt AM, et al. Self-expanding metallic stents for relieving malignant colorectal obstruction: a systematic review. Ann Surg. 2007;246(1):24–30.
76. Kye BH, et al. Comparison of long-term outcomes between emergency surgery and bridge to surgery for malignant obstruction in right-sided Colon Cancer: a multicenter retrospective study. Ann Surg Oncol. 2016;23(6):1867–74.
77. Targownik LE, et al. Colonic stent vs. emergency surgery for management of acute left-sided malignant colonic obstruction: a decision analysis. Gastrointest Endosc. 2004;60(6):865–74.
78. Serpell JW, et al. Obstructing carcinomas of the colon. Br J Surg. 1989;76(9):965–9.
79. Mella J, et al. Population-based audit of colorectal cancer management in two UK health regions. Colorectal Cancer working group, Royal College of Surgeons of England clinical epidemiology and audit unit. Br J Surg. 1997;84(12):1731–6.
80. Sagar J. Colorectal stents for the management of malignant colonic obstructions. Cochrane Database Syst Rev. 2011;11:CD007378.
81. Jimenez-Perez J, et al. Colonic stenting as a bridge to surgery in malignant large-bowel obstruction: a report from two large multinational registries. Am J Gastroenterol. 2011;106(12):2174–80.
82. Cheung HY, et al. Endolaparoscopic approach vs conventional open surgery in the treatment of obstructing left-sided colon cancer: a randomized controlled trial. Arch Surg. 2009;144(12):1127–32.
83. Hurwitz H, et al. Bevacizumab plus irinotecan, fluorouracil, and leucovorin for metastatic colorectal cancer. N Engl J Med. 2004;350(23):2335–42.
84. Grothey A, et al. Bevacizumab beyond first progression is associated with prolonged overall survival in metastatic colorectal cancer: results from a large observational cohort study (BRiTE). J Clin Oncol. 2008;26(33):5326–34.
85. van den Berg MW, et al. Long-term results of palliative stent placement for acute malignant colonic obstruction. Surg Endosc. 2015;29(6):1580–5.
86. Abelson JS, et al. Long-term Postprocedural outcomes of palliative emergency stenting vs stoma in malignant large-bowel obstruction. JAMA Surg. 2017;152(5):429–35.
87. Keranen I, et al. Outcome of patients after endoluminal stent placement for benign colorectal obstruction. Scand J Gastroenterol. 2010;45(6):725–31.
88. Suzuki N, et al. Colorectal stenting for malignant and benign disease: outcomes in colorectal stenting. Dis Colon Rectum. 2004;47(7):1201–7.
89. Pommergaard HC, et al. A clinical evaluation of endoscopically placed self-expanding metallic stents in patients with acute large bowel obstruction. Scand J Surg. 2009;98(3):143–7.
90. Levine RA, Wasvary H, Kadro O. Endoprosthetic management of refractory ileocolonic anastomotic strictures after resection for Crohn's disease: report of nine-year follow-up and review of the literature. Inflamm Bowel Dis. 2012;18(3):506–12.
91. Gianotti L, et al. A prospective evaluation of short-term and long-term results from colonic stenting for palliation or as a bridge to elective operation versus immediate surgery for large-bowel obstruction. Surg Endosc. 2013;27(3):832–42.
92. Sloothaak DA, et al. Oncological outcome of malignant colonic obstruction in the Dutch stent-in 2 trial. Br J Surg. 2014;101(13):1751–7.
93. Kim HJ, et al. Oncologic safety of stent as bridge to surgery compared to emergency radical surgery for left-sided colorectal cancer obstruction. Surg Endosc. 2013;27(9):3121–8.

Lower GI Bleeds

25

Katherine A. Kelley and Karen J. Brasel

Introduction

Lower gastrointestinal bleeding (LGIB) is the most common reason for GI bleeding, accounting for 30–40% of cases with patients reporting these symptoms [1]. The annual incidence is approximately 35–41 cases per 100,000 people in developed countries [2], and the average age of presentation is 63–77 years [3]. Mortality is estimated at 1.47% [2]. There is a rising incidence of this disease, likely due to the aging population of the United States and an increase in use of anticoagulants. LGIB has been reported as the most common diagnosis leading to hospitalization with greater than 500,000 discharges in 2012 at a cost of nearly five billion dollars [1].

A LGIB is defined as any bleeding below the ligament of Treitz. Hematochezia is the most common presenting symptom (55.5%), followed by maroon stool (16.7%), and melena (11.0%) [4]. It is important to note that these symptoms may also occur with rapid upper gastrointestinal bleeds. Recent literature has also cited "middle" gastrointestinal bleeds as a separate entity defined as bleeding from the small bowel. For the purpose of this chapter, we will discuss the manage-

ment of colonic and rectal acute bleeding. LGIB can also be subclassified into severe, moderate, and occult bleeds. Occult bleeding is slow and chronic and normally presents with microcytic hypochromic anemia. Stool is often guaiac positive. Moderate GI bleeds present with melena or hematochezia, but the patients remain hemodynamically normal. Severe GI bleeds are defined by melena or hematochezia with tachycardia, low urine output, and other signs of poor perfusion.

As a brief review, circulation to the colon and rectum is supplied via the superior mesenteric artery (SMA), inferior mesenteric artery (IMA), and internal iliac arteries, which are all branches of the aorta. The SMA branches include the ileocolic artery, right colic artery, and middle colic artery. The IMA supplies the left colic artery, the sigmoid artery, and the superficial rectal artery. The rectum is supplied by the superficial rectal artery and the middle and inferior rectal arteries, branches of the internal iliac, and the pudendal arteries, respectively. The SMA and IMA are connected via the marginal artery of Drummond, which may be a vital collateral in older individuals with vascular disease.

The majority of LGIBs will spontaneously resolve without intervention. Individuals needing hospital admission are those with ongoing or severe bleeding, with a transfusion requirement greater than two units of packed red blood cells (pRBCS), and those with significant comorbidities who require hemodynamic monitoring.

K. A. Kelley · K. J. Brasel (✉)
Department of Surgery, Oregon Health and Sciences
University, Portland, OR, USA
e-mail: brasel@ohsu.edu

© Springer International Publishing AG, part of Springer Nature 2019
C. V. R. Brown et al. (eds.), *Emergency General Surgery*, https://doi.org/10.1007/978-3-319-96286-3_25

Table 25.1 Risk factors that predict severity of lower GI bleed

Risk factors		
Heart rate >100 beats/min		
Systolic blood pressure ≤115 mmHg		
Syncope		
Non-tender abdominal exam		
Rectal bleeding in first 4 h		
Aspirin use (>81 mg)		
>2 comorbid illnesses		
Low risk	Moderate risk	High risk
0 factors	1–3 factors	> 3 factors
Likelihood of severe bleeding[a]		
9%	43%	84%

Adapted from [5]

[a]Severe bleeding defined as continued bleeding in the first 24 h or recurrent bleeding after 24 h of stability

Table 25.2 Common etiologies for lower gastrointestinal bleeding and their frequency

Etiology	Frequency
Diverticular bleeding	30–65%
Angiodysplasia	4–15%
Hemorrhoids	4–12%
Ischemic colitis	4–11%
Inflammatory bowel disease	3–15%
Colorectal neoplasia	2–11%
Post-polypectomy bleeding	2–7%
Rectal ulcer	0–8%

Multiple predictors of likelihood of bleeding severity have been identified: abnormal vital signs, syncope, non-tender abdominal exam, bleeding within 4 h of presentation, aspirin use, more than two comorbid diseases, initial hematocrit less than 35%, and gross blood on rectal exam [5, 6]. These factors can be used to stratify patients requiring admission. Additionally, multiple risk calculators have been designed to identify individuals at greater risk of morbidity and mortality [5, 7] (Table 25.1).

Etiology

There are multiple etiologies of LGIB, the most common cause of which is diverticular bleeding, while the following occur at lower frequencies: angiodysplasia, hemorrhoids, ischemic colitis, inflammatory bowel disease (IBD), neoplasia, post-polypectomy bleeding, and rectal ulcer (Table 25.2) [8].

Colonic Sources

Diverticulosis is a condition when multiple false diverticula of the colonic wall occur where the penetrating vessels perforate the circular muscle fibers. Diverticulosis is common in the aging population, but only a small proportion of these individuals will develop severe bleeding. The patient will likely present with painless hematochezia. Angiodysplasia is the degeneration of normal blood vessels that have a propensity to bleed. The right colon is most frequently involved. Patients with angiodysplasia are older with multiple comorbidities and will often present with occult bleeding or painless hematochezia [3]. Ischemic colitis is due to reduced mesenteric blood flow secondary to hypoperfusion, which most commonly affects the splenic flexure and leads to necrosis, sloughing, and then bleeding of the colonic wall. Patients commonly have concomitant cardiovascular disease and present with crampy abdominal pain and eventual hematochezia. A linear ulceration may be observed at the antimesenteric border on an endoscopy. IBD includes both Crohn's disease and ulcerative colitis. Crohn's disease is associated with transmural inflammation of the gastrointestinal tract and can involve the GI tract from the mouth to the perianal region. Ulcerative colitis is intermittent inflammation limited to the mucosal layer of the colon. It commonly involves the rectum and may extend in a proximal and continuous fashion to involve other parts of the colon. Both can present with hematochezia. Neoplasms are associated with slow bleeding and commonly demonstrate microcytic anemia. Patients may present with changes in bowel habits and weight loss. Left-sided cancers are more likely to present with hematochezia, while right-sided cancers will have hemoccult-positive stools. Post-polypectomy bleeding is often common and will be observed in individuals with recent colonoscopy. Infectious etiologies of lower GI bleeding are also possible. A majority of these individuals with colonic bleeding sources improve with conservative management [3].

Anorectal Sources

Anorectal disease, such as hemorrhoids and anal fissures, can present with bleeding and make up about 15% of cases. Anal fissures are tears in the anal mucosa, but do not typically develop significant bleeds. Individuals with hemorrhoids, which are distended anal arteriovenous duplexes, of either internal or external plexi, can develop profuse painless bleeding. Solitary rectal ulcers are the result of ischemic changes from the pressures exerted on the prolapsed tissues during defecation. Most anorectal sources of LGIBs can easily be identified on anoscopy.

Initial Assessment

Upon presentation to the hospital, a complete history and physical examination should be performed, and concurrent resuscitation should be initiated (Fig. 25.1). A history should include the following details: the amount of blood, color of the blood, frequency and duration of bleeding, history of gastroesophageal reflux disease (GERD), prior GI bleeding, weight loss, use of blood thinners, use of alcohol, recent colonoscopy, history of cancer, coagulopathy, colitis, IBD, or radiation therapy. The physical examination includes vital signs and abdominal and rectal exams. Anoscopy should be performed to rule out hemorrhoidal bleeding, rectal ulcers, or fissures. A complete blood cell count, metabolic panel, coagulopathy panel, as well as a type and cross should be collected. A CBC will help differentiate the chronicity of the blood loss (microcytic anemia suggests chronic blood loss). Additionally, a serum nitrogen/creatinine ratio of more than 30 increases the likelihood of upper GI bleed (UGIB) [10].

Resuscitation during the initial assessment includes placement of two large-bore IVs, monitoring, and IV fluid resuscitation. A nasogastric (NG) tube should be placed. NG lavage of blood or "coffee grounds" suggests an UGIB with need for subsequent upper endoscopy. LGIB resuscitation recommendations are based on multiple randomized controlled trials in UGIB that recommend early resuscitation. This

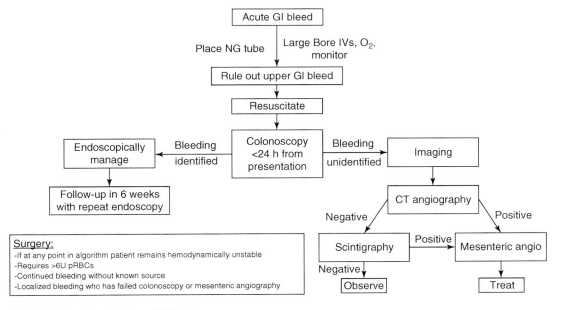

Fig. 25.1 Algorithm for lower GI bleeds

approach reduces mortality. Patients should be transfused to a goal hemoglobin greater than seven. Multiple studies have identified an improved mortality with restrictive resuscitation (Hb >7) rather than liberal (Hb >9) use of blood transfusion, which has predicted a slightly higher survival and reduced recurrence of bleeding [11, 13]. One may consider use of liberal transfusion (Hb >9) in individuals with massive bleeding, significant comorbid illness, or possible delay in receiving therapeutic interventions. We also recommend a platelet goal greater than 50,000 in individuals who may require endoscopic management and control of severe bleeding.

Diagnostic/Therapeutic Assessment

Colonoscopy

Colonoscopy remains the preferred tool for initial assessment of a LGIB. It can be used to identify, diagnose, and treat bleeding relatively efficiently and safely. Both insertion and withdrawal of the endoscope should be carefully performed; when done well, colonoscopy has a diagnostic yield of 91% [8]. As stated earlier, esophagogastroduodenoscopy should be performed in individuals who present with signs and symptoms consistent with UGIB. Various studies have reported conflicting results regarding the optimal timing of colonoscopy. Urgent colonoscopy is more likely to identify the stigmata of recent bleeding, but has no effect on length of stay, ICU stay, transfusion requirement, or mortality [14, 15]. According to American College of Gastroenterology (ACG) recommendations, at least 4 liters of polyethylene glycol solution, or the equivalent, should be administered over a period of 4 h prior to performing the colonoscopy. It should be administered at a rate of approximately 1 liter every 30–45 min and may be administered via an NG tube if there is a high risk of aspiration [3]. Patients should be without food for at least 8 h prior to colonoscopy but may have clear liquids until 2 h prior to intervention.

The most frequent endoscopic intervention used for management of LGIB is thermal contact plus injection therapy [8]. Epinephrine solution in a dilution of 1:10,000 or 1:20,000 is injected in aliquots of 1–2 mL at the site of active bleeding or around a nonbleeding visible vessel. The visible vessel may also be treated effectively by using a 10–15 J heater probe or bipolar coagulation (10–16 W), with 2–3-s pulse applications. Diverticular bleeding is appropriately managed with this approach [16]. Angiodysplasia can be treated effectively with argon plasma ablation therapy with a low risk of recurrence [17]. The argon beam is easy to apply and is able to treat large surface areas with a predictable depth of penetration. Lower power settings of 30–45 W at 1 L/minute argon flow rate are used to decrease the risk for perforation in the thin-walled right side of the colon. The probe should be held between 1 and 3 mm away from the mucosal surface and applied at 1–2-s pulses [3]. Endoscopic clip placement is an alternative treatment option. Clips can be deployed over a bleeding vessel at the neck of the diverticulum or to oppose the walls and close the diverticular orifice. This management strategy has a low risk of recurrence [18]. Post-polypectomy bleeding is best treated with mechanical clip or contact thermal therapy with the addition of epinephrine injection as indicated. Endoscopic band ligation for diverticular bleeding is a novel treatment strategy that may be limited by inadequate suction of diverticula with small orifices or large domes.

Endoscopic interventions carry a 0.3–0.6% complication rate, suggesting these strategies are feasible and safe [8]. Placement of a tattoo should be performed in order to assess the area at later intervals or if surgical intervention is eventually required. If there is evidence of recurrent bleeding, colonoscopy may be attempted again. Individuals with ischemic colitis, inflammatory ulcerative colitis, or colorectal neoplasms are generally not amenable to endoscopic hemostasis, and if bleeding persists, surgical management should be discussed.

Imaging

In individuals who cannot be prepped or stabilized for colonoscopy or have failed localization on colonoscopy, computed tomographic angiog-

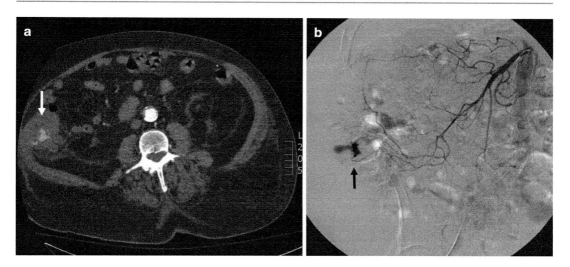

Fig. 25.2 Sample images from concurrent use of CTA and therapeutic angiography for LGIB. (**a**) Blush is noted in the ascending colon on CTA (white arrow); (**b**) contrast extravasation is noted from the SMA on angiography (black arrow)

Table 25.3 Efficacy of imaging strategies for LGIB

Imaging strategy	Rate of bleeding	Diagnostic yield	Therapeutic efficacy	Risk of early rebleed	Rate of complications
Radionuclide scan	0.1–0.5 ml/min	40–73%	NA	NA	Rare
CTA	0.3 ml/min	24–94%	NA	NA	0–11%
Angiography	0.5 ml/min	23–72%	14–100%	1–57%	0–60%

raphy (CTA) with the potential addition of radio-nuclide technetium-99 m-labeled red-cell scintigraphy is indicated. CTA has a sensitivity of 91–92% and can detect bleeding rate of 0.3 mL/minute (Table 25.3). It is considered more sensitive, reduces the total number of imaging procedures, and is more precise at locating the bleed than other imaging strategies. Successful identification of bleeding source will most likely lead to mesenteric angiography; however, in institutions lacking interventional radiology capabilities, it can be used to guide surgical management (Fig. 25.2).

The addition of scintigraphy can also localize bleeding and improve the diagnostic yield of CTA by 2.4 times, [20]. It can detect bleeding rates of 0.1–0.5 ml/minute (Table 25.3). Based on a retrospective review of 160 patients, individuals with immediate blush on scintigraphy require immediate angiography. If blush was seen within 2 min, the positive predictive value was 75%, while those who had a blush that appeared greater

than 2 min later, there was a negative predictive value of 93% [19]. The study is positive in 38% of patients, with an accuracy rate of 30% [21].

The above strategies are used to determine if there is a benefit to utilizing mesenteric angiography. CTA can localize bleeding in 24–94% of select cases [22], but angiography alone is overall less sensitive and may have a positive yield of only 35% [23]. When angiography is used in combination with CTA, there is 100% accuracy [24]. In patients who are hemodynamically normal, a mesenteric angiogram can detect bleeding at a rate of 0.5 mL/min (Table 25.3). In practice, the SMA, IMA, and the celiac are investigated. Angiographic interventions include selective vasopressin infusion and super selective angio-embolization. Embolization with micro-coils, polyvinyl alcohol particles, glue, Gelfoam, vascular plugs, or water-insoluble gelatin may improve the success rate of this technique and decrease the occurrence of adverse events. Embolization can be safely performed with a low risk of morbidity [25]. Side effects include fever and abdominal pain. Adverse events of bowel infarction, nephrotoxicity, and groin hematoma may occur in up to 17% of individuals but are individually too infrequent to quantify [24, 26].

Operative Management

Surgery may be needed to control bleeding in 10–25% of patients with active bleeding that persists despite resuscitation and endoscopic/angiographic interventions, recurrent bleeding, or requiring greater than six units of PRBCS in 24 h. Individuals with an identified source of bleeding are candidates for segmental colectomies; however, they have a higher risk of recurrent bleeding than those who undergo a total colectomy [27]. In individuals without an identified bleeding source, despite complete intestinal evaluation, subtotal abdominal colectomies may be necessary. Segmental colectomies in patients without an identified bleeding source but suggested external pathology are discouraged as the mortality rate is higher due to the risk of rebleed [29]. In individuals who do not require surgery initially, approximately 10% will require surgical management following either a rebleed or the need for elective resection of diverticular disease [28].

Outcomes

Following management of LGIB, poor outcomes are associated with creatinine greater than 1.7 mg/dL, age over 60 years, abnormal hemodynamic parameters on presentation, and persistent bleeding within the first 24 h [9]. Multiple scoring systems have been designed to predict hospital outcomes for patients with acute lower GI bleeds [30]. Those with higher risk of in-hospital mortality are those with intestinal ischemia, comorbid illness, active malignancy, bleeding during a separate cause of hospitalization, coagulopathy, hypocalcemia, transfusion, and male

gender. Colorectal polyps and hemorrhoidal bleeding are associated with the lowest risk of mortality [31, 32]. Recurrent bleeding is anticipated in approximately 21% of patients and will require readmission. Individuals on anticoagulation and those with active malignancy have the highest risk of recurrence.

Other Circumstances

Coagulopathy

Patients presenting with LGIB are frequently on blood thinners for various diseases. These therapies include aspirin, clopidogrel, warfarin, direct thrombin inhibitors, and factor Xa inhibitors. These interventions have been associated with an increased incidence of LGIB. [33, 34]. Conversely, individuals on heparin or low molecular weight heparin deep venous thrombosis (DVT) prophylaxis only have a 0.2% risk of GI bleeds. [39]. GI bleeding in individuals on the former medications may be managed by cessation of the product and reversal with either vitamin K, fresh frozen plasma (FFP), or PCC. Direct thrombin inhibitors can be stopped as the half-lives of the drugs are usually 12–24 h and will be reversed by the time endoscopy is performed [35]. In cases of severe bleeding, use of specific reversal agents, such as idarucizumab for dabigatran and andexanet alfa for factor Xa inhibitors, may be used [35].

For individuals with drug-eluting cardiac stents, short-term discontinuation of a clopidogrel with continued aspirin therapy is safe greater than 12 months from stent placement but is tolerated if under this time frame [36]. Following LGIB management and bleeding cessation, continuation of aspirin is associated with an increased risk of recurrent LGIB, but reduced risk of serious cardiovascular events and death. Providers must therefore discuss the risks and benefits of this therapy [37]. Use of a PPI or histamine H_2 receptor antagonist should be encouraged, as it reduces the risk of upper GI bleeding, when compared with no therapy [38].

Occult GI bleeding

In patients who have an obscure GI bleed, capsule endoscopy can be used to identify middle GI bleeds with a sensitivity of 95% and specificity of 75% [40]. Push enteroscopy or double-balloon enteroscopy may be attempted in hemodynamically normal patients. Additionally, intraoperative enteroscopy/colonoscopy can be considered in individuals who are hemodynamically unstable and require operative intervention without identified bleeding source. Additional endoscopic interventions include topical hemostasis agents that are currently under study and may provide options for treatment [41], as well as endoscopic band ligation of diverticular hemorrhage [42].

Conclusions

Acute LGIB is a frequent cause of hospitalization. The most common etiologies are diverticular bleeding, angiodysplasia, and hemorrhoids. The main goals of patient care are to stabilize, localize, and treat. Localization can be completed with either urgent colonoscopy or CTA with appropriate interventions as available. Colectomy is reserved for those patients who continue to bleed following these interventions, those who remain hemodynamically abnormal, or those requiring greater than six units of pRBCs. The management of this field continues to evolve with the advancement of endoscopic and angiographic interventions, but surgery remains a safe definitive treatment in many cases.

References

1. Peery AF, Crockett SD, Barritt AS, Dellon ES, Eluri S, Gangarosa LM, Jensen ET, Lund JL, Pasricha S, Runge T, Schmidt M, Shaheen NJ, Sandler RS. Burden of Gastrointestinal, Liver, and Pancreatic Diseases in the United States. Gastroenterology. 2015;149:1731–41. e3.
2. Laine L, Yang H, Chang SC, Datto C. Trends for incidence of hospitalization and death due to GI complications in the United States from 2001 to 2009. Am J Gastroenterol. 2012;107:1190–5. quiz 1196.
3. Committee ASOP, Pasha SF, Shergill A, Acosta RD, Chandrasekhara V, Chathadi KV, Early D, Evans JA, Fisher D, Fonkalsrud L, Hwang JH, Khashab MA, Lightdale JR, Muthusamy VR, Saltzman JR, Cash BD. The role of endoscopy in the patient with lower GI bleeding. Gastrointest Endosc. 2014;79:875–85.
4. Gayer C, Chino A, Lucas C, Tokioka S, Yamasaki T, Edelman DA, Sugawa C. Acute lower gastrointestinal bleeding in 1,112 patients admitted to an urban emergency medical center. Surgery. 2009;146:600–6. discussion 606-7.
5. Strate LL, Saltzman JR, Ookubo R, Mutinga ML, Syngal S. Validation of a clinical prediction rule for severe acute lower intestinal bleeding. Am J Gastroenterol. 2005;100:1821–7.
6. Velayos FS, Williamson A, Sousa KH, et al. Early predictors of severe lower gastrointestinal bleeding and adverse outcomes: a prospective study. Clin Gastroenterol Hepatol. 2004;2:485–90.
7. Aoki T, Nagata N, Shimbo T, Niikura R, Sakurai T, Moriyasu S, Okubo H, Sekine K, Watanabe K, Yokoi C, Yanase M, Akiyama J, Mizokami M, Uemura N. Development and Validation of a Risk Scoring System for Severe Acute Lower Gastrointestinal Bleeding. Clin Gastroenterol Hepatol. 2016;14:1562–1570.e2.
8. Strate LL, et al. The role of colonoscopy and radiological procedures in the management of acute lower intestinal bleeding. Clin Gastroenterol Hepatol. 2010;8(4):333–43.
9. Newman J, Fitzgerald JE, Gupta S, Von Roon AC, Sigurdsson HH, Allen-Mersh TG. Outcome predictors in acute surgical admissions for lower gastrointestinal bleeding. Color Dis. 2012;14:1020–6.
10. Srygley FD, Gerardo CJ, Tran T, Fisher DA. Does this patient have a severe upper gastrointestinal bleed? JAMA. 2012;307:1072–9.
11. Baradarian R, Ramdhaney S, Chapalamadugu R, Skoczylas L, Wang K, Rivilis S, Remus K, Mayer I, Iswara K, Tenner S. Early intensive resuscitation of patients with upper gastrointestinal bleeding decreases mortality. Am J Gastroenterol. 2004;99:619–22.
12. Villanueva C, Colomo A, Bosch A, Concepcion M, Hernandez-Gea V, Aracil C, Graupera I, Poca M, Alvarez-Urturi C, Gordillo J, Guarner-Argente C, Santalo M, Muniz E, Guarner C. Transfusion strategies for acute upper gastrointestinal bleeding. N Engl J Med. 2013;368:11–21.
13. Odutayo A, Desborough MJ, Trivella M, Stanley AJ, Doree C, Collins GS, Hopewell S, Brunskill SJ, Kahan BC, Logan RF, Barkun AN, Murphy MF, Jairath V. Restrictive versus liberal blood transfusion for gastrointestinal bleeding: a systematic review and meta-analysis of randomised controlled trials. Lancet Gastroenterol Hepatol. 2017;2:354–60.
14. Green BT, Rockey DC, Portwood G, Tarnasky PR, Guarisco S, Branch MS, Leung J, Jowell P. Urgent colonoscopy for evaluation and management of acute lower gastrointestinal hemorrhage: a randomized controlled trial. Am J Gastroenterol. 2005;100:2395–402.
15. Seth A, Khan MA, Nollan R, Gupta D, Kamal S, Singh U, Kamal F, Howden CW. Does Urgent Colonoscopy Improve Outcomes in the Management of Lower Gastrointestinal Bleeding? Am J Med Sci. 2017;353:298–306.

16. Jensen DM, Machicado GA, Jutabha R, Kovacs TO. Urgent colonoscopy for the diagnosis and treatment of severe diverticular hemorrhage. N Engl J Med. 2000;342:78–82.

17. Olmos JA, Marcolongo M, Pogorelsky V, Herrera L, Tobal F, Davolos JR. Long-term outcome of argon plasma ablation therapy for bleeding in 100 consecutive patients with colonic angiodysplasia. Dis Colon Rectum. 2006;49:1507–16.

18. Kaltenbach T, Watson R, Shah J, Friedland S, Sato T, Shergill A, Mcquaid K, Soetikno R. Colonoscopy with clipping is useful in the diagnosis and treatment of diverticular bleeding. Clin Gastroenterol Hepatol. 2012;10:131–7.

19. Ng DA, Opelka FG, Beck DE, Milburn JM, Witherspoon LR, Hicks TC, Timmcke AE, Gathright JB. Predictive value of technetium Tc 99m-labeled red blood cell scintigraphy for positive angiogram in massive lower gastrointestinal hemorrhage. Dis Colon Rectum. 1997;40:471–7.

20. Gunderman R, Leef J, Ong K, Reba R, Metz C. Scintigraphic screening prior to visceral arteriography in acute lower gastrointestinal bleeding. J Nucl Med. 1998;39:1081–3.

21. Feuerstein JD, Ketwaroo G, Tewani SK, Cheesman A, Trivella J, Raptopoulos V, Leffler DA. Localizing Acute Lower Gastrointestinal Hemorrhage: CT Angiography Versus Tagged RBC Scintigraphy. AJR Am J Roentgenol. 2016;207(3):578–84.

22. Jaeckle T, Stuber G, Hoffmann MH, Jeltsch M, Schmitz BL, Aschoff AJ. Detection and localization of acute upper and lower gastrointestinal (GI) bleeding with arterial phase multi-detector row helical CT. Eur Radiol. 2008;18(7):1406–13.

23. Browder W, Cerise EJ, Litwin MS. Impact of emergency angiography in massive lower gastrointestinal bleeding. Ann Surg. 1986;204:530–6.

24. Zahid A, Young CJ. Making decisions using radiology in lower GI hemorrhage. Int J Surg. 2016;31:100–3.

25. Koh DC, Luchtefeld MA, Kim DG, Knox MF, Fedeson BC, Vanerp JS, Mustert BR. Efficacy of transarterial embolization as definitive treatment in lower gastrointestinal bleeding. Colorectal Dis. 2009;11(1):53–9.

26. Yi WS, Garg G, Sava JA. Localization and definitive control of lower gastrointestinal bleeding with angiography and embolization. Am Surg. 2013;79:375–80.

27. Farner R, Lichliter W, Kuhn J, Fisher T. Total colectomy versus limited colonic resection for acute lower gastrointestinal bleeding. Am J Surg. 1999;178:587–91.

28. Mcguire HH. Bleeding colonic diverticula. A reappraisal of natural history and management. Ann Surg. 1994;220(5):653.

29. Baker R, Senagore A. Abdominal colectomy offers safe management for massive lower GI bleed. Am Surg. 1994;60(8):578–81. discussion 582.

30. Kollef MH, O'brien JD, Zuckerman GR, Shannon W. BLEED: a classification tool to predict outcomes in patients with acute upper and lower gastrointestinal hemorrhage. Crit Care Med. 1997;25:1125–32.

31. Sengupta N, Tapper EB, Patwardhan VR, Ketwaroo GA, Thaker AM, Leffler DA, Feuerstein JD. Risk factors for adverse outcomes in patients hospitalized with lower gastrointestinal bleeding. Mayo Clin Proc. 2015;90:1021–9.

32. Strate LL, Ayanian JZ, Kotler G, Syngal S. Risk factors for mortality in lower intestinal bleeding. Clin Gastroenterol Hepatol. 2008;6:1004–10.

33. Casado Arroyo R, Polo-Tomas M, Roncales MP, Scheiman J, Lanas A. Lower GI bleeding is more common than upper among patients on dual antiplatelet therapy: long-term follow-up of a cohort of patients commonly using PPI co-therapy. Heart. 2012;98:718–23.

34. Abraham NS, Hartman C, Richardson P, Castillo D, Street RL, Naik AD. Risk of lower and upper gastrointestinal bleeding, transfusions, and hospitalizations with complex antithrombotic therapy in elderly patients. Circulation. 2013;128:1869–77.

35. Cheung KS, Leung WK. Gastrointestinal bleeding in patients on novel oral anticoagulants: Risk, prevention and management. World J Gastroenterol. 2017;23:1954–63.

36. Eisenberg MJ, Richard PR, Libersan D, Filion KB. Safety of short-term discontinuation of antiplatelet therapy in patients with drug-eluting stents. Circulation. 2009;119:1634–42.

37. Chan FK, Leung Ki EL, Wong GL, Ching JY, Tse YK, Au KW, Wu JC, Ng SC. Risks of bleeding recurrence and cardiovascular events with continued aspirin use after lower gastrointestinal hemorrhage. Gastroenterology. 2016;151:271–7.

38. Abraham NS, Hlatky MA, Antman EM, Bhatt DL, Bjorkman DJ, Clark CB, Furberg CD, Johnson DA, Kahi CJ, Laine L, Mahaffey KW, Quigley EM, Scheiman J, Sperling LS, Tomaselli GF. ACCF/ACG/AHA 2010 expert consensus document on the concomitant use of proton pump inhibitors and thienopyridines: a focused update of the ACCF/ACG/AHA 2008 expert consensus document on reducing the gastrointestinal risks of antiplatelet therapy and NSAID use. Am J Gastroenterol. 2010;105:2533–49.

39. Leonardi MJ, Mcgory ML, Ko CY. The rate of bleeding complications after pharmacologic deep venous thrombosis prophylaxis: a systematic review of 33 randomized controlled trials. Arch Surg. 2006;141(8):790–7. discussion 797–9.

40. Hartmann D, Schmidt H, Bolz G, Schilling D, Kinzel F, Eickhoff A, Huschner W, Moller K, Jakobs R, Reitzig P, Weickert U, Gellert K, Schultz H, Guenther K, Hollerbuhl H, Schoenleben K, Schulz HJ, Riemann JF. A prospective two-center study comparing wireless capsule endoscopy with intraoperative enteroscopy in patients with obscure GI bleeding. Gastrointest Endosc. 2005;61:826–32.

41. Barkun AN, Moosavi S, Martel M. Topical hemostatic agents: a systematic review with particular emphasis on endoscopic application in GI bleeding. Gastrointest Endosc. 2013;77:692–700.

42. Ishii N1, Setoyama T, Deshpande GA, Omata F, Matsuda M, Suzuki S, Uemura M, Iizuka Y, Fukuda K, Suzuki K, Fujita Y. Endoscopic band ligation for colonic diverticular hemorrhage. Gastrointest Endosc. 2012;75(2):382–7.

Ischemic Colitis

26

Dirk C. Johnson and Kimberly A. Davis

Introduction

Ischemic colitis (IC) is the most common form of ischemic injury to the gastrointestinal tract. Its annual incidence is approximately 1.6 patients per 100,000 and has remained constant for decades [75]. IC is the etiology of acute lower GI bleeding in 9–24% of hospitalized patients and affects up to 18/100,000 hospitalized patients [10]. Often IC is transient with reversible clinical symptoms. There are two common subtypes of IC: severe (15%) and more commonly mild-moderate (85%). Severe IC has transmural necrosis and is often associated with multisystem organ failure (MOF). The other variety rarely presents with MOF [84]. Most cases occur spontaneously, although some may occur after a cardiac event or in the postoperative period, commonly after aortic and cardiac surgery [89].

Ischemic colitis affects a wide variety of patients especially the elderly. It is poorly studied despite being relatively common. As the population ages, it will likely be more commonly encountered.

D. C. Johnson (✉)
Department of General Surgery, Trauma and Acute Medical Care, Yale University, New Haven, CT, USA
e-mail: Dirk.johnson@yale.edu

K. A. Davis
Department of Surgery, Yale School of Medicine, New Haven, CT, USA

History

In 1948, Thomson first reported a case of colonic ischemia which gives insight to the difficulty in diagnosing ischemic colitis (IC). In his seminal description, he alluded that the relative rarity of large bowel ischemia in comparison with small bowel ischemia was the prevailing sentiment of that time [87]. In the following decade, colon ischemia was more commonly recognized and became associated with abdominal aortic operations [59, 80]. A transient variant of IC was defined in the early 1960s and called "reversible vascular occlusion of the colon" by Boley [6]. Soon thereafter, an expanded clinical description including endoscopic and histological findings was reported [52]. However, it is Marston who is credited with putting IC in its broader clinical context [58].

Anatomy

Colonic perfusion is autoregulated but has significant influence from extrinsic factors as well as intrinsic demands such as motility, metabolism, and humoral elements [32]. The colon has less blood flow and comparatively less vascular redundancy than small bowel making it more vulnerable to ischemia [29]. The typical vascular supply of the colon includes flow from the both the superior mesenteric artery (SMA) and the inferior mesenteric artery (IMA). The SMA usu-

© Springer International Publishing AG, part of Springer Nature 2019
C. V. R. Brown et al. (eds.), *Emergency General Surgery*, https://doi.org/10.1007/978-3-319-96286-3_26

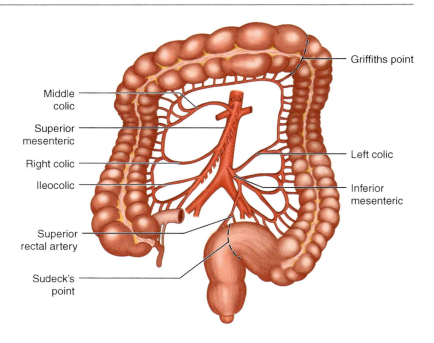

ally divides into left and right branches with the right eventually giving rise to ileocolic, right colic, and middle colic arteries. The left colon is supplied by the IMA and its branches left colic and sigmoid arteries. The IMA is half the caliber or the SMA at their origins from the aorta. Other branches of the IMA along with branches of the internal iliac arteries perfuse the rectum and anal canal [76].

Mesenteric blood supply is highly collateralized in general. In the colon, the main collaterals are the marginal artery of Drummond (MAD) and the meandering artery of Moskowitz. The MAD is the most important redundancy between the SMA and IMA. It runs a short distance from the mesenteric border of the colon and is fed from a network of tributaries from the right, middle, and left colic and sigmoidal arteries [47]. The MAD is more reliably found on the left as compared to the right where it is poorly developed in up to 75% of people. Gradual stenosis of the SMA or IMA may be compensated by dilation of MAD or the meandering artery (of Moskowitz), formerly known as the arc of Riolan. The arc of Riolan and the meandering artery of Moskowitz are vaguely defined vessels that form connections between the middle and left colic arteries and are found near the base of the colonic

mesentery. They represent some confusion, and it has been proposed that their distinction should be abolished [50]. The rectum has dual bloody supply from both the IMA and internal iliac arteries; it is rarely found to be ischemia [34].

There are two notable points of vulnerability in the colonic blood supply: Griffith's point and Sudeck's point [Fig. 26.1]. Griffith's point is where the limits of the middle colic and left colic distributions meet at the splenic flexure. In this area, the marginal artery of Drummond is underdeveloped in up to 30% of patients or absent in as many 5% of the population [60, 83]. Less commonly affected is Sudeck's point, which is at the territorial confluence of the sigmoidal artery and the superior rectal arteries but distal to the last at the level of the rectosigmoid junction [72, 76]. Both points have less redundancy and more reliance on the larger arteries leaving them unprotected during episodes of reduced flow. Both points of poor collateral circulation are referred to as a "watershed" areas [83]. The most commonly affected segment is the left colon (32.6%), followed by the distal colon (24.6%), right colon (25.2%), and entire colon (7.3%). The frequencies of dominant hepatic and splenic flexure involvement were much lower at 1.23 and 4.8%, respectively. The sigmoid was involved in 20.8% of all cases [9].

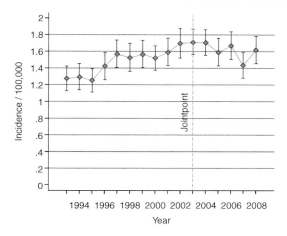

Fig. 26.2 Annual incidence for IC for patients requiring colectomy in the USA. (Sadler. *Can J Gastroenterol Hepatol* 2014 [75])

Epidemiology

IC is the most common form of gastrointestinal ischemia comprising as much as 60% of an intestinally ischemia. It is likely underreported leaving the true incidence unclear and understudied [Fig. 26.2]. The rate may be increasing or may represent better recognition [90]. A large series of IC cases found evidence to suggest the most cases of IC may occur in outpatient settings suggesting that hospitalized patients may be in the minority [54]. The estimates in general populations range from 4.5 to 44 hospitalizations per 100,000 person-years [38, 54, 90]. The largest US study estimated the incidence at approximately 15 hospitalizations for 100,000 person-years [54]. Most studies agree there is a strong female predominance especially in younger patients [54, 82]. There is speculation that oral contraceptive use may be a risk factor of IC in young women [20]. The classic patient is both elderly and female [9, 38, 54, 64, 79].

Pathophysiology and Risk Factors

IC occurs when the blood flow the colon is inadequate to meet demand. The disease process is flow based and not related to anatomic arterial occlusion. There is an abrupt decrease of perfusion to the colonic wall due to hypovolemia lead-ing to inadequate flow in small arterioles [7, 9]. Hypoperfusion can be from many causes including anatomic restrictions to flow, hypovolemia, underlying hematologic disorders, vasculitides, and the use of drugs (prescribed or illicit).

There are a multitude of documented risk factors that should raise clinician's suspicion of IC. Chronic diseases including cardiovascular disorders and atherosclerosis can lead low flow states and are associated with vasoactive medications and hypovolemia. Chronic renal failure requiring hemodialysis and chronic constipation are also associated with IC [32]. Acute infectious causes have been reported [44, 66]. In younger patients, underlying vasculitides, hypercoagulable states, strenuous exercise resulting in hypovolemia, and illicit drug use may cause IC [14, 20, 46, 51, 56, 85]. Postsurgical patients, particularly after cardiac and aortic operations, are at risk. A history of prior operations including cardiac, aortic, or gastrointestinal exists in almost half of patients [67].

Underlying Chronic Disease States

End-stage renal disease requiring dialysis is a recognized risk factor for the development of IC. The rapid exchange of body fluids and the presence of hypotension that occurs during hemodialysis may cause contraction of the mesenteric arteries, especially the superior mesenteric artery, thereby inducing IC of the right colon [13].

Prescription Medications

The literature reports more than 20 different agents related cases of IC. Antihypertensive agents account for 12.5% of all reports of medication-induced IC. Chemotherapeutic drugs (9%), immunosuppressive agents (5%), and anticoagulants (3%) have also been associated. Other common classes of prescription drug are lipid-lowering agents (3%), platelet aggregation inhibitors (2%), antidiabetics (2%), acid-suppressive agents (3%), and supplements, probiotics, or enzymes (6%). Mental health agents have also been indicted with antipsychotics (4%) more common than antidepressants (2%) [5].

Constipation is a rare but reported cause of IC Ischemic especially in patients with irritable bowel syndrome (IBS). Some cases are associated with alosetron, a drug used to treat refractory diarrhea-predominant IBS. The proposed mechanism is related to elevated intraluminal pressure reducing blood flow resulting in segmental colonic wall ischemia [3, 30]. Constipation along with smoking was the most common risk factor identified in young otherwise healthy IC patients, although not occurring statistically more often than in older patients [46]. In the IBS population, the relative risk for IC was 2.78 times higher for patients with constipation alone [81]. Laxative use is a confounding in this group. The impact of cathartics has not been studied as it relates to IC in the IBS population but may increase to incidence of perforation. Two medications for treatment of irritable bowel syndrome, tegaserod and alosetron, have each been removed from the US market at least in part due to their association with IC [5].

Bleeding Disorders

Abnormal clotting is observed in 28–74% of patients with IC [25]. While not surprising, hypercoagulable states like antiphospholipid antibody syndrome and factor V Leiden mutation are overrepresented present in patients with IC. These disease states are tenfold more common in IC than in the general population [89]. Other blood dyscrasias are associated with IC which include systemic lupus erythematosus, polycythemia vera, antithrombin deficiency, protein C and S deficiencies, and paroxysmal nocturnal hemoglobinuria [42, 62].

Postsurgical Patients

A common iatrogenic cause of IC is surgery on the abdominal aorta. IC can be a severe adverse event after both open and endovascular abdominal aortic aneurysm repair. Fortunately the prevalence is low (2–3%), but the mortality rate is high (>50%) [4, 61, 70]. Surgical disruption of flow through the IMA during aortic reconstruction without adequate collaterals from the MAD is the etiology in these patients. IC is more common following repair of ruptured aortas (9%) and open repairs (1.9 vs 0.5% endovascular) [70]. Irrespective of the operative technique, IC is associated with elevated rates of morbidity and double to quadruple mortality rates [30, 70]. Risk factors for postoperative IC following aneurysm repair include pre-existing renal failure, rupture, suprarenal extension, diabetes, bleeding dyscrasias, and significant intraoperative blood loss necessitating transfusion [61].

Intraabdominal hypertension has been identified as an important mechanism behind colonic hypoperfusion after ruptured AAA repair [22]. IMA reimplantation and restoration of flow to the hypogastric artery in high-risk patients may reduce the rates of postoperative IC, but this remains controversial [61].

IC after cardiac surgery with extracorporeal circulation is an infrequent but highly lethal complication with an incidence of <1% and mortality range of 30–100% [1, 57]. The inflammatory changes from cardiopulmonary bypass can compromise the barrier typically provided by colonic mucosa in the normal state. Furthermore, intraoperative hypothermia and vasoconstrictive medications may exacerbate colonic ischemia [1, 88] Long cross-clamp times, need for intra-aortic balloon pumps, and elevated serum lactate are risk factors for developing IC [33, 35]. Depressed cardiac output and consequent splanchnic hypoperfusion can lead to an irreversible ischemic insult. Serum lactate levels above 5 mmol associated with metabolic acidosis should raise suspicion for mesenteric ischemia, although due to lack of specificity, their utility is debated [33, 37].

Younger Patients and Athletes

A retrospective study of IC in young Japanese patients suggested smoking and uremia were more significant risk factors than in elderly patients. [46]. Autoimmune vasculitis, myointimal hyperplasia of mesenteric vein, and infectious colitis are other risk factors for IC in younger patients [18, 36]. Hormonal therapy with estrogens and oral contraceptives pills have long been associated with some thrombotic risks, and IC is among them [63].

Long-distance running is connected to IC, particularly in younger patients, and has been dubbed "runner's colitis" [14, 24, 56]. It can occur even after relatively short runs [40]. Runners tend to develop their ischemia in the cecum and right colon. Hypoperfusion is related to the duration and intensity of activity, insufficient previous training, dehydration, hypovolemia from perspiration and high temperatures, polycythemia, and hyponatremia [14, 40, 56]. Most cases improve with nonoperative management [14].

Cocaine, well known for its vasoconstrictive properties, has been identified as a cause of IC particularly in young people as having methamphetamines [51]. Patients with cocaine although typically younger have a significantly higher mortality than matched controls [26]. Chronic use of both drugs can induce ischemia via activation of adrenergic receptors [39].

Diagnosis

There is no typical clinical presentation of IC. Common findings include the abrupt onset of crampy often mild abdominal pain, generally in the left lower quadrant. The pain may be associated with lower GI bleeding and the urge to defecate. More severe cases of IC may present with distention, anorexia, nausea, and vomiting. Signs of impending sepsis may be present in severe cases. Most patients have insidious symptoms and no clear precipitating factor. Because of the wide differential for this constellation of symptoms, diagnosis is often delayed as a workup ensues [64]. Laboratory findings are nonspecific and therefore of limited clinical value. Commonly patients will present with leukocytosis and metabolic acidosis. Lactic dehydrogenase acidosis, base deficit, and leukocytosis may be present in more severe or advanced cases but should be considered relatively late signs [60, 89]. Experimentally, lactate isomer assays for D-lactate have been shown to be more specific, but this is not widely available in clinical practice [71]. Recent studies have offered serum procalcitonin levels as corollary of colonoscopic findings, and additional data point to guide therapeutic decisions in postoperative ischemic colitis [17].

IC is a spectrum of disease, including reversible colopathy with submucosal or intramural hemorrhage, transient colitis, chronic colitis, stricture, gangrene, and fulminant pancolitis. Complete recovery is likely for mild cases where the ischemia is confined to the mucosa, the most vulnerable layer of the colon. Severe cases affecting additional layers of the colonic wall may have long-term sequela such as scarring and strictures. Transmural ischemia can lead to gangrene, perforation, peritonitis, and sepsis [60].

IC can be divided based on its vascular distribution in to left and right variants with tendency toward subtle changes in clinical presentation. Left IC is more typically associated with shock, coagulation disorders, aortic operations, and cardiac disease. It is more likely to present with hematochezia than right IC. In contrast, right IC less often presents with hematochezia but more often associated with SMA stenosis and end-stage renal disease [12, 31, 72]. A subset of right IC can have a presentation that mimics a mass in the proximal colon especially in elderly women [45].

Imaging Studies

Plain Radiography

X-rays of the abdomen are of low yield in diagnosing IC especially mild or early cases. When obtained early in the disease course, a nonspecific gas pattern or distended loops consistent with an ileus should be expected. If necrosis and perforation is suspected, an upright abdominal film can identify pneumoperitoneum and indication for an emergency operation. Between these extremes phase, mucosal thickening from edema or hemorrhage can be seen and is frequently described as "thumbprinting." Pneumatosis is rarely seen but when present is highly suggestive of ischemia but is seen in other disease states (i.e., infectious colitis and any immunosuppressant therapy) [19, 74, 89]. The diagnostic accuracy of plain radiographs may be augmented by the instillation of barium into the colon. Suggestive BE findings are thumbprinting, pseudopolyps, sacculation, tubular narrowing, and a ragged, saw-toothed irregularity of the mucosa. This practice is largely of historical interest in the acute diagnosis of IC, as barium installation impedes endoscopic evaluation and may cause perforation [89].

Sonography

Ultrasonography can detect colonic wall edema and suggests IC with appropriate clinical correlation. Segmental thickening of large bowel longer than 10 cm, in symptomatic patients older 50 years, is highly correlated (87.5%PPV) with endoscopic findings of IC [55]. According to Lopez et al., abdominal sonography has a high positive predictive value in detecting IC (PPV 87.5%). The sensitivity of ultrasound for detecting thickening has been demonstrated to be high (93%) [73]. The ease of repeating examinations affords the opportunity to follow disease progression. However, typically limitations of the technology related to overlying bowel gas and operator experience are factors, as is the low sensitivity in states of hypoperfusion with color Doppler sonography [89].

Computerized Tomography (CT)

CT is an accurate imaging tool for the evaluation of abdominal pain of all types including patients suspected to have IC symptoms. Mild to moderate IC manifests as thickened bowel walls, luminal dilatation, adjacent fat stranding, and occasionally ascites [89]. Stratified attenuation or the double halo or target signs may be present. In this pattern, two (double halo) or three (target) concentric and symmetric layers of alternating densities can be distinguished in edematous colon images with intravenous contrast enhancement [86] [Fig. 26.3]. The degree of inflammation, edema, or bleeding can influence the heterogeneity of the colonic thickening which is most often circumferential [2, 74, 79, 86]. Segments of abnormally thick walls of 8–9 mm are not uncommon [2, 28]. Acute mesenteric arterial occlusion may be identified by CT, but due to lack of reperfusion, the bowel wall is paper thin [11, 28, 41].

Angiography

Angiographic evaluation is generally not indicated in the diagnosis of IC, because IC is

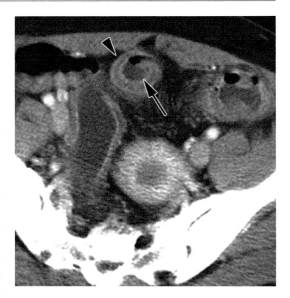

Fig. 26.3 Transverse CT demonstrates the double halo, or target, sign with inner (mucosa, arrow) and outer (muscularis propria, arrowhead) rings of high attenuation separated by a ring of low attenuation, which represents submucosa with edema [86]

related to perfusion and flow abnormalities more commonly than to fixed anatomic abnormalities. If a fixed lesion is suspected, abnormalities of the mesenteric vasculature may be better seen with CT angiogram due to its ability to identify luminal irregularities from atherosclerosis and thrombi [48, 79]. It is infrequently employed but can help elucidate the etiology of IC [48, 79]. The potential increase in information gained from a CT angiography must be weighed against the greater risks. Those additional risks include radiocontrast-induced nephropathy, additional radiation, and higher cost as compared to contrast-enhanced CT without proven clinical benefit [79]. Formal digital subtraction angiography may show mesenteric artery occlusion, increased arterial caliber, or other more subtle findings but is seldom helpful in the diagnosis [25].

Endoscopy

Lower GI endoscopy is the gold standard to establish the diagnosis, as the first part of the colon to lose perfusion is the antimesenteric mucosa. Early endoscopy should be considered when CT scan findings are suspicious [29]. Colonoscopy should be avoided in patients with signs of diffuse peritonitis. When done in acute IC, colonoscopy should be performed with minimal insufflation to avoid excessive distension of the colon, which could worsen the existing ischemia of the wall. CO_2 insufflation is preferable, as CO_2 is rapidly absorbed and exerts a vasodilating action [89]. Bowel preparation prior to colonoscopy is not indicated, as this may induce toxic dilation or perforation of the colon [60].

Colonoscopy findings are dependent on the phase and extent of ischemia. Early ischemia of the mucosa appears pale, friable, or edematous alone but can have petechial hemorrhages, erosions, and patches of erythema, with or without ulcerations and bleeding [Fig. 26.4]. A single linear ulcer or strip of mucosal inflammation running along the antimesenteric border is associated with mild

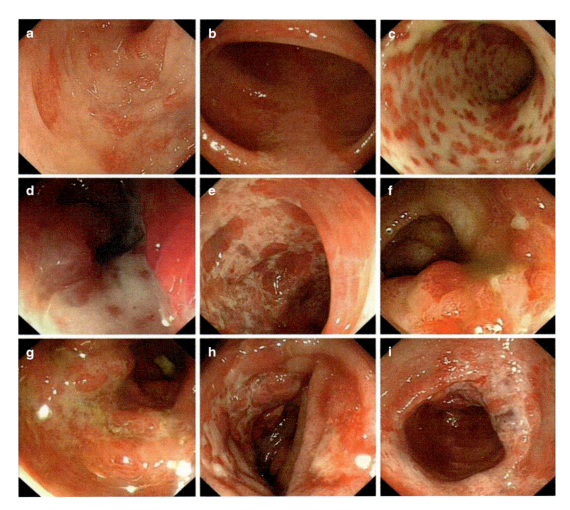

Fig. 26.4 Endoscopic findings of ischemic colitis. (**a**) Patchy erythema and mucosal congestion in rectosigmoid junction. (**b**) A single linear ulcer running along the longitudinal axis of the descending colon. (**c**) Petechial hemorrhages interspersed with pale areas in the descending colon. (**d**) Cyanotic, edematous mucosa with scattered ulceration in the sigmoid colon. (**e**) Pseudomembranes with purple-hemorrhagic nodules in the descending colon. (**f**) Congestive mucosa and pseudopolyps in the descending colon. (**g**) Mucosal edema, exudate and pseudotumor-like in the descending colon. (**h**) Bluish-black mucosal nodules with mucosal congestion and hemorrhage in the ascending colon approaching hepatic flexure. (**i**) Lumen structure and mucosal granularity in the descending colon [92]

Table 26.1 Favier endoscopic classification

Stage	Endoscopic findings	Mortality
Stage 1	Ischemia limited to the mucosa with petechiae and small ulcerations with intervening healthy mucosa	0%
Stage 2	Ischemia extending to the muscularis mucosa with large ulcerations	(−) MOF = 0%
		(+) MOF = 53%
Stage 3	Transmural ischemia with necrosis of the muscularis and possible perforation	(−) MOF = 17%
		(+) MOF = 66%

cases. Later findings are bluish-black mucosal nodules with a dark or dusky background. More rarely pseudopolyps, pseudotumor-like, and pseudomembranes are found. Chronic IC has a much different appearance with strictures, abnormal haustrations, and granular-appearing mucosa [92].

The Favier endoscopic classification grades the extent of colonic ischemic and standardizes disease severity [15] [Table 26.1]. Unfortunately, none of these endoscopic findings are unique for ischemia. Segmental abnormalities with abrupt transition between normal and diseased mucosa with normal rectum can help distinguish ischemia from other conditions such as IBD [27, 92].

When biopsies are taken, the nonspecific pathological findings include erosion, granulation tissue hyperplasia, bleeding in the lamina propria, and macrophages with hemosiderin pigmentation in the submucosa [30, 92]. Advanced ischemia shows epithelial loss, inflammatory cells, and submucosal congestion within the specimens [89].

Critically Ill Patients

Patients in intensive care units can present as mammoth diagnostic challenges. Altered sensorium from sepsis or sedation, mechanical ventilation, and heavy narcotic analgesia may obscure signs and symptoms. Furthermore, active comorbid conditions like cardiac, respiratory, and renal failure may make transportation to definitive testing difficult or impossible. This may result in delay of the diagnosis and adversely affect outcomes.

Endoscopy in the ICU is the most useful test for critically ill patients with hematochezia where IC is suspected. Bedside upper endoscopy is widely accepted and used as an early diagnostic test for upper gastrointestinal bleeding in the ICU setting. In contrast, lower endoscopy for hematochezia is much less widely used, studied, and accepted [23].

Nonoperative Management

Medical management is appropriate for mild to moderate IC. Since hypovolemia and hypoperfusion are the core pathophysiologic derangements, the primary goal is to restore normal tissue oxygenation before the target cells are beyond salvage [60, 63]. All management strategies typically start with bowel rest to decrease metabolic demands associated with digestion. Oral intake should be restricted to essential medications. Total parenteral nutrition may be required depending on the severity of the disease and the time to symptom resolution, which generally takes 8–14 days [8, 72]. Any precipitating factors such as medications should be discontinued immediately [89]. Broad-spectrum antibiotics are widely recommended, but there is very little scientific evidence for their use [10]. Coverage for enteric aerobic and anaerobic flora designed to treat translocation of bacteria from the weakened mucosa and consequent bacteremia is standard. Clinicians should adhere to the principles of antibiotics stewardship and tailor antimicrobial coverage and discontinue coverage as soon as it is appropriate.

After successful medical management of moderate to severe cases, endoscopy should be performed every 3–4 months to assess for sequela of IC. Structuring is a common finding and colonoscopy can diagnose the condition and allow for mechanical dilatation. Chronic colitis resulting from continuous colon ischemia or unhealed areas of ischemic mucosa should be treated with elective colectomy [43, 89].

Surgical Management

Indications for operative intervention may be urgent or delayed. Surgical intervention is required in 20% of cases [49]. Indications for immediate operative intervention include the presence of diffuse peritonitis on exam, evidence of necrosis on CT imaging (pneumatosis, portal venous air, intraperitoneal air, megacolon), or endoscopic visualization (irreversible necrosis of the colonic mucosa and muscularis) [62, 65]. Surgery is also indicated in patients with less severe endoscopic evidence of ischemia, if there is evidence of MOF or if the patient fails to improve within 24–48 h of maximal medical management. In this population, laparoscopy can be helpful as it can detect the presence of transmural gangrene of the affected part of the large bowel, with/without perforation and peritonitis [69, 23]. Delayed operative intervention may be indicated for ongoing diarrhea, continued lower GI bleeding, or persistent colitis despite 14 days of treatment. Chronic indications for surgery include symptomatic colonic strictures and protein-losing colopathy.

In the operating room, determining the extent of resection can be a challenge, but all gangrenous bowel must be resected. This is most often done via midline laparotomy. The external appearance of healthy serosa may obscure underlying submucosal infarction. An intraoperative colonoscopy can be used when there is a question [34]. Other intraoperative tools to evaluate the perfusion of the colon include Doppler ultrasonography, photoplethysmography, oxygen electrodes, pulse oximetry of transcolonic oxygen saturation, and fluorescein. The most common method, universally applicable evaluation, is direct inspection by the bowel in question to verify adequacy of the surgical margins [89]. As many as 25% of patients may need an additional resection [78].

Resectional procedures may be done also in cases of chronic ischemia, i.e., chronic segmental colitis with recurrent sepsis, and colonic strictures causing obstructive symptoms. Patients who have developed a stricture after an acute episode of IC or have a stricture as a result from chronic ischemia may be treated with segmental colectomy [43, 89].

Outcomes

The prognosis after an episode of IC is related mainly to the degree of ischemic insult to the mural tissues [89]. Most cases are mild and of short duration resolving rapidly with nonoperative management. These cases have an excellent prognosis, and two-thirds or more of these patients can be successfully managed without an operation [23]. Complete clinical recovery can be expected within 2 weeks, with improvement of mucosal findings [89]. The overall mortality for IC is 22%, which rises to 39% for severe cases requiring a partial or total colectomy [21, 75, 91].

Overall predictors of poor outcomes include male gender, tachycardia, a lack of rectal bleeding, peritonitis, septic shock, and location of ischemia in the right colon [68, 82]. Severe comorbidities, such as liver disease, renal disease, and congestive heart failure, increase mortality. Lower socioeconomic status also portends toward a worse prognosis and likely represents poorer overall health status [75].

Approximately 20% of patients will need emergency surgical intervention, and this portends a poor prognosis [43, 49, 75, 77, 89]. The majority of postoperative deaths occur within 30 days of surgery [53, 89]. Pre-existing cardiac failure (ejection fraction of <20%), acute kidney injury, metabolic acidosis and a pressor requirement, previous history of cardiovascular surgery, ASA score ≥ 4, and surgical delay ≥3 days are independent risk factors for postoperative mortality [67, 75].

For most patients, the long-term prognosis for IC is favorable. Recurrence rates are about 3% within 1 year and increase yearly to nearly 10% at 5 years. Survival rate 5 years after admission for IC is 69% and most of the deaths are unrelated to IC [16].

Conclusion

Ischemic colitis has a variable and nonspecific presentation and makes the diagnosis difficult, even for seasoned providers. Clinical suspicion should be piqued by the presence of identified risk factors that can lead to earlier recognition of this potentially lethal disease. CT and colonoscopy are the best initial tools to evaluate for IC. Most cases respond with nonoperative management, but surgery may be needed. Prompt diagnosis and treatment are of vital importance but must start with clinical suspicion of this often-insidious condition.

Key Points

- IC is the most common type of intestinal ischemia.
- The mechanism of ischemic colitis is typically hypoperfusion.
- Presenting symptoms are abdominal pain and tenderness followed by hematochezia.
- Focal vascular lesions are unusual; therefore angiography has a limited role.
- Computed tomography is an excellent screening tool.
- Colonoscopy is the diagnostic gold standard and is safe when performed carefully.
- Most cases can be treated with supportive care.
- Twenty percent of patients will require surgery despite medical management because of peritonitis, full-thickness necrosis, MOF, or clinical deterioration.
- Severe cases managed nonoperatively should be monitored for late complications.

References

1. Arif R, Farag M, Zaradzki M, Reissfelder C, Pianka F, Bruckner T, Kremer J, Franz M, Ruhparwar A, Szabo G, Beller CJ, Karck M, Kallenbach K, Weymann A. Ischemic colitis after cardiac surgery: can we foresee the threat? PLoS One. 2016;11(12):e0167601. https://doi.org/10.1371/journal.pone.0167601.
2. Balthazar EJ, Yen BC, Gordon RB. Ischemic colitis: CT evaluation of 54 cases. Radiology. 1999;211(2):381–8. https://doi.org/10.1148/radiology.211.2.r99ma28381.
3. Beck IT. Possible mechanisms for ischemic colitis during alosetron therapy. Gastroenterology. 2001;121(1):231–2.
4. Becquemin JP, Majewski M, Fermani N, Marzelle J, Desgrandes P, Allaire E, Roudot-Thoraval F. Colon ischemia following abdominal aortic aneurysm repair in the era of endovascular abdominal aortic repair. J Vasc Surg. 2008;47(2):258–63 discussion 263. https://doi.org/10.1016/j.jvs.2007.10.001.
5. Bielefeldt K. Ischemic colitis as a complication of medication use: an analysis of the Federal Adverse Event Reporting System. Dig Dis Sci. 2016;61(9):2655–65. https://doi.org/10.1007/s10620-016-4162-x.
6. Boley SJ, Schwartz S, Lash J, Sternhill V. Reversible vascular occlusion of the colon. Surg Gynecol Obstet. 1963;116:53–60.
7. Brandt L, Boley S, Goldberg L, Mitsudo S, Berman A. Colitis in the elderly. A reappraisal. Am J Gastroenterol. 1981;76(3):239–45.
8. Brandt LJ, Feuerstadt P. Beyond low flow: how I manage ischemic colitis. Am J Gastroenterol. 2016;111(12):1672–4. https://doi.org/10.1038/ajg.2016.456.
9. Brandt LJ, Feuerstadt P, Blaszka MC. Anatomic patterns, patient characteristics, and clinical outcomes in ischemic colitis: a study of 313 cases supported by histology. Am J Gastroenterol. 2010;105(10):2245–52 quiz 2253. https://doi.org/10.1038/ajg.2010.217.
10. Brandt LJ, Feuerstadt P, Longstreth GF, Boley SJ, Gastroenterology, A. C. O. ACG clinical guideline: epidemiology, risk factors, patterns of presentation, diagnosis, and management of colon ischemia (CI). Am J Gastroenterol. 2015;110(1):18–44 quiz 45. https://doi.org/10.1038/ajg.2014.395.
11. Cappell MS, Mahajan D, Kurupath V. Characterization of ischemic colitis associated with myocardial infarction: an analysis of 23 patients. Am J Med. 2006;119(6):527.e521–9. https://doi.org/10.1016/j.amjmed.2005.10.061.
12. Chang HJ, Chung CW, Ko KH, Kim JW. Clinical characteristics of ischemic colitis according to location. J Korean Soc Coloproctol. 2011;27(6):282–6. https://doi.org/10.3393/jksc.2011.27.6.282.
13. Choi SR, Jee SR, Song GA, Park SJ, Lee JH, Song CS, Park HU. Predictive factors for severe outcomes in ischemic colitis. Gut Liver. 2015;9(6):761–6. https://doi.org/10.5009/gnl15167.
14. Cohen DC, Winstanley A, Engledow A, Windsor AC, Skipworth JR. Marathon-induced ischemic colitis: why running is not always good for you. Am J Emerg Med. 2009;27(2):255.e255–7. https://doi.org/10.1016/j.ajem.2008.06.033.
15. Colin R, Balmes JL, Favier C. Endoscopy in the diagnosis of regressive ischemic colitis. Chirurgie. 1974;100(1):49–51.
16. Cosme A, Montoro M, Santolaria S, Sanchez-Puertolas AB, Ponce M, Durán M, Cabriada JL, Borda N, Sarasqueta C, Bujanda L. Prognosis and follow-up of 135 patients with ischemic colitis over a five-year period. World J Gastroenterol. 2013;19(44):8042–6. https://doi.org/10.3748/wjg.v19.i44.8042.
17. Cossé C, Sabbagh C, Fumery M, Zogheib E, Mauvais F, Browet F, Rebibo L, Regimbeau JM. Serum procalcitonin correlates with colonoscopy findings and can guide therapeutic decisions in postoperative ischemic

colitis. Dig Liver Dis. 2017;49(3):286–90. https://doi.org/10.1016/j.dld.2016.12.003.

18. Costa MN, Saiote J, Pinheiro MJ, Duarte P, Bentes T, Ferraz Oliveira M, Ramos J. Segmental colitis caused by idiopathic myointimal hyperplasia of mesenteric veins. Rev Esp Enferm Dig. 2016;108(12):821–6. https://doi.org/10.17235/reed.2016.4051/2015.

19. Cuschieri J, Florence M, Flum DR, Jurkovich GJ, Lin P, Steele SR, Symons RG, Thirlby R, Collaborative, S. Negative appendectomy and imaging accuracy in the Washington state surgical care and outcomes assessment program. Ann Surg. 2008;248(4):557–63. https://doi.org/10.1097/SLA.0b013e318187aeca.

20. Deana DG, Dean PJ. Reversible ischemic colitis in young women. Association with oral contraceptive use. Am J Surg Pathol. 1995;19(4):454–62.

21. Díaz Nieto R, Varcada M, Ogunbiyi OA, Winslet MC. Systematic review on the treatment of ischaemic colitis. Color Dis. 2011;13(7):744–7. https://doi.org/10.1111/j.1463-1318.2010.02272.x.

22. Djavani K, Wanhainen A, Valtysson J, Björck M. Colonic ischaemia and intra-abdominal hypertension following open repair of ruptured abdominal aortic aneurysm. Br J Surg. 2009;96(6):621–7. https://doi.org/10.1002/bjs.6592.

23. Doulberis M, Panagopoulos P, Scherz S, Dellaporta E, Kouklakis G. Update on ischemic colitis: from etiopathology to treatment including patients of intensive care unit. Scand J Gastroenterol. 2016;51(8):893–902. https://doi.org/10.3109/00365521.2016.1162325.

24. Eichner ER. Ischemic colitis in athletes. Curr Sports Med Rep. 2011;10(5):242–3. https://doi.org/10.1249/JSR.0b013e31822d354b.

25. Elder K, Lashner BA, Al Solaiman F. Clinical approach to colonic ischemia. Cleve Clin J Med. 2009;76(7):401–9. https://doi.org/10.3949/ccjm.76a.08089.

26. Elramah M, Einstein M, Mori N, Vakil N. High mortality of cocaine-related ischemic colitis: a hybrid cohort/case-control study. Gastrointest Endosc. 2012;75(6):1226–32. https://doi.org/10.1016/j.gie.2012.02.016.

27. Favier C, Bonneau HP, Tran Minh V, Devic J. Endoscopic diagnosis of regressive ischemic colitis. Endoscopic, histologic and arteriographic correlations. Nouv Presse Med. 1976;5(2):77–9.

28. Fernandes T, Oliveira MI, Castro R, Araújo B, Viamonte B, Cunha R. Bowel wall thickening at CT: simplifying the diagnosis. Insights Imaging. 2014;5(2):195–208. https://doi.org/10.1007/s13244-013-0308-y.

29. Feuerstadt P, Brandt LJ. Colon ischemia: recent insights and advances. Curr Gastroenterol Rep. 2010;12(5):383–90. https://doi.org/10.1007/s11894-010-0127-y.

30. FitzGerald JF, Hernandez Iii LO. Ischemic colitis. Clin Colon Rectal Surg. 2015;28(2):93–8. https://doi.org/10.1055/s-0035-1549099.

31. Flobert C, Cellier C, Berger A, Ngo A, Cuillerier E, Landi B, Marteau P, Cugnenc PH, Barbier JP. Right

colonic involvement is associated with severe forms of ischemic colitis and occurs frequently in patients with chronic renal failure requiring hemodialysis. Am J Gastroenterol. 2000;95(1):195–8. https://doi.org/10.1111/j.1572-0241.2000.01644.x.

32. Gandhi SK, Hanson MM, Vernava AM, Kaminski DL, Longo WE. Ischemic colitis. Dis Colon Rectum. 1996;39(1):88–100.

33. Ghosh S, Roberts N, Firmin RK, Jameson J, Spyt TJ. Risk factors for intestinal ischaemia in cardiac surgical patients. Eur J Cardiothorac Surg. 2002;21(3):411–6.

34. Green BT, Tendler DA. Ischemic colitis: a clinical review. South Med J. 2005;98(2):217–22. https://doi.org/10.1097/01.SMJ.0000145399.35851.10.

35. Groesdonk HV, Klingele M, Schlempp S, Bomberg H, Schmied W, Minko P, Schäfers HJ. Risk factors for nonocclusive mesenteric ischemia after elective cardiac surgery. J Thorac Cardiovasc Surg. 2013;145(6):1603–10. https://doi.org/10.1016/j.jtcvs.2012.11.022.

36. Guillén-Paredes MP, Martínez-Fernández J, Valero Navarro G. Segmental intestinal necrosis in a young patient. Rev Esp Enferm Dig. 2017;109(9):666. https://doi.org/10.17235/reed.2017.4880/2017.

37. Hasan S, Ratnatunga C, Lewis CT, Pillai R. Gut ischaemia following cardiac surgery. Interact Cardiovasc Thorac Surg. 2004;3(3):475–8. https://doi.org/10.1016/j.icvts.2004.04.003.

38. Higgins PD, Davis KJ, Laine L. Systematic review: the epidemiology of ischaemic colitis. Aliment Pharmacol Ther. 2004;19(7):729–38. https://doi.org/10.1111/j.1365-2036.2004.01903.x.

39. Holubar SD, Hassinger JP, Dozois EJ, Masuoka HC. Methamphetamine colitis: a rare case of ischemic colitis in a young patient. Arch Surg. 2009;144(8):780–2. https://doi.org/10.1001/archsurg.2009.139.

40. Horta D, Puig V, Melcarne L. Ischemic colitis in an athlete: running is not always good for you. Rev Esp Enferm Dig. 2016;108(7):443. https://doi.org/10.17235/reed.2016.4184/2015.

41. Iacobellis F, Berritto D, Fleischmann D, Gagliardi G, Brillantino A, Mazzei MA, Grassi R. CT findings in acute, subacute, and chronic ischemic colitis: suggestions for diagnosis. Biomed Res Int. 2014;2014:895248. https://doi.org/10.1155/2014/895248.

42. Iannella I, Candela S, Di Libero L, Argano F, Tartaglia E, Candela G. Ischemic necrosis with sigmoid perforation in a patient with systemic lupus erythematosus (SLE): case report. G Chir. 2012;33(3):77–80.

43. Jin NC, Kim HS, Kim DH, Song YA, Kim YJ, Seo TJ, Park SY, Park CH, Joo YE, Choi SK, Rew JS. A comparison of clinical characteristics between medically-treated patients and surgically-treated patients with ischemic colitis. Clin Endosc. 2011;44(1):38–43. https://doi.org/10.5946/ce.2011.44.1.38.

44. Kendrick JB, Risbano M, Groshong SD, Frankel SK. A rare presentation of ischemic pseudomem-

branous colitis due to Escherichia coli O157:H7. Clin Infect Dis. 2007;45(2):217–9. https://doi.org/10.1086/518990.

45. Khor TS, Lauwers GY, Odze RD, Srivastava A. "Mass-forming" variant of ischemic colitis is a distinct entity with predilection for the proximal colon. Am J Surg Pathol. 2015;39(9):1275–81. https://doi.org/10.1097/PAS.0000000000000438.

46. Kimura T, Shinji A, Horiuchi A, Tanaka N, Nagaya T, Shigeno T, Nakamura N, Komatsu M, Umemura T, Arakura N, Matsumoto A, Tanaka E. Clinical characteristics of young-onset ischemic colitis. Dig Dis Sci. 2012;57(6):1652–9. https://doi.org/10.1007/s10620-012-2088-5.

47. Kornblith PL, Boley SJ, Whitehouse BS. Anatomy of the splanchnic circulation. Surg Clin North Am. 1992;72(1):1–30.

48. Korotinski S, Katz A, Malnick SD. Chronic ischaemic bowel diseases in the aged--go with the flow. Age Ageing. 2005;34(1):10–6. https://doi.org/10.1093/ageing/afh226.

49. Kwak HD, Kang H, Ju JK. Fulminant gangrenous ischemic colitis: is it the solely severe type of ischemic colitis? Int J Color Dis. 2017;32(1):147–50. https://doi.org/10.1007/s00384-016-2700-9.

50. Lange JF, Komen N, Akkerman G, Nout E, Horstmanshoff H, Schlesinger F, Bonjer J, Kleinrensink GJ. Riolan's arch: confusing, misnomer, and obsolete. A literature survey of the connection(s) between the superior and inferior mesenteric arteries. Am J Surg. 2007;193(6):742–8. https://doi.org/10.1016/j.amjsurg.2006.10.022.

51. Linder JD, Mönkemüller KE, Raijman I, Johnson L, Lazenby AJ, Wilcox CM. Cocaine-associated ischemic colitis. South Med J. 2000;93(9):909–13.

52. Littman L, Boley SJ, Schwartz S. Sigmoidoscopic diagnosis of reversible vascular occlusion of the colon. Dis Colon Rectum. 1963;6:142–6.

53. Longo WE, Ballantyne GH, Gusberg RJ. Ischemic colitis: patterns and prognosis. Dis Colon Rectum. 1992;35(8):726–30.

54. Longstreth GF, Yao JF. Epidemiology, clinical features, high-risk factors, and outcome of acute large bowel ischemia. Clin Gastroenterol Hepatol. 2009;7(10):1075–1080.e1071-1072 quiz 1023. https://doi.org/10.1016/j.cgh.2009.05.026.

55. López E, Ripolles T, Martinez MJ, Bartumeus P, Blay J, López A. Positive predictive value of abdominal sonography in the diagnosis of ischemic colitis. Ultrasound Int Open. 2015;1(2):E41–5. https://doi.org/10.1055/s-0035-1559775.

56. Lucas W, Schroy PC. Reversible ischemic colitis in a high endurance athlete. Am J Gastroenterol. 1998;93(11):2231–4. https://doi.org/10.1111/j.1572-0241.1998.00621.x.

57. Mangi AA, Christison-Lagay ER, Torchiana DF, Warshaw AL, Berger DL. Gastrointestinal complications in patients undergoing heart operation: an analysis of 8709 consecutive cardiac surgical patients. Ann Surg. 2005;241(6):895–901. discussion 901-894.

58. Marston A, Pheils MT, Thomas ML, Morson BC. Ischaemic colitis. Gut. 1966;7(1):1–15.

59. Mckain J, Shumacker HB. Ischemia of the left colon associated with abdominal aortic aneurysms and their treatment. AMA Arch Surg. 1958;76(3):355–7.

60. Misiakos EP, Tsapralis D, Karatzas T, Lidoriki I, Schizas D, Sfyroeras GS, Moulakakis KG, Konstantos C, Machairas A. Advents in the diagnosis and Management of Ischemic Colitis. Front Surg. 2017;4:47. https://doi.org/10.3389/fsurg.2017.00047.

61. Moghadamyeghaneh Z, Sgroi MD, Chen SL, Kabutey NK, Stamos MJ, Fujitani RM. Risk factors and outcomes of postoperative ischemic colitis in contemporary open and endovascular abdominal aortic aneurysm repair. J Vasc Surg. 2016;63(4):866–72. https://doi.org/10.1016/j.jvs.2015.10.064.

62. Mohanapriya T, Singh KB, Arulappan T, Shobhana R. Ischemic colitis. Indian J Surg. 2012;74(5):396–400. https://doi.org/10.1007/s12262-012-0425-8.

63. Mosińska P, Fichna J. Ischemic colitis: current diagnosis and treatment. Curr Drug Targets. 2015;16(3):209–18.

64. Mosli M, Parfitt J, Gregor J. Retrospective analysis of disease association and outcome in histologically confirmed ischemic colitis. J Dig Dis. 2013;14(5):238–43. https://doi.org/10.1111/1751-2980.12045.

65. Moszkowicz D, Mariani A, Trésallet C, Menegaux F. Ischemic colitis: the ABCs of diagnosis and surgical management. J Visc Surg. 2013;150(1):19–28. https://doi.org/10.1016/j.jviscsurg.2013.01.002.

66. Muldoon J, O'Riordan K, Rao S, Abecassis M. Ischemic colitis secondary to venous thrombosis. A rare presentation of cytomegalovirus vasculitis following renal transplantation. Transplantation. 1996;61(11):1651–3.

67. Noh M, Yang SS, Jung SW, Park JH, Im YC, Kim KY. Poor prognostic factors in patients who underwent surgery for acute non-occlusive ischemic colitis. World J Emerg Surg. 2015;10:12. https://doi.org/10.1186/s13017-015-0003-z.

68. O'Neill S, Elder K, Harrison SJ, Yalamarthi S. Predictors of severity in ischaemic colitis. Int J Color Dis. 2012;27(2):187–91. https://doi.org/10.1007/s00384-011-1301-x.

69. Othman M, El-Majzoub N, Khoury G, Barada K. Laparoscopy rather than colonoscopy for the diagnosis and treatment of fulminant ischemic colitis. Int J Color Dis. 2014;29(11):1443–4. https://doi.org/10.1007/s00384-014-1919-6.

70. Perry RJ, Martin MJ, Eckert MJ, Sohn VY, Steele SR. Colonic ischemia complicating open vs endovascular abdominal aortic aneurysm repair. J Vasc Surg. 2008;48(2):272–7. https://doi.org/10.1016/j.jvs.2008.03.040.

71. Poeze M, Froon AH, Greve JW, Ramsay G. D-lactate as an early marker of intestinal ischaemia after ruptured abdominal aortic aneurysm repair. Br J Surg. 1998;85(9):1221–4. https://doi.org/10.1046/j.1365-2168.1998.00837.x.

72. Rania H, Mériam S, Rym E, Hyafa R, Amine A, Najet BH, Lassad G, Mohamed TK. Ischemic colitis in five points: an update 2013. Tunis Med. 2014;92(5):299–303.

73. Ripollés T, Simó L, Martínez-Pérez MJ, Pastor MR, Igual A, López A. Sonographic findings in ischemic colitis in 58 patients. AJR Am J Roentgenol. 2005;184(3):777–85. https://doi.org/10.2214/ajr.184.3.01840777.

74. Romano S, Romano L, Grassi R. Multidetector row computed tomography findings from ischemia to infarction of the large bowel. Eur J Radiol. 2007;61(3):433–41. https://doi.org/10.1016/j.ejrad.2006.11.002.

75. Sadler MD, Ravindran NC, Hubbard J, Myers RP, Ghosh S, Beck PL, Dixon E, Ball C, Prusinkiewicz C, Heitman SJ, Kaplan GG. Predictors of mortality among patients undergoing colectomy for ischemic colitis: a population-based United States study. Can J Gastroenterol Hepatol. 2014;28(11):600–4.

76. Sakorafas GH, Zouros E, Peros G. Applied vascular anatomy of the colon and rectum: clinical implications for the surgical oncologist. Surg Oncol. 2006;15(4):243–55. https://doi.org/10.1016/j.suronc.2007.03.002.

77. Scharff JR, Longo WE, Vartanian SM, Jacobs DL, Bahadursingh AN, Kaminski DL. Ischemic colitis: spectrum of disease and outcome. Surgery. 2003;134(4):624–9 discussion 629-630. https://doi.org/10.1016/S0039.

78. Schneider TA, Longo WE, Ure T, Vernava AM. Mesenteric ischemia. Acute arterial syndromes. Dis Colon Rectum. 1994;37(11):1163–74.

79. Sherid M, Sifuentes H, Samo S, Sulaiman S, Husein H, Tupper R, Spurr C, Vainder J, Sridhar S. Risk factors of recurrent ischemic colitis: a multicenter retrospective study. Korean J Gastroenterol. 2014;63(5):283–91.

80. Smith RF, Szilagyi DE. Ischemia of the colon as a complication in the surgery of the abdominal aorta. Arch Surg. 1960;80:806–21.

81. Suh DC, Kahler KH, Choi IS, Shin H, Kralstein J, Shetzline M. Patients with irritable bowel syndrome or constipation have an increased risk for ischaemic colitis. Aliment Pharmacol Ther. 2007;25(6):681–92. https://doi.org/10.1111/j.1365-2036.2007.03250.x.

82. Sun D, Wang C, Yang L, Liu M, Chen F. The predictors of the severity of ischaemic colitis: a systematic review of 2823 patients from 22 studies. Color Dis. 2016;18(10):949–58. https://doi.org/10.1111/codi.13389.

83. Sun MY, Maykel JA. Ischemic colitis. Clin Colon Rectal Surg. 2007;20(1):5–12. https://doi.org/10.1055/s-2007-970194.

84. Theodoropoulou A, Koutroubakis IE. Ischemic colitis: clinical practice in diagnosis and treatment. World J Gastroenterol. 2008;14(48):7302–8.

85. Theodoropoulou A, Sfiridaki A, Oustamanolakis P, Vardas E, Livadiotaki A, Boumpaki A, Paspatis G, Koutroubakis IE. Genetic risk factors in young patients with ischemic colitis. Clin Gastroenterol Hepatol. 2008;6(8):907–11. https://doi.org/10.1016/j.cgh.2008.03.010.

86. Thoeni RF, Cello JP. CT imaging of colitis. Radiology. 2006;240(3):623–38. https://doi.org/10.1148/radiol.2403050818.

87. Thomson FB. Ischaemic infarction of the left colon. Can Med Assoc J. 1948;58(2):183–5.

88. Tofukuji M, Stahl GL, Metais C, Tomita M, Agah A, Bianchi C, Fink MP, Sellke FW. Mesenteric dysfunction after cardiopulmonary bypass: role of complement C5a. Ann Thorac Surg. 2000;69(3):799–807.

89. Washington C, Carmichael JC. Management of ischemic colitis. Clin Colon Rectal Surg. 2012;25(4):228–35. https://doi.org/10.1055/s-0032-1329534.

90. Yadav S, Dave M, Edakkanambeth Varayil J, Harmsen WS, Tremaine WJ, Zinsmeister AR, Sweetser SR, Melton LJ, Sandborn WJ, Loftus EV. A population-based study of incidence, risk factors, clinical spectrum, and outcomes of ischemic colitis. Clin Gastroenterol Hepatol. 2015;13(4):731–738.e731–736 quiz e741. https://doi.org/10.1016/j.cgh.2014.07.061.

91. Yngvadottir Y, Karlsdottir BR, Hreinsson JP, Ragnarsson G, Mitev RUM, Jonasson JG, Möller PH, Björnsson ES. The incidence and outcome of ischemic colitis in a population-based setting. Scand J Gastroenterol. 2017;52(6–7):704–10. https://doi.org/10.1080/00365521.2017.1291718.

92. Zou X, Cao J, Yao Y, Liu W, Chen L. Endoscopic findings and clinicopathologic characteristics of ischemic colitis: a report of 85 cases. Dig Dis Sci. 2009;54(9):2009–15. https://doi.org/10.1007/s10620-008-0579-1.

Ogilvie's Syndrome

27

Morgan Schellenberg and Kazuhide Matsushima

Introduction

Ogilvie's syndrome is a condition wherein the colon becomes dilated without a mechanical cause of obstruction. It is also known as acute colonic pseudo-obstruction. Ogilvie's syndrome is the eponymous term, named after William Heneage Ogilvie, a Chilean surgeon born in the 1800s who first described the condition. This original description was based on two of his patients, both with retroperitoneal tumors invading the celiac plexus, who had acute colonic obstruction without a mechanical cause [1]. Because of the involvement of the celiac plexus, he postulated that a disorder of sympathetic innervation was the likely precipitant of this condition. With further study of the condition over the past century, it now appears that acute pseudo-obstruction of the colon is likely the result of parasympathetic, and not sympathetic, dysfunction [2], but the pathophysiology remains incompletely understood. Most agree that the condition is related to autonomic dysfunction within the gastrointestinal tract, with decreased parasympathetic tone to the colon resulting in colonic dilation that mimics obstruction but without a mechanical obstruction. Alternate theories suggest that the pathophysiology involves decreased splanchnic blood flow [3–5] or decreased systemic levels of prostaglandin E [3, 6, 7].

Epidemiology

Ogilvie's syndrome occurs almost exclusively among hospitalized or institutionalized patients with a precipitating event. Patients are commonly elderly, with a mean age of 64–74 years [8, 9]. The risk factors for Ogilvie's syndrome are extensive (Table 27.1). According to a large case series (n = 1027), the most frequent inciting events are surgery, cardiorespiratory disease, and nonoperative trauma [8]. Of the surgical precipitants, orthopedic and obstetric surgical patients seem to be at especially high risk. In addition to typically being hospitalized patients of advanced age with a predisposing event, these patients frequently have underlying medical disorders. These can be neurologic, for example, dementia; metabolic, such as diabetes mellitus, hypokalemia, or uremia; oncologic; or infectious, such as from cytomegalovirus or herpes zoster [3, 10] (Table 27.1). Certain medications, including tricyclic antidepressants, alpha agonists, calcium channel blockers, laxatives, and especially narcotics, can precipitate or worsen colonic pseudo-obstruction. Because advanced age, immobility, polypharmacy, and medical comorbidities are risk factors, Ogilvie's syndrome is

M. Schellenberg · K. Matsushima (✉)
Division of Trauma and Surgical Critical Care,
LAC+USC Medical Center, Los Angeles, CA, USA
e-mail: kazuhide.matsushima@med.usc.edu

© Springer International Publishing AG, part of Springer Nature 2019
C. V. R. Brown et al. (eds.), *Emergency General Surgery*, https://doi.org/10.1007/978-3-319-96286-3_27

Table 27.1 Etiologies and risk factors for Ogilvie's syndrome

	Etiologies and risk factors
Neurologic	Dementia/delirium Parkinson's disease Cerebrovascular accident (CVA)
Respiratory	Pneumonia Chronic obstructive pulmonary disease (COPD) Need for mechanical ventilation
Cardiovascular	Arrhythmia Myocardial infarction (MI) Congestive heart failure (CHF)
Gastrointestinal	Intra-abdominal infection Intra-abdominal hematoma Trauma Gastrointestinal bleeding Abdominal compartment syndrome
Metabolic/endocrine	Uremia Diabetes mellitus (DM) Electrolyte abnormalities Need for dialysis
Musculoskeletal	Immobility
Surgical	Pelvic/hip surgery Cesarean section Abdominal surgery
Pharmacologic	Opioids Laxatives Anticholinergic medications Dopamine agonists

especially common in the intensive care unit (ICU).

Presentation

Patients with Ogilvie's syndrome present with symptoms similar to those seen with mechanical bowel obstruction, including nausea, vomiting, abdominal pain, and obstipation. The differential diagnosis is broad but should include any type of mechanical large bowel obstruction. Mechanical causes of large bowel obstruction include, most commonly, a colonic mass; diverticular disease, including stricture; and colonic volvulus, typically sigmoid or cecal. Other less common causes of mechanical large bowel obstruction include inflammatory bowel disease and hernias. In addition to these mechanical causes, toxic megacolon must be considered. This can occur as a result of

chronic or severe inflammatory bowel disease (IBD) or from an infectious colitis, such as *C. difficile*. Although toxic megacolon can also occur after ischemic or collagenous causes of colitis, these are rare etiologies [11]. While toxic megacolon and Ogilvie's syndrome present similarly radiographically, these entities can often be easily distinguished clinically because patients with toxic megacolon are typically quite sick, with diffuse abdominal pain and signs of systemic toxicity, while patients with Ogilvie's syndrome are often systemically well. The clinical history is also typically discriminating, with patients with toxic megacolon having antecedent signs and symptoms of IBD or infectious colitis.

When assessing a patient for potential Ogilvie's syndrome, the differential diagnosis must be kept in mind, and questions should be targeted toward narrowing the differential diagnosis, searching for a suggestive history, the presence of constitutional or extraintestinal symptoms, past medical and surgical history, and medications. Physical examination begins with vital signs and general inspection. Although mild tachycardia may occur with Ogilvie's syndrome, related to poor oral intake and resultant volume depletion, marked tachycardia, hypotension, or fever should raise concern for perforation. Visual inspection typically reveals a markedly distended abdomen. Mild diffuse tenderness can be expected, but peritonitis is concerning for perforation. The clinician should note the presence or absence of abdominal wall hernias.

Investigations

Laboratory Investigations

If the history and physical examination are concerning for Ogilvie's syndrome, the next steps are laboratory and imaging investigations. Laboratory evaluation should begin with a complete blood count, complete metabolic panel, and measurement of the serum lactate. Hemoconcentration may be evident, with an elevated white blood cell count or hematocrit. A marked leukocytosis should raise concerns for an underlying infectious etiology or perforation. The metabolic panel should be inspected for electrolyte abnormalities, particularly hypokalemia, hypomagnesemia, and hypocalcemia. There may also be evidence of prerenal acute kidney injury. Finally, serial measurements of the serum lactate can be a useful reflection of the degree of bowel ischemia.

Imaging Investigations

Patients with abdominal pain and distension typically undergo an abdominal X-ray (AXR) as the initial imaging investigation. Findings of colonic dilation can be due to mechanical or pseudo-obstruction (Fig. 27.1). Patients who have an incompetent ileocecal valve may also show small bowel dilation. Importantly, the AXR is not specific for the diagnosis of Ogilvie's syndrome and cannot rule out a mechanical obstruction. The value of AXR in this setting is twofold. It should be inspected for free air and pneumatosis, which indicate hollow viscus perforation and bowel

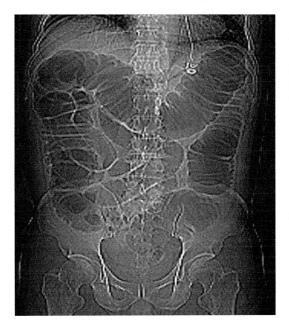

Fig. 27.1 Abdominal X-ray of a patient with Ogilvie's syndrome. Dilation of the colon and small bowel is demonstrated

ischemia, respectively, and are triggers for exploratory laparotomy in the appropriate clinical setting. Secondly, the AXR should be inspected for alternate diagnoses, such as a sigmoid volvulus, which presents with colonic dilation and a typical "coffee bean" sign.

Patients with a physical examination showing peritonitis with free air demonstrated on AXR should be brought directly to the operating room for exploratory laparotomy. Other patients with stable vital signs and a history, physical examination, and AXR consistent with large bowel obstruction without evidence of perforation should next undergo a computed tomography (CT) scan of the abdomen and pelvis. The CT scan should be inspected for colonic dilation and signs of bowel ischemia or perforation (Fig. 27.2). Additionally, the CT scan should be used to exclude a mechanical cause for the colonic dilation. Findings suggestive of malignancy, including colorectal lesions and signs of metastases, should be sought, as well as alternate diagnoses including hernias, volvuli, and diverticular disease (Fig. 27.3). Intravenous (IV) contrast should be used unless contraindicated, since IV contrast allows the clinician and radiologist to assess the bowel wall for viability. Oral contrast is of limited additional value and is typically forgone. Rectal contrast is not used routinely but can be helpful to define or exclude a colorectal mass in rare cases where CT scan is equivocal for mechanical obstruction [12].

Ogilvie's syndrome tends to affect the cecum and right colon principally because the bowel wall is thinnest in these locations. Measurements should be taken of the maximum diameter of the transverse colon and cecum on abdominal imaging. Diameters greater than 9 cm and 12 cm, respectively, have been shown to indicate impending perforation [3, 13].

A diagnosis of Ogilvie's syndrome is one of exclusion. In particular, mechanical causes of colonic obstruction must be ruled out. Historically, contrast enemas were performed to exclude an obstructing lesion. CT scan now has sufficient sensitivity (96%) to rule out an obstruction lesion, and therefore contrast enemas to exclude distal obstruction in Ogilvie's syndrome

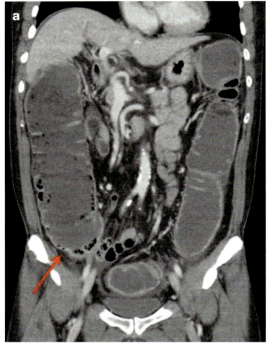

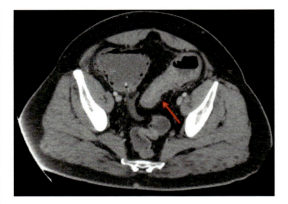

Fig. 27.3 CT scan of a patient with a large bowel obstruction due to sigmoid colon diverticular stricture. The CT scan of a patient with colonic dilation must be inspected for causes of mechanical obstruction, including diverticular disease (arrow)

tion, contrast enemas may help relieve pseudo-obstruction osmotically by stimulating the evacuation of intraluminal contents [15]. However, concerns about inducing perforation in patients with marked colonic distension limit the clinical utility of contrast enemas in Ogilvie's syndrome.

Management

Once alternate diagnoses have been excluded, the management of Ogilvie's syndrome is performed in a stepwise fashion and aims to prevent colonic distension to the point of colonic ischemia, necrosis, or perforation. Treatment begins with supportive measures, including intravenous fluid administration, nasogastric (NG) and rectal tube placement, electrolyte repletion, treatment of any precipitating conditions, and cessation of causative medications. If these measures are unsuccessful, decompression should be attempted either pharmacologically with neostigmine or endoscopically. Surgery is reserved for cases that are refractory to supportive treatment and pharmacologic or endoscopic decompression and for patients with evidence of perforation or ischemia.

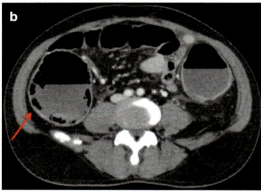

Fig. 27.2 CT scan of a patient with Ogilvie's syndrome. Colonic dilation and pneumatosis (arrow) of the cecum and ascending colon are noted

are rarely necessary [12]. If used, water-soluble contrast (e.g., gastrografin) is preferred because of the risks of barium peritonitis if perforation has not been excluded. Although barium allows for a more detailed assessment of the mucosa than gastrografin, this advantage is rarely relevant in this clinical scenario [14]. In addition to excluding a mechanical cause for colonic obstruc-

Supportive Treatment

Many patients with Ogilvie's syndrome will resolve after a brief period of supportive treatment consisting of bowel rest, early ambulation, intravenous fluids, electrolyte replacement, and discontinuation of inciting medications, particularly narcotics. Bowel rest should involve the placement of a NG tube as well as a rectal tube.

Close clinical monitoring is a hallmark of initial supportive management, with serial abdominal examinations and frequent re-evaluation of vital signs in order to detect the development of peritonitis, tachycardia, hypotension, or fever in a timely fashion. Any of these signs can indicate perforation and the need for surgical intervention. Some advocate for serial AXRs at 12–24-h intervals in order to track cecal diameter and inspect for evidence of perforation [16].

Because of the concern for mucosal and ultimately full-thickness ischemia and perforation as the result of marked and persistent colonic distension, most clinicians consider pharmacologic or endoscopic decompression once the patient has been treated with supportive measures for 24–48 h or if the cecal diameter approaches 12 cm on AXR. The precise timing is not well defined by the current literature, although the available evidence suggests that supportive treatment alone will resolve the pseudo-obstruction in up to 70% of patients by a median time of 1.6 days [17, 18]. For patients who fail supportive management alone, the choice of decompression strategies remains controversial and largely depends on the institutional resources and patient factors.

Pharmacologic Decompression: Neostigmine

Neostigmine is a reversible acetylcholinesterase inhibitor that exerts its effects on the gastrointestinal tract by increasing the availability of acetylcholine and activating muscarinic receptors in the mucosa and smooth muscle. This, in turns, causes muscle contraction, which allows for the elimination of colonic gas and stool and thereby resolves colonic pseudo-obstruction. To relieve pseudo-obstruction, 2 mg is typically given by slow IV pushover several minutes. Neostigmine can be expected to exert its effects rapidly, with a median response time of 4 min but ranging upward of 30 min [19]. If a single 2 mg dose of neostigmine does not resolve symptoms, it can be redosed twice at 3-h intervals as necessary (for a maximum total dose of 6 mg) [10, 20–22].

Because of its mechanism of action, neostigmine can have important cardiac effects. Consequently, patients should be placed on a cardiac monitor prior to drug administration. Although they seldom occur (<7%) [19], bradycardia and hypotension should be anticipated and treated with atropine and IV fluid bolus if they occur. Cardiac monitoring and close clinical evaluation should continue for at least 30 min after administration, which is often best achieved in an ICU setting.

In addition to the potential cardiac effects, other side effects are neurologic (seizures, tremors, restlessness); respiratory (bronchoconstriction); and gastrointestinal (nausea, vomiting, diarrhea, abdominal pain). Because of the side effect profile of neostigmine, it should not be used to decompress patients with Ogilvie's syndrome who have a history of cardiac disease (bradycardia, rate-controlling medications such as beta-blockers, or recent myocardial infarction), asthma, or peptic ulcer disease.

In patients without these contraindications, neostigmine is an excellent option to relieve pseudo-obstruction. In fact, major gastroenterology guidelines recommend neostigmine as the decompression method of choice among patients who fail supportive therapy alone [14]. A recent meta-analysis showed neostigmine to be approximately 90% effective in treating Ogilvie's syndrome [19], although some individual studies reported success rates as low as 35–49% [23, 24] or as high as 91% [22].

Endoscopic Decompression

Colonoscopy can be used to decompress the colon in Ogilvie's syndrome. Evacuation of the colonic gas using a standard colonoscope resolves colonic pseudo-obstruction in 75–90% of cases [24]. Although there is some concern about the risk of perforation with endoscopy in the setting of acute distension, studies show the risk of perforation is no different after colonoscopy as compared to either neostigmine or the natural history of untreated Ogilvie's syndrome (all approximately 4%) [24]. Proponents of the endoscopic decompression first strategy, followed by neostigmine administration if this fails, argue that colonoscopy is more successful than neostigmine after a single intervention (75–81% vs 36–49%) [23, 24]. Additionally, endoscopy avoids the side effect profile of neostigmine, which can be significant especially in terms of its cardiovascular risks in the elderly and comorbid population typically affected by Ogilvie's syndrome. However, colonoscopy does require endoscopy equipment, trained nurses, and an endoscopist.

Leaving a rectal tube at the completion of the endoscopic decompression is a key maneuver to allow for continued decompression and prevent recurrence. One study showed that leaving a rectal tube in place increased the success of endoscopic decompression from 25% to 80% [25]. It is unclear where the rectal tube should be ideally positioned to achieve decompression. Some authors advocate for placing the decompressive tube in the cecum or right colon to achieve maximum benefit, but this can be technically challenging.

No studies comparing cost-effectiveness between endoscopic and pharmacologic decompression have yet been done. Additionally, specific patient populations that may respond better to one decompression strategy over the other have not yet been well defined. One recent study shows that advanced age and male gender predicted poor response to endoscopic decompression [23]. However, no patient factors or inciting etiologies were predictive of failure or success with neostigmine administration [23].

It is likely that there are subgroups of patients who will respond better to decompression with one technique versus the other, but these groups are currently undefined. At this time, it is clear that patients with bradycardia or hypotension should not receive neostigmine, and therefore

that endoscopic decompression should be attempted if conservative measures fail. In the absence of cost data and further information about rates of response to therapy among specific subgroups, the decision between endoscopic and pharmacologic decompression for most patients is guided by resource availability and clinician preference. If a patient does not respond to decompression by one method, the other technique of decompression should be attempted next.

Surgery

Surgery is indicated for patients with perforation, impending perforation, and those who fail management with supportive treatment, endoscopic decompression, and neostigmine. A precise and universally accepted definition of impending perforation is lacking but is considered by most to be a cecal diameter >9–12 cm. At that degree of distension, the cecal and ascending colonic walls are so thin that perforation is imminent.

Prior to intubation, the NG tube must be confirmed to be in proper position in the stomach and connected to wall suction to minimize the risks of aspiration on induction. It is prudent to treat these patients as though they have a full stomach and perform a rapid sequence induction for intubation. Perioperative antibiotics should be administered prior to skin incision. The operation should begin with an exploration of the abdomen to confirm the absence of a colonic mass, evidence of malignancy, or other precipitating factors such as a large retroperitoneal hematoma or intra-abdominal abscess.

The surgical procedure of choice for the management of pseudo-obstruction is controversial. There are many surgical options (proximal diversion alone, segmental colectomy, and subtotal colectomy) and no high-quality data to guide the decision-making. Practically, the surgeon must evaluate the status of the entire colon before planning the surgical approach. Serosal tears, evidence of ischemia, and sites of perforation must be noted. In a poor surgical candidate without perforation or compromise of bowel wall integrity, an ostomy might be the simplest, quickest, and most prudent course of action.

Perforation or ischemia, which occurs in up to 15% of all patients with Ogilvie's syndrome [3], necessitates resection. A segmental resection can be considered if the colonic distension and compromised area are relatively limited. In general, a subtotal colectomy is preferred for Ogilvie's syndrome that requires operative intervention. A primary anastomosis with or without proximal diversion or an end ileostomy can be considered.

Prognosis

Ogilvie's syndrome tends to recur after treatment. Recurrence rates after either pharmacologic or endoscopic decompression approach 40% within the first few days of treatment [3, 26]. One study showed that polyethylene glycol (PEG) solution administration after the achievement of colonic decompression resulted in a significantly lower rate of pseudo-obstruction recurrence within the first 7 days [27]. Data on sustained response to treatment beyond 7 days are very limited. Avoidance of risk factors (such as immobility, electrolyte abnormalities, and precipitating medications) is likely the best approach to preventing recurrence.

Surgery is infrequently required, with only approximately 6% of patients requiring operative intervention [28]. However, the need for surgery significantly increases the risk of mortality among patients with Ogilvie's syndrome, from 14% to 30% for patients managed nonoperatively to 30–50% among those managed operatively [3].

Conclusions

Ogilvie's syndrome, or acute colonic pseudo-obstruction, most commonly affects patients >60 years of age and occurs after an inciting event, including orthopedic surgery, nonoperative trauma, and cardiorespiratory failure. Patients typically present with abdominal pain, distension, and obstipation. The diagnosis of Ogilvie's syndrome is one of exclusion. CT scan of the abdomen and pelvis can reliably exclude a mechanical large bowel obstruction, and contrast enemas are rarely necessary. The management of Ogilvie's syndrome begins with supportive therapy, including NG and rectal tube decompression, IV fluids, correction of electrolyte abnormalities, and ambulation. If this fails to resolve the pseudo-obstruction within 24–48 h, either pharmacologic decompression with neostigmine or endoscopic decompression should be attempted next. In patients with a cardiac history, neostigmine should be avoided because of its risks of bradycardia and hypotension. Patients who fail one method of decompression should next receive the other method of decompression before being deemed to have failed nonoperative management. Surgical management is indicated for patients with perforation or ischemia and for those who have failed treatment with supportive measures and decompression.

References

1. Ogilvie H. Large-intestine colic due to sympathetic deprivation: a new clinical syndrome. Br Med J. 1948;2:671–2.
2. Maloney N, Vargas HD. Acute intestinal Pseudo-obstruction (Ogilvie's syndrome). Clin Colon Rectal Surg. 2005;18(2):96–101.
3. Pereira P, Djeudji F, Leduc P, Fanget F, Barth X. Ogilvie's Syndrome - Acute Colonic Pseudo-Obstruction. J Visc Surg. 2015;152:99–105.
4. Desouches G, Bastien J, Joublin M. Acute idiopathic dilatation and perforation of the cecum in a patient with streptococcal septicemia. Gastroenterol Clin Biol. 1978;2(2):185–8.
5. Bardsley D. Pseudo-obstruction of the large bowel. Br J Surg. 1974;61(12):963–9.
6. Nadrowski L. Paralytic ileus: recent advances in pathophysiology and treatment. Curr Surg. 1983;40(4):260–73.
7. Bachulis BL, Smith PE. Pseudoobstruction of the Colon. Am J Surg. 1978;136(1):66–72.
8. Wegener M, Borsch G. Acute colonic Pseudo-obstruction (Ogilvie's syndrome): presentation of 14 of our own cases and analysis of 1027 cases reported in the literature. Surg Endosc. 1987;1(3):169–74.
9. Bode WE, Beart RW Jr, Spencer RJ, Culp CE, Wolff BG, Taylor BM. Colonoscopic decompression for acute Pseudoobstruction of the Colon (Ogilvie's syndrome): report of 22 cases and review of the literature. Am J Surg. 1984;147(2):243–5.

10. Chudzinski AP, Thompson EV, Ayscue JM. Acute Colonic Pseudoobstruction. Clin Colon Rectal Surg. 2015;28:112–7.
11. Autenrieth DM, Baumgart DC. Toxic Megacolon. Inflamm Bowel Dis. 2012;18(3):584–91.
12. Jaffe T, Thompson WM. Large bowel obstruction in the adult: classic radiographic and CT findings, etiology, and mimics. Radiology. 2015;275(3):651–63.
13. Vanek VW, Al-Salti M. Acute Pseudo-obstruction of the Colon (Ogilvie's syndrome): an analysis of 400 cases. Dis Colon Rectum. 1986;29(3):203–10.
14. Harrison ME, Anderson MA, Appalaneni V, Banerjee S, Ben-Menachem T, Cash BD, Fanelli RD, Fisher L, Fukami N, Gan SI, Ikenberry SO, Jain R, Khan K, Krinsky ML, Maple JT, Shen B, Guilder TV, Baron TH, Dominitz JA. The role of endoscopy in the Management of Patients with known and suspected colonic obstruction and Pseudo-obstruction. Gastrointest Endosc. 2010;71(4):669–79.
15. Schermer CR, Hanosh JJ, Davis M, Pitcher DE. Ogilvie's syndrome in the surgical patient: a new therapeutic modality. J Gastrointest Surg. 1999;3(2):173–7.
16. Johnson CD, Rice RP, Kelvin FM, Foster WL, Williford ME. The radiologic evaluation of gross Cecal distension: emphasis on Cecal ileus. Am J Roentgenol. 1985;145(6):1211–7.
17. De Giorgio R, Barbara G, Stanghellini V, Tonini M, Vasina V, Cola B, Corinaldesi R, G B, De Ponti F. Review article: the pharmacological treatment of acute colonic Pseudo-obstruction. Aliment Pharmacol Ther. 2001;15(11):1717–27.
18. Sloyer AF, Panella VS, Demas BE, Shike M, Lightdale CJ, Winawer SJ, Kurtz RC. Ogilvie's syndrome: successful management without colonoscopy. Dig Dis Sci. 1988;33(11):1391–6.
19. Valle RGL, Godoy FL. Neostigmine for acute colonic Pseudo-obstruction: a meta-analysis. Ann Med Surg. 2014;3:60–4.
20. White L, Sandhu G. Continuous neostigmine infusion versus bolus neostigmine in refractory Ogilvie's syndrome. Am J Emerg Med. 2011;29(5):576.e1–3.
21. Paran H, Silverberg D, Mayo A, Shwartz I, Neufeld D, Freund U. Treatment of acute colonic Pseudo-obstruction with neostigmine. J Am Coll Surg. 2000;190(3):315–8.
22. Ponec RJ, Saunders MD, Kimney MBN. Neostigmine for the treatment of acute colonic Pseudo-obstruction. N Engl J Med. 1999;341(3):137–41.
23. Peker KD, Cikot M, Bozkurt MA, Ilhan B, Kankaya B, Binboga S, Seyit H, Alis H. Colonoscopic decompression should be used before neostigmine in the treatment of Ogilvie's syndrome. Eur J Trauma Emerg Surg. 2017;43:557–66.
24. Tsirline VB, Zemlyak AY, Avery MJ, Colavita PD, Christmas AB, Heniford BT, Sing RF. Colonoscopy is superior to neostigmine in the treatment of Ogilvie's syndrome. Am J Surg. 2012;204:849–55.
25. Geller A, Petersen BT, Gostout CJ. Endoscopic decompression for acute colonic Pseudo-obstruction. Gastrointest Endosc. 1996;44:144–50.
26. Loftus CG, Harewood GC, Baron TH. Assessment of predictors of response to neostigmine for acute colonic Pseudo-obstruction. Am J Gastroenterol. 2002;97:3118–22.
27. Sgouros SN, Vlachogiannakos J, Vassiliadis K, Bergele C, Stefanidis G, Nastos H, Avgerinos A, Mantides A. Effect of polyethylene glycol electrolyte balanced solution on patients with acute colonic Pseudo obstruction after resolution of colonic dilation: a prospective, randomised, placebo controlled trial. Gut. 2006;55:638–42.
28. Ross SW, Oommen B, Wormer BA, Walters AL, Augenstein VA, Heniford BT, Sing RF, Christmas AB. Acute colonic Pseudo-obstruction: defining the epidemiology, treatment, and adverse outcomes of Ogilvie's syndrome. Am Surg. 2016;82:102–11.

Colon Volvulus

28

Rebecca E. Plevin and Andre R. Campbell

Colonic volvulus occurs when a portion of the large intestine becomes twisted around its mesentery, occluding the intestinal lumen and causing a bowel obstruction. If the colon twists 360° or more around the axis, the vascular supply may become obstructed leading to ischemia and perforation. Congenital conditions in children, such as malrotation or Hirschsprung's disease, can lead to colonic volvulus. More often, though, it is an acquired condition that occurs in adults and increases in frequency with older age.

Volvulus accounts for approximately 10–15% of large bowel obstructions in the United States, making it the third most common cause of large bowel obstructions in Americans [1]. Rates of volvulus are higher worldwide, particularly in a region termed the "volvulus belt" which includes South America, the Middle East, India, Africa, and Russia [2–4]. In these regions, volvulus accounts for as much as 50% of large bowel obstructions. The sigmoid colon is the site of torsion in approximately two thirds of patients. The remaining cases involve the cecum (15–30%), transverse colon (2–5%), or splenic flexure (1%) [5, 6].

R. E. Plevin
Department of Surgery, Zuckerberg San Francisco General Hospital, University of California San Francisco, San Francisco, CA, USA

A. R. Campbell (✉)
Department of Surgery, University of California San Francisco, San Francisco, CA, USA
e-mail: Andre.Campbell@ucsf.edu

Etiology and Pathophysiology

Volvulus usually occurs in an elongated segment of colon connected to a long mesentery and a narrow mesenteric base. The long segment of colon is prone to twisting around its mesenteric pedicle, particularly if the base of the mesentery is narrow. This results in bowel obstruction, dilation, and ischemia and perforation if not promptly treated.

Conditions associated with elongation of the colon predispose a patient to sigmoid volvulus. The rate of sigmoid volvulus in the United States increases with advanced age, with the average patient being between 60 and 80 years old [6]. Chronic constipation, frequent laxative or enema use, and spinal cord injury are common risk factors. Men are more prone to sigmoid volvulus than women. This has been attributed through anatomic studies to the finding that the male sigmoid mesentery is longer than it is wide, while the reverse is true in women [7]. Psychiatric disease, and particularly disease treated with psychotropic medications, is also associated with higher rates of sigmoid volvulus [8]. This is likely due to the constipating effects of many psychotropic medications. Patients living in the "volvulus belt" who develop the condition, in contrast, are typically younger (40–50 years of age) and healthier than volvulus patients in the United States.

The term "cecal volvulus" may actually refer to one of several clinical entities. Despite the

© Springer International Publishing AG, part of Springer Nature 2019
C. V. R. Brown et al. (eds.), *Emergency General Surgery*, https://doi.org/10.1007/978-3-319-96286-3_28

name, cecal volvulus more frequently involves torsion of a mobile ascending colon distal to the ileocecal valve. However, there are occasional true cases of cecal volvulus where a mobile cecum and ascending colon twist around the colonic mesentery. Patients who develop cecal volvulus are younger; the typical cecal volvulus patient in the United States is 40–60 years old and is more often female. Cecal *bascule* is a similar but distinct clinical entity where the cecum folds anteriorly on itself, causing an obstruction. Cecal bascule occurs in patients with adhesive bands anterior to the cecum or ascending colon. These bands form a fixed point over which the cecum folding occurs. Cecal bascule may occur intermittently and then resolve, causing symptoms of intermittent obstruction.

Transverse colon and splenic flexure volvulus are rare clinical entities described largely in case reports. The transverse colon mesentery tends to be broad, short, and well fixated to the retroperitoneum, making the transverse colon an unlikely site for torsion. When transverse colon volvulus does occur, it is usually in the setting of underlying pathophysiology that causes lengthening of the mesentery (e.g., chronic constipation or neuropsychiatric disorders), lack of colonic fixation at the splenic or hepatic flexures, or congenital malrotation [9, 10]. Splenic flexure volvulus is even less common. It occurs in patients who lack retroperitoneal fixation of the splenic flexure or who have undergone surgery with transection of these points of fixation [11, 12].

Sigmoid Volvulus

Presentation

Symptoms of volvulus occur along a spectrum ranging from intermittent or chronic dysmotility to frank perforation. Patients with sigmoid volvulus often describe a long history of constipation and symptoms of acute or subacute bowel obstruction. A careful history and physical exam can help suggest a colonic obstruction, but imaging studies are typically necessary to precisely localize the site and etiology of the patient's

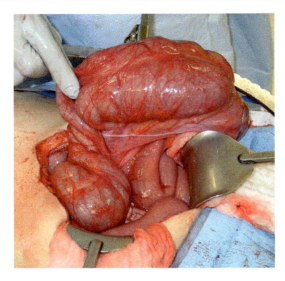

Fig. 28.1 Dilated sigmoid colon with visible twisting secondary to sigmoid volvulus

symptoms. As the colon torses, its lumen occludes and the colon distends (Fig. 28.1). Venous drainage is obstructed much earlier than the arterial inflow, and as a result, patients may not present with the sudden onset of acute abdominal pain that is seen with mesenteric ischemia. Instead, they often report slow-onset cramping abdominal pain that worsens, becomes constant, and is accompanied by progressive distention. Obstipation is common. Because the sigmoid colon can spontaneously detorse, patients may report symptoms that were relieved by an explosive episode of large volume diarrhea, only to later recur. Vomiting is often absent or is a late finding due to the distal location of the obstruction. When present, it typically occurs after several days of symptoms and is feculent.

On physical exam, patients who have been symptomatic for several days are distended, tympanic, and have diffuse, mild tenderness throughout the abdomen. With late presentations, arterial occlusion and transmural pressure on the colon wall secondary to intraluminal distention produce tissue ischemia. Symptoms in this setting range from focal to diffuse peritonitis. Hemodynamic abnormalities, severe pain, or rebound tenderness should alert the clinician to the possibility of intestinal ischemia. If untreated, these patients can progress to frank tissue necrosis, perforation, and sepsis.

Diagnosis

Radiographic studies are invaluable in diagnosing sigmoid volvulus. An upright or left lateral decubitus X-ray is obtained to look for free air beneath the diaphragm, which suggests perforation and mandates the need for urgent exploration. The classic finding on abdominal X-ray in sigmoid volvulus is the "bent inner tube sign." The twisted sigmoid colon becomes dilated, with its apex pointing toward the right upper quadrant and the twisted segment of colon in the left lower quadrant. Gas is typically absent from the rectum, and an air-fluid level may be present in the colon. Plain abdominal radiograph is sufficient to diagnose sigmoid volvulus in nearly 2/3 of patients [13].

In the past, contrast enema was performed when the plain X-ray was nondiagnostic. It shows the pathognomonic "bird's beak" narrowing of the colon at the distal obstruction site, with contrast enema present distal to the obstruction and absent in the proximal colon. Contrast enema should only be performed in patients without signs of perforation. Today, a CT scan is most often obtained if the plain abdominal X-ray fails to elucidate a diagnosis. CT has nearly 100% accuracy for diagnosis of sigmoid volvulus and is therefore of great utility [14]. Classic CT scan findings include a closed-loop colonic obstruction and a mesenteric "whirl" where the colonic vasculature becomes twisted around the mesenteric axis (Fig. 28.2).

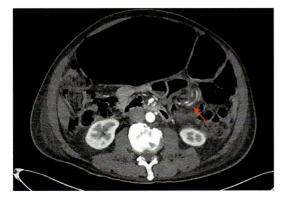

Fig. 28.2 62-year-old man with sigmoid volvulus. CT scan demonstrates dilated sigmoid colon and mesenteric "whirl sign" (arrow)

Management

Management of sigmoid volvulus has two aims: to relieve the obstruction and to prevent recurrence. Endoscopic detorsion was first described in 1947 by Bruusgaard [15] and continues to be the initial treatment for sigmoid volvulus today. In the stable patient, endoscopic decompression relieves the obstruction and allows definitive surgery to be performed electively once the patient has been resuscitated and medically optimized. Endoscopy is only appropriate in patients without signs of perforation or colonic ischemia; patients with these signs should undergo urgent operative exploration. Endoscopic detorsion can be performed with a rigid or flexible sigmoidoscope or colonoscope. Detorsion with a rigid sigmoidoscope was classically performed with the patient positioned on their hands and knees. However, this can be difficult for patients, particularly the elderly or those with significant abdominal pain. Instead, flexible sigmoidoscopy is performed with the patient in the left lateral decubitus position. The mucosa is examined for signs of bowel ischemia such as ulceration or necrosis. If these are encountered, the procedure is aborted and the patient prepared for surgery. If the colon mucosa appears healthy, the endoscope is gently advanced until a rush of air and feces (often quite dramatic) occurs as the colon detorses. A rectal tube is advanced past the site of torsion to prevent recurrent volvulus and to facilitate decompression of the proximal bowel. An abdominal radiograph is obtained to confirm successful detorsion. If the procedure is unsuccessful, the patient is taken to the operating room.

Endoscopic decompression is successful in 80% of patients, but without surgical treatment, approximately 70% will have a recurrence. Aggressive resuscitation and optimization are crucial to operative success. In the elderly patient population with multiple medical comorbidities, careful attention is paid to cardiopulmonary status, renal function, and fluid balance. The patient should undergo formal bowel preparation and complete colonoscopy in order to identify any neoplasms at the site of torsion or in the proximal colon. There is ongoing debate about whether bowel preparation is necessary in patients who have had a recent colonoscopy (and thus do not require bowel preparation for this purpose). Bowel preparation has been the standard for elective colon resection, but recent data suggests that it may be unnecessary and may adversely impact outcomes. In addition, studies have demonstrated that patients with penetrating colon trauma can undergo resection and primary anastomosis without increased infection rates. Thus, it is likely safe to omit bowel preparation in patients who do not require it for preoperative colonoscopy.

In the past, patients with sigmoid volvulus were sometimes treated with pexy of the sigmoid colon to the pelvic sidewall, which was thought to decrease the risk of recurrent volvulus. This operation takes less time than colon resection and was thus attractive in fragile patients with medical comorbidities. Unfortunately, the recurrence rate with sigmoidopexy is unacceptably high (up to 50%), and thus we do not recommend this procedure.

If endoscopic detorsion is unsuccessful or there is concern for colon necrosis, the involved colon should be resected without detorsion to avoid releasing inflammatory mediators from the necrotic bowel into the circulation. To minimize spillage in patients who did not undergo bowel preparation, an intestinal clamp is placed on the proximal colon. The proximal and distal resection sites are identified. The mesentery in the specimen is divided prior to colon resection using either the clamp-and-tie technique or the LigaSure. The colon is then divided and passed off the field. If there is no concern for colonic ischemia on preoperative endoscopy, the colon can be detorsed prior to resection.

Colostomy Versus Primary Anastomosis

If the volvulus is successfully detorsed and an elective operation performed, primary colon anastomosis is appropriate provided the patient is hemodynamically stable, is well nourished, and does not have signs of colon necrosis. A temporary protective ileostomy can decrease the complications associated with anastomotic leak. Primary anastomosis is sometimes performed in patients who require surgery in the acute setting,

but we feel that these patients should all have a protective diverting ostomy. Sigmoid resection with end colostomy (Hartmann's procedure) is used in patients who are hemodynamically unstable or show systemic signs of sepsis. Hartmann's procedure is generally also indicated in patients who have necrotic colon at the time of surgery and are nutritionally depleted or immunosuppressed or those who have fecal incontinence at baseline.

Laparoscopic management of sigmoid volvulus has been successfully performed in recent years, and research demonstrates that the laparoscopic approach is safe [16]. However because there is limited intraperitoneal working space in patients with a hugely dilated colon, we recommend open surgery when the colon cannot be detorsed preoperatively. In patients who undergo endoscopic decompression and bowel preparation, the same resection options exist by the laparoscopic approach as for the open. Advantages to laparoscopic surgery are that it is better tolerated in patients with severe pulmonary disease and may convey a lower risk of wound complications in those at high risk of infection or dehiscence. The experience and skill of the surgeon is of paramount importance when deciding whether to attempt laparoscopic management.

Cecal Volvulus

Presentation

As discussed above, patients with cecal volvulus are typically younger and more often female than patients with sigmoid volvulus. In cecal volvulus, the ascending colon and cecum are mobile and have minimal attachments to the retroperitoneum. This mobility allows the ascending colon and cecum to rotate around the mesenteric axis, causing a true volvulus, or allows the cecum to fold up anteriorly on itself, causing a cecal bascule.

Cecal volvulus and bascule are difficult to diagnose because the symptoms are often nonspecific. Patients with a true cecal volvulus may describe sudden right-sided abdominal pain, distention, and tenderness to palpation. The symptoms of a cecal volvulus are more acute than those of a sigmoid volvulus, so these patients may seek medical attention earlier. Patients with cecal bascule often present with intermittent obstructive symptoms as the bascule folds and unfolds upon itself. This can make the clinical diagnosis of cecal bascule challenging. Ischemia or perforation should be suspected in patients who present with localized or general peritonitis.

Diagnosis

Radiographic studies are helpful in the diagnosis of cecal volvulus and bascule. However, up to 15% of cecal volvulus are only diagnosed at laparotomy [17]. An upright or left lateral decubitus X-ray is obtained to evaluate for free air below the diaphragm. In cecal volvulus the classic finding on abdominal X-ray is an air-filled, ahaustral cecum that extends from the right lower quadrant to the mid-abdomen or left upper quadrant. CT scan is useful when the diagnosis is unclear from plain X-rays. CT scan shows a dilated ileum and cecum with abrupt cutoff in the right lower quadrant. A "whirl sign" may be visible as the cecum, ascending colon, and mesentery swirl around the vascular pedicle [18].

In cecal bascule, the mobile distal portion of the cecum folds cephalad and anteriorly, causing an intermittent obstruction of the colon lumen. It can be difficult to appreciate a cecal bascule on X-ray, and abdominal CT scan will only reveal the process if performed while the cecum is obstructed.

Management

Colonoscopic decompression is rarely successful in cecal volvulus. As a result, surgery is the treatment of choice. Right hemicolectomy with primary ileocolic anastomosis is effective and has low morbidity and mortality, making it ideal in all patients who are able to tolerate the operation. Hemicolectomy is preferred to ileocectomy

because in many cases the volvulized segment involves the ascending colon. The recurrence rate after right hemicolectomy with primary anastomosis is less than 10% [19]. In a true cecal bascule, ileocectomy and primary anastomosis are appropriate if the ascending colon is appropriately fixed to the retroperitoneum. Detorsion and cecopexy or cecostomy were used in the past for frail patients who could not tolerate a long operation. Approximately 1/3 of these patients will have a recurrence, though, so these procedures are not recommended.

Colon resection with primary anastomosis is appropriate in many cases of emergent cecal volvulus. Even in patients with cecal perforation or gangrene, primary anastomosis is preferred because it has lower rates of anastomotic leak (0–9%) and mortality (0–23%) than resection with diversion [19, 20]. Hemodynamically unstable patients, however, should undergo resection and end ileostomy in order to decrease operative time. As with sigmoid volvulus, a necrotic cecum should not be detorsed prior to resection in order to avoid reperfusion injury and worsening acidosis. Instead, the proximal and distal points of resection are identified, bowel clamps are applied, and the mesentery is transected. The colon and ileum are transected last, and the specimen is passed directly off the field to avoid spillage. Creation of an end ileostomy should also be considered in patients at high risk of anastomotic leak, including those who use steroids or suffer from severe malnutrition.

Transverse Colon and Splenic Flexure Volvulus

Volvulus of the transverse colon or splenic flexure is rare, representing less than 5% of volvulus cases. When these conditions do occur, the presentation depends on the acuity with which the volvulus develops. Acute, complete volvulus leads to sudden onset of severe abdominal pain, nausea, vomiting, and abdominal distention. More chronic or incomplete volvulus presents with intermittent obstructive symptoms and abdominal pain. CT scan is diagnostic, demonstrating a volvulized loop of colon with a mesenteric "whirl." The treatment for volvulus of the transverse colon or splenic flexure is resection of the involved segment. Primary anastomosis is performed in the clinically stable patient without signs of sepsis; unstable patients should undergo colostomy placement and mucous fistula or creation of a long Hartmann's pouch.

Summary

Colonic volvulus accounts for one in every ten cases of colonic obstruction in the United States. Chronic constipation and conditions that worsen constipation are the most common risk factor. Sigmoid volvulus is treated with colonic decompression followed by resection, while cecal volvulus and transverse colon volvulus are treated with resection. Management decisions, including whether or not to perform a primary anastomosis or colostomy, are based on the anatomic location of the volvulus, hemodynamic stability of the patient, and viability of the involved colon.

References

1. Ballantyne GH, et al. Volvulus of the colon. Incidence and mortality. Ann Surg. 1985;202(1):83–92.
2. Schagen van Leeuwen JH. Sigmoid volvulus in a West African population. Dis Colon Rectum. 1985;28(10):712–6.
3. Saidi F. The high incidence of intestinal volvulus in Iran. Gut. 1969;10(10):838–41.
4. De U. Sigmoid volvulus in rural Bengal. Trop Doct. 2002;32(2):80–2.
5. Ballantyne GH. Review of sigmoid volvulus: history and results of treatment. Dis Colon Rectum. 1982;25(5):494–501.
6. Lal SK, et al. Sigmoid volvulus an update. Gastrointest Endosc Clin N Am. 2006;16(1):175–87.
7. Bhatnagar BN, et al. Study on the anatomical dimensions of the human sigmoid colon. Clin Anat. 2004;17(3):236–43.
8. Ballantyne GH. Sigmoid volvulus: high mortality in county hospital patients. Dis Colon Rectum. 1981;24(7):515–20.
9. Walczak DA, et al. Volvulus of transverse colon as a rare cause of obstruction - a case report and literature review. Pol Przegl Chir. 2013;85(10):605–7.
10. Liolios N, et al. Volvulus of the transverse colon in a child: a case report. Eur J Pediatr Surg. 2003;13(2):140–2.
11. Mittal R, et al. Primary splenic flexure volvulus. Singapore Med J. 2007;48(3):e87–9.
12. Ballantyne GH. Volvulus of the splenic flexure: report of a case and review of the literature. Dis Colon Rectum. 1981;24(8):630–2.
13. Mangiante EC, et al. Sigmoid volvulus. A four-decade experience. Am Surg. 1989;55(1):41–4.
14. Levsky JM, et al. CT findings of sigmoid volvulus. AJR Am J Roentgenol. 2010;194(1):136–43.
15. Bruusgaard C. Volvulus of the sigmoid colon and its treatment. Surgery. 1947;22(3):466–78.
16. Liang JT, Lai HS, Lee PH. Elective laparoscopically assisted sigmoidectomy for the sigmoid volvulus. Surg Endosc. 2006;20(11):1772–3.
17. Grossmann EM, et al. Sigmoid volvulus in Department of Veterans Affairs Medical Centers. Dis Colon Rectum. 2000;43(3):414–8.
18. Rappaport A, et al. The whirl sign in caecal volvulus: a decisive diagnostic clue. JBR-BTR. 2007;90(6):532–4.
19. Madiba TE, Thomson SR. The management of cecal volvulus. Dis Colon Rectum. 2002;45(2):264–7.
20. Tuech JJ, et al. Results of resection for volvulus of the right colon. Tech Coloproctol. 2002;6(2):97–9.

The Treatment of Peri-Rectal Abscesses for the Emergency General Surgeon

29

Emily Miraflor and Gregory Victorino

Peri-Rectal Abscess

At first appearances, the treatment of a peri-rectal abscess seems quite simple: drainage. However, there are some patient-related factors and anatomic subtleties that can make what is often perceived as a simple problem more complex. Advance knowledge of some of these factors can make the complex scenarios simpler and also prevent morbidity to the patient in the long term. With changing practice patterns, the acute care surgeon or on-call surgeon is increasingly called upon to manage peri-rectal infections [8] so it is important to be aware of which peri-rectal abscesses may require more advance planning and which can be simply drained without further evaluation. This chapter will offer practical guidelines to manage these patients.

Anatomy

In order to treat peri-rectal abscesses appropriately, it is important to understand the potential spaces in which these abscesses occur and the relationship of those potential spaces to the

sphincter musculature. The easiest conceptual model used to understand anal sphincter anatomy is the "funnel within a funnel" model (Fig. 29.1). The inner funnel is made up of the rectum and the distal thickened circular muscle layer that comprises the internal anal sphincter (IAS). The outer funnel is the pelvic floor also known as the levator ani muscles which tapers to the external anal sphincter (EAS). During dissection, the IAS will appear white with circularly oriented muscle fibers since it is made up of autonomically innervated smooth muscle. In contrast, the EAS is made up of skeletal muscle so it will be redder in appearance, like skeletal muscle found in other parts of the body. The EAS travels further distally than the IAS; thus the intersphincteric groove is apparent only when the EAS is mildly effaced. The entire space is confined by the bones of the

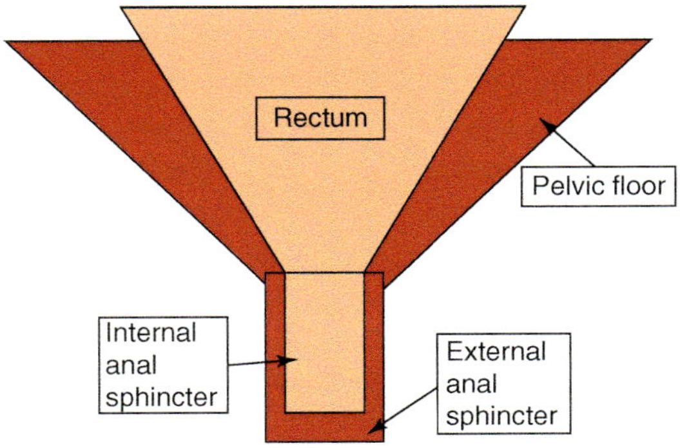

E. Miraflor
Department of Surgery, UCSF-East Bay Surgery Program, Oakland, CA, USA

G. Victorino (✉)
UCSF Medical Center, San Francisco, CA, USA
e-mail: gregory.victorino@ucsfmedctr.org

Fig. 29.1 Schematic of the relationships between the rectum, the pelvic floor, and the sphincter complexes

© Springer International Publishing AG, part of Springer Nature 2019
C. V. R. Brown et al. (eds.), *Emergency General Surgery*, https://doi.org/10.1007/978-3-319-96286-3_29

Fig. 29.2 Potential spaces surrounding the rectum, pelvic floor, and sphincter complexes (IAS, internal anal sphincter; EAS, external anal sphincter)

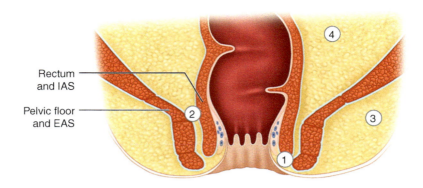

Rectum and IAS

Pelvic floor and EAS

1 - Peri-anal and submucosal
    space
2 - Internsphincteric space
3 - Ischiorectal space
4 - supralevator space

pelvis, laterally the ischium and posteriorly the sacrum. The anterior border is the vagina in females and the prostate in males.

Using this model the potential spaces where abscess can occur become easier to visualize (Fig. 29.2). A perianal abscess occurs just beneath the skin adjacent to the anal opening. An ischiorectal abscess forms in the space between the funnels and the ischium in the ischiorectal fat pad. An intersphincteric abscess occurs between the two funnels, and a supralevator abscess occurs above the level of the pelvic floor between the rectum and the levator ani complex. At the posterior midline, there are two potential spaces where abscesses can form that are important to be aware of due to their role in the formation of horseshoe abscesses (Fig. 29.3). These are the superficial and deep posterior anal spaces. The superficial posterior anal space (SPAS) is bordered by the skin distally, the anal coccygeal ligament superiorly, the anal canal anteriorly, and fat posteriorly. The deep posterior anal space (DPAS) is confined by the levator ani superiorly, the anococcygeal ligament inferiorly, the anal canal anteriorly, and the sacrum posteriorly. Since the superior and inferior borders of the SPAS and DPAS are strong connective tissue structures, when abscesses form in these spaces, the path of least resistance for the spread of purulent fluid is

into the contiguous lateral tissue planes of the ischiorectal spaces (Fig. 29.4).

Etiology

The majority of peri-rectal abscesses will have originated from an infected anal gland. Anal glands are located near the dentate line and produce lubricating mucous which protects the anoderm during defecation. If the outflow tract of the gland becomes obstructed with debris, bacterial infection can ensue and abscesses form. The abscess may remain local, in the perianal space, or it may extend into one of the potential spaces described above. A small minority of abscesses are not due to infected anal glands but instead are caused by Crohn's disease, skin infections, trauma, sexually transmitted diseases, or complications of radiation [1, 4, 12].

It is important to note that abscesses in the supralevator space have two potential etiologies. They can arise from an infected anal gland within the intersphincteric space where the purulence has ascended into the supralevator space, or they can come from an abdominal process such as diverticulitis, appendicitis, or a tubo-ovarian abscess where the purulence has descended from the abdomen into the supralevator space. The proper manage-

Fig. 29.3 Relationship of the superficial and deep posterior anal spaces to the coccyx, rectum, and anococcygeal ligament

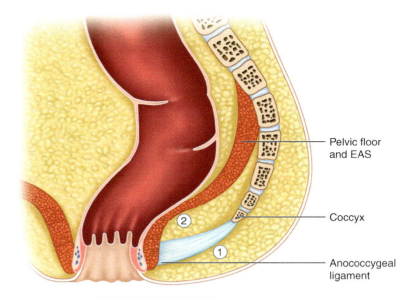

1 - Superficial posterior anal space
2 - Deep posterior anal space

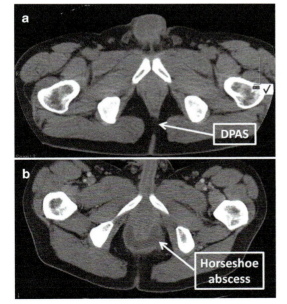

Fig. 29.4 (**a**) CT scan showing the ischiorectal spaces in continuity with the deep posterior anal space (DPAS). (**b**) CT scan of a horseshoe abscess that started in the deep posterior anal space and tracked laterally into the ischiorectal spaces

ment of supralevator abscesses depends on determining the etiology of the infection, and this is explained in more detail below [4].

Evaluation

One goal of the initial evaluation of a patient with a suspected peri-rectal abscess is to determine whether the patient can be categorized as having a simple abscess or a complex abscess. This classification scheme can help guide treatment, since a simple abscess can be readily drained either in the clinic, in the emergency room, or in the operating room without additional medical therapy, whereas, a complex abscess may require a more extensive workup, a specific drainage strategy, and an antibiotic therapy in addition to surgical drainage.

A simple abscess is one that is readily apparent on examination, confined to a single peri-rectal space, and located inferior to the pelvic floor in a patient with no prior history of

Table 29.1 Characteristics of simple versus complex peri-rectal abscesses

Simple abscesses	Complex abscesses
First occurrence	Recurrent or history of prior anorectal procedures
Readily apparent on physical exam	Not apparent on exam
Confined to a single peri-rectal space	Involves more than one peri-rectal space
Located below the pelvic floor (levator ani)	Located above the pelvic floor (supralevator)
No history of inflammatory bowel disease	Accompanied by severe cellulitis or necrotic tissues
No immunocompromised state	Immunocompromised by diabetes, neutropenia, or immunosuppressants
	Prior diagnosis of inflammatory bowel disease

abscesses, inflammatory bowel disease, or other immunocompromising states. A complex abscess has any of the following features: not apparent on external examination, involves more than one peri-rectal space (e.g., an intersphincteric abscess that has tracked cephalad into the supralevator space), located superior to the pelvic floor, or presents with simultaneous necrosis. A patient with a recurrent abscess or who is immunocompromised by diabetes, neutropenia, or HIV should also be placed into the complex category. Patients with inflammatory bowel disease can have simple abscesses, but since they are often immunocompromised or affected by other peri-rectal pathologies, abscesses in this population should be treated as complex (Table 29.1).

Presentation and History

Nearly every patient with a peri-rectal abscess will present with pain. A retrospective study of patients with a peri-rectal abscess who presented to the emergency room found that 99% of them had a chief complaint of pain [7]. The pain is typically described as constant and throbbing in nature. Swelling was less common and found only in 46% of patients. About 25% had active drainage or a fever. A little over one third had a prior abscess. Patients with peri-rectal abscesses

predictably report worsening of pain with bowel movements [7].

In addition to eliciting a history related to the suspicion of a peri-rectal abscess, it is important to also determine the patient's baseline continence status to gas, liquid, and solid stools. A history of prior anorectal pathology or procedures should be sought, including obstetric tears. Prior medical history that indicates an impaired immune response should be determined. On review of symptoms, it is important to ask about urinary retention since that may be a sign of a more severe infection concerning for pelvic sepsis.

The majority of peri-rectal abscesses can be detected on external anal physical exam, with only a minority (about 10%) discovered solely on internal digital rectal exam findings [7]. Typical findings include asymmetric swelling, tenderness, warmth, cellulitis and fluctuance. Spontaneous drainage may be present. A patient with a peri-rectal abscess is unlikely to tolerate anoscopy and it is generally unrevealing.

Laboratory Studies and Imaging

Laboratory studies are often ordered prior to the request for surgical evaluation. In most cases they do not help to confirm or rule out the diagnosis. While a normal white blood cell count neither rules in nor rules out an infectious process, other lab values may help with some treatment decisions. For instance, the chemistry panel may reveal poorly controlled diabetes, or it may show renal insufficiency that would affect medication or imaging choices. If labs have not been obtained, and the clinical situation is straightforward, it is safe to omit laboratory testing prior to surgical intervention.

If there is strong clinical suspicion for a peri-rectal abscess based on physical exam, imaging is not necessary. In fact, surprisingly, the sensitivity of computed tomography (CT) scan to detect abscesses is not very high at just 77%, so a CT will miss about one in four abscesses. The sensitivity is even lower in patients with a compromised immune system. This was determined by a retrospective study where the authors reviewed the imaging of patients who had a known abscess. They concluded that in the situation where the clinical findings were equivocal and a CT scan didn't show an abscess, it is still worthwhile to perform an examination under anesthesia to evaluate for an abscess since the sensitivity of CT is less than perfect [2].

Other investigators have attempted to use endoanal or transperineal ultrasound to localize fluid collections in the setting of ambiguous clinical exams. For the purposes of identifying an abscess, transperineal ultrasound was found to be equivalent to endoanal ultrasound [11]. Although, it is also feasible to localize peri-rectal abscesses at the bedside using the curvilinear ultrasound probe and attempts can be made at aspirating the collection under ultrasound guidance [3], this should not replace standard operative incision and drainage since a risk factor for recurrence of peri-rectal abscesses is inadequate primary drainage [7]. Additionally, many patients with a peri-rectal abscess will not tolerate bedside ultrasonography and therefore may require examination under anesthesia and drainage in the operating room if an abscess is found to be the source of their pain.

Magnetic resonance imaging (MRI) is not necessary for the patient with a simple abscess. However, patients with more complicated presentations, recurrent abscesses, or suspected fistulas are good candidates for MRI to help guide therapy. MRI is useful to identify additional fluid collections or fistulas with unusual trajectories [11].

Treatment

After obtaining the patient's history, performing a physical exam, and evaluating available laboratory data or imaging, an assessment should be made about whether the patient has a simple abscess or a complex abscess (Table 29.1). If the abscess is readily apparent on examination and appears to be confined to a single peri-rectal space located below the pelvic floor in a patient without any immunocompromising condition or history of inflammatory bowel disease, then simple incision and drainage is all that is needed. Depending on the patient's tolerance and the surgeon's comfort,

this can be done in the clinic, in the ER with light sedation, or in the operating room. The operating room is the ideal venue as the examination and drainage can be performed with ample analgesia and the adequacy of the drainage can be ensured.

Method of Drainage for a Simple Abscess

Roughly half of patients who undergo incision and drainage of a perianal abscess will develop a persistent drainage tract at the site of the incision. Thus when we drain an abscess, we may be creating a future fistula-in-ano. For this reason it is important to plan your incision in such a way that the simplest possible fistula tract is created. Rather than making the incision over the area of maximal fluctuance, it is critically important that the incision should be made in the area of fluctuance, but as close as possible to the sphincter complex without being in the sphincter complex [4]. This will create a simple short fistula tract should the area fail to heal. Since postoperative antibiotics are not necessary in the case of simple abscesses, there is no need to obtain wound cultures or tissue cultures at the time of drainage.

Generally, there are few loculations in peri-rectal abscesses. The surgeon should refrain from aggressive attempts to disrupt loculations, especially in the region of the sphincters and the rectum. Instruments, including the Yankauer suction tip should never be pointed toward the sphincter or the rectum. In the inflamed state, imprudent instrumentation of the area can result in an iatrogenic rectal perforation and the subsequent development of an extra-sphincteric fistula (a fistula that travels from the rectum, outside of the sphincter complex out onto the perianal skin).

Some authors advocate for routine inspection of the anal canal, looking for an internal opening of a fistula that is feeding the abscess cavity. This can be done by injecting hydrogen peroxide into the abscess cavity while looking in the anal canal for an internal opening. When the internal opening is identified, some suggest that a primary fistulotomy in this area should be performed in order to prevent an abscess recurrence and prevent a future fistula. The problem with this practice is that while it is true that some patients do go on to form a fistula, not all patients will form a fistula. In fact, less than 50% of abscess sufferers go on to have a fistula-in-ano. Thus about half the patients are over treated using this approach and undergo an unnecessary sphincterotomy that may impair their continence as they age. Therefore, in the case of a simple abscess, it is not necessary to look for an internal opening or perform a primary fistulotomy [11], and doing so may cause harm.

If there is concern that the cavity will close prior to complete drainage of the local sepsis, it is acceptable to place a small open drain such as a mushroom catheter, a Malecot catheter, or a Penrose drain into the cavity that should be removed in a few days. Routine packing of the wound by the patient or their caregiver does not facilitate wound healing or prevent recurrence. In fact an improperly packed or over-packed abscess cavity may damage the sphincters, further arguing against wound packing. Initial wound packing for hemostasis is an acceptable practice, and this packing should be removed on the first postoperative day [11].

With regard to postoperative care, antibiotic therapy is unnecessary after drainage of a simple abscess in an immunocompetent patient, [11]. Typically drainage itself affords significant pain relief. Postoperative analgesia is best performed with a multimodality therapy including acetaminophen, nonsteroidal anti-inflammatories, and opiate. A bowel regiment should be given, and if a bowel movement does not occur within 72 h of surgery, a gentle laxative is recommended to avoid impaction. Soaking in a warm tub (sitz baths) can offer symptomatic relief but it is not required. Soaks or showers are recommended after bowel movements to facilitate good hygiene. If a drain was placed at the time of surgery, it should be removed within a few days.

Method of Drainage for a Complex Abscess

Patients with a complex abscess (Table 29.1) should be drained in the same manner as those with simple abscesses with some modifications.

In the case of a recurrent abscess (especially one with a short interval to recurrence such as less than a month) or an abscess that appears to involve more than one peri-rectal space, it is prudent to obtain imaging to better determine the locations of the fluid collections and facilitate complete drainage. If imaging shows a supralevator collection, the source of the collection needs to be determined since supralevator collections can be due to either descending pelvic processes such as a tubo-ovarian abscess or diverticulitis or due to an ascending peri-rectal process such as an intersphincteric abscess. Supralevator abscesses that are derived from pelvic processes are better served with an interventional radiology-placed drain, whereas supralevator abscesses that originate from a peri-rectal abscess can be drained through the perineum.

Patients with complicated abscesses are more likely to require postoperative antibiotics due to surrounding cellulitis or the presence of an immunocompromising condition such as AIDS or medications that impair the immune system, like biologic therapies in the inflammatory bowel disease population. Thus, it is reasonable to obtain wound cultures in this population. A small portion of these cultures will return with MRSA rather than enteric flora so culture data in this instance may change therapy. MRSA abscesses tend to have high failure rates with drainage alone, so having culture information may explain why an abscess recurred if it was found to be infected with MRSA [1].

Candidates for postoperative antibiotic therapy are patients with immune compromising conditions such as AIDS, leucopenia, poorly controlled diabetes, or medication-induced immunosuppression from steroids or biologic therapies directed at inflammatory bowel disease. Peri-rectal infections with surrounding cellulitis are another indication for postoperative antibiotics. Unless there is strong suspicion for MRSA or culture data proving the presence of MRSA, antibiotics directed toward enteric flora is all that is required.

Patients with inflammatory bowel disease are at higher risk of abscess recurrence, and they are often on medications that impair their immune system. In this case, if an internal opening is easily identified, a draining seton should be placed to prevent abscess recurrence and worsening local sepsis [4] (PR Fleshner personal communication). There are many acceptable ways to place a seton. The ideal seton is loose enough to prevent painful constriction of the sphincter muscles and has a low profile that prevents discomfort. Vessel loops are often used as a seton, and when secured to itself with a silk tie, they have a flat profile that is more comfortable to the patient than when it is tied into bulky knots (Fig. 29.5). Placing a seton will likely result in a fistula that will need to be dealt with at a later stage, but the benefits of preventing another infection in an immunocompromised patient often outweigh the risks. If the subsequent fistula is a low transsphincteric fistula, a simple fistulotomy can be performed in the future with good results.

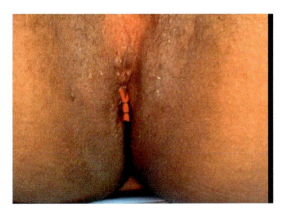

Fig. 29.5 Seton secured placed through a fistula-in-ano and secured to itself. The flat profile improves tolerability

Special Situations

Horseshoe Abscesses

While horseshoe abscesses can occur either from the anterior or posterior midline and track into the lateral ischiorectal spaces, they more commonly occur posteriorly (Fig. 29.4). They usually originate in the deep posterior anal space which lies between the anococcygeal ligament and the pelvic floor. Adequate drainage requires entry into the deep posterior anal space and into the lateral ischiorectal spaces. First an incision through the skin just outside of the sphincter complex, between the external anal sphincter and the coccyx, is made. The anococcygeal ligament is a tough connective tissue structure, so the surgeon will need to take a clamp to pop through this ligament and enter the space. Upon entry into the space, purulent fluid should be immediately drained. The lateral spaces will need to be drained as well. This can be accomplished with counterincisions into the ischiorectal spaces or by feeding a Penrose drain into both spaces from the deep postanal space to facilitate drainage in the postoperative period [12] (Fig. 29.6). While typically depicted in the prone position, horseshoe abscesses can be drained adequately in the lithotomy position as well.

Fournier's Gangrene

Fournier's gangrene is an extensive, necrotizing, soft tissue infection that can arise from neglected perianal infections, often in the setting of poorly

Fig. 29.6 Drainage method for horseshoe abscesses. An incision is made through the anococcygeal ligament to drain fluid from the deep postanal space (DPAS). Counterincisions are made into the ischiorectal fossa to drain purulent fluid that tracked laterally

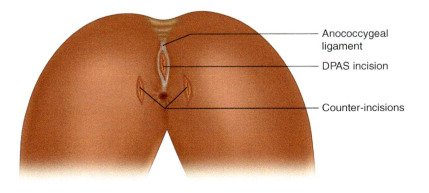

controlled diabetes. It can present with the usual signs of sepsis such as fever, tachycardia, and hypotension along with pelvic pain or urinary retention. Physical examination may show erythema or necrosis of the perianal tissues. Imaging is not necessary, but if a CT is done, there may be large amounts of soft tissue gas or extensive soft tissue inflammation demonstrated by fat stranding (Fig. 29.7). Expeditious operative debridement is the key to successful treatment. Repeated debridement may be necessary to control the disease. The sphincters are usually spared, but if they are involved, diversion should be performed. The choices for diversion include a diverting loop ileostomy, a diverting transverse colostomy, or a sigmoidostomy. Of the three choices, the best option, if future reversal is anticipated, is diverting loop ileostomy because it is the easiest to reverse and has the lowest rate of stomal complications such as retraction, ischemia, prolapse, and herniation. The least attractive option is a

transverse colostomy due to increased rates of prolapse and herniation as well as pouching problems. A transverse colostomy is also more difficult to close. An end sigmoidostomy with a Hartmann's pouch is a good option if the sphincters are severely compromised because a permanent sigmoidostomy results in fewer physiologic derangements than an ileostomy and its output is easier to manage [6]. If the sphincters are uninvolved, it is possible to avoid a diverting ostomy altogether and still provide adequate wound care. This can be accomplished with a "medical colostomy" using a low residue diet and antidiarrheals [9]. Alternatively a rectal tube device can be used to contain stool [5], but in order for this technique to work, the patient must be placed on a bowel regimen that will produce liquid stools. Additionally, rectal tubes when left in place long term can complicate nursing care, cause patient discomfort, and if the balloon is overinflated result in rectal necrosis.

Neutropenic Patients

Neutropenic patients, those with absolute neutrophil counts of less than 500/mm^3, can develop peri-rectal infections that do not become suppurative because they do not have sufficient neutrophil activity to produce a purulent fluid collection. When evaluating a neutropenic patient, an internal examination should be avoided. The examination should be limited to the perianal skin due to the theoretical risk of causing an infection during the examination. If there is strong suspicion for a fluid collection, imaging should be performed. Any fluid collections identified are promptly drained, and antibiotic therapy is continued until neutropenia and symptoms resolve [10].

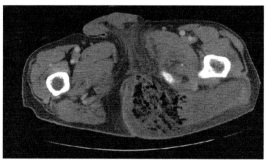
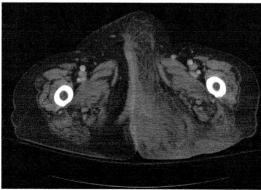

Fig. 29.7 Computed tomography findings of patients who had Fournier's gangrene. Extensive soft tissue gas or inflammation should raise concern for Fournier's gangrene

Summary

Peri-rectal abscesses are common problems faced by the emergency general surgeon. Drainage of simple abscesses can be easily performed. Complex abscesses still require drainage, but treatment should be augmented with antibiotics, and in the case of immunocompromised patients, it is reasonable to place setons. Knowledge of the peri-rectal spaces and ligaments can aid in the identification and treatment of complex abscesses including horseshoe abscesses.

References

1. Brown SR, Horton JD. Perirectal abscess infections related to MRSA. J Surg Res. 2009;66:264–6.
2. Caliste X, Nazir S. Sensitivity of computed tomography in detection of peri-rectal abscess. Am Surg. 2011;77:166–8.
3. Chandwani D, Shih R. Bedside ultrasound in the evaluation of perirectal abscesses. Am J Emerg Med. 2004;22:315.
4. Corman M. Corman's Colon and Rectal surgery. In: Corman M, editor. Corman's Colon and Rectal surgery. 6th ed. Philadelphia: Wolters Kluwer; 2013. p. 367–81.
5. Goh M, Chew M. Nonsurgical faecal diversion in the management of severe perianal sepsis: a retrospective evaluation of the flexible faecal management system. Singap Med J. 2014;55(12):635–9.
6. Hendren S, Hammond K. Clinical practice guidelines for ostomy surgery. Dis Colon Rectum. 2015;58:375–87.
7. Marcus RH, Stine RJ. Perirectal abscess. Ann Emerg Med. 1995;25:597–603.
8. Pottenger BC, Galante JM. Modern acute care surgeon: characterization of an evolving surgical niche. J Trauma Acute Care Surg. 2014;78:120–5.
9. Robertson HD. Use of an elemental diet as a nutritionally complete medical colostomy. South Med J. 1983;76(8):1005–7.
10. Steele SL, Hull TR. The ASCRS textbook of colon and rectal surgery. 3rd ed. New York: Springer; 2016.
11. Vogel JD, Johnson EK. Clinical practic guidelins for the management of anorectal abscess. Dis Colon Rectum. 2016;59:1117–33.
12. Whiteford MH. Perianal abscess and fistula disease. Clin Colon Rectal Surg. 2007;20:102–9.

Diagnosis and Treatment of Acute Hemorrhoidal Disease and the Complications of Hemorrhoidal Procedures

30

James M. Tatum and Eric J. Ley

Overview of Hemorrhoids

Hemorrhoids, colloquially "piles," are common and range in severity from inconvenience (Napoleon at Waterloo) to fatal (David Livingston in Africa) [1]. They represent one of medicine's oldest problems, one which we are fortunate enough to now understand and possess multiple options for treatment.

Anatomy

Hemorrhoids are the sinusoidal vascular cushions composed of the anastomoses of the arterioles of the terminal branches of the superior rectal and hemorrhoidal systems as well as the smaller branches of the middle and inferior hemorrhoidal arteries and their respective venous drainage system [2, 3]. There are three hemorrhoidal plexuses, predictably found in the anal canal at three positions: laterally on the left and on the right at anterior and posterior positions. Each hemorrhoidal plexus extends under both

anorectal mucosa above the dentate line proximally (internal hemorrhoid) and under the somatically innervated anoderm distal to the dentate line (external hemorrhoid) [4]. The non-pathologic hemorrhoid functions as a vascular "cushion," both adding mass to the anal canal, serving to maintain continence in time of increased intraabdominal pressure as they expand during Valsalva, and functioning in sensing between solid bowel movement and flatus [2, 3].

The vascular anatomy of the anal canal is particularly important in patients with portal hypertension. There are connections between the superior anal vein, which ordinarily has portal drainage, and the middle and inferior rectal veins, which drain into the systemic venous circulation, making the anal canal a notable site for portal systemic shunting. The congestion of portal venous hypertension found in cirrhosis or other disease of increased portal hypertension can result in anorectal varicosities of these anastomoses [5]. These varices are of clinical concern given their propensity for troublesome bleeding in the cirrhotic patient. It should be clear that these anorectal varices are clinically and anatomically distinct from hemorrhoids and that confusing them can have fatal consequences for the patient [5].

A key point to remember about the anatomy of hemorrhoids is that they are not innately pathological; they are not the same as anorectal varices and are often vaguely described by both

J. M. Tatum · E. J. Ley (✉)
Department of Surgery, Cedars Sinai Medical Center, Los Angeles, CA, USA
e-mail: Eric.Ley@cshs.org

patients and junior trainees. The perineum merits careful examination by an experienced clinician capable of distinguishing between prolapse, fissure, mass, papilloma, polyp, abscess, fistula, melanoma, inflammatory bowel disease, varices with an acute or chronic pathology, and any of a variety of other conditions [2]. *The single most important consideration when considering perineal anatomy is that someone familiar with it performs or supervises the clinical examination to avoid misdiagnosis and mistreatment.*

Pathophysiology of Disease

The hemorrhoid cushions become pathological and present to the clinician when they experience venous congestion or clot with subsequent prolapse with or without incarceration or strangulation, bleeding from ulceration, thrombosis, or pain [2, 6]. Factors contributing to pathological hemorrhoid conditions include habitual straining during bowel movements to achieve complete rectal emptying. Western low-fiber diets are often linked to this behavior and the disease [2].

Epidemiology

Many people suffer from enlarged hemorrhoids although the exact number is unknown as it is often a self-limited condition or one for which patients do not seek medical care. The prevalence is estimated to be more than 4% of the adult US population [7]. Hemorrhoids are more common in Caucasians with the highest prevalence between ages 45 and 65 years. Hemorrhoids in the young are uncommon, and alternative explanations for bleeding must be dutifully sought if the diagnosis is not certain.

Diagnoses and Evaluation of Hemorrhoid Disease

Classification

Hemorrhoids are first classified by position relative to the dentate line, proximal being internal and distal being external. The site of origin determines the involvement of the superior vs. inferior hemorrhoidal plexus, respectively, but more importantly it determines symptoms. External hemorrhoids underlie somatically innervated skin and when thrombosed are associated with dramatic and incapacitating pain. Internal hemorrhoids are covered by mucosa and are relatively painless. Hemorrhoids may involve both the internal and external components at any of the three anatomic locations; these are referred to as "mixed" hemorrhoids.

Internal hemorrhoids are graded on a four-tier scale by severity of prolapse as shown in Fig. 30.1. Grade I hemorrhoids are defined by non-prolapsing prominent vessels, Grade II as prolapsing when bearing down with spontaneous reduction, Grade III prolapse with bearing down requiring manual reduction, and Grade IV as non-reducible prolapse [4]. Bleeding may occur from hemorrhoids of any grade.

Symptoms

Hemorrhoids are asymptomatic in more than 40% of people with pathological hemorrhoids. The most common symptoms are bleeding and pain [8].

Symptoms of Internal Hemorrhoids
Grades I–III internal hemorrhoids often present with complaints of bleeding on toilet paper or spotting in the toilet after a bowel movement. Other symptoms include pruritus, incontinence, difficulty cleaning the perineum after bowel

Fig. 30.1 Illustration of Grades I–IV internal hemorrhoids

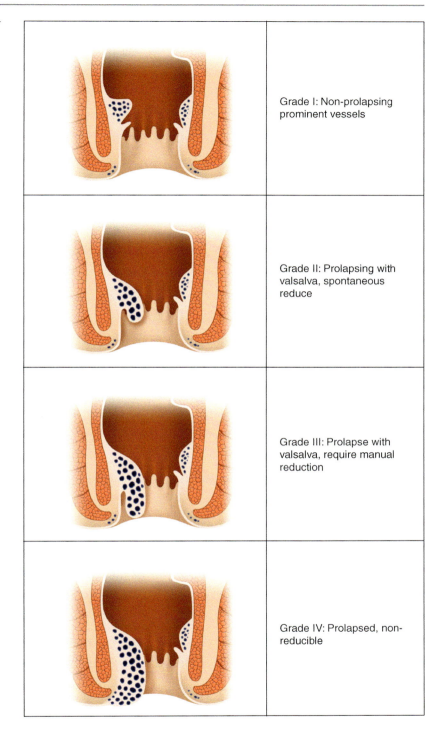

Grade I: Non-prolapsing prominent vessels

Grade II: Prolapsing with valsalva, spontaneous reduce

Grade III: Prolapse with valsalva, require manual reduction

Grade IV: Prolapsed, non-reducible

movement, or concern of prolapse. Grade IV internal hemorrhoids present with more prominent complaints of the same symptoms. Thrombosed internal hemorrhoids can present with pain or more commonly symptoms of discomfort, difficulty completely evacuating, or anal leakage. The prolapsed Grade IV hemorrhoid can become incarcerated or strangulated with subsequent thrombosis, necrosis, and bleeding.

Symptoms of External Hemorrhoids

External hemorrhoids are not graded. In the absence of thrombosis, external hemorrhoids often go unnoticed in the absence of bleeding. Thrombosis of an external hemorrhoid (TEH) is excruciating. If not evacuated, the TEH pains will generally abate over a few days [2, 8].

Initial Evaluation

Hemorrhoids can usually be diagnosed with an oral history and a physical examination. In general, any anorectal condition, especially those involving bleeding, require a digital rectal examination and often anoscopy on first presentation. The one exception to this rule is in patients with prominent pain and no external signs of thrombosed or prolapsing hemorrhoids. Provided these patients have minimal signs of bleeding, infection, or inflammatory bowel disease, the diagnosis of anal fissure can be considered. If anal fissure is the most likely diagnosis from history and visual examination, the DRE may be *delayed* until a later date and treatment of the fissure has commenced. Care must always be taken in performing DRE or anoscopy on patient with end-stage liver disease as it may cause intractable bleeding. All other patients require a DRE +/− anoscopy for the initial diagnosis of hemorrhoids. Anoscopy is superior to flexible sigmoidoscopy for initial diagnosis as the hollow barrel of the side-viewing endoscopy which allows hemorrhoids to be viewed from the sidewall which facilitates careful inspection and a specific diag-

Table 30.1 American Society of Colon and Rectal Surgeons practice parameters

1. The evaluation of patients with hemorrhoids should include a directed history and physical examination
Grade of recommendation: strong recommendation based on low-quality evidence **1C**[a]

Source: Rivadeneira et al. [7]
[a]Recommendations made using GRADE system [9]

nosis [7]. These examinations are aided by proper patient positioning: knee to chest while in prone jackknife or left lateral position [3] (Table 30.1).

Diagnostic Procedures, Imaging, and Laboratory Testing

Laboratory tests are not indicated unless there is a clinical concern of anemia from blood loss, concern for pelvic sepsis, or diagnostic uncertainty regarding soft tissue infection or abscess of the perineum. We do recommend coagulation tests in patients with end-stage liver disease or on oral anticoagulants and will also consider them in pregnant patients with bleeding from pathological hemorrhoids.

Imaging is rarely indicated in the setting of uncomplicated hemorrhoidal disease, and when indicated it is used to aid in the evaluation of pelvic sepsis or to evaluate for diagnoses other than hemorrhoids such as abscess, necrotizing soft tissue infection, or rectal malignancy. Imaging studies to be considered in this setting include CT scan of the abdomen and pelvis, intrarectal ultrasonography, or barium enema.

Endoscopy

Formal endoscopic (colonoscopy or sigmoidoscopic) evaluation of the colon is indicated in selected patients with hemorrhoidal bleeding including those with iron deficiency anemia, + fecal occult blood test, age ≥ 50 years in patients without colonoscopy within 10 years, and age ≥ 40 years in those with a concerning family history and no recent colonoscopy and those with symptoms or signs concerning for inflammatory bowel disease or malignancy [7] (Table 30.2).

Table 30.2 American Society of Colon and Rectal Surgeons practice parameters

2. Complete endoscopic evaluation of the colon is indicated in select patients with hemorrhoids and rectal bleeding
Grade of recommendation: strong recommendation based on moderate-quality evidence **1B**[a]

Source: Rivadeneira et al. [7]
[a]Recommendations made using GRADE system [9]

Table 30.3 American Society of Colon and Rectal Surgeons practice parameters

3. Dietary modification consisting of adequate fluid and fiber intake is the primary first-line nonoperative therapy for patients with symptomatic hemorrhoid disease
Grade of recommendation: strong recommendation based on moderate-quality evidence **1B**[a]

Source: Rivadeneira et al. [7]
[a]Recommendations made using GRADE system [9]

Nonoperative Treatment of Hemorrhoid Disease

Hemorrhoids amenable to nonoperative therapy rarely present to the acute care surgeon as their acute management and disposition are well within the scope of practice of the emergency room physician or primary care provider. On the occasion when nonoperative hemorrhoids present to the surgeon, there are multiple noninvasive options that can be considered and recommended; these interventions are also part of the treatment of those who do require an acute intervention.

Lifestyle Modifications

The avoidance of constipation with adequate hydration and fiber intake is of paramount importance both in preventing trauma to the hemorrhoidal plexus and preventing prolapse [2, 4]. Diarrhea can be equally problematic for those with Grades III–IV as continence is compromised as is the ability to maintain good hygiene. Adequate dietary fiber is again of paramount importance. Sitz baths are an equally important mechanism of hygiene, especially in those with Grades III–IV or external hemorrhoids (Table 30.3).

Oral Medications

Oral fiber supplements should be recommended at a dose that optimizes stool consistency and regularity. European studies have examined the use of micronized and purified flavonoid with or without anti-inflammatory medications to treat hemorrhoid symptoms [4]. These medications are not approved by the Food and Drug Administration for use in the United States.

Topical Treatments

Multiple over-the-counter remedies exist to treat hemorrhoids and hemorrhoid symptoms. There are no studies that support the use of over-the-counter therapy to reduce either bleeding or prolapse; however, some have been shown to reduce symptoms and inflammation [4]. Topical corticosteroids can be used, with caution, over a short duration to reduce inflammation. Other over-the-counter devices, creams, ointments, or gels may be recommended for use at the patients' discretion, and we have found, anecdotally, that gels with a local anesthetic do improve patients' symptoms. The most effective topical therapy is warm water during a sitz bath or shower to maintain good hygiene and minimize trauma.

Operative Treatment of External Hemorrhoid Disease

Thrombosed External Hemorrhoids (TEH)

TEH frequently present as an acutely painful, sometimes bleeding, anal mass. Thrombosis generally occurs after unusually intense straining from lifting, prolonged sitting, or constipation.

These are sometimes amenable to conservative treatment with oral analgesia, sitz baths, and the application of topical anesthetics +/− topical nifedipine. Pain will generally resolve over a 2–3-day period and swelling will resolve in 7–10 days [10].

If the patient presents within 72 h (ideally ≤48 h) of thrombosis, surgical evacuation may be considered. Patients with severe ulceration and bleeding, rupture, or signs concerning for infection should undergo excision within 72 h of symptom onset. This procedure should be performed through an elliptical incision overlying the thrombosed hemorrhoid in a radial orientation to the anus after a four-finger stretch of the anus and rectum [6]. The thrombosed hemorrhoidal plexus is ligated and excised. We prefer to perform this procedure in the operating room under general anesthesia. The wound is generally left open and the specimen is always sent to pathology. Antibiotics can be prescribed at the discretion of the surgeon; we recommend them when there is concern of infection prior to surgery as well as in patients with diabetes and in those with obvious poor hygiene. Bedside incision and evacuation of the TEH do provide symptomatic relief if done early. This relief is frequently complicated by recurrence or re-bleeding; however, rates of recurrence after excision and incision considered together are lower than after conservative management [10]. Rubber band ligation of a TEH will result in excruciating pain on the part of the patient. Rubber band application to an external hemorrhoid is contraindicated in all cases.

Patients with resolved TEH often develop skin tags which can be troubling in terms of hygiene or appearance. These may be excised by a non-acute care surgeon in an elective setting (Table 30.4).

Table 30.4 American Society of Colon and Rectal Surgeons practice parameters

5. Most patients with thrombosed external hemorrhoids benefit from surgical excision within 72 h of the onset of symptoms
Grade of recommendation: strong recommendation based on low-quality evidence **1C**[a]

Source: Rivadeneira et al. [7]
[a]Recommendations made using GRADE system [9]

Non-thrombosed External Hemorrhoids

In the absence of thrombosis or frank hemorrhage, external hemorrhoids should not be operated on in an acute setting. Large or troubling external hemorrhoids may be considered for excision in an elective setting, usually by a colorectal surgeon experienced in this nonstandard procedure.

Operative Treatment of Internal Hemorrhoids (Fig. 30.2)

Thrombosed Internal Hemorrhoids

Thrombosis of internal hemorrhoids may occur, usually as a complication in a prolapsed Grades III–IV hemorrhoid. Surgery is rarely recommended unless there is true strangulation. Surgical treatment if necessary is a formal excision hemorrhoidectomy of some, or all, of the diseased hemorrhoidal plexuses.

Internal Hemorrhoids

Office-Based Procedures

Sclerotherapy: Sclerotherapy of Grades I–II internal hemorrhoids is accomplished in the non-anesthetized patient with no other anal or rectal pathology by the application of a variety of sclerosing agents into the hemorrhoid while avoiding the hemorrhoidal vein [2]. Potential complications include abdominal pain, impotence, nerve injury, and hepatic abscess. We do not recommend that this procedure be performed in an acute setting by a non-expert.

Infrared coagulation: Heat is applied to Grades I–II internal hemorrhoid resulting in coagulation and eventual obliteration. If an external component is present, then anesthesia is required.

Rubber band ligation: Application of a rubber band at the base of the internal hemorrhoid results in ischemic necrosis and amputation of the plexus. The procedure can be accompanied by pain, increasing in amount as proximity to the dentate line increases. Rubber bands may not be

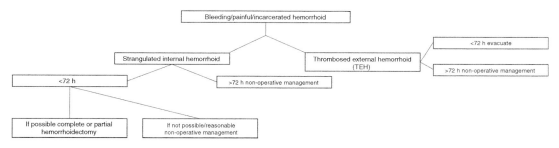

Fig. 30.2 Decision algorithm for acute painful hemorrhoids

Table 30.5 American Society of Colon and Rectal Surgeons practice parameters

4. Most patients with grades I, II, and III hemorrhoid disease in whom medical treatment fails may be effectively treated with office-based procedures, such as banding, sclerotherapy, and infrared coagulation. Hemorrhoid banding is typically the most effective option
Grade of recommendation: strong recommendation based on moderate-quality evidence **1B**[a]

Source: Rivadeneira et al. [7]

[a]Recommendations made using GRADE system [9]

applied distal to (or ideally within 1 cm of) the dentate line. There is a risk of hemorrhage as the banded hemorrhoid sloughs 1–2 weeks post procedure. Rubber band ligation requires only simple mechanical equipment which is intuitive to use and should be part of the scope of practice of the acute care surgeon. This is our preferred method of intervention if called to address bleeding internal hemorrhoids.

Other local interventions have been described including cryotherapy and diathermy. These treatments are beyond the scope of an acute care surgery text (Table 30.5).

Operative Treatment of Internal Hemorrhoids

Multiple Procedures for the Operative Treatment of Internal or Mixed Hemorrhoids: Each requires specialized knowledge, and each has potentially devastating complications to the surrounding tissue and patient. Catastrophic bleeding from an internal hemorrhoid should nearly always be amenable to local therapies such as banding or simple open hemorrhoidectomy. Attempting to perform a complex operative procedure in an acute setting is not recommended without the

consultation of a colorectal surgeon first. Antibiotics are not required prior to the performance of hemorrhoidectomy; however, we do administer them to patients with signs of infection, diabetics, and smokers as hemorrhoidectomy in these patients is associated with a higher risk of postoperative complications [11].

Closed Hemorrhoidectomy: Local anesthesia mixed with epinephrine is used to infiltrate the anal submucosa. A plane is developed between the internal sphincter and the hemorrhoidal tissue which is then excised and the pedicle ligated. All incisions are closed both internally and on the skin. Complications may include incontinence, pelvic sepsis, or hemorrhage.

Open Hemorrhoidectomy: It is similar to closed hemorrhoidectomy without submucosal or skin closure. Both procedures have a risk of subsequent stenosis of the anal canal, and care must be taken to leave bridging tissue between hemorrhoid plexuses. Open hemorrhoidectomy is sometimes indicated in a subacute setting to treat necrotic hemorrhoids or those with intractable bleeding not amenable to other interventions. You must remember to liberally dilate the anal canal before performance of these procedures to reduce the risk of subsequent stenosis.

Harmonic/LigaSure Hemorrhoidectomy: Planes are developed in the same fashion as the above procedures, and dissection/resection is achieved with the energy device of the surgeons choosing. This is our preferred method to treat intractable bleeding of necrotic internal hemorrhoids in the acute setting.

Stapled Hemorrhoidopexy: Use of modified circular stapler is used to resect a segment of the rectal mucosa and submucosa after approximation with a purse-string suture. We do not recom-

Table 30.6 American Society of Colon and Rectal Surgeons practice parameters

6. Surgical hemorrhoidectomy should be reserved for patients who are refractory to office procedures, who are unable to tolerate office procedures, who have large external hemorrhoids, or who have combined internal and external hemorrhoids with significant prolapse (grades III to IV)
Grade of recommendation: strong recommendation based on moderate-quality evidence **1B**[a]

Source: Rivadeneira et al. [7]
[a]Recommendations made using GRADE system [9]

mend this device for use in the acute setting or by a non-colorectal surgeon. The procedure can lead to incontinence or infection. If the patient's hemorrhoids are accompanied by significant rectal prolapse, the patient deserves to have consultation with a colorectal surgery prior to any non-emergent procedure (Table 30.6).

Complications of Hemorrhoid Surgery

The acute care surgeon may occasionally encounter patients who have undergone recent intervention for external or internal hemorrhoids. Acute problems can range from urinary retention or bleeding accompanying sloughing of internal hemorrhoids following banding or other office-based procedures. The dreaded complication is pelvic sepsis following stapled hemorrhoidectomy. More chronic problems such as stenosis of the anal canal may also present with acute on chronic colonic obstruction.

The bleeding after banding, sclerotherapy, or thermal procedure is usually self-limited requiring only supportive care; however, we have on occasion needed to take a patient to the operating room for exam under anesthesia and intervention. Colonoscopy with endoscopic ligation can also be considered if available at your facility [12]. Chronic anal stenosis with colon obstruction can be temporized with either dilatation or more dramatically with colon diversion in the operating room. A barium enema or CT scan should precede any operative intervention if possible.

Stapled hemorrhoidectomy can be complicated by severe complications including pelvic sepsis, necrotizing soft tissue infection, rectal

necrosis, or pelvic abscess. Any of these complications can be rapidly fatal if not diagnosed early and treated aggressively. Prompt diagnosis, resuscitation, and treatment which may include operative exploration, drainage and/or, resection may be necessary. A high index of suspicion should be maintained by the acute care surgeon when consulted on the patient who recently underwent operative hemorrhoidectomy.

Acknowledgments We would like to acknowledge Rex Chung, MD of the Department of Surgery at Cedars-Sinai Medical Center, for his contribution of illustrations to this chapter.

References

1. Welling DR, Wolff BG, Dozois RR. Napoleon at waterloo. Dis Colon Rectum. 1988;31:303–5.
2. Kaidar-Person O, Person B, Wexner SD. Hemorrhoidal disease: a comprehensive review. J Am Coll Surg. 2007;204:102.
3. Sanchez C, Chinn B. Hemorrhoids. Clin Colon Rectal Surg. 2011;24:005.
4. Lohsiriwat V. Hemorrhoids: from basic pathophysiology to clinical management. World J Gastroenterol. 2012;18:2009.
5. Khalloufi Al K. Management of rectal varices in portal hypertension. World J Hepatol. 2015;7:2992.
6. Hardy A, Cohen C. The acute management of haemorrhoids. Ann R Coll Surg Engl. 2014;96:508.
7. Rivadeneira DE, Steele SR, Ternent C, Chalasani S, Buie WD, Rafferty JL, Standards Practice Task Force of The American Society of Colon and Rectal Surgeons. Practice parameters for the Management of Hemorrhoids (revised 2010). Dis Colon Rectum. 2011;54:1059.
8. Migaly J, Sun Z. Review of hemorrhoid disease: presentation and management. Clin Colon Rectal Surg. 2016;29:022.
9. Brochard L, Abroug F, Brenner M, Broccard AF, Danner RL, Ferrer M, et al. An official ATS/ERS/ESICM/SCCM/SRLF statement: prevention and Management of Acute Renal Failure in the ICU patient. Am J Respir Crit Care Med. 2010;181:1128.
10. Greenspon J, Williams SB, Young HA, Orkin BA. Thrombosed external hemorrhoids: outcome after conservative or surgical management. Dis Colon Rectum. 2004;47:1493.
11. Nelson DW, Champagne BJ, Rivadeneira DE, Davis BR, Maykel JA, Ross HM, et al. Prophylactic antibiotics for hemorrhoidectomy. Dis Colon Rectum. 2014;57:365.
12. Davis KG, Pelta AE, Armstrong DN. Combined colonoscopy and three-quadrant Hemorrhoidal ligation: 500 consecutive cases. Dis Colon Rectum. 2007;50:1445.

Spontaneous Pneumothorax

31

Jaye Alexander Weston and Anthony W. Kim

History

Jean Marc Gaspard Itard first coined the term pneumothorax in 1803, when he described five cases where free air was found in the chest after traumatic events [1]. It was not until 1819 that Rene Laennec first described the clinical features of a pneumothorax where he theorized existing lung blebs and unprovoked rupture were the cause of a spontaneous pneumothorax [2]. The term pneumothorax is derived from the Greek words *pneuma,* relating to air, and *thorakos* relating to the breastplate or chest. It is better known today as a collection of air outside the lung within the pleural cavity between the parietal and visceral pleura. There are several types of pneumothorax owing to the etiology of this entity including spontaneous, traumatic, and iatrogenic pneumothorax. We will focus on the spontaneous pneumothorax for the remainder of this chapter specifically discussing traditional approaches to this disease process.

Spontaneous pneumothorax can be further divided into primary and secondary, which relates to the causes of each. Primary spontaneous pneumothorax (PSP) is a localized rupture of a bleb in otherwise normal lungs without an inciting traumatic event. A secondary spontaneous pneumothorax (SSP) occurs due to underlying pulmonary disease such as COPD. Other diseases causing SSP include HIV-related infection *Pneumocystis carinii* pneumonia, Langerhans cell granulomatosis, and lymphangioleiomyomatosis, among several other disease processes.

Epidemiology

The incidence of age-adjusted primary spontaneous pneumothorax has been reported at 7.4/100,000 a year for males and 1.2/100,000 for females. In comparison, the incidence of secondary spontaneous pneumothorax is 6.3/100,000 for males and 1.2/100,000 for females [3]. PSP typically occurs in tall, thin, young males usually between the ages of 10 and 30 years. Although PSP is not associated with overt lung disease, a predominant risk factor is smoking cigarettes, which has been reported to increase the risk by as much as 20-fold [4]. The peak incidence of SSP is in elderly individuals over the age of 60 years, paralleling the diseases it is most associated with such as COPD [5].

J. A. Weston · A. W. Kim (✉)
Division of Thoracic Surgery, Keck University School of Medicine of the University of Southern California, Los Angeles, CA, USA
e-mail: anthony.kim@med.usc.edu

© Springer International Publishing AG, part of Springer Nature 2019
C. V. R. Brown et al. (eds.), *Emergency General Surgery*, https://doi.org/10.1007/978-3-319-96286-3_31

Pathophysiology

Primary Spontaneous Pneumothorax

PSP is categorized as not being associated with apparent lung disease; however, it is often associated with subpleural bullae that rupture leading to pneumothorax (Fig. 31.1). The evidence of subpleural bullae has been found in 76–100% of patients undergoing video-assisted thoracoscopic surgery [6]. The matter in which bullae develop is presumed to be due to degradation of elastic fibers in the lung parenchyma. Smoking appears to play a significant role in the influx of neutrophils and macrophages that create an imbalance of protease enzymes that lead to the destruction of the elastic fibers. The resultant bullae produce an inflammatory destruction of the small airways leading to an air leak into the lung interstitium. Once enough pressure builds up, a rupture occurs in the visceral pleura allowing air to escape that creates a separation between the parietal and visceral pleura, defined as a pneumothorax.

Secondary Spontaneous Pneumothorax

The pathophysiology for SSP is dependent on the disease process that leads to the development of the pneumothorax. COPD, which is the most common cause of SSP, leads to pneumothorax in the similar manner as the subpleural bullae in PSP (Fig. 31.2). The airway inflammation and elastin destruction leads to an increase in alveolar pressure that moves from the interstitium toward the hilum. The build of pressure in the hilum leads to pneumomediastinum and eventually a violation of the parietal pleura [6]. In comparison, *P. carinii* leads to a pneumothorax by rupturing the alveolus directly due to necrosis of the lung from infection [7].

Clinical Presentation

The presenting symptoms of a spontaneous pneumothorax are usually pleuritic chest pain and sudden onset of dyspnea [8]. The chest pain associated with pneumothorax is often described as sharp or stabbing in nature. The degree of symptoms is dependent on whether it is a PSP or SSP. SSPs are often more symptomatic because they already have a compromised pulmonary reserve, whereas PSPs are less symptomatic due to the fact that these patients are otherwise typically young and healthy. Additionally, patients with SSP may provide an additional history supporting the presumed diagnosis of exerting themselves or engaging in an activity that may be associated with a mechanism of injury that involves a Valsalva maneuver.

The physical examination findings associated with a pneumothorax can be decreased breath

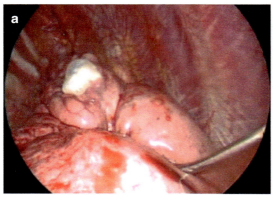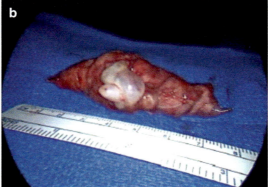

Fig. 31.1 Primary spontaneous pneumothorax: (**a**) intraoperative image of apical bleb, (**b**) image of resected ruptured bleb

Fig. 31.2 Secondary spontaneous pneumothorax: (**a**) intraoperative image of apical bullae with anthracotic and diseased lung, (**b**) image of resected bullae

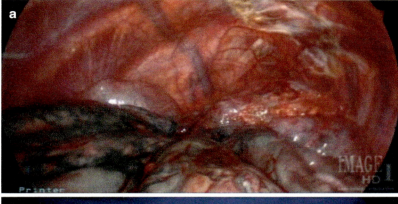

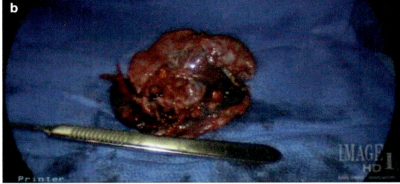

sounds on the side of the pneumothorax, hyper-resonance to percussion, and decreased chest wall movement on the affected side [9]. Additional measurements used clinically may include arterial blood gas and oxygen saturations, which often demonstrate an increased A-A gradient and slightly diminished oxygen saturations on room air, respectively.

Imaging

The clinical diagnosis of a spontaneous pneumothorax can be confirmed with imaging. The most common imaging modality used is a posterior-anterior chest radiograph that reveals a less than 1 mm area of visceral pleura that is displaced if a pneumothorax is present. The radiograph is able to diagnose most pneumothoraces but is of limited utility when the pneumothorax develops in the anterior chest or costophrenic angle. Also, radiographs can lead to false positives in individuals with extremely large bullae appearing as

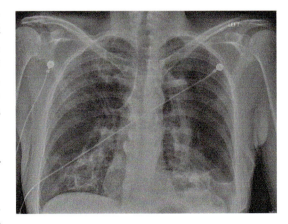

Fig. 31.3 Chest radiograph of a large left bullae mimicking left pneumothorax. Careful inspection reveals concave lining of bullae superiorly

a pneumothorax (Fig. 31.3). Nevertheless, chest radiographs are an excellent imaging modality alone to detect and make clinical decisions in more obvious large and symptomatic pneumothoraces (Fig. 31.4). In fact, it is important to understand that when presented with a patient who has clinical suspicion of a pneumothorax and who evolves into developing tension physiology, it is imperative that an emergent intervention such as decompression be performed without waiting for a confirmatory imaging study.

In this era of medicine, computed tomography (CT) scans are sensitive and accurate in diagnosing a pneumothorax. CT scans allow for the detection of small pneumothoraces and the esti-

mation of size and can differentiate between bullous lungs that may appear as a pneumothorax on simple chest radiograph (Fig. 31.5). In addition, CT scan may be a preferred imaging modality in elderly individuals or people with history of smoking to rule out malignancy as potential cause of pneumothorax or coincident disease due to the shared risk factor of tobacco use.

Treatment

The goal of therapy for a pneumothorax is removing the air from the pleural space and preventing recurrence. The management of a pneumothorax is dependent on the degree of symptoms and type of pneumothorax. The options include observation, aspiration of air from the pleural space, chest tube placement, pleurodesis (mechanical and chemical), and operative surgical bleb resection and pleurodesis via video-assisted thoracoscopy or thoracotomy approach. The more invasive therapies generally are reserved for those patients who are symptomatic from a spontaneous pneumothorax, have a large pneumothorax, or have not responded to observation.

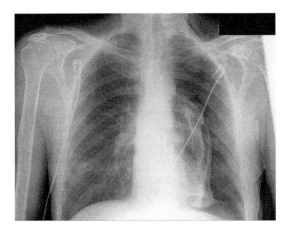

Fig. 31.4 Chest radiograph of a large left pneumothorax

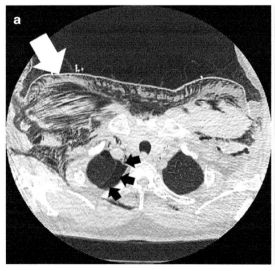
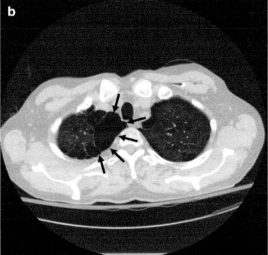

Fig. 31.5 CT scan images of (**a**) right apical pneumothorax with small thick black arrows denoting apical pneumothorax and large white arrow denoting subcutaneous emphysema, (**b**) right apical bullae with small thin black arrows denoting bullae

Observation

A small pneumothorax is defined as less than 15% of the hemithorax or less than 3 cm in distance between the apex and the cupola [10]. Despite this ostensibly objective criterion, the designation of a small pneumothorax still remains at the discretion of the managing clinician. A small pneumothorax can present with minimal clinical symptoms, and the patient can be observed if they are asymptomatic and the small pneumothorax is found incidentally on chest imaging. It is often recommended that in this context, a patient should be observed for 3–6 h in the clinical setting. A repeat chest radiography also should be performed to monitor for an interval change in size. If the repeat chest radiograph demonstrates interval improvement in size of the pneumothorax, then the patient can be discharged with follow-up and a repeat chest radiograph as an outpatient [10]. The body will naturally reabsorb the air from the pleural space, allowing small pneumothoraces to be observed. There are two methods that can increase the rate of resolution of a pneumothorax noninvasively, and these include supplemental oxygen and use of incentive spirometry. The use of supplemental oxygen works by increasing the partial pressure of oxygen and increasing the gradient of nitrogen absorption; it has been shown to increase the rate of reabsorption by a factor of four in comparison to room air alone in the observation setting [11, 12]. In addition, incentive spirometry has been shown to improve resolution of the pneumothorax by making the patient sustain maximal inspiration, which can aide in the absorption of air in the pleural space [13].

Aspiration

Another technique used to re-expand the lung following pneumothorax is aspiration. Simple aspiration is defined as the removal of pleural air via a needle or cannula followed by immediate removal once there is evidence of improvement in the pneumothorax [9]. Obviously, relief from the symptoms warranting the aspiration also confirms the success of the procedure, and the lack thereof may suggest the inadequate removal of air or another etiology for the symptoms. This technique can be applied to a pneumothorax that may range from small to large as long as the patient is stable clinically. Access into the pleural cavity is achieved employing the Seldinger technique at the level of the second intercostal space in the midclavicular line. A needle is used to gain access over the superior portion of the rib followed by wire placement and catheter placement. The catheter is then connected to a three-way stopcock or valved system that allows for syringe removal of pleural air akin to how a thoracentesis is performed. Response to aspiration is monitored by a post-aspiration chest radiograph. If the pneumothorax has resolved, the catheter can be removed. If there is only interval improvement of the pneumothorax following aspiration, the catheter then should be transitioned to functioning as a small tube thoracostomy, exchanged for a pigtail catheter, or up-sized to a larger bore chest tube [14].

Tube Thoracostomy

The most common method used to treat both PSP and SSP is via chest tube placement. It is the suggested method of choice for any large pneumothorax, defined as greater than 3 cm from the apex to cupola and for any symptomatic patients [10]. The choice of chest tube utilized can vary from small-bore catheters that are often less than or equal to 14 French (Fr) to large chest tubes ranging up to 36 Fr. Once placed, the tube thoracostomy can be connected to either a Heimlich valve or pleural evacuation system. Suction on these latter systems is not absolutely required, and placing it to a water seal chamber mode should allow for adequate lung expansion to the chest wall.

The small-bore catheters are often inserted in a similar manner as described for simple aspiration. A needle is inserted in the second intercostal space in the midclavicular line. The catheter is then directed apically and can be connected to a Heimlich valve. A Heimlich valve is a device with a one-way valve that is attached to the end of the catheter. It will allow air to exit the pleural space and prevent it from reentering. Alternatively, the small-bore type may be connected to a more conventional water-seal pleural evacuation system. The catheters are used routinely in emergency rooms because of the ease of access and improved patient comfort which is comparable to large-bore chest tubes.

The large-bore chest tubes vary in size as previously described, but most commonly range from 16 Fr to 28 Fr for a PSP or SSP. A chest tube is inserted in the anterior axillary line either in the fourth or fifth intercostal space and directed to the apex of the chest wall. The chest tube is then connected to a water-seal pleural evacuation system and placed to either water-seal mode or controlled suction to -20 cm of water (-20 cm H_2O).

Management of a catheter or large-bore chest tube after placement is dependent on the provider, reliability of the patient, and immediate effect of placement on the size of the pneumothorax. Ideally, upon placement of a tube thoracostomy, there is a complete resolution of a pneumothorax demonstrated by chest radiograph. It is common practice to watch the patient for 24–48 h monitoring for air leaks and continued resolution of pneumothorax. However, if a patient is reliable and immediate improvement in the clinical symptoms and pneumothorax size is noted, the patient can be transitioned to a Heimlich valve and discharged home with close follow-up. There is a theoretical increased risk of infecting the pleural space with this strategy, and, therefore, it requires a highly compliant patient for this approach. If the pneumothorax does not have immediate improvement, the tube thoracostomy can remain on water seal or then be connected to suction at -20 cm H_2O. There is controversy over the use of suction for a pneumothorax versus leaving the chest tube to water seal with reasonable and rationale arguments for either option. Ultimately, the clinical circumstances should dictate the appropriate modality to eliminate any residual entrapped air. Once the lung is completely annealed to the chest wall and there is no air leak seen in the water seal chamber, the tube is often removed. The success rate for tube thoracostomy is usually >90% for PSP, but with each subsequent reoccurrence, the rate of success drops significantly reaching <20% success rate for a third time occurrence [15]. This reason is why the use of pleurodesis becomes an important adjunct to ensure resolution for recurrences.

Pleurodesis

Following the placement of a tube thoracostomy, an additional adjunct in the treatment of pneumothorax is the use of pleurodesis. Pleurodesis is a technique used to create symphysis between the parietal and visceral pleura to facilitate intentional adherence of the lung to the chest wall internally. From a broad perspective, there are two methods of pleurodesis: (1) chemical and (2) mechanical (mechanical pleurodesis will be discussed in the subsequent operative intervention section).

The most common agents used to perform chemical pleurodesis include sterile grade talc and pharmaceutical or antiseptic solution. There are a number of pharmaceutical or antiseptic solutions that can be employed including more commonly doxycycline, tetracycline, bleomycin, and betadine [10]. The success rates range from 75% to 92% as evidenced by the recurrence rates of pneumothoraces ranging from 8% to 25% [16, 17]. Due to the relatively high recurrence rates, it is generally preferred to reserve chemical pleurodesis for patients that are suboptimal operative candidates.

The recommended dosing of talc is 2 grams because at higher doses such as 5 grams, commonly used for malignant pleural effusions, there is the possibility of inducing adult respiratory distress syndrome [18]. The incidence of this complication has been reported to be minimal at 0.15–0.71% [19]. The occurrence is believed to be associated with small particulate size that facilitates the systemic absorption of talc. Consequently, talc formulations with larger particulate size have been employed to ameliorate this risk [20]. Nevertheless, prior to its use, the potential of this complication must be included in the informed consent discussion.

Despite the success of talc pleurodesis, the adverse effect profile has rendered it as the alternative pleurodesis choice at many institutions. Other primary chemical agents such as doxycycline are often the preferred agent of choice for chemical pleurodesis. The dosing of doxycycline for bedside pleurodesis is usually 500–1500 mg, which is infused with 1% lidocaine due to pain associated with the medication. Surgical dogma once perpetuated the belief that patients should shift position to allow for the spread of the agent throughout the chest cavity; however, technetium-labeled agents evaluated on nuclear imaging following pleurodesis have demonstrated no difference in dispersion of the agent in the pleural cavity with maneuvers such as deep breathing with incentive spirometry [21]. After the sclerosing agent is allowed to dwell in the chest following a finite period of time such as 1–2 h, the chest tube is then placed on suction for 48 h to maximize the apposition of the visceral and parietal pleural surfaces. Daily chest radiographs and frequent monitoring for air leaks are useful adjuncts. Typically, the dwell time will require that the chest tube is clamped near its entry point following the instillation of the agent. This approach is acceptable when the air leak has resolved and the pleurodesing is being performed to prevent further recurrences. However, in some circumstances, when there is an active air leak, clamping the tube may be contraindicated due to the possibility of creating a tension pneumothorax. In this case, the tubing of the chest tube should simply be elevated over the chest of the patient to allow for gravity to facilitate the dwelling of the agent in the chest while simultaneously allowing for the air to escape.

The use of CT imaging following pleurodesis should be limited and interpreted with caution following the instillation of sclerosing agents, because the inflammatory process may be interpreted erroneously as an infectious process, such as an empyema. Often times, owing to the intentional inflammatory reaction induced by the sclerosing agent, a fever may accompany a pleurodesis for several days, sometimes with very high temperatures. Since infections of the pleural space can occur, clinical judgment should be exercised in discerning if a truly infectious process is ongoing versus the aforementioned response. More long-term sequelae of pleurodesis, particularly with talc pleurodesis, are the inflammatory reactions that may remain durable and longer lasting. This phenomenon can affect the interpretation of other imaging studies such as positron emission tomography (PET) scans if obtained for other reasons.

Surgical Therapy

Surgery for the treatment of spontaneous pneumothorax is used frequently when conservative or less invasive methods do not meet with success. Indications for treatment include failure of complete lung expansion despite 5–7 days of chest tube placement, large or persistent air leaks over a predetermined time period, recurrence of spontaneous pneumothorax, and synchronous or metachronous bilateral spontaneous pneumothorax [9]. Additionally, professions at risk for developing issues from pressure differentials at work such as airline pilots and scuba divers should also be considered for definitive intervention even after a first time occurrence of a spontaneous pneumothorax [22].

The goals of surgery are to ensure complete lung expansion, remove associated bullae, and perform adequate pleurodesis to prevent recurrence. The preferred surgical method used for treatment of spontaneous pneumothorax is video-assisted thoracoscopic surgery (VATS) as compared to an open thoracotomy [9, 10]. Some studies have suggested slightly better prevention of recurrence, as low as 1%, with an open thoracotomy approach, but other meta-analysis have largely shown no difference [23]. The primary differences between the VATS and open modalities remain the better postoperative pain control, shorter hospital lengths of stay, and improved total economic cost that favors the use of VATS as the surgical technique of choice.

The VATS approach may be performed using a variety of incision strategies including a single-incision approach. Classically, a three-port technique in which a double lumen endotracheal tube is utilized for single lung ventilation is employed. During the procedure, the lung is carefully inspected to look for bullae, which are most commonly located at the apical segments of the upper lobes and superior segments of the lower lobes. If no bullae are seen on visual inspection, then the attention is often turned to searching for an air leak which can be aided by submerging the lung under saline and inflating the lung gently in a controlled manner to look for air bubbles in a systematic manner. The areas involved with blebs or air leaks are then resected using a standard thoracoscopic stapler. If a uniportal approach is used, a 1.5–2 cm incision is made in the midaxillary line at the sixth intercostal space where all three instruments are inserted through a wound retractor in the same plane. Some argue there is improved postoperative pain with a single incision compared to the three-port incision [24]. Other locations for the single-incision approach are acceptable as well and most likely depend on both surgeon comfort and experience in determining the optimal approach for a specific patient.

The other objective of surgical intervention is to create fusion between the visceral and parietal surfaces of the pleura to prevent recurrence. This can be done either by pleurodesis (both mechanical and chemical) or by parietal pleurectomy. Mechanical pleurodesis is the most common method performed at the time of surgery because of the ease of taking a Bovie scratch pad and aggressively irritating the parietal pleura. The abrasion from the scratch pad creates an inflammatory response that will lead to symphysis between the parietal and visceral pleura upon lung expansion. Additionally, some surgeons will elect to also perform a chemical pleurodesis at the time of VATS with either talc or doxycycline. Furthermore, the other method of choice to prevent recurrence at time of surgery is a pleurectomy, which is the removal of the parietal pleura. Data suggesting the advantages of either pleurectomy or pleurodesis over the other in terms of lower recurrence rates are lacking, and, often, they are performed in conjunction with one another based on surgeon preference.

Conclusions

Spontaneous pneumothorax is a commonly encountered disease process seen in an emergency setting. It is important for the healthcare team to be familiar with the diagnoses and treatment of PSP and SSP. CT scans can confirm the diagnosis, but starting with a chest radiograph to guide therapy is reasonable in many clinical circumstances. The treatment options remain vast and depend on the presentation of the patient and the type of pneumothorax. If simple tube thoracostomy fails or recurrent pneumothorax is seen, it is recommended that a thoracic surgeon or pulmonologist be consulted for assistance in the management of this patient.

References

1. Myers JA. Simple spontaneous pneumothorax. Dis Chest. 1954;26:420–41.
2. Driscoll PJ, Aronstam EM. Experiences in the management of recurrent spontaneous pneumothorax. J Thorac Cardiovasc Surg. 1961;42:174–8.
3. Melton LJ, Hepper NG, Offord KP. Incidence of spontaneous pneumothorax in Olmsted County, Minnesota: 1950 to 1974. Am Rev Respir Dis. 1979;120:1379–82.
4. Gobbel WG, Rhea WG, Nelson IA, Daniel RA. Spontaneous pneumothorax. J Thorac Cardiovasc Surg. 1963;46:331–45.
5. Primrose WR. Spontaneous pneumothorax: a retrospective review of aetiology, pathogenesis, and management. Scott Med J. 1984;29:15–20.
6. Sahn SA, Heffner JE. Spontaneous pneumothorax. N Engl J Med. 2000;342(12):868–74.
7. Eng RH, Bishburg E, Smith SM. Evidence for destruction of lung tissue during pneumocystis carinii infection. Arch Intern Med. 1987;147:746–9.
8. Seremetis MG. The management of spontaneous pneumothorax. Chest. 1970;57:65–8.
9. MacDuff A, Arnold A, Harvey J. Management of spontaneous pneumothorax: British Thoracic Society pleural disease guideline 2010. Thorax. 2010;65(Suppl 2):ii18–31.
10. Baumann MH, Strange C, Heffner JE, et al. Management of spontaneous pneumothorax: an American College of Chest Physicians Delphi consensus statement. Chest. 2001;119:590–602.
11. Northfield TC. Oxygen therapy for spontaneous pneumothorax. BMJ. 1971;4:86–8.
12. Hill RC, DeCarlo DP Jr, Hill JF, Beamer KC, Hill ML, Timberlake GA. Resolution of experimental pneumothorax in rabbits by oxygen therapy. Ann Thorac Surg. 1995;59:825–8.

13. Pribadi RR, Singh G, Rumende CM. The role of incentive spirometry in primary spontaneous pneumothorax. Acta Med Indones. 2016;48(1):54–7.
14. Ayed AK, Chandrasekaran C, Sukumar M. Aspiration versus tube drainage in primary spontaneous pneumothorax: a randomised study. Eur Respir J. 2006;27:477–82.
15. Jain SK, Al-Kattan KM, Hamdy MG. Spontaneous pneumothorax: determinants of surgical intervention. J Cardiovasc Surg. 1998;39:107–11.
16. Light RW, O'Hara VS, Moritz TE, et al. Intrapleural tetracycline for the prevention of recurrent spontaneous pneumothorax: results of a Department of Veterans Affairs cooperative study. JAMA. 1990;264:2224–30.
17. Almind M, Lange P, Viskum K. Spontaneous pneumothorax: comparison of simple drainage, talc pleurodesis, and tetracycline pleurodesis. Thorax. 1989;44:627–30.
18. Rinaldo JE, Owens GR, Rogers RM. Adult respiratory distress syndrome following intra-pleural instillation of talc. J Thorac Cardiovasc Surg. 1983;85:523–6.
19. Sahn SA. Talc should be used for pleurodesis. Am J Respir Crit Care Med. 2000;162(6):2023–4.
20. Bridevaux JM, Tschopp G, Cardillo G, et al. Short-term safety of thorascopic talc pleurodesis for recurrent primary spontaneous pneumothorax: a prospective European multicentre study. Eur Respir J. 2011;38:770–3.
21. Vargas FS, Teixeira LR, Coelho IJ, Braga GA, Terra-Filho M, Light RW. Distribution of pleural injectate. Effect of volume of injectate and animal rotation. Chest. 1994;106(4):1246–9.
22. Gygax-Genero M, Manen O, Chemsi M, et al. Treatment specifics for spontaneous pneumothorax in flight personnel. Rev Pneumol Clin. 2010;66(5):302–7.
23. Barker A, Maratos EC, Edmonds L, Lim E. Recurrence rates of video-assisted thoracoscopic versus open surgery in the prevention of recurrent pneumothorax: a systemic review of randomised and non-randomised trials. Lancet. 2007;370:329–50.
24. Bertolaccini L, Pardolesi A, Brandolini J, Solli P. Uniportal video-assisted thoracic surgery for pneumothorax and blebs/bullae. J Visc Surg. 2017;3:107.

Empyema

32

Neil Venardos and John D. Mitchell

Introduction

Empyema is a combination of two Greek words. The first is a prefix "en" meaning within, and the second is "pyema," which means accumulation of pus. An empyema can describe a collection of purulent material anywhere in the body; however empyema thoracis more specifically describes a collection of pus within the pleural cavity. Imhotep, the Egyptian physician, described pleural infection around 3000 BC; however Hippocrates was the first to describe surgical drainage of empyema by trephination [1].

The current incidence has been estimated to be around 65,000 patients per year in the United States, carrying a mortality of 20% and mean hospitalization duration of around 15 days [2]. However, the incidence of pleural infection in adults is increasing. Finley et al. [3] found an increasing incidence of pneumonia, as did Grijalva et al. [4]. The latter study found that the overall incidence of parapneumonic empyema-related hospitalization rates increased from 3.04 per 100,000 in 1996 to 5.98 per 100,000 in 2008.

Patients at risk for pleural infection mirror those for pneumonia. These patients often have diabetes mellitus, immunosuppression, GERD, alcohol and drug abuse, and history of aspiration or poor oral hygiene [5]. Patients with empyema present with symptoms similar to those who have pneumonia. They typically have cough, fever, dyspnea, pleuritic chest pain, and sputum production. Unfortunately these symptoms do not help differentiate pneumonia from patients with empyema [6]. Findings on physical examination may include fever, crackles, egophony, decreased breath sounds, and fremitus. These findings are often not detectable; thus it is essential to obtain imaging in these patients. The RAPID score can be used to predict which patients with pleural infections have worse outcomes [7]. Any patient with persistent signs of sepsis after 2 or 3 days of treatment for their pneumonia has a high likelihood of having an associated pleural infection and should be appropriately imaged. Furthermore, any patient who begins to show signs of sepsis after an intrathoracic procedure should undergo workup for possible pleural infection.

Etiology

Empyema most frequently is the result of a parapneumonic effusion, making up between 40% and 60% of the total cases diagnosed each year. Postsurgical empyemas make up another 20–30% of cases, most often resulting from lung resections, esophagectomies, and mediastinal procedures. Posttraumatic empyemas make up for

N. Venardos · J. D. Mitchell (✉)
Division of Cardiothoracic Surgery, University of Colorado School of Medicine, Aurora, CO, USA
e-mail: john.mitchell@ucdenver.edu

most of the other cases, accounting for most of the remaining 5–10% of all empyemas [8].

Diagnosis

Initial imaging should begin with chest radiograph, and the lateral film can assist in identifying effusions not present on posteroanterior imaging. Pleural ultrasound has emerged as an important next step in further characterization of the effusion. Ultrasound can identify septations and guide needle placement for aspiration and/or pleural catheter placement [9].

Definitive evaluation of chest effusions is provided by CT scanning with intravenous contrast. CT scanning can identify bronchogenic carcinoma, endobronchial foreign body, or esophageal pathology. Loculated empyemas can be distinguished from pleural-based lung abscesses. Particular imaging characteristics include parietal pleural thickening and pleural enhancement in 86% and 96% of patients, respectively. A "split pleura sign" is encountered when both the visceral and parietal pleura enhance concomitantly. This sign can be seen in up to 68% of empyemas [10]. Air bubbles can indicate pleural space infection. If the pleural fluid thickness is less than 2–2.5 cm, the effusion may respond to antibiotics alone.

Pleural fluid analysis is critical for further management of patients with pleural effusions. The presence of pus, positive gram stain, positive culture [11], or pleural pH < 7.2 [12] suggests the presence of an empyema, and a chest tube should be placed. Other important predictors of need for tube thoracostomy include pleural fluid glucose <40 mg/dL or LDH value >1000 IU/L. Culture should be obtained during initial aspiration – not from the tube later on. The most commonly identified organisms were categorized by Maskell et al. [5]. The following table groups these bacteria into community-acquired and hospital-acquired organisms.

Staging of Empyema

Empyema occurs in three stages, defined by the American Thoracic Society back in 1964 [13]. The first stage is considered to be exudative.

Fluid moves into the pleural space due to increased vascular permeability. This fluid is free-flowing and does not typically contain bacterial organisms. Most effusions of this type do not require drainage [11]. Without treatment, the effusion may progress to stage 2, which is referred to as the fibrinopurulent stage. Fibrin is deposited over the visceral and parietal surfaces of the lung, and the fluid itself becomes purulent. The pleural space may become loculated as more fibrin becomes deposited. The pleural fluid at this stage has a low pH (<7.2), glucose (<2.2 mmol/L), and LDH level (<1000 IU/L). The third and final stage is reached when a solid fibrous pleural peel has formed, encasing the underlying lung. The lung cannot completely expand at this point without removal of the peel.

Management of Acute (Early) Empyema

Management of pleural infection begins with adequate medical care of the patient undergoing the workup. A thoracic surgeon should be involved early in the care of these patients, as sepsis can develop in patients with untreated infection of the pleural space. In addition, unless there are clear contraindications, the patient should be placed on thrombosis prophylaxis, nutrition should be optimized, and blood cultures should be drawn [14]. Only patients with high likelihood of bronchial obstruction as a cause for the empyema should undergo bronchoscopy.

In addition to obtaining cultures, antibiotic therapy must be started early and targeted at the most common offending organisms (see prior section). Choice of antibiotic should be guided by culture data, local resistance patterns, antimicrobial stewardship policies, and the agent's pharmacologic properties. For patients with community-acquired empyema with low risk for methicillin-resistant *Staphylococcus aureus* infection, a second or third (non-pseudomonal) cephalosporin such as ceftriaxone or an aminopenicillin with beta-lactamase inhibitor (ampicillin/sulbactam) provides good coverage. Metronidazole should be added if suspicion for anaerobic infection is high [14]. Duration of treatment for empyema is variable depending on the organism and response to treatment, but at least 2 weeks of antibiotic therapy should be pursued [15]. Overall duration of therapy is a matter of debate.

Antibiotics may be started while arranging for pleural fluid sampling, and complete drainage of the pleural cavity is critical for successful treatment [12]. Indications for chest tube placement include frank pus on aspiration, positive direct gram stain or culture, pH <7.2, glucose <400 mg/L, LDH >1000 IU/mL, total protein >3 g/mL, and WBC >15,000 cells/mm^3 [11]. Other indications for early chest tube drainage include loculation on imaging, which may be associated with worse outcomes [16]. For effusions with no or minimal septations, placement of a small-bore (<14Fr) drainage catheter is now considered an acceptable option for first-line therapy in these patients [7, 14]. Drains of this caliber must be regularly flushed for effective drainage of the space, as blockage rates can be as high as 64% in patients with empyema [17]. Patients with more complicated effusions or frank pus on aspiration should receive tube thoracostomy drainage. Patients not responding to initial therapy require repeat pleural fluid sampling, further drainage procedures, or surgical therapy [15].

Once adequate drainage has been achieved, many patients will clinically improve, and no further therapy outside of completion of the appropriate antibiotic course is warranted. Early stage empyema (stage I or II) can be treated by either fibrinolytics or early video-assisted thoracoscopic surgery. Fibrinolytics have been in use since 1945 for pleural infections, but the clinical effectiveness of these drugs is not clear. These chemicals are thought to encourage lysis of septations to allow improved drainage via the catheter. Streptokinase is the most widely studied of these agents. Maskell et al. [18] published a randomized controlled trial evaluating streptokinase and found no reduction in the need for surgical intervention, no mortality reduction, and no reduction in hospital stay. Wait et al. [19] compared chest tube and fibrinolytic therapy with video-assisted thoracoscopic surgery (VATS). The authors found a higher treatment success rate, shorter chest tube duration, shorter hospital stay, and lower average cost with the VATS [19].

However, the MIST2 trial demonstrated that the combination of tPa and DNase had improved pleural drainage and reduced hospital stay. In addition, there was a 3/4 reduction in the need for surgical intervention at 3 months [20]. At this time it is difficult to synthesize prior studies of tPA and DNase therapy for empyema, since empyema patients are generally a particularly heterogeneous group of patients. As of now, the AATS and BTS guidelines recommend against the routine use of fibrinolytics in patients who are reasonable surgical candidates [14, 15].

Video-assisted thoracoscopic surgery (VATS) is the preferred first-line approach in all patients with stage II acute empyema. This approach is also preferred for patients who fail antibiotic/chest tube management. The two goals of surgical therapy are as follows: (1) complete removal of infection from the pleural space and (2) re-expansion of the lung. VATS should be defined as the absence of rib spreading in order to complete the procedure. In a large series, success with VATS was reported to be between 80% and 85% [21]. This study found that the success of VATS depended upon the length of preoperative symptoms. The choice of VATS vs. open decortication depends on multiple factors, including the patient's ability to tolerate one-lung ventilation, coagulopathy, local resources and expertise, and imaging characteristics. VATS has certainly shown a benefit vs. open surgery for other procedures such as lobectomy for cancer. One such study showed a reduction in postoperative pain, length of stay, blood loss, respiratory compromise, and complications [22]. There are few drawbacks to choosing a VATS-first approach in appropriately selected patients, as the procedure can typically be converted to an open procedure during the same trip to the operating room. Fears about longer operating times and learning curves have slowly been dying out. A review of 14 studies by Chambers et al. [23] demonstrated a clear benefit of VATS over open surgery for empyema. Granted this review included mostly single-institution retrospective cohort studies, the findings show that VATS affords shorter length of stay, less pain, and lower morbidity. Unfortunately, these studies are inherently flawed, as the distinction between stage II and III empyema is often not made until the time of surgery. The authors of any of these publications may also have been more biased toward one operation or the other.

The technique of video-assisted thoracoscopic decortication has been described [24]. The procedure begins with general anesthesia using lung isolation. This can be accomplished with the use of a bronchial blocker or a double-lumen endotracheal tube. The two principles of this procedure are to fully debride the cavity and completely remove the fibrous peel from the parietal/visceral surfaces. Two or three incisions can be utilized. A 1 cm incision located in the eighth intercostal space in the midaxillary line serves as the camera port. An additional 3–4 cm incision located anteriorly in the fifth intercostal space is utilized as an access port. Alternatively, this access incision can be made smaller, and an additional port can be placed posteriorly in the fifth or sixth intercostal space to assist with instrument handling. Instruments are carefully introduced under thoracoscopic guidance, and the lung is decorticated. The peel is removed from the surface of the lung using a combination of sharp and blunt dissection, taking care to avoid the lung parenchyma beneath. Electrocautery is utilized to control chest wall bleeding. At the end of the procedure, a chest tube (or multiple chest tubes) is placed using direct thoracoscopic guidance. Critical elements of postoperative care include early mobilization, aggressive chest physiotherapy, continuous chest tube suction for at least 48 h, and expeditious chest tube removal once the cavity has been fully evacuated and lung expansion achieved. Complications related to VATS surgery most frequently include atelectasis, prolonged air leak, reintubation, ventilator dependence, need for tracheostomy, and need for blood transfusion [24].

Management of Chronic Empyema

The final stage of empyema is heralded by the formation of a solid fibrous pleural peel, primarily caused by the actions of fibroblasts. These rinds trap the lung, creating persistent pleural spaces which have the potential to remain infected. Three types of surgical techniques are used to treat the chronic empyema. These include decortication and debridement, space obliteration, and open drainage [25]. The choice of technique involves an assessment of the source of infection, lung expansion, space filling options, and the health of the patient.

The workhorse operation for chronic empyema in patients medically fit for surgery is open decortication performed via thoracotomy [26] (Fig. 32.1). The procedure is becoming less common as more pulmonary infections are treated earlier on in the disease course. These procedures involve carefully peeling off the fibrous rind from the visceral and parietal pleurae. Necrotic lung parenchyma can be resected if this is the source of sepsis or hemoptysis. An epidural can often be placed, and no data supports increased risk of epidural abscess; however placement of an epidural should be a patient-specific decision. The approach is typically through a standard or muscle-sparing posterolateral thoracotomy [28]. An incision is made over the sixth rib. The sixth rib is removed and the pleura exposed. Dissection is carried through the extrapleural plane using sharp and blunt dissection in an anterior and posterior direction. The apex is dissected, carefully avoiding the subclavian vessels. The same concern is taken at the hilum, avoiding tearing large vessels or injury to the phrenic nerve. The pleura is then mobilized off the diaphragm. The visceral peel is then removed from the lung using a knife to begin dissection, and then the plane between the lung and peel is developed using a peanut sponge. Complete decortication often includes empyemectomy or

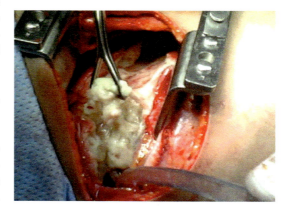

Fig. 32.1 Open thoracotomy and decortication. Note removal of the thick peel from the surface of the lung. (Figure from Hajjar et al. [27])

Table 32.1 Empyema Bacteriology

Type of pneumonia	Organisms
Community-acquired	*Streptococcus* spp. (~52%) *S. milleri* *S. pneumoniae* *S. intermedius* *Staphylococcus aureus* (~11%) Gram-negative aerobes (9%) *Enterobacteriaceae* *E. coli* Anaerobes (20%) *Fusobacterium* spp. *Bacteroides* spp. *Peptostreptococcus* spp. Mixed
Hospital-acquired	Staphylococci Methicillin-resistant *S. aureus* (MRSA) (25%) *S. aureus* (10%) Gram-negative aerobes (17%) *E. coli* *Pseudomonas aeruginosa* *Klebsiella* spp. Anaerobes (8%)

Table adapted from Davies et al. [14]

removal of the thick purulent collection within its surrounding rinds. Chest tubes are placed anteriorly, posteriorly, and along the diaphragm in order to thoroughly evacuate the space.

Surgical resection of the lung must be included with decortication when the underlying lung is destroyed or when associated areas of severe cavitary disease/bronchiectasis are identified on preoperative CT scan. Resection options include decortication with lobectomy or pneumonectomy. Extrapleural pneumonectomy is a final option for patients who have all underlying lobes involved. This procedure is particularly difficult and involves dissection of thick, fibrous peel off of multiple critical structures. In addition, the bronchial stump is at particularly high risk for breakdown, forming fistulas and recurrent empyemas [29].

Beyond decortication, space filling procedures should be performed when the lung cannot expand to fill the space or the destroyed lung has to be removed during the operation. Pedicled muscle flaps are ideal for this purpose. These adjuncts are particularly useful when a bronchopleural fistula is encountered [30]. An intercostal muscle flap is one option. Extrathoracic muscle options typically used include latissimus dorsi, serratus anterior, and pectoralis major flaps [30]. Other flaps

including omentum can be used as well, with the understanding that omental pedicle transposition requires entry into the abdominal cavity, raising the risk of infection. These muscle flaps can be performed at the first operation or later on after this initial infection has been dealt with.

Another space-obliterating technique is thoracoplasty. These procedures were originally used on tuberculosis patients prior to development of drugs active against tuberculosis. These procedures involve removal of portions of the ribs and chest wall, compressing the chest cavity. Procedures such as pleural tenting and the Schede thoracoplasty are somewhat morbid and disfiguring. These procedures are reserved for the most severe cases after flap or open window techniques have been exhausted [31].

In patients who are debilitated and not good candidates for the decortication, flap placement, or thoracoplastic procedures, a better option is the open thoracic window [32]. This procedure involves marsupialization of the infected pleural cavity. These patients typically have chronic contamination resulting from a bronchopleural fistula, making attempts to close down and sterilize the space difficult. This procedure is described in more detail below (see "Bronchopleural fistula" section). Wound VAC dressings have also been applied to close the infected cavity down, and some institutions have found success with this technique [33]. This technique must be used with caution, since significant portions of the patient's functioning parenchyma can be sucked down and rendered nonfunctional.

Chest tube drainage left in chronic empyema cavities is another effective way to deal with a stage III empyema. The tube can be placed during the first surgery or as a stand-alone measure to drain infection in deconditioned patients who cannot tolerate operation.

A few special situations deserve mention. One is empyema necessitans. In his unfortunate situation, empyema expresses through the chest wall and presents as an enlarging chest wall abscess. This situation can be managed with closed decortication or open drainage procedures [34].

Another special situation is a post-pneumonectomy empyema. This scenario complicates up to 15% of cases after pneumonectomy

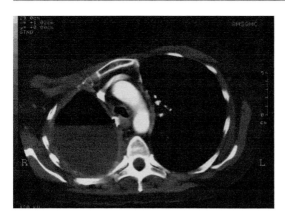

Fig. 32.2 CT scan image of a patient who developed a bronchopleural fistula after undergoing right-sided pneumonectomy. The air-fluid interface is noted at the level of the right main stem stump closure. (Figure from Zanotti et al. [36])

[35]. Bronchopleural fistula is frequently encountered in these patients, occurring in about eight out of ten post-pneumonectomy empyema cases. These infections can be challenging to manage. Of particular importance is an acute presentation in post-pneumonectomy patients, which can result in acute respiratory compromise, as the contralateral bronchus fills with chest fluid (Fig. 32.2). The patient should be immediately positioned in the lateral decubitus position until drainage can be obtained. The next section discusses broader management strategies for patients with BPF.

Management of Bronchopleural Fistula

Empyema can be complicated by bronchopleural fistula (BPF), which provides a constant source of contamination in the pleural space. The lung is not expandable in these situations, trapped by a thickened fibrous peel. The etiology of BPF can range from a dehiscence of a bronchial closure after pulmonary resection or an anastomotic dehiscence after bronchoplastic resection. Predisposing factors have been defined for patients undergoing anatomic lung resection. These risk factors include malnutrition, immunosuppression, radiation therapy, poorly controlled pulmonary/pleural infection, smoking, and chemotherapy [36]. Other risk factors for this dreaded

complication include right pneumonectomy, completion pneumonectomy, diminished pulmonary reserve, and extended lymph node dissection. BPF typically presents as persistent air leak, new evidence of pneumomediastinum, a decrease in the fluid level in the ipsilateral pleural cavity, or a new air-fluid level at the height of the bronchial stump after pneumonectomy or lung resection. CT scanning can suggest the presence of BPF, but bronchoscopy is better for diagnosing and characterizing the fistula. Occasionally, surgical exploration must be necessary for diagnosis.

Management of the bronchopleural fistula depends on the etiology, chronicity, and health of the underlying lung, along with the patient's nutritional status. Endobronchial treatment has been described for BPF; however, success rates are low [37]. Definitive management in medically optimized patients with ideal nutritional status typically is performed via posterolateral thoracotomy. Next, the bronchial stump is resected back to healthy tissue, and the stump is over-sewn with absorbable suture. Finally, soft tissue autologous buttressing is performed to reinforce the closure. Flaps such as the latissimus dorsi, pectoralis major, or intercostal muscle can be used. In patients without these options, free flaps can be used [38]. Omental transposition can be used for this as well, and this can be a particularly good option for a poorly controlled infection within the chest [39]. Creation of an open thoracostomy window is an acceptable treatment strategy for empyema with a persistent BPF. The original procedure, as described by Leo Eloesser [32], involved the excision of two to three ribs along with creation of a U-shaped flap with marsupialized skin edges. A modified version of this procedure is used today, whereby a window is created using an inverted U-shaped muscle flaps. This allows dependent drainage of the pleural space and resolution of the infection.

Patients can even be sent home after resolution of sepsis with wound care and packing changes as the space granulates. When appropriate granulation tissue has formed, primary chest closure using the Clagett procedure is one option for these patients [40]. This procedure involves filling the residual cavity with antibiotics such as neomycin and polymyxin B mixed with saline. Next, a watertight closure of the thoracostomy opening is achieved by excising excessive skin, mobilizing the serratus muscle, and sewing the opening closed in layers. This procedure can be quite effective when performed in the right setting, achieving success in up to 80% of patients in one series [41]. Failure of a Clagett requires reversion back to the Eloesser flap with or without space obliteration procedures (Figs. 32.3 and 32.4).

Fig. 32.3 This figure shows a cross section of the empyema cavity and the modified Eloesser flap. Note the tongue flap attached to the base of the empyema cavity. (Figure from *Sabiston and Spencer Surgery of the Chest*, 8th edition [42])

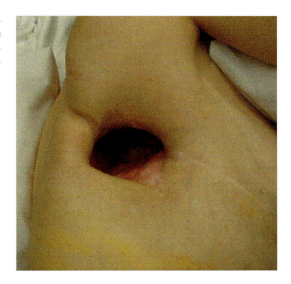

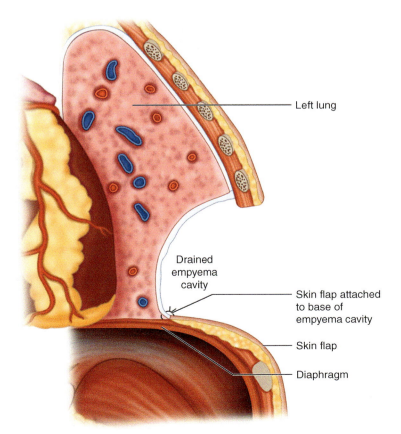

Fig. 32.4 This is a patient with a matured Eloesser located just above the diaphragm. The serratus muscle is preserved under the superior skin flap. (Figure from Zanotti et al. [36])

Pediatric Considerations

For the pediatric population, current guidelines recommend tube thoracostomy with or without fibrinolytics for the initial treatment of patients with empyema. If the patient fails to respond to therapy, VATS debridement should be the next step in management.

Traumatic Empyema

Empyema may complicate the hospital course of up to 26% of patients with posttraumatic retained hemothorax [43]. Identified risk factors for formation of empyema in trauma patients include duration of tube thoracostomy, length of intensive care unit stay, pulmonary contusion, laparotomy, and retained hemothorax [44]. These empyemas may be approached in similar matter as described for empyema of other etiologies; however, earlier operative intervention may be warranted in lower-risk patients [45, 46].

References

1. Christopoulou-Aletra H, Papavramidou N. "Empyemas" of the thoracic cavity in the Hippocratic Corpus. Ann Thorac Surg. 2008;85(3):1132–4. https://doi.org/10.1016/j.athoracsur.2007.11.031.
2. Molnar TF. Current surgical treatment of thoracic empyema in adults. Eur J Cardiothorac Surg. 2007;32(3):422–30. https://doi.org/10.1016/j.ejcts.2007.05.028.
3. Finley C, Clifton J, Fitzgerald JM, Yee J. Empyema: an increasing concern in Canada. Can Respir J. 2008;15(2):85–9.
4. Grijalva CG, Zhu Y, Nuorti JP, Griffin MR. Emergence of parapneumonic empyema in the USA. Thorax. 2011;66(8):663–8. https://doi.org/10.1136/thx.2010.156406.
5. Maskell NA, Batt S, Hedley EL, Davies CWH, Gillespie SH, Davies RJO. The bacteriology of pleural infection by genetic and standard methods and its mortality significance. Am J Respir Crit Care Med. 2006;174(7):817–23. https://doi.org/10.1164/rccm.200601-074OC.
6. Dean NC, Griffith PP, Sorensen JS, McCauley L, Jones BE, Lee YCG. Pleural effusions at first ED encounter predict worse clinical outcomes in patients with pneumonia. Chest. 2016;149(6):1509–15. https://doi.org/10.1016/j.chest.2015.12.027.
7. Rahman NM, Kahan BC, Miller RF, Gleeson FV, Nunn AJ, Maskell NA. A clinical score (RAPID) to identify those at risk for poor outcome at presentation in patients with pleural infection. Chest. 2014;145(4):848–55. https://doi.org/10.1378/chest.13-1558.
8. Chapman SJ, Davies RJO. The management of pleural space infections. Respirology. 2004;9(1):4–11. https://doi.org/10.1111/j.1440-1843.2003.00535.x.
9. Stavas J, vanSonnenberg E, Casola G, Wittich GR. Percutaneous drainage of infected and noninfected thoracic fluid collections. J Thorac Imaging. 1987;2(3):80–7.
10. Waite RJ, Carbonneau RJ, Balikian JP, Umali CB, Pezzella AT, Nash G. Parietal pleural changes in empyema: appearances at CT. Radiology. 1990;175(1):145–50. https://doi.org/10.1148/radiology.175.1.2315473.
11. Light RW, Girard WM, Jenkinson SG, George RB. Parapneumonic effusions. Am J Med. 1980;69(4):507–12.
12. Heffner JE, Brown LK, Barbieri C, DeLeo JM. Pleural fluid chemical analysis in parapneumonic effusions. A meta-analysis. Am J Respir Crit Care Med. 1995;151(6):1700–8. https://doi.org/10.1164/ajrccm.151.6.7767510.
13. Andrews NC, Parker EF, Shaw RR, Wilson NJ, Webb WR. Management of nontuberculous empyema: a statement of the subcommittee on surgery. Am Rev Respir Dis. 1962;85:935–6.
14. Davies HE, RJO D, CWH D, BTS Pleural Disease Guideline Group. Management of pleural infection in adults: British Thoracic Society Pleural Disease Guideline 2010. Thorax. 2010;65(Suppl 2):ii41–53. https://doi.org/10.1136/thx.2010.137000.
15. Shen KR, Bribriesco A, Crabtree T, et al. The American Association for Thoracic Surgery consensus guidelines for the management of empyema. J Thorac Cardiovasc Surg. 2017;153(6):e129–46. https://doi.org/10.1016/j.jtcvs.2017.01.030.
16. Huang HC, Chang HY, Chen CW, Lee CH, Hsiue TR. Predicting factors for outcome of tube thoracostomy in complicated parapneumonic effusion for empyema. Chest. 1999;115(3):751–6.
17. Davies HE, Merchant S, McGown A. A study of the complications of small bore "Seldinger" intercostal chest drains. Respirology. 2008;13(4):603–7. https://doi.org/10.1111/j.1440-1843.2008.01296.x.
18. Maskell NA, Davies CWH, Nunn AJ, et al. U.K. controlled trial of intrapleural streptokinase for pleural infection. N Engl J Med. 2005;352(9):865–74. https://doi.org/10.1056/NEJMoa042473.
19. Wait MA, Sharma S, Hohn J, Dal Nogare A. A randomized trial of empyema therapy. Chest. 1997;111(6):1548–51.
20. Rahman NM, Maskell NA, West A, et al. Intrapleural use of tissue plasminogen activator and DNase in pleural infection. N Engl J Med. 2011;365(6):518–26. https://doi.org/10.1056/NEJMoa1012740.

21. Luh S-P, Chou M-C, Wang L-S, Chen J-Y, Tsai T-P. Video-assisted thoracoscopic surgery in the treatment of complicated parapneumonic effusions or empyemas. Chest J. 2005;127(4):1427. https://doi.org/10.1378/chest.127.4.1427.

22. Farjah F, Backhus LM, Varghese TK, et al. Ninety-day costs of video-assisted thoracic surgery versus open lobectomy for lung cancer. Ann Thorac Surg. 2014;98(1):191–6. https://doi.org/10.1016/j.athoracsur.2014.03.024.

23. Chambers A, Routledge T, Dunning J, Scarci M. Is video-assisted thoracoscopic surgical decortication superior to open surgery in the management of adults with primary empyema? Interact Cardiovasc Thorac Surg. 2010;11(2):171–7. https://doi.org/10.1510/icvts.2010.240408.

24. Tong BC, Hanna J, Toloza EM, et al. Outcomes of video-assisted thoracoscopic decortication. ATS. 2010;89:220–5. https://doi.org/10.1016/j.athoracsur.2009.09.021.

25. Shiraishi Y. Surgical treatment of chronic empyema. Gen Thorac Cardiovasc Surg. 2010;58(7):311–6. https://doi.org/10.1007/s11748-010-0599-6.

26. Martella AT, Santos GH. Decortication for chronic postpneumonic empyema. J Am Coll Surg. 1995;180(5):573–6.

27. Hajjar WM, Ahmed I, Al-Nassar SA, et al. Video-assisted thoracoscopic decortication for the management of late stage pleural empyema, is it feasible? Ann Thorac Med. 2016;11(1):71–8. https://doi.org/10.4103/1817-1737.165293.

28. Thurer RJ. Decortication in thoracic empyema. Indications and surgical technique. Chest Surg Clin N Am. 1996;6(3):461–90.

29. Okano T, HE W. Some problems in extrapleural pneumonectomy for tuberculous empyema and destroyed lung. J Thorac Surg. 1958;35(4):523–31.

30. Miller JI. The history of surgery of empyema, thoracoplasty, Eloesser flap, and muscle flap transposition. Chest Surg Clin N Am. 2000;10(1):45–53. viii

31. Pomerantz BJ, Cleveland JC, Pomerantz M. The Schede and modern thoracoplasty. Oper Tech Thorac Cardiovasc Surg. 2000;5(2):128–34. https://doi.org/10.1053/otct.2000.5076.

32. Eloesser L. Of an operation for tuberculous empyema. Ann Thorac Surg. 1969;8(4):355–7.

33. Sziklavari Z, Ried M, Zeman F, et al. Short-term and long-term outcomes of intrathoracic vacuum therapy of empyema in debilitated patients. J Cardiothorac Surg. 2016;11(1):148. https://doi.org/10.1186/s13019-016-0543-7.

34. Akgül AG, Örki A, Örki T, Yüksel M, Arman B. Approach to empyema necessitatis. World J Surg. 2011;35(5):981–4. https://doi.org/10.1007/s00268-011-1035-5.

35. Ng CSH, Wan S, Lee TW, Wan IYP, Arifi AA, Yim APC. Post-pneumonectomy empyema: current management strategies. ANZ J Surg. 2005;75(7):597–602. https://doi.org/10.1111/j.1445-2197.2005.03417.x.

36. Zanotti G, Mitchell JD. Bronchopleural fistula and empyema after anatomic lung resection. Thorac Surg Clin. 2015;25(4):421–7. https://doi.org/10.1016/j.thorsurg.2015.07.006.

37. Jiang F, Huang J, You Q, Yuan F, Yin R, Xu L. Surgical treatment for bronchopleural fistula with omentum covering after pulmonary resection for non-small cell lung cancer. Thorac Cancer. 2013;4(3):249–53. https://doi.org/10.1111/j.1759-7714.2012.00161.x.

38. Takanari K, Kamei Y, Toriyama K, Yagi S, Torii S. Management of postpneumonectomy empyema using free flap and pedicled flap. Ann Thorac Surg. 2010;89(1):321–3. https://doi.org/10.1016/j.athoracsur.2009.02.094.

39. Okada M, Tsubota N, Yoshimura M, Miyamoto Y, Yamagishi H, Satake S. Surgical treatment for chronic pleural empyema. Surg Today. 2000;30(6):506–10. https://doi.org/10.1007/s005950070116.

40. OT C, JE G. A procedure for the management of postpneumonectomy empyema. J Thorac Cardiovasc Surg. 1963;45:141–5.

41. Zaheer S, Allen MS, Cassivi SD, et al. Postpneumonectomy empyema: results after the Clagett procedure. Ann Thorac Surg. 2006;82(1):279–87. https://doi.org/10.1016/j.athoracsur.2006.01.052.

42. Sabiston DC, Sellke FW, Del Nido PJ, Swanson SJ. Sabiston & Spencer surgery of the chest. Philadelphia: Saunders; 2010.

43. DuBose J, Inaba K, Okoye O, et al. Development of posttraumatic empyema in patients with retained hemothorax. J Trauma Acute Care Surg. 2012;73(3):752–7. https://doi.org/10.1097/TA.0b013e31825c1616.

44. Eren S, Esme H, Sehitogullari A, Durkan A. The risk factors and management of posttraumatic empyema in trauma patients. Injury. 2008;39(1):44–9. https://doi.org/10.1016/j.injury.2007.06.001.

45. Navsaria PH, Vogel RJ, Nicol AJ. Thoracoscopic evacuation of retained posttraumatic hemothorax. Ann Thorac Surg. 2004;78(1):282–5. https://doi.org/10.1016/j.athoracsur.2003.11.029.

46. Bar I, Stav D, Fink G, Peer A, Lazarovitch T, Papiashvilli M. Thoracic empyema in high-risk patients: conservative management or surgery? Asian Cardiovasc Thorac Ann. 2010;18(4):337–43. https://doi.org/10.1177/0218492310375752.

Incarcerated Inguinal Hernias

33

Shirin Towfigh

Inguinal hernias have been treated surgically since the age of ancient Egypt [1]. At that time, it became apparent that life-threatening hernias require an operation. The indications for surgical treatment of inguinal hernias have since evolved immensely. Options for repair of inguinal hernias are varied. On the one hand, most minimally symptomatic inguinal hernias can be safely observed [2]. On the other extreme, *strangulated* inguinal hernias are life-threatening and must be treated emergently. The *incarcerated* inguinal hernia, however, can be a diagnostic and therapeutic dilemma. There has been no clinical trial studying incarcerated inguinal hernias. We have no widely accepted treatment algorithm for its treatment. The surgeon can be left wondering if his or her decision to observe or to operate was indeed the most correct one. This chapter will focus on the treatment algorithm for incarcerated inguinal hernias in the adult population.

Definitions

An incarcerated inguinal hernia is one in which the contents are no longer reducible. Reducibility can be subjective. Patients may report incidents of incarceration, which self-resolve. Should these patients be treated like a patient with no history

of inguinal hernia incarceration? Patients may present with irreducible inguinal hernia contents to the emergency room, yet the physician may be able to reduce the contents. Should they still be treated as if they have an incarcerated hernia? Lastly, patients may have a minimally symptomatic incarcerated inguinal hernia that no one can reduce. The clinical algorithm may be different for each of these situations.

The timing of the incarceration is of importance. Though patients may present with an acutely incarcerated inguinal hernia, others may have chronically incarcerated hernias. Again, the clinical scenario may be different for each of these. In one study, 1/3 of patients with incarcerated inguinal hernia who underwent an emergent operation were asymptomatic prior to their presentation [3].

Lastly, the amount of pain and other clinical symptoms that are associated with the incarceration is of importance. For example, an acutely incarcerated inguinal hernia with 10/10 pain may be treated differently than an acutely incarcerated inguinal hernia without any pain.

A strangulated inguinal hernia is technically not the same as an incarcerated one. By definition, a strangulated hernia includes ischemic contents. The ischemia may be reversible in some situations, but there must be some evidence of ischemia to inherit the label of strangulation. Irreducibility is typical in such situations, but it is not a prerequisite. In other words, almost all strangulated hernias are also incarcerated. That said, there is a spectrum

S. Towfigh
Beverly Hills Hernia Center, Beverly Hills, CA, USA

© Springer International Publishing AG, part of Springer Nature 2019
C. V. R. Brown et al. (eds.), *Emergency General Surgery*, https://doi.org/10.1007/978-3-319-96286-3_33

of presentation. An incarcerated inguinal hernia can evolve into a strangulated one. Also, it may be difficult to discern one vs the other. In most studies addressing incarcerated inguinal hernias, strangulated hernias are addressed as a subset of the incarcerated hernias, and so the two diagnoses are addressed as one entity [3–5]. This can confuse the surgeon, as these studies make no clinical distinction between the two presentations. In this chapter, we will tease out the scenario of the obviously strangulated inguinal hernias and focus the bulk of our discussion on the non-strangulated incarcerated inguinal hernia.

Inguinal hernias include direct and indirect inguinal hernias. Their content may include fat (most commonly), the intestine, and/or a nearby organ. Femoral hernias are infra-inguinal and share in the myopectineal orifice but are not the same as inguinal hernias (Fig. 33.1). Their presentation and risks for incarceration are quite different than inguinal hernias. In this chapter, we will discuss femoral hernias separately from inguinal hernias.

Strangulated Hernias

All strangulated hernias must be operated on emergently as a lifesaving procedure. If left untreated, all patients with strangulated hernias will die. There are situations in which patients with strangulated hernias do not undergo any operation. These are typically rare situations wherein the patient wishes to forego any interventions, even if life-saving, or the patient's clini-

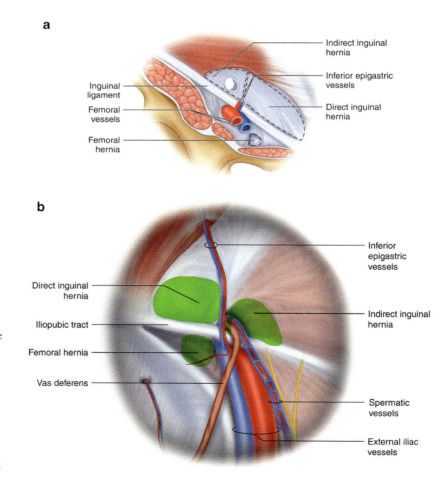

Fig. 33.1 The myopectineal orifice. Note the anatomy of the various hernias as they relate to the inguinal ligament/iliopubic tract and the vessels. (**a**) Myopectineal orifice from anterior or open view, right groin. (**b**) Myopectineal orifice from retroperitoneal or laparoscopic view, right groin

cal situation is so critical that an operation will not improve the expected mortality, such as in a patient with end-stage liver failure.

Strangulated inguinal hernias present with severe symptoms. These may include signs of sepsis (fever, shock), intestinal obstruction (vomiting), constant unrelenting pain, acute abdomen, and skin changes overlying a firm mass in the groin (erythema, edema, exfoliation, blistering). Imaging is often not necessary to confirm a diagnosis. However, in modern day, it is not uncommon to have a CT scan or X-ray ordered and completed prior to surgical consultation. Imaging findings would show signs consistent with ischemia and/or infarction: pneumatosis, edema, free fluid, and free gas.

The general teaching is that intestinal infarction can occur within 6 h of mesenteric occlusion. Thus, time is of the essence. One small study showed that delay in operating 12 or more hours after onset of systems will result in higher risk for intestinal resection [6].

As with any emergent operation, the goal is to save the patient's life. Thus, in the situation of a strangulated inguinal hernia, the goal is not to repair the hernia. The hernia is not the life-threatening issue. The focus should primarily be to address the ischemia. This may require fat and/or intestinal resection.

Depending on the patient's clinical situation, the operation can be performed as a single-stage procedure or may need to be performed in multiple stages. The safest decision is always the best decision.

The first stage is resection of the strangulated contents. In one scenario, the patient may be floridly septic and in shock. The best intraoperative decision would be to rapidly excise the infarcted intestine and leave the patient in discontinuity, with an open abdomen. The hernia is not repaired at this stage. In the case of a damage control situation, the acute abdomen should be treated as one would any other situation involving mesenteric ischemia. These situations are nicely addressed in detail in the "Mesenteric Ischemia" and "Ischemic Colitis" chapters of this book. Once the patient is clinically stable, the hernia repair can be addressed. In this scenario of an unstable

patient, definitive hernia repair may not even occur at the primary admission.

The timing of the hernia repair would depend on the clinical situation of the patient. We have no tools to predict the risk of re-incarceration or re-strangulation if a hernia is not definitively repaired. This assessment has never been studied. There is no rule that the hernia must be repaired within days or even during the same admission as the strangulation episode. That said, most surgeons tend to repair the hernia at the same time or within days of the first-stage operation of a strangulated hernia.

I do not agree that a hernia should undergo definitive repair if the patient is unfit for the operation. Rushing to repair a hernia in a sub-optimal setting—such as when the patient remains critically ill, septic, and malnutritioned—may result in a higher risk of complications related to the repair. Complications and morbidity after an emergency operation are also significantly higher than after an elective operation [3, 7, 8].

The top two complications include infection and recurrence. Both can significantly complicate options and outcomes for future hernia repairs, sometimes spiraling the patient toward a poor quality of life with risks for giant hernias and chronic pain.

We know that "putting some stitches" in a hernia will not hold the repair. More often, it may tear the tissue, which will make the subsequent hernia larger. It may entrap a nerve if poorly placed. A bona fide tissue repair involves quite a bit of tissue dissection and rearrangement. I do not recommend that in the face of infection, edema, and/or poor nutrition. If or when that hernia repair recurs, the surgeon loses the chance at offering the same repair electively.

The use of biologic or absorbable mesh prosthetics has been promoted in situations of gross contamination or prior contamination. The recurrence rates are higher when using biologic mesh in an emergent situation than with elective repairs, and surgical site infection remains a problem [9, 10]. Some of the data regarding biologic mesh outcome must be extracted from the ventral hernia population, as the outcome of biologic mesh in inguinal hernias has not been well studied [11, 12]. The most recent meta-analysis looking at use of biologic mesh in ventral hernias reports a pooled 30% hernia recurrence rate when implanted in contaminated fields, 9% recurrence rate in potentially contaminated fields, plus a 50% surgical site complication rate [13]. It is also quite costly. Nevertheless, it is an option.

The use of nonabsorbable synthetic mesh in a grossly contaminated field has been reported. There are a few small population reports showing where patients had reasonable outcomes after synthetic mesh implants in contaminated fields. Larger studies in the ventral hernia population have not supported this practice, even if using macroporous lightweight mesh [14–16]. It is also not my practice to place synthetic mesh in a contaminated field. The morbidity of dealing with a mesh infection is too high for me to consider it a valid option in my practice.

If the patient is unfit for a definitive repair, and the surgeon is concerned for early recurrence of a strangulation event, my recommendation is to consider plugging the hernia defect with an absorbable product, such as a sheet of an absorbable hemostatic agent. This would temporarily reduce the risk of any content reentering the defect.

Risk Stratification

Treatment of strangulated hernias is basically straightforward: operate. Meanwhile, the case of the incarcerated (non-strangulated) inguinal hernia has many shades of gray. As such, the surgeons should stratify the treatment plan based on the hernia's risk for progression to a strangulated inguinal hernia.

An incarcerated inguinal hernia may vary from being asymptomatic and non-obstructing to painful and obstructing. Those that are symptomatic may share many clinical findings with a strangulated inguinal hernia. These may include nausea, constant or colicky pain, overlying skin changes such as erythema, warmth over the hernia site, and intestinal obstruction. In general, if any of these findings are notable in a patient with an incarcerated inguinal hernia, the risk of pro-

gression to strangulation is real. Urgent surgical treatment is recommended. Early attention to this category of incarcerated inguinal hernia can be lifesaving [7].

Secondarily, the incarcerated inguinal hernia should be stratified based on the patient's quality of life. For example, if a patient has a chronically incarcerated inguinal hernia that is minimally symptomatic, then urgent surgical attention may not significantly improve his or her quality of life. A better choice may be elective repair, under controlled perioperative circumstances, with improved outcome. Watchful waiting may even be an option in the asymptomatic or minimally symptomatic patient with incarcerated inguinal hernia. That said, none of the watchful waiting trials included incarcerated inguinal hernias in their study population [2, 17].

Diagnosis

The first level of diagnosis of an incarcerated inguinal hernia is clinical. The patient may notice a bump or mass in the groin. This is more commonly appreciated in nonobese patients [18]. If there are symptoms, they tend to be focused at the level of the herniation. The timing of the symptoms is important, as those with shorter period of symptoms are at higher need for emergent attention [19, 20]. Obstructive symptoms, such as nausea, bloating, and vomiting, are common when the intestine is involved. However, most incarcerated inguinal hernias involve only fat.

In some patients, an intestinal obstruction may be the only sign of an incarcerated inguinal hernia; thus, physical examination should always include a hernia examination [8]. This is more commonly missed among non-surgeons than surgeons, with up to 1/3 of the bowel obstructions being missed as due to inguinal hernia [21].

Findings of overlying erythema, warmth, and hypesthesia are concerning as they may be suggestive of ischemia and impending strangulation.

Imaging can be an important adjunct to physical examination, especially if there is a question about content and its viability [8]. X-rays can show intestinal obstruction and sometimes gas below the inguinal ligament. CT scan is the most common imaging modality. Use of both oral and IV contrast would be ideal, as it will best identify intestinal content, evaluate for intestinal wall edema and perfusion, and more clearly show any free fluid and gas within the hernia defect.

Laboratory testing is minimal for evaluation of an incarcerated inguinal hernia. If there is concern for ischemia, then a CBC is warranted. An elevation in WBC in the setting of an incarcerated inguinal hernia should be treated as an urgent matter, with impending strangulation if treatment is not offered in a timely manner.

Nonoperative Treatment Options

In an acutely incarcerated inguinal hernia, selective reduction of the incarcerated inguinal hernia is an option if there is no suggestion of nonviable tissue, especially the intestine. In an early study, 80% of patients with incarcerations were deemed appropriate candidates for reduction [22]. Of those, 2/3 were successfully reduced. The majority of the patients who had successful reductions (62%) required medications, whereas 38% could be reduced by the physician's skill alone.

Reduction of an incarcerated inguinal hernia should be considered if (a) there is no clinical finding suggestive of strangulation and (b) the patient is symptomatic from the incarceration. If the inguinal hernia is asymptomatic or minimally symptomatic and has been chronically incarcerated, then attempts at reduction are not typically necessary. It will not improve outcome.

If the asymptomatic or minimally symptomatic inguinal hernia is acutely incarcerated, it may be to the patient's benefit reduce it. This will reduce the risk of edema and progression to needing an emergent operation. Also, it will help maintain the integrity of the inguinal canal. As these patients may have recurrent incarceration episodes, it may be helpful to educate the patient about how to reduce their hernia.

The technique to reduce an inguinal hernia involves some basic knowledge of anatomy. Most will be indirect inguinal hernias, implying a long,

narrow, often oblique canal as opposed to the wide short canal of the direct hernia. The contents of the hernia should be lengthening to accommodate the inguinal canal prior to reducing them into the abdomen. This form of manual reduction is referred to as taxis. It requires skill rather than force and should be used judiciously. To quote from Dr. Joseph Parrish's [23] essay:

> Now let common sense speak on this subject. What can be more irrational than to apply force to a tender bowel already in a state of inflammation? What more likely plan to hurry on the bowel to mortification, and the patient to death? I lay it down as a principle that all force in such a case is improper— arte non vi should be the maxim of the surgeon.

When reducing an incarcerated inguinal hernia, the surgeon must be aware of the risk of *reduction en masse* [24]. This is the scenario in which the hernia sac is seemingly reduced from the defect but intestinal obstruction remains. The cause is usually a stricture at the neck of the hernia sac, wherein the incarcerated contents remain entrapped within the hernia sac, and the peritoneal sac is reduced intraperitoneally. Thus, in many situations, observation is necessary after reduction of an incarcerated inguinal hernia with obstruction. Surgical intervention is mandated if the obstruction does not resolve.

Operative Treatment Options

The options for a patient with incarcerated inguinal hernia are plenty and dependent more so on the skill of the surgeon. Most incarcerated inguinal hernias can be approached via open or laparoscopic approach. Neither has been shown to be superior to the other [8]. The safest approach is the best approach, and that may differ based on the experience of the surgeon.

The open approach for an incarcerated inguinal hernia can be via inguinal, low transverse, or laparotomy approach. The primary goals must be to reduce the incarcerated content, assess for viability of the content, and release any obstruction. Thus, it is alright to make two incisions, inguinal and laparotomy, as necessary to assure that those goals are met.

Assuming the patient is stable and there is no gross contamination of the field, the inguinal hernia repair can be performed at the same setting. This can be performed via open or laparoscopic approach. Also, both a mesh and non-mesh tissue repair can be performed. There is little contraindication to synthetic mesh implantation in the setting of incarcerated non-strangulated inguinal hernia, assuming there is no intestinal resection, as these are considered clean wound classes. In the situation where there has been reversible intestinal ischemia, one can argue there has been bacterial translocation, and so the site of the hernia is potentially contaminated. Many studies have confirmed the safety of synthetic mesh placement in a potentially contaminated situation [25, 26]. Monofilament macroporous lightweight mesh is preferred in these situations, as the risk of mesh infection may be lower [8]. Judicious use of antibiotics perioperatively would be prudent nevertheless.

If an open approach is chosen, I prefer the posterior approach as opposed to the common anterior approach. Variations of this approach have been described by many surgeons, including Arthur Cheatle, AK Henry, Renee Stoppa, Lloyd Nyhus, and Robert Condon [27]. I prefer the technique described by Nyhus and Condon. The surgeon starts with a low transverse incision two fingerbreadths cephalad to the inguinal ligament. This is basically a one-sided transverse laparotomy. With this incision, the surgeon can gain intraperitoneal access to reduce the hernia contents and assess their viability. Any sac-related stricture or adhesions can be released. Intestinal resection can be performed if necessary. Since this is a low incision, the surgeon has direct access to the inguinal canal for the hernia repair. It is a bit more difficult to repair an inguinal hernia from a low midline incision. At this point, the peritoneum can be closed, and an extraperitoneal approach can be taken to reduce the hernia sac and expose the hernia defect. In the extraperitoneal space, similar to that seen with the laparoscopic approach, the surgeon has a choice of mesh placement or tissue-based repair. The tissue repair is an iliopubic tract repair, wherein the transversalis arch is sewn down to the iliopubic tract (Fig. 33.2).

The laparoscopic approach can be considered in a hemodynamically stable patient. The approach begins intraperitoneally, with the goal of reducing the contents from the hernia. In the case of intestinal obstruction, it is very important to assure that entry is performed safely, such as with open Hasson technique. This may reduce the risk of intestinal injury as the abdomen will be distended with dilated loops of the intestine abutting the abdominal wall. Secondly, the herniated intestine may be edematous and friable. To reduce the risk of bowel injury during its reduction from the hernia defect, it is safest to tug on the distal decompressed intestine and not the dilated thin-walled edematous proximal intestine. If intestinal resection is necessary, then that can be performed in laparoscopic or open fashion, depending on the surgeon's skill. Hernia repair can then be performed as a transabdominal preperitoneal approach with mesh, if considered safe.

Morbidity and Mortality

The mortality risk associated with elective hernia surgery is negligible, regardless of age [7]. Death is rarely part of the discussion when consenting for this operation. However, mortality associated with emergency hernia surgery is quite high. Nilsson et al. [7] reported the standardized mortality ratio (SMR) after emergency hernia surgery to be 6.18 for men and 8.68 for women. This is in part due to increased age and comorbidities [3, 7, 20]. Patients undergoing an emergency hernia operation are about 10 years older than those undergoing an elective operation. Other reasons include need for more complex operations, such as bowel resection or laparotomy, at the time of emergency hernia surgery. A bowel resection increases the SMR to 22.29 [7].

It is recommended, therefore, that all attempts be made to prevent need for an emergency operation. For example, symptomatic inguinal hernias with intermittent incarceration should be considered for elective repair. Also, those with acute symptoms should be more likely to undergo elective repair than those with chronic symptoms.

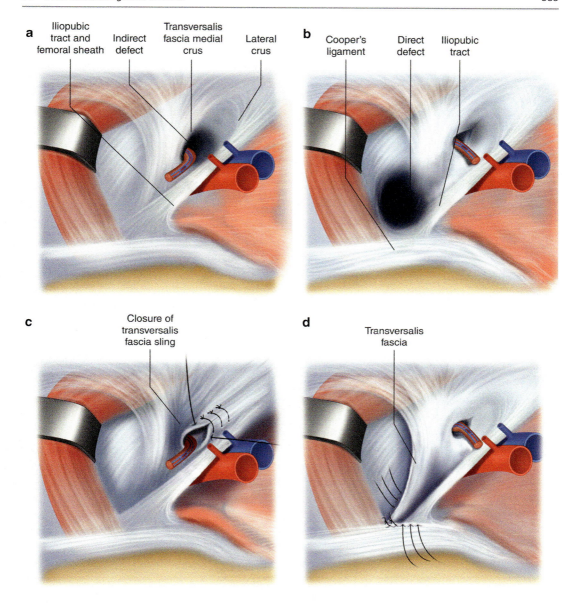

Fig. 33.2 Posterior approach iliopubic tract repair, right groin. (**a**) Myopectineal orifice with indirect inguinal hernia. (**b**) Myopectineal orifice with direct inguinal hernia. (**c**) Iliopubic tract repair of indirect inguinal hernia, approximating lateral transversalis arch to iliopubic tract. (**d**) Iliopubic tract repair of direct inguinal hernia, approximating medial transversalis arch to Cooper's ligament and iliopubic tract

One small population retrospective study suggests that patients with less than 3 months of symptoms should be considered a priority, as they are at highest risk for need for emergent operation [19]. A later study considered the same risk in patients with less than 1 year of symptoms [20].

Further risk factors for poor outcome include delay in treatment. This may be delay in presentation or delay in operation. Most studies suggest need for bowel resection, and thus increase in morbidity and mortality, peaks if obstructive symptoms lasted 48 h or longer [4, 20] (Table 33.1).

Table 33.1 Morbidity and mortality are increased among incarcerated/strangulated adult groin hernia patients with the following risk factors (with Permission from The HerniaSurge Group) [8]

Age > 65 years, especially octogenarians
Prolonged symptom duration
Delay to admission, diagnosis, and surgery
Prolonged time from admission to start surgery
Incarceration for more than 24 h
Symptom duration of 3 or more days
Bowel obstruction
Lack of health insurance
Associated midline laparotomy for exploration after incarcerated/strangulated hernia reduction
Femoral hernia, especially right-sided
Female gender

The Case of the Incarcerated Femoral Hernia

Like inguinal hernias, femoral hernias occur within the myopectineal orifice. However, they are very different in epidemiology and presentation than an inguinal hernia. Women are more likely than men to have incarcerated femoral hernias by a factor of 7 [28]. We know that femoral hernias have the highest incidence of incarceration, strangulation, and associated mortality of all hernias [8, 29]. Accordingly, women have a higher risk of mortality from emergency hernia surgery [7].

Femoral hernias are at highest risk for incarceration and strangulation [28]. Over 1/3 of femoral hernias present for the first time as an intestinal obstruction and/or strangulation [30]. Accordingly, intestinal resection is also more frequent with femoral hernias (23% vs 5% for emergent inguinal hernias). Those who present with strangulated intestine are also at higher risk for sepsis and death. Women who present emergently with a femoral hernia have a 4% 30-day mortality rate [31].

Timely diagnosis is prudent, as a delay in diagnosis greater than 6 h correlated with worse outcome [28]. Thus, the workup for intestinal obstruction in a female, especially older than 65 years, should rule out femoral hernia. Also, based on the known high risk for strangulation

and mortality, it is recommended that femoral hernias be repaired electively, even if asymptomatic [8]. Watchful waiting is discouraged.

Femoral hernias are hard to diagnose clinically, as the femoral space is small, and so they don't commonly present with a bulging mass. Furthermore, due to the stiff confines of the canal (lacunar ligament, Cooper's ligament, iliopubic tract), it is very difficult to reduce a femoral hernia.

The philosophy behind treatment of a femoral hernia is no different than that of inguinal hernias. The surgical approach is more commonly posterior, as the anterior transinguinal and infrainguinal approaches have been shown to be limiting. This can be performed via open or laparoscopic approach, as described above.

References

1. Legutko J, Pach R, Solecki R, et al. The history of treatment of groin hernia. Folia Med Cracov. 2008;49(1–2):57–74.
2. Fitzgibbons RJ, Giobbie-Harder A, Gibbs JO, Dunlop DD, et al. Watchful waiting vs repair of inguinal hernia in minimally symptomatic men: a randomized clinical trial. JAMA. 2006;295(3):285–92.
3. Ohana G, Manevwitch I, Weil R, et al. Inguinal hernia: challenging the traditional indication for surgery in asymptomatic patients. Hernia. 2004;8:117–20.
4. Kulah B, Kulacoglu IH, Oruc MT, et al. Presentation and outcome of incarcerated external hernias in adults. Am J Surg. 2001;181:101–4.
5. Alvarez JA, Baldonedo RF, Bear IG, et al. Incarcerated groin hernias in adults: presentation and outcome. Hernia. 2014;8:121–6.
6. Tanaka N, Uchida N, Ogihara H, et al. Clinical study of inguinal and femoral incarcerated hernias. Surg Today. 2010;40:1144–7.
7. Nilsson H, Stylianidis G, Haapamäki M, et al. Mortality after groin hernia surgery. Ann Surg. 2007;245(4):656.
8. The HerniaSurge Group. International guidelines for groin hernia management. Hernia. 2018;22(1):1–165. https://doi.org/10.1007/s10029-017-1668-x.
9. Itani KMF, Rosen M, Vargo D, et al. Prospective study of single-stage repair of contaminated hernias using a biologic porcine tissue matrix: the RICH Study. Surgery. 2012;152(3):498–505.
10. Bellows CF, Shadduck P, Helton WS, et al. Early report of a randomized comparative clinical trial of Strattice™ reconstructive tissue matrix to lightweight synthetic mesh in the repair of inguinal hernias. Hernia. 2014;18(2):221–30.

11. Ansaloni L, Catena F, Coccolini F, et al. Inguinal hernia repair with porcine small intestine submucosa: 3-year follow-up results of a randomized controlled trial of Lichtenstein's repair with polypropylene mesh versus Surgisis Inguinal Hernia Matrix. Am J Surg. 2009;198(3):303–12.

12. Bochicchio GV, Jain A, McGonigal K, et al. Biologic vs synthetic inguinal hernia repair: 1-year results of a randomized double-blinded trial. J Am Coll Surg. 2014;218(4):751–7.

13. Atema JJ, de Vries FEE, Boermeester MA. Systematic review and meta-analysis of the repair of potentially contaminated and contaminated abdominal wall defects. Am J Surg. 2016;212(5):982–95.

14. Choi JJ, Palaniappa NC, Dallas KB, et al. Use of mesh during ventral hernia repair in clean-contaminated and contaminated cases: outcomes of 33,832 cases. Ann Surg. 2012;255:176–80.

15. Carbonell AM, Criss CN, Cobb WS, et al. Outcomes of synthetic mesh in contaminated ventral hernia repairs. J Am Coll Surg. 2013;217(6):991–8.

16. Brahmbhatt R, Martindale R, Liang MK. Jumping the gun? Evaluating the evidence for synthetic mesh in contaminated hernia repairs. J Am Coll Surg. 2014;218(30):498–9.

17. O'Dwyer PJ, Norrie J, Alani A, et al. Observation or operation for patients with an asymptomatic inguinal hernia: a randomized clinical trial. Ann Surg. 2006;244(2):167.

18. Rosemar A, Angerras U, Rosengren A. Body mass index and groin hernia: a 34-year follow-up study in Swedish men. Ann Surg. 2008;247:1064–8.

19. Gallegos NC, Dawson J, Jarvis M, et al. Risk of strangulation in groin hernias. Br J Surg. 1991;78:1171–3.

20. Rai S, Chandra SS, Smile SR. A study of the risk of strangulation and obstruction in groin hernias. Aust N Z J Surg. 1998;68:650–4.

21. McEntee G, Pender D, Mulvin D, et al. Current spectrum of intestinal obstruction. Br J Surg. 1987;74:976–80.

22. Kauffman HM, O'Brien DP. Selective reduction of incarcerated inguinal hernia. Am J Surg. 1970;119(6):660–73.

23. Parrish J. Practical observations on strangulated hernia: and some of the diseases of the urinary organs. Philadelphia: Key and Biddle; 1836. 261 p.

24. Corner EM, Howitt AB. The reduction en masse of strangulated and non-strangulated herniæ. Ann Surg. 1908;47(4):573–87.

25. Atila K, Guler S, Inal A, et al. Prosthetic repair of acutely incarcerated groin hernias: a prospective clinical observational cohort study. Langenbeck's Arch Surg. 2010;395(5):563–8.

26. Sawayama H, Kanemitsu K, Okuma T, et al. Safety of polypropylene mesh for incarcerated groin and obturator hernias: a retrospective study of 110 patients. Hernia. 2014;18(3):399–406.

27. Nyhus LM. The posterior (preperitoneal) approach and iliopubic tract repair of inguinal and femoral hernias—an update. Hernia. 2003;7(2):63–7.

28. Kurt N, Oncel M, Ozkan Z. Risk and outcome of bowel resection in patients with incarcerated groin hernias: retrospective study. World J Surg. 2003;27:741–3.

29. Beadles CA, Meagher AD, Charles AG. Trends in emergent hernia repair in the United States. JAMA Surg. 2015;150(3):194–200.

30. Dahlstrand U, Wollert S, Nordin P, et al. Emergency femoral hernia repair: a study based on a national register. Ann Surg. 2009;249(4):672–6.

31. Koch A, Edwards A, Haapaniemi S, et al. Prospective evaluation of 6895 groin hernia repairs in women. Br J Surg. 2005;92(12):1553–8.

Incarcerated Umbilical and Ventral Hernia Repair

Molly R. Deane and Dennis Y. Kim

Introduction

Ventral herniorrhaphies are commonly performed procedures worldwide. Approximately 175,000 umbilical hernia repairs are performed annually in the USA, where umbilical and epigastric hernias comprise 10% of all primary hernias [1]. Ventral hernia repairs are much more common with an estimated 350,000–500,000 open and laparoscopic procedures performed annually in the USA [2]. Left untreated, both types of hernias may ultimately result in life-threatening complications including incarceration and strangulation. Of the 2.3 million inpatient abdominal hernia repairs performed between 2001 and 2010 in the USA, approximately one-fourth were performed emergently [3].

Etiologies and Presentation

Ventral hernias occur as a result of defects in the abdominal wall fascia and muscles through which preperitoneal or intraperitoneal contents may protrude. Ventral hernias may be classified on the basis of whether or not they are primary, also known as true, ventral hernias (nonincisional).

M. R. Deane · D. Y. Kim (✉)
Department of Surgery, Harbor-UCLA Medical Center, Torrance, CA, USA
e-mail: dekim@dhs.lacounty.gov

These are further classified based upon their location or the plane of tissue through which the defect occurs. *Epigastric hernias* are midline abdominal hernias occurring between the umbilicus and xiphoid process. The defect is typically small and occurs as a result of incomplete fusion of the midline due to a lack of decussating fibers. Multiple defects may be encountered and incarceration is uncommon. *Spigelian hernias* are rare hernias which occur through the Spigelian fascia – a section of the aponeurosis between the semilunar line and the lateral border of the rectus muscle extending from the eighth costal cartilage to the pubis. The majority of these hernias occur at or above the arcuate line and may be difficult to diagnose on physical examination [4]. Patients often present with incarceration or strangulation. *Parastomal hernias* occur as a result of the creation of a defect in the abdominal wall through which the bowel is brought out to create the stoma.

Umbilical hernias may be congenital or acquired. In children, these hernias occur as a result of delayed or incomplete closure of the umbilical ring, which usually occurs by the age of 5. In children, the majority of umbilical hernias are asymptomatic, and the standard approach to management is observation with the expectation of spontaneous closure. Common indications for umbilical hernia repair include failure to close by 5 years of age, large hernias, and concerns over the appearance of the umbilicus and abdomen. Although uncommon, incarceration, which may

© Springer International Publishing AG, part of Springer Nature 2019
C. V. R. Brown et al. (eds.), *Emergency General Surgery*, https://doi.org/10.1007/978-3-319-96286-3_34

manifest with abdominal pain, distension, bilious emesis, and a tender mass over the umbilicus, warrants immediate exploration and repair.

Acquired umbilical hernias develop in adulthood and occur as a result of increases in intra-abdominal pressure as may occur in the setting of obesity, chronic cough, or recurrent heavy lifting. Pregnancy, ascites, and other processes resulting in increased abdominal distension may also contribute to the development of an umbilical hernia. In adulthood, umbilical hernias occur more commonly in women than in men. These hernias often contain omentum and preperitoneal fat.

Incisional hernias are by far the most common ventral hernias encountered and occur at the site of a previous incision. Approximately 10–15% of incisions will develop a hernia over time, and careful attention to closure techniques is paramount to reducing incisional hernias [5]. Development of a postoperative wound infection, immunosuppression, and obesity are associated with an increased risk for an incisional hernia as is the need for emergent surgery. The majority of these hernias manifest in the early postoperative period. The most common type of ventral hernia is a midline incisional hernia, comprising approximately 90%. Trocar or laparoscopic port site hernias may occur in 0.5–1.0% of patients [6].

Umbilical and ventral hernias are both susceptible to complications, the most concerning of which are incarceration and strangulation. *Incarceration* occurs when the contents of a hernia are irreducible due to a narrowed opening, adhesions to the hernia sac, or both. A *Richter's hernia* is an example of an incarcerated hernia in which a portion of the antimesenteric border becomes incarcerated in the fascial defect with the potential for obstruction or strangulation. *Strangulation* involves compromised blood supply to the contents of the hernia with progression to ischemia and perforation.

Clinical Presentation

Evaluation of a patient with a suspected incarcerated ventral hernia begins with a detailed history and physical examination in conjunction with active resuscitative efforts. Symptoms of increasing or intractable pain, nausea, and vomiting should be sought, in addition to the presence of fevers, chills, and other constitutional symptoms. Operative risk stratification including an assessment of medical comorbidities, medications, functional status, and frailty should be performed. Additionally, details should be sought regarding previous surgeries, the indications for those surgeries, and the development of complications postoperatively. For patients with a known ventral hernia, duration, changes in size over time, and the ability to reduce the hernia may be important factors to consider when embarking upon the decision to repair a ventral hernia acutely.

A focused physical examination should be performed to identify local and systemic complications. The presence of surgical scars, location, and contents of the hernia, as well as the size of the fascial defect, should be sought during the exam. The presence of the systemic inflammatory response syndrome, particularly when accompanied by the presence of erythematous skin changes overlying the hernia, palpation tenderness, or peritonitis, is highly suggestive of strangulation with resultant sepsis. Strangulation should be identified expeditiously as delays to operative intervention can lead to progressive bowel compromise and further complications including shock with resultant organ dysfunction. Early detection of progression from incarceration to strangulation remains a challenge.

Diagnosis

Diagnostic imaging in the form of plain radiographs or contrast-enhanced CT scans, with or without oral contrast, may provide additional information regarding the presence of a bowel obstruction, ischemia, and perforation. Bowel obstruction is diagnosed based on the presence of distended or dilated loops of bowel. A transition point can often be identified at or near the neck of the hernia in these patients (Fig. 34.1). Findings suggestive of bowel ischemia on CT scan include bowel wall thickening, reduced wall enhancement, mesenteric stranding, pneumatosis intestinalis, and the presence of ascites or free fluid (Figs. 34.2 and 34.3). The presence of fluid in the hernia sac has been associated with an increased risk for surgical site infections [7]. The sensitivity of CT to identify bowel ischemia varies widely, and results should be interpreted in light of findings from the history and physical exam. Additional information provided by CT includes the presence of additional hernia defects, status of the abdominal wall musculature, and the presence of loss of domain. All of these variables should be incorporated into the surgical decision-

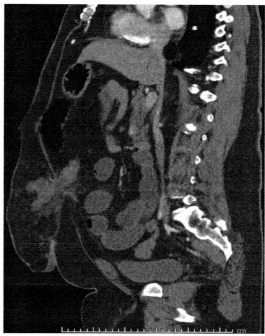

Fig. 34.3 Sagittal CT demonstrating incarcerated umbilical hernia with free fluid in dependent portion of the hernia sac

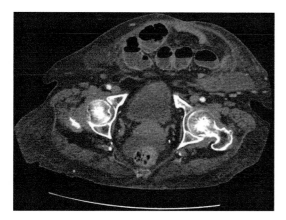

Fig. 34.1 Axial CT demonstrating dilated and collapsed small bowel within a large recurrent ventral hernia. Note also the presence of free fluid

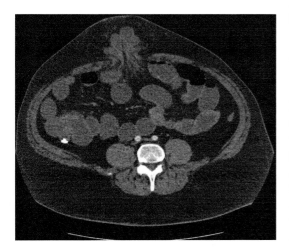

Fig. 34.2 CT scan demonstrating the presence of an incarcerated umbilical hernia with resultant small bowel obstruction

making process. It should be emphasized that the diagnosis of incarcerated or strangulated ventral hernia is primarily established on the basis of history and clinical exam findings. Lab values including an elevated white blood cell count, the presence of a bandemia, and lactic acidosis may be suggestive of bowel strangulation.

Management

For patients with an incarcerated ventral hernia complicated by bowel obstruction, nasogastric tube decompression in conjunction with fluid resuscitation should be undertaken prior to operative intervention. The aggressiveness of fluid resuscitation is determined by the patient's overall volume and metabolic status. For patients in whom strangulation is suspected, early goal-directed therapy should be instituted with an emphasis on source control. Early administration of broad-spectrum antibiotics to cover for common enteric pathogens as well as skin flora should be provided in addition to fluids, while arrangements are made for emergent surgical intervention.

Surgical Technique

The choice of operative approach is largely dictated by patient anatomy and physiology, surgeon experience, and the presence of complications associated with the incarcerated hernia. Key factors to consider are outlined in Table 34.1. In emergency general surgery patients presenting with strangulated ventral hernias and hemodynamic instability due to septic and/or cardiogenic shock, we recommend a damage control or staged approach to management. Source control and avoidance of iatrogenic injury are the guiding principles of the first stage, in conjunction with active and aggressive resuscitation. Infected mesh should be excised, and nonviable or compromised bowel should be resected and the patient left in discontinuity followed by temporary closure and admission to the intensive care unit. During the second stage, invasive hemodynamic monitoring, optimization of oxygen delivery, and support of end-organ dysfunction in a goal-directed fashion should continue until key endpoints are achieved such as reversal of acidosis, correction of the base deficit, and repletion of volume deficits. In the final stage, patients are brought back to the operating room where the gastrointestinal tract is placed back into continu-

Table 34.1 Factors determining approach to repair of an incarcerated ventral hernia

Factors	Management options and considerations
Hemodynamic status of patient	Definitive repair (stable) versus damage control or staged approach (unstable)
Operative approach	Open versus laparoscopic
Wound classification	Clean, clean-contaminated, contaminated, dirty
Type of repair	Primary (tissue) versus mesh
Selection of mesh	Synthetic, biologic, biosynthetic
Location of mesh insertion	Onlay, inlay, sublay, underlay

ity and final definitive closure or serial partial closures are performed.

Open Repair

Incarcerated Umbilical Hernia

The majority of patients presenting with an incarcerated ventral hernia will undergo an open herniorrhaphy, with or without the use of mesh. Patients should be positioned supine on the operating room table with arms abducted at 90°. Following induction with a general anesthetic, patients are widely prepped and draped. Perioperative parenteral antibiotics should be administered prior to skin incision.

For patients with an uncomplicated incarcerated umbilical hernia, injection of local anesthetic along the skin and subcutaneous tissue of the inferior umbilical ridge or depression should be performed. A semilunar incision is then made along the inferior aspect of the umbilicus, and the subcutaneous tissues are sharply cleared from the surrounding fascia and umbilical stalk. A Kelly or curved hemostat can be used to develop a window around the stalk, which is then divided. The hernia sac is identified and freed from surrounding tissues and the umbilical skin using a combination of sharp and blunt dissection. The neck of the hernia is identified, and the surrounding fascia is cleared circumferentially for 1.5–2.0 cm followed by opening of the hernia sac and inspection of hernia contents to ensure viability. The contents of the hernia are then reduced and the hernia sac excised ensuring that enough remains to allow for re-approximation and closure using an absorbable 2-0 or 3-0 suture. The undersurface of the fascial defect is also cleared of any adhesions on the peritoneal surface. Defects less than 2–3 cm in size can be primarily repaired in a transverse fashion without the use of mesh using interrupted permanent 0 sutures. Careful attention should be paid to hemostasis, ensuring adequate bites of fascia both above and below the defect. The umbilicus should then be secured or tacked to the fascia using a 3-0 absorbable suture being careful not to buttonhole the skin. The skin is closed with a running absorbable subcuticular suture and a cotton ball placed in the umbilicus which is then covered with a waterproof transparent dressing.

For larger umbilical defects (>2–3 cm), consideration should be given to placement of a mesh plug or patch to reduce tension at the site of the repair and the risk for recurrence. In patients in whom the potential for bowel resection and more extensive procedures may be required, a vertical incision which skirts around the umbilicus may be employed, as opposed to the standard curvilinear incision, as this incision may be extended superiorly or inferiorly as needed. Decisions regarding the type and location of mesh placement are discussed below. The authors' preference is to place mesh in the sublay or retrorectus position whenever feasible.

Incarcerated Ventral Hernia

Patients undergoing repair of an incarcerated ventral hernia should be positioned, prepped, and draped in a similar fashion to patients undergoing an incarcerated umbilical hernia repair. Depending on the location of the ventral hernia(s), a generous vertical or transverse incision can be made directly over the hernia itself or along the midline. If unsightly scars are present along or in the path of the incision, these can be excised during the process of entry into the abdomen. The hernia sac and peritoneum are then dissected free from the surrounding tissues, and the neck of the hernia is dissected circumferentially from the surrounding fascia which should be cleared for a distance of 3–4 cm. The sac is then incised to allow for inspection of the contents of the hernia and to ensure viability. Fluid present within the sac may be cultured at this time. The contents of the hernia are then reduced into the peritoneal cavity, or interventions such as omentectomy or bowel resection are carried out as dictated. If the contents of the hernia are not readily reducible, the fascial defect should be sharply elongated to allow return of the hernia contents into the peritoneal cavity. The peritoneum is reapproximated, and the decision to place a mesh and the location of mesh placement are made.

Defects larger than 2–3 cm should be repaired with mesh to decrease the risk of recurrence.

Even among patients with contaminated abdominal wall defects, synthetic mesh placed in a sublay fashion within the retrorectus space with approximation of the fascia ventral to the mesh appears to have similar outcomes to patients undergoing repair with a biologic mesh [8]. Judicious use and placement of subcutaneous drains are required to decrease the risk for postoperative seroma formation.

Whenever possible, bridging of ventral hernias or placement of mesh in an inlay position should be avoided as such repairs do not provide optimal mechanical stabilization of the abdominal wall and the lack of fascial overlap precludes mesh-tissue integration or ingrowth, which may ultimately increase the risk of infection and recurrence. In patients with large or complex ventral hernias in whom primary fascial reapproximation cannot be achieved, advanced myofascial release techniques should be employed. Both an anterior component separation technique and a transversus abdominis muscle release (TAR), a modification of the classic retrorectus muscular Stoppa repair technique, are reasonable surgical options. Patients with *loss of domain* (variably defined as ≥50% of the abdominal viscera residing outside of the abdominal cavity) will often require the use of these techniques during the reconstruction of their complex abdominal wall hernias.

Traditionally, an anterior component release involves the development of large skin flaps that allow for the identification of the linea semilunaris which is then incised 2–3 cm lateral to it, being careful to limit the incision to the external oblique aponeurosis and avoiding the internal oblique and transversus abdominis fascia. A plane is then developed between the external oblique and the internal oblique laterally to the posterior axillary line, superiorly toward the costal margin, and inferiorly to the inguinal ligaments. This mobilization results in each ipsilateral complex being able to be advanced toward the midline 4 cm in the upper abdomen, 8 cm at the waist, and 3 cm in the lower abdomen [9]. Component separation can be a useful and low-cost option for repair of large midline abdominal wall hernias.

For patients with complex abdominal wall hernias or those requiring complex abdominal wall reconstruction, we advocate for repair using the TAR technique or posterior component separation. Briefly, following a midline laparotomy and meticulous adhesiolysis with reduction of contents into the abdominal cavity, the retrorectus space is entered by sharply incising the posterior rectus sheath just lateral to the midline. The linea semilunaris is then identified, and the posterior rectus sheath is incised medial to the neurovascular bundles supplying the rectus muscles to reveal the underlying transversus abdominis muscle (Figs. 34.4 and 34.5) [10]. The muscle is then divided allowing entry into the space between the transversus abdominis and the transversalis fascia, which is developed laterally and posteriorly as well as superiorly and inferiorly. This allows for medialization and closure of the peritoneum and transversalis fascia over which a large mesh can be placed and fixated in the retrorectus space followed by re-approximation of the anterior rectus sheath over the mesh (Figs. 34.6 and 34.7) [10].

Selection of Mesh and Location of Placement

With the exception of very small ventral hernias (<2-3 cm), mesh should be employed in order to reduce recurrence. Various types of mesh are available for use, and they have widely varying properties which lead to different indications for use. Heavyweight meshes have thick polymers, small pore size, and high tensile strength which, in combination with the profound tissue reaction, leads to a dense scar. Lightweight meshes are composed of thinner filaments and have larger pores making them more flexible and inducing less of a foreign body reaction which, in some cases, has led to higher rates of recurrence. Different meshes have different shrinkage properties, and the amount of shrinkage correlates with density so that heavyweight meshes with smaller pores have more shrinkage due to increased scar. Overall scar tissue shrinks to ~60% of the surface area of the original wound [11, 12].

In addition to factors such as wound class, the risk of infection is also related to mesh characteristics such as type of filament and pore size. It has been advocated that if synthetic mesh placement is being considered in a contaminated field, a lightweight macroporous mesh should be used as it may have a lower risk of infection and also because there are data demonstrating the possibility of eradication of infection in this type of mesh without removal [13]. A recent prospective, multi-institutional study of surgical and quality-of-life outcomes comparing heavyweight, midweight,

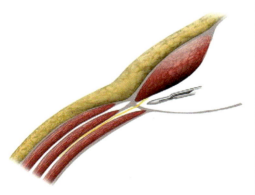 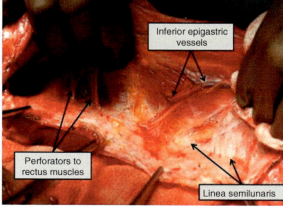

Fig. 34.4 The posterior rectus sheath is incised about 0.5–1 cm medial to the anterior/posterior rectus sheath junction to expose the underlying transversus abdominis muscle. Note the perforator nerves that are preserved during retromuscular dissection and subsequent posterior component release

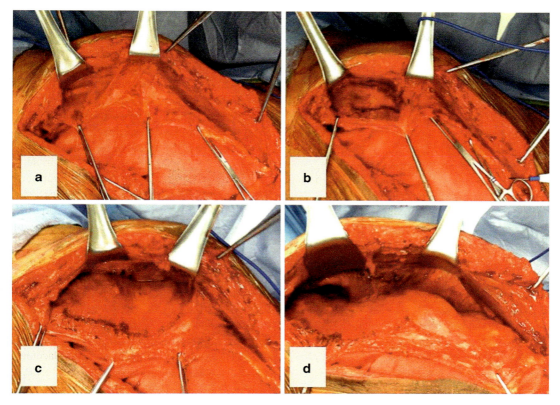

Fig. 34.5 Sequential steps of the TAR technique: (**a**) exposure of the posterior rectus fascia, (**b**) incision of the posterior rectus sheath and the underlying transversus abdominis muscle, (**c**) further division of the posterior sheath/transversus abdominis with development of the lateral space, and (**d**) dissection caudal to the arcuate line of Douglas toward the space of Retzius

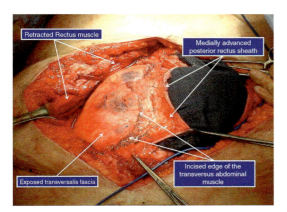

Fig. 34.6 Transversus abdominis muscle release allows for posterior component separation with entrance to the space between the transversalis fascia and the divided transversus abdominis muscle. This sublay space is sufficient for significant prosthetic reinforcement of a visceral sac

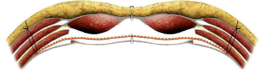

Fig. 34.7 The anterior rectus sheaths then are reapproximated in the midline ventral to the mesh to re-create the linea alba

and lightweight mesh in open ventral hernia repair demonstrated that midweight mesh had fewer surgical site infections (SSIs) and decreased length of hospital stay, whereas lightweight mesh was associated with worse quality of life at 6 and 12 months postoperatively [14].

Biomaterials or biologic meshes may have a lower risk of infection over time but come at a much higher cost than traditional, synthetic mesh products. As such, insertion or use of these meshes is typically reserved for contaminated and dirty wounds. Due to degradation and host remodeling, it has been proposed that these meshes may become vascularized and largely replaced by host tissues thereby potentially decreasing the risk of permanent mesh infection. Biologic materials are processed leading to a scaffold of porous extracellular matrix which undergoes remodeling and incorporation by the host. Some biologic meshes have been processed to have additional cross-linking, such as those chemically processed with glutaraldehyde, and this slows degradation in the hopes of leading to a stronger host collagen framework; however, this is controversial [15]. The biologic meshes (Table 34.2) are classified based upon species of origin, source of collagen matrix, decellularization process, whether they are cross-linked, storage requirements, and need for rehydration at the time of use [16].

Mesh may be placed in a variety of locations. Typically, this involves placement in an onlay, inlay, sublay, or underlay/intraperitoneal location. *Onlay* repairs involve placement of the mesh over the anterior fascia and usually require development of skin flaps. As discussed earlier, an *inlay* placement involves placement of mesh between the fascial edges. *Sublay* mesh placement in the retrorectus space is considered by many to be the ideal location for mesh placement.

Underlay placement involves placement of the mesh in the peritoneal cavity below the peritoneum. This is the typical location of mesh placement when performing a laparoscopic ventral or umbilical hernia repair. Placement within the peritoneal cavity necessitates the use of a hybrid or dual-layer mesh with an absorbable nonadherent surface positioned toward the abdominal contents to decrease the potential for adhesions.

Wound Classification

The amount of bacterial burden in the wound is the most significant risk factor for postoperative infection. The Centers for Disease Control and Prevention (CDC) wound classification predicts the relative probability that a given wound will become infected, and the World Society of Emergency Surgery has developed guidelines for mesh use based upon wound class. For CDC class I and II wounds, use of synthetic mesh is recommended for incarcerated hernias, with or without intestinal resection, provided there is no gross spillage. In these groups, there was no statistically significant difference in the rate of deep incisional SSIs or return to OR in 30 days compared to nonmesh patients. However, the rate of recurrence was lower in hernias repaired with mesh [16]. For CDC class III and IV wounds, additional factors determine the type of repair and mesh used. Small her-

Table 34.2 Types of biologic mesh

Brand name	Company	Type	Species	Additional cross-link	Sterilized
Alloderm®	LifeCell	Dermis	Human	No	No
Allomax™	CR Bard	Dermis	Human	No	Yes
FlexHD™	MTF	Dermis	Human	No	No
Collamend™	CR Bard	Dermis	Porcine	Yes	Yes
Permacol™	Covidien	Dermis	Porcine	Yes	Yes
Strattice®	LifeCell	Dermis	Porcine	No	Yes
Surgimend®	TEI	Dermis	Bovine, fetal	No	Yes
XenMatrix™	CR Bard	Dermis	Porcine	No	Yes
Surgisis®	Cook	Intestinal Submucosa	Porcine	No	Yes
Periguard®	Synovis	Pericardium	Bovine	Yes	Yes
Tutopatch®	Tutogen	Pericardium	Bovine	No	Yes
Veritas®	Synovis	Pericardium	Bovine	No	Yes
BioA®	WL Gore	Synthetic bioabsorbable		N/A	Yes
TIGR®	Novus Scientific	Synthetic bioabsorbable		N/A	Yes

nia defects (<3 cm) should be repaired primarily, and, when not possible, a biologic mesh may be used. In contaminated or dirty fields, there are data supporting the use of a biologic matrix over a synthetic mesh; however, studies are of low quality with conflicting results [8, 17, 18]. The use of synthetic mesh in clean contaminated and contaminated cases has been demonstrated to be comparable to biologic mesh repairs in terms of outcomes.

Laparoscopic Repair

Minimally invasive techniques can be successfully employed in the repair of incarcerated or strangulated hernias. Prior to establishing pneumoperitoneum, it is important to assess the size of the defect and mark out the borders of the hernia in order to assist with the selection of an appropriately sized mesh. Access to the peritoneal cavity can be achieved using an open Hasson technique or via a closed technique using a Veress needle at Palmer's point or with the aid of a dilating optical trocar. Following insufflation and establishment of adequate pneumoperitoneum, reduction of hernia contents followed by evaluation of bowel viability will dictate the next operative steps. An appropriately sized composite- or dual-coated mesh can then be fixated using a combination of tacks and transfascial sutures ensuring 4–5 cm of overlap circumferentially.

For patients with strangulated hernias where viability needs to be addressed and bowel resection performed, the feasibility of laparoscopy is decreased and surgeon dependent. Hemodynamically unstable patients may not be able to tolerate pneumoperitoneum. Additionally, as an underlay repair is typically performed in patients undergoing laparoscopic repair, the presence of strangulation and a dirty field may mandate an open repair and placement of mesh in an extraperitoneal location.

Special Circumstances

Cirrhotic patients with ascites and an incarcerated ventral hernia present a unique management challenge. In the absence of incarceration and provided that the liver disease is not advanced (child's B or C), several groups have advocated for elective repair of umbilical hernias in order to prevent complications of ascitic leak or incarceration. When cirrhotic patients present with incarceration or strangulation, emergent operation is required. Protein loss and large fluid shifts should be anticipated and repleted via infusion of albumin in a similar fashion to patients undergoing a large-volume paracentesis (6–8 g/L). Whenever possible a primary tissue repair should be performed. If mesh is required, consideration should be given to a biologic mesh. Placement of an intraperitoneal drain is optional and may help prevent rapid accumulation of tense ascites with the potential for ascitic leak and hernia recurrence. Alternatively, paracentesis may be performed as required, while optimization of medical therapy takes place. Occasionally, transjugular intrahepatic portosystemic shunt (TIPS) may be required for refractory ascites.

Postoperative Course

Postoperatively, subcutaneous drain output should be monitored and drains removed when there is <30 cc output in a 24-h period. Placement of an abdominal binder is suggested but not required. Duration of antibiotic therapy will depend on the presence or absence of contamination, and pharmacologic venous thromboembolism prophylaxis should be administered in the immediate postoperative period. Glucose control along with dietary modification, weight loss, and smoking cessation are important modifications that may prevent wound-healing complications and hernia recurrence.

Acknowledgements The authors would like to acknowledge Elsevier and RightsLink® for granting permission for the use of figures from a previously published article [10].

References

1. Rutkow IM. Epidemiologic, economic, and sociologic aspects of hernia repair in the United States in the 1990s. Surg Clin N Am. 1998;78(6):941–51.

2. SAGES Webmaster. Laparoscopic ventral hernia repair patient information from SAGES. http://www.sages.org/publications/patient-information. 2015. Accessed 10 Oct 2017.
3. Beadles CA, et al. Trends in emergent hernia repair in the United States. JAMA Surg. 2015;150(3):194–200.
4. Richards AT. Spigelian hernias. Op Tech Gen Surg. 2004;6(3):228–39.
5. Le Huu Nho R. Incidence and prevention of ventral incisional hernia. J Visc Surg. 2012;149(5 Suppl):e3–14.
6. Chatzimavroudis G, et al. Trocar site hernia following laparoscopic cholecystectomy: a 10-year single center experience. Hernia. 2017; https://doi.org/10.1007/s10029-017-1699-3. Epub 2017 Oct 25.
7. Loftus TJ, et al. Computed tomography evidence of fluid in the hernia sac predicts surgical site infection following mesh repair of acutely incarcerated ventral and groin hernias. J Trauma Acute Care Surg. 2017;83(1):170–4.
8. Carbonell AM, et al. Outcomes of synthetic mesh in contaminated ventral hernia repairs. J Am Coll Surg. 2013;217(6):991–8.
9. Nguyen VT, Shestak KC. "Separation of anatomic components" method of abdominal wall reconstruction. Op Tech Gen Surg. 2006;8(4):183–91.
10. Novitsky YW, et al. Transversus abdominis muscle release: a novel approach to posterior component separation during complex abdominal wall reconstruction. Am J Surg. 2012;204(5):709–16.
11. Brown CN, Finch JG. Which mesh for hernia repair? Ann R Coll Surg Engl. 2010;92(4):272–8.
12. Klosterhalfen B, et al. The lightweight and large porous mesh concept for hernia repair. Expert Rev Med Devices. 2005;2(1):103–17.
13. Amid PK, et al. Biomaterials for "tension-free" hernioplasties and principles of their applications. Minerva Chir. 1995;50(9):821–6.
14. Groene SA, et al. Prospective, multi-institutional surgical and quality-of-life outcomes comparison of heavyweight, midweight, and lightweight mesh in open ventral hernia repair. Am J Surg. 2016;212(6):1054–62.
15. Hunter JD 3rd, Cannon JA. Biomaterials: so many choices, so little time. What are the differences? Clin Colon Rectal Surg. 2014;27(4):134–9.
16. Dunne JR, et al. Abdominal wall hernias: risk factors for infection and resource utilization. J Surg Res. 2003;111(1):78–84.
16. Choi JJ, et al. Use of mesh during ventral hernia repair in clean-contaminated and contaminated cases: outcomes of 33,832 cases. Ann Surg. 2012;255(1):176–80.
17. Harth KC, et al. Biologic mesh use practice patterns in abdominal wall reconstruction: a lack of consensus among surgeons. Hernia. 2013;17(1):13–20.
18. Bondre IL, et al. Suture, synthetic, or biologic in contaminated ventral hernia repair. J Surg Res. 2016;200(2):488–94.

Paraesophageal Hernia and Gastric Volvulus

35

K. Conley Coleman and Daniel Grabo

Introduction

Hiatal hernias are a relatively common incidental finding on radiographic or endoscopic evaluation with estimates of incidence ranging from 10% to 50% for the general population [1]. A paraesophageal hernia is a rare type of hiatal hernia that mainly affects older adults (age 65–75 years). Medical management of reflux symptoms is the mainstay of therapy for a hiatal hernia. However, surgical management is often required for the management of failed medical therapy in hiatal hernia and in complicated paraesophageal hernia (gastric volvulus, bleeding, or obstruction).

Classification and Etiology

The most common type of hiatal hernia is type I, or a sliding hiatal hernia, which accounts for about 95% of all hiatal hernias with the remaining 5% being true paraesophageal (types II, III, and IV) hernias [2]. Hiatal hernias are classified as follows:

I. Type I, also called a sliding hiatal hernia, occurs when the gastroesophageal (GE) junction ascends into the thorax through the esophageal hiatus, pulling the cardia of the stomach up as well. This occurs due to a laxity in the phrenoesphageal ligament.

II. Type II is a true paraesophageal hernia, where the GE junction resides in the abdomen but a portion of the stomach fundus herniates through the hiatus into the thorax. This is commonly due to a combination of phrenoesphageal ligament laxity and widening of the esophageal hiatus.

III. Type III occurs as a combination of type I hiatal and II paraesophageal hernias. The GE junction ascends into the thorax as well as the fundus of the stomach herniating in parallel thought the hiatus.

IV. Type IV is when an organ other than the stomach herniates through the hiatus into the thorax. This is most commonly the colon, but can be the spleen, or small bowel as well.

Trauma, congenital malformations, and iatrogenic factors, such as complications from surgical dissection, have all been implicated in the development of hiatal hernias [3]. Type I hiatal hernias result from the progressive disruption of the GE junction and as such a portion of the gastric cardia herniates upward. Type II, III, and IV paraesophageal hernias can result in displacement of the greater curvature of the stomach into the thorax due to hernia enlargement and laxity in the gastrocolic and gastrosplenic ligaments. The GE junction, however, often remains fixed in the

K. Conley Coleman · D. Grabo (✉)
Department of Surgery, West Virginia University, Morgantown, WV, USA
e-mail: daniel.grabo@hsc.wvu.edu

abdomen, and this results in the herniated stomach rotating around its longitudinal axis.

Gastric volvulus can occur if the stomach rotates around its long or short axis, resulting in organoaxial or mesenteroaxial, respectively. Organoaxial volvulus occurs when the stomach rotates around its long axis as drawn from the GE junction to the pylorus where as mesenteroaxial volvulus occurs when the stomach rotates around a perpendicular line drawn from the lesser curvature to the greater curvature. Gastric volvulus is more common in persons age > 50 years and in those with diaphragmatic defects. Gastric volvulus can be classified as primary or secondary gastric volvulus [4]. Primary gastric volvulus is due to abnormalities occurring with the gastric ligaments which allows the stomach to twist. More common, however, is secondary gastric volvulus which occurs as the result of anatomic abnormalities not associated with gastric ligamentous distention. These are usually due to paraesophageal hernias or diaphragmatic hernias but also can be due to diaphragmatic eventration and phrenic nerve paralysis.

Acute gastric volvulus can be a surgical emergency if the stomach becomes rotated in such a way as to cause ischemia. Unfortunately, acute gastric volvulus is associated with mortality rates that range from 30% to 50% [4]. In this circumstance emergent, surgical intervention is warranted to prevent gastric necrosis. Quick diagnosis along with appropriate perioperative management and surgical therapies is the key to minimizing the risk of the morbidity and mortality that is associated with gastric necrosis. Chronic or intermittent gastric volvulus is less severe in nature; however, chronic rotation of the stomach can result in gastric ulceration, bleeding, and anemia.

Clinical Presentation and Diagnosis

Hiatal Hernia

While most patients with small type I hiatal hernias are asymptomatic, as the hernia enlarges, symptoms of gastroesophageal reflux (GERD) including heartburn, regurgitation, and dysphagia can occur [5]. A hiatal, type I, hernia is suspected based on symptoms consistent with GERD. Complications are rare and are usually related to reflux. Barium swallow, upper endoscopy, and esophageal manometry are utilized in the diagnosis; however, a full discussion of these modalities is outside the scope of this emergency surgery chapter.

Paraesophageal Hernia

Paraesophageal (types II, III, IV) hernias are often asymptomatic or result in only vague, intermittent symptoms of epigastric/substernal pain, postprandial fullness, regurgitation, and dysphagia. Complications of paraesophageal hernias are due to mechanical problems and include gastric volvulus, bleeding from ulcerations and erosions in the herniated organs, and respiratory complications [6].

Gastric Volvulus

Acute gastric volvulus and strangulated paraesophageal hernias have similar clinical histories. Symptoms typically involve severe epigastric abdominal pain and/or lower chest pain. Intractable vomiting often occurs as well and can often be unproductive. Borchardt's triad is often a finding associated with acute gastric volvulus and consists of chest pain, vomiting with inability to produce emesis, and the inability to pass a nasogastric tube. Development of gastric ischemia and necrosis will be manifested by severe abdominal pain and peritonitis. Chronic or subacute gastric volvulus usually causes vague or subclinical symptoms such as mild upper abdominal discomfort, dysphagia, and heartburn.

Findings on examination will depend on the severity of the obstruction and ischemia. Depending on the degree of volume depletion, the patient may present in a spectrum from mild tachycardia to hypovolemic shock. If gastric outlet obstruction is present, the stomach can become dilated and filled with fluid resulting in upper abdominal distention.

Laboratory findings may show electrolyte derangements consistent with multiple episodes of vomiting. Hypokalemia may be present as well as a hypochloremic metabolic alkalosis. Elevation in the white blood cell count can be present as well, and persistent elevation after gastric decompression may indicate gastric ischemia and possible perforation. An elevation in lactate may be present and could point toward the presence of gastric ischemia.

Radiographic finding in the acute settings may show a classic large, spherical air-filled density in the chest with an air-fluid level present on plain film; see Fig. 35.1. If acute gastric volvulus is suspected, computer tomography (CT) scan should be obtained to evaluate the stomach in relation to surrounding structures in three dimensions. CT scan in an acute gastric volvulus can show a dilated stomach positioned in the chest. It may also demonstrate the esophagus and stomach rotating around one another, a swirl sign, best seen in the transverse plane. CT scan can also be used to detect other pathology occurring such as free air, free fluid, other anatomic abnormalities, diaphragmatic defects, and pneumatosis of the stomach. Finally, CT scan can also aid in ruling out other pathologic causes as the source. See Fig. 35.2a, b demonstrating CT findings of a patients with incarcerated paraesophageal hernias.

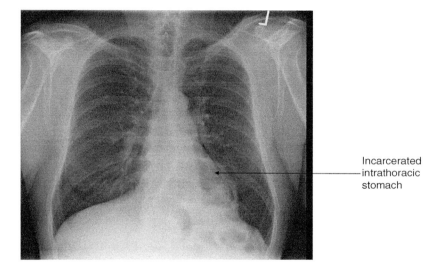

Fig. 35.1 PA chest X-ray demonstrating acute incarcerated paraesophageal hernia

Incarcerated intrathoracic stomach

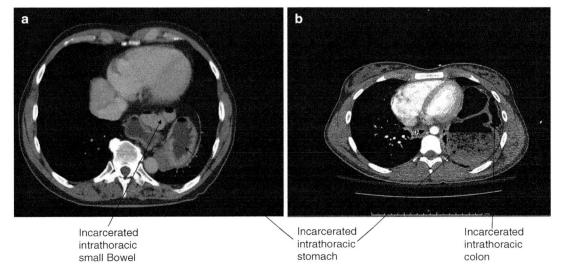

Incarcerated intrathoracic small Bowel

Incarcerated intrathoracic stomach

Incarcerated intrathoracic colon

Fig. 35.2 (**a**) Type IV paraesophageal hernia with intrathoracic stomach and small bowel and (**b**) the stomach and colon

Fig. 35.3 Contrast esophogram demonstrating chronic hiatal hernia with portion of intrathoracic stomach as well as intra-abdominal

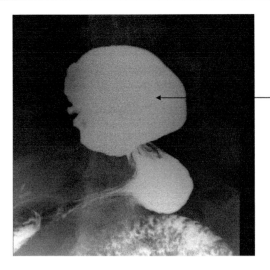

Incarcerated intrathoracic stomach

Radiographs in the chronic setting of gastric volvulus often demonstrate abnormal positioning of the stomach in the chest. Additional contrast-enhanced imaging (upper gastrointestinal series) and endoscopy are often used to confirm the diagnosis. See Fig. 35.3 demonstrating incarcerated paraesophageal hernia with intrathoracic and intra-abdominal stomach.

Management

Asymptomatic type I hiatal hernias do not require surgical intervention. Medical management of GERD is the mainstay of therapy. The role of surgery in the management of GERD is reserved for failure of medical therapy, intractable symptoms, and progression of disease.

The prophylactic correction of asymptomatic paraesophageal hernias remains controversial as the annual risk of developing acute symptoms requiring emergent surgery is less than 2% [5]. This risk decreases exponentially after 65 years, and the mortality rate from elective paraesophageal hernia repair is approximately 1.4% [5]. Elective repair, however, is required in patients with a paraesophageal hernia and subacute symptoms, such as GERD refractory to medical therapy, dysphagia, postprandial pain, early satiety, and anemia.

Options for repair include surgical approaches transabdominally or transthoracically often uti-

lizing laparoscopic or video-assisted techniques, alone or in combination. The optimal operative approach remains controversial and varies by surgeon preference and experience. Laparoscopic repair of PEH is associated with overall low morbidity and mortality (30 day 1.7% and 0.8%, respectively) and an estimated 10% recurrence rate [7, 8]. Regardless of approach, the principles of surgical repair of PEH remain the same and vary by incision of choice, body cavity approach, and order in which they are performed. However, they include the following:

- Dissection of the hiatus, removal of hernia sac, and reduction and derotation of the stomach.
- Esophageal mobilization with at least 3–4 cm intra-abdominal length (the use of Collis gastroplasty to gain additional esophageal length).
- Closure of hiatal defect with primary suture repair and selective use of mesh (biologic or permanent) which has been shown to be effective in reducing recurrences.
- Fundoplication, most often Nissen-type, benefits patients who have preexisting GERD.
- Anterior gastropexy with suture or gastrostomy tube can be used to reduce the risk of recurrence.

Surgical repair is required in patients with symptoms resulting from paraesophageal hernias. *Emergent repair is required* in patients with gastric volvulus, uncontrolled bleeding, strangulation, perforation, obstruction, or respiratory compromise that results from a paraesophageal hernia. Paraesophageal hernias that present as an emergency are associated with a high mortality.

Preoperative Considerations and Resuscitation

Light et al. present a useful and comprehensive management algorithm for acute gastric volvulus in *surgical* endoscopy in 2016 [4]. Once the diagnosis is confirmed, initial management should focus on stabilization and resuscitation. Fluid resuscitation with isotonic crystalloid and/or blood therapy (if bleeding/anemic) should be started along with correction of any electrolyte derangement. The addition of broad spectrum antibiotics early on after the diagnosis is made or strongly suspected is important as well. Concomitantly, immediate gastric decompression should be performed with placement of a nasogastric tube. Decompression of the stomach will provide symptomatic alleviation and can sometimes result in spontaneous reduction of the volvulus. Gastric decompression improves perfusion to the gastric wall which allows for further medical optimization as the need to emergently go to the operating room is abated.

If an NG tube cannot be passed, endoscopic assistance can be performed for decompression. If endoscopic assistance is needed, this is best preformed in patients in which an airway has been secured via endotracheal tube intubation. Minimal insufflation should be used during the endoscopy. Once the esophagoscope is successfully in the stomach, gastric contents can be suctioned to provide decompression, and an NG tube can then be placed.

Once a successful NG tube is placed and gastric decompression is obtained, repeat abdominal radiographic imagining should be obtained to confirm placement of the tube and decompression of the stomach. Once confirmed, the NG tube should remain in the stomach to prevent reaccumulation of fluid and repeated distention of

the stomach. If gastric decompression cannot be obtained via nasogastric tube placement or endoscopy, immediate surgical decompression should be performed.

Endoscopic Therapy

Endoscopic derotation is often used as first-line therapy to manage patients with idiopathic or primary gastric volvulus and in patients who are poor surgical candidates with secondary (paraesophageal hernia-related) gastric volvulus [4]. The placement of a percutaneous endoscopic gastrostomy (PEG) tube aids in fixing the stomach to its normal position. The addition of a second PEG tube may prevent future rotation of the stomach. One PEG is placed into the gastric body; the other is placed more distal in the stomach.

Surgical Therapy

Surgical repair of secondary gastric volvulus, most commonly the result of paraesophageal hernia, consists of reducing and derotating the stomach, removal of nonviable gastric tissue, repair of anatomic defects, and gastric fixation. Open or laparoscopic surgical techniques can be used, and the approach largely depends on the preference and experience of the surgeon. Traditionally, acute gastric volvulus is managed via an open surgical approach; however, observational studies suggest that a laparoscopic approach may be preferred to open surgery because of the advantages of shorter hospital stay and reduced perioperative morbidity [9].

Via an upper midline laparotomy, the stomach is reduced from the hernia sac. This is typically accomplished initially by gentle downward traction of the stomach starting anteriorly. Lysis of adhesions between the stomach/omentum and the hernia sac is often necessary prior to delivery of the stomach into the abdomen where it can be manually derotated.

Obvious ischemic areas of the stomach necessitate gastric resection in the form of partial or rarely subtotal gastrectomy. Consideration should be given to a second-look operation to see if the appearance of the stomach improves over 12–36 h. Repair of an associated anatomic defect, such as a paraesophageal hernia, is often necessary to reduce the risk of recurrence.

After the stomach is reduced and derotated, the hernia sac needs to be completely excised. The distal esophagus is mobilized, and an antireflux procedure is often performed. Closure of the defect, with or without mesh, is performed.

Gastric fixation is accomplished in one of two ways. Simple direct suturing of the anterior stomach to the abdominal wall or placement of gastrostomy tube effectively tethers the anterior wall of the stomach to the posterior aspect of the abdominal wall. Gastric fixation via PEG tube placement, while routinely performed along with endoscopic derotation, is not required following repair of anatomic diaphragm defects.

For the patient with severe metabolic derangements who might not be suited for definitive repair, a staged approach is another option. The priority is control of sepsis which includes at least a few of the initial principles of surgical management: reduction of the hernia contents, derotation of the volvulized stomach and other organs, and resection of nonviable tissue. Once this has been accomplished, determination if the patient can tolerate definitive repair must be made. Alternatively, leaving the patient in temporary discontinuity with NG decompression in place, abdominal packing on raw surface and temporary abdominal closure devices is a useful alternative. After this abbreviated "damage control" operation in which the source of sepsis has been controlled, the patient can be taken to the ICU for hemodynamic and metabolic optimization as well as the recruitment of consultants for definitive repair if needed [10].

Postoperative Management

Patients should be admitted postoperatively to an appropriate level of care for their clinical condition. Scheduled antiemetics can be administered to help prevent postoperative nausea and vomiting [11]. A nasogastric tube can also be left in place postoperatively to provide gastric decompression and help prevent postoperative nausea and vomiting.

In 24–48 h, a barium swallow study should be obtained to evaluate the hernia repair, determine the presence of an esophageal leak, and assess gastric emptying. If the barium swallow is negative, a clear liquid diet can be started and advanced to a low-residue diet as tolerated. Those undergoing a laparoscopic repair can typically be discharged on postoperative day 2 [9]. If an open repair is preformed, return of bowel function should occur prior to discharging the patient.

Recurrence

While recurrence of unrepaired gastric volvulus is common, there are few data that report on recurrence following repair. Recurrence of surgically corrected gastric volvulus indicates failure of anatomic repair or inadequate fixation of the stomach to the abdominal wall.

Summary

Although type I hiatal hernias are more common, they rarely result in a surgical emergency. Paraesophageal hernias occur less frequently; however, they can present with devastating complications. A quick and accurate diagnosis of strangulated paraesophageal hernia/gastric volvulus is crucial to providing appropriate, timely therapy.

If strangulation or volvulus is present or there are symptoms of obstruction, bleeding, perforation, or respiratory distress, emergent operative intervention is indicated. Appropriate fluid and blood component resuscitation with attention to electrolyte derangements, broad-spectrum antibiotics, NG decompression, and urgent surgical repair should be undertaken immediately.

Whether proceeding in an open or laparoscopic manner, the core principles of operative repair of a paraesophageal hernia remain the same:

- Dissection around the hiatus and complete reduction of the hernia sac (and stomach derotation if volvulus is present)
- Dissection of the intrathoracic esophagus until adequate (3–4 cm) intra-abdominal length is obtained
- Hiatal defect repair
- Antireflux and gastric fixation procedure

If transfer to a tertiary care center with a high-volume foregut practice is not possible, then, keeping in mind these principles, one should proceed with a safe operation that has as its primary aim to achieve source control of sepsis by reducing the hernia, detorsing the volvulized stomach, and resecting necrotic tissue.

Gastric volvulus and strangulated paraesophageal hernia represent a surgical emergency and should be treated as such. Once diagnosed, quick action and appropriate operative intervention can prevent a potential catastrophic condition.

References

1. Dean C, Etienne D, Carpentier B, et al. Hiatal hernias. Surg Radiol Anat. 2012;34:291–9.
2. Schieman C, Grondin SC. Paraesophageal hernia: clinical presentation, evaluation, and management controversies. Thorac Surg Clin. 2009;19:473–84.
3. Stylopoulos N, Rattner DW. The history of hiatal hernia surgery: from Bowditch to laparoscopy. Ann Surg. 2005;241:185.
4. Light D, Links D, Griffin M. The threatened stomach: management of the acute gastric volvulus. Surg Endosc. 2016;30:1847–52.
5. Stylopoulos N, Gazelle GS, Rattner DW. Paraesophageal hernias: operation or observation? Ann Surg. 2002;236:492.
6. Bawahab M, Mitchell P, Church N, et al. Management of acute paraesophageal hernia. Surg Endosc. 2009;23:255–9.
7. Luketich JD, Nason KS, Christie NA, et al. Outcomes after a decade of laparoscopic giant paraesophageal hernia repair. J Thorac Cardiovasc Surg. 2010;139:395–404. 404.e391
8. Rathore MA, Andrabi SI, Bhatti MI, et al. Metaanalysis of recurrence after laparoscopic repair of paraesophageal hernia. JSLS. 2007;11:456–60.
9. Yates RB, Hinojosa MW, Wright AS, et al. Laparoscopic gastropexy relieves symptoms of obstructed gastric volvulus in highoperative risk patients. Am J Surg. 2015;209:875–80.
10. Stawicki SP, Brooks A, Bilski T, et al. The concept of damage control: extending the paradigm to emergency general surgery. Injury. 2008;39:93–101.
11. Puri V, Kakarlapudi GV, Awad ZT, et al. Hiatal hernia recurrence: 2004. Hernia. 2004;8:311–7.

Extremity Compartment Syndrome

36

Col (Ret) Mark W. Bowyer

Pathophysiology/Epidemiology

CS has been found wherever a compartment is present: the hand, forearm, upper arm, abdomen, buttock, and entire lower extremity. The pathophysiology of CS is relatively straightforward. Groups of muscles and their associated nerves and vessels are surrounded by thick fascial layers that define the various compartments of the extremities which are of relatively fixed volume. Compartment syndrome occurs either when compartment size is restricted or compartment volume is increased. Several conditions have been implicated in causing CS [1–32] and are detailed in Table 36.1.

As the pressure within the compartment (from blood, fluid, or external pressure) increases, the tissue perfusion decreases, and cellular metabolism is impaired, leading to cellular death. If this pressure is not relieved in a timely fashion (reported to be 4–6 h but may be less (as little as an hour) in a patient with shock), irreversible damage will occur. Polytrauma patients with hypotension can sustain irreversible injury at lower compartment pressures than patients with normal blood pressures, and a very high index of suspicion should be maintained in this group.

The leg (calf) is the area that is most commonly affected accounting for 68% in a large civilian series (Branco), followed by the forearm (14%), and the thigh (9%) [33]. In a review of 294 combat injured soldiers undergoing 494 fas-

Table 36.1 Factors implicated with the development of acute limb compartment syndrome [1–32]

Restriction of compartment size	Increased compartment volume
	From hemorrhage:
	Fractures
Casts	Vascular injury
Splints	Drugs (anticoagulants)
Burn eschar	Hemophilia; sickle cell
Tourniquets	*From muscle edema/ swelling*:
Tight dressings	Crush – Trauma, drugs, or alcohol
Fracture reduction	Rhabdomyolysis/blast injury
Closure of fascial defects	Sepsis
Incomplete skin release	Exercise induced
Military antishock trousers	Envenomation or bee sting
Prolonged extrication trapped limb	Massive resuscitation
Localized external pressure	Intra-compartmental fluid infusion
Long leg brace	Phlegmasia cerulea dolens
Automated BP monitoring	Electrical burns
Malpositioning on OR table	Reperfusion injury
	Postpartum eclampsia

C. M. W. Bowyer
Uniformed Services University of the Health
Sciences, Bethesda, MD, USA
e-mail: mark.bowyer@usuhs.edu

© Springer International Publishing AG, part of Springer Nature 2019
C. V. R. Brown et al. (eds.), *Emergency General Surgery*, https://doi.org/10.1007/978-3-319-96286-3_36

ciotomies, Ritenour et al. reported the calf as the most common site (51%) followed by the forearm (22.3%), thigh (8.3%), upper arm (7.3%), hand (5.7%), and foot (4.8%) [34].

Certain injury patterns have been associated with higher likelihood of needing fasciotomy. Blick et al. found a close association between grade of fracture, degree of comminution, and risk of development of CS in a retrospective review of 198 open tibia fractures [35]. Abouezzi et al. found a 28% incidence of fasciotomy in patients with peripheral vascular injuries treated at a Level I trauma center. They determined that injury to popliteal vessels was more likely (62% cases) to result in fasciotomy than above the knee vascular injury (19% cases) [36]. This finding was echoed by Gonzalez et al. [37] who reported that CS of the lower extremity was more likely to be associated with penetrating injuries below the knee (94%) than above the knee. Another study evaluated femoral vascular injuries in particular and found that the rates of fasciotomy depended on whether there was isolated arterial (13% fasciotomy) or venous injury (3% fasciotomy), or a combination (38% fasciotomy) [38].

Branco et al. [33] found that incidence of fasciotomy varied widely by mechanism of injury (0.9% after motor vehicle collision to 8.6% after a gunshot wound). Additionally the need for fasciotomy was related to the type of injury ranging from 2.2% incidence for patients with closed fractures up to 41.8% in patients with combined venous and arterial injuries. The study by Branco identified ten risk factors associated with the need for fasciotomy after extremity trauma: Young males, with penetrating or multi-system trauma, requiring blood transfusion, with open fractures, elbow or knee dislocations, or vascular injury (arterial, venous, or combined) are at the highest risk of requiring a fasciotomy after extremity trauma [33].

Diagnosis

The diagnosis of compartment syndrome is a clinical diagnosis. The classically described five "Ps" – *pain*, pallor, paresthesias, paralysis, and

pulselessness – are pathognomonic of compartment syndrome. However, *these are usually late signs, and extensive and irreversible injuries may have taken place by the time they are manifested.* The most important symptom of CS is *pain greater than expected due to the injury alone.* Remember that the loss of pulse is a late finding, and the presence of pulses does not rule out CS! *The presence of open wounds does* not *exclude CS.* In fact, the worst open fractures are actually more likely to have a CS.

In actual practice, tissue pressure (compartment pressure) measurements have a limited role in making the diagnosis of CS. However, in polytrauma patients associated with head injury, drug and alcohol intoxication, intubation, spinal injuries, use of paralyzing drugs, extremes of age, unconsciousness, or low diastolic pressures, measuring compartment pressures may be of use in determining the need for fasciotomy. The pressure threshold for making the diagnosis of CS is controversial. A number of authors recommend 30 mm Hg [39, 40], and others cite pressures as high as 45 mm Hg [41]. Ouellete [42] recommended that an ICP of 15–25 should be used in patients with clinical signs and greater than 25 for those without. Many surgeons use the "Delta-P" system. The compartment pressure is subtracted from the patient's diastolic blood pressure to obtain the Delta-P with muscle was at risk when the ICP was within 10–30 mmHg of the diastolic pressure [43]. If the Delta-P is less than 30, the surgeon should be concerned that a CS may be present. Other factors to consider when considering fasciotomy are length of time of transport to definitive care and ability to do serial exams.

Compartment syndrome is a first and foremost a clinical diagnosis, and a patient manifesting with signs and symptoms of a CS should be operated on expeditiously. In patients with polytrauma, CS should be a diagnosis of exclusion, and one should have a low threshold for performing fasciotomy especially in patients with vascular trauma. The safest approach is to err on the side of early and aggressive intervention, and if one thinks of about doing a fasciotomy, it should be done. The reliance on clinical examination with a low threshold for fascial release may result in unwarranted fasciotomies, but it avoids the grave consequences of a missed diagnosis.

Treatment of Compartment Syndrome

The definitive treatment of compartment syndrome is *early and aggressive fasciotomy*. In patients with vascular injury who require fasciotomy in conjunction with a vascular repair, it makes great sense to perform the fasciotomy *before* doing the repair. The rationale for this is that the ischemic compartment is likely to already be tight and thus will create inflow resistance to your vascular repair, making it susceptible to early thrombosis. The remainder of this chapter will detail the relevant anatomy, landmarks, step-by-step surgical techniques, and pitfalls associated with fasciotomy of the extremities most commonly affected by CS.

Lower Leg Fasciotomy

The lower leg (calf) is the most common site for CS requiring fasciotomy. The leg has four major tissue compartments bounded by investing muscle fascia (see Fig. 36.1).

It is important to understand the anatomical arrangement of these compartments as well as some key structures within each compartment in order to perform a proper four-compartment fas-

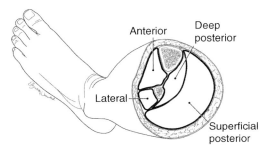

Fig. 36.1 The cross-sectional anatomy of the midportion of the left lower leg depicting the four compartments that must be released when performing a lower leg fasciotomy

ciotomy. It is not necessary to remember the names of all the muscles in each compartment, but it is useful to remember that the anterior compartment contains the anterior tibial artery and vein and the common peroneal nerve (recently renamed the common fibular nerve), the lateral compartment the superficial peroneal (recently renamed the superior fibular) nerve (which must not be injured), the superficial posterior compartment the soleus and gastrocnemius muscles, and the deep posterior compartment the posterior tibial and peroneal vessels and the tibial nerve.

When dealing with a traumatically injured extremity, there is absolutely no role for getting fancy. The use of a single incision for four-compartment fasciotomy of the lower extremity is mentioned to condemn it. Attempts to make cosmetic incisions should also be condemned, and the mantra should be "bigger is better." Compartment syndrome of the lower extremity dictates *two-incision four-compartment fasciotomy* with *generous* skin incisions [29, 44].

There are several key features that will enable a successful two-incision four-compartment fasciotomy. One of the key steps is proper placement of the incisions. As extremities needing fasciotomy are often grossly swollen or deformed, marking the key landmarks will aid in placement of the incisions. It is useful to mark the patella and the tibial tuberosity as well as the tibial spine which serves as a reliable midpoint between the incisions. The lateral malleolus and fibular head are the landmarks used to identify the course of the fibula on the lateral portion of the leg (Fig. 36.2). The lateral incision is marked just anterior (~1 fingerbreadth) to the line of the fibula or *a finger in front of the fibula*. It is important to stay anterior to the fibula as this minimizes the chance of damaging the superficial peroneal (superior fibular) nerve and helps to correctly identify the intermuscular septum between the anterior and lateral compartments.

The medial incision is made one thumb breadth below the palpable medial edge of the tibia or *a thumb below the tibia* (Fig. 36.3). The extent of the skin incision should be to a point approximately three fingerbreadths below the tibial tuberosity and above the malleolus on

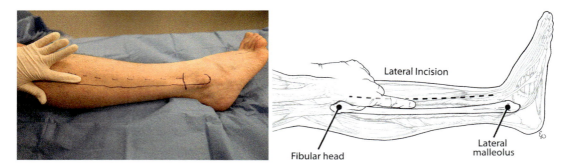

Fig. 36.2 The fibular head and lateral malleolus (on the right lower leg) are used as reference points to mark the edge of the fibula, and the lateral incision (*dotted line*) is marked one finger in front of this (*a finger in front of the fibula*)

either side. It is very important to mark the incisions on both sides prior to opening them, as the landmarks of the swollen extremity will become rapidly distorted once the incisions are made.

The Lateral Incision of the Lower Leg

The lateral incision (Fig. 36.2) is made *one finger in front of the fibula* and should in general extend from three fingerbreadths below the head of the fibula down to three fingerbreadths above the lateral malleolus. The exact length of the skin incision will depend on the clinical setting. Care must be taken to make sure that it is long enough so that the skin does not serve as a constricting band. The skin and subcutaneous tissue are incised to expose the fascia encasing the lateral and anterior compartments. Care should be taken to avoid the lesser saphenous vein and peroneal (fibular) nerve when making these skin incisions.

Once the skin flap is raised, the intermuscular septum is identified. This is the structure that divides the anterior and lateral compartments. In the swollen or injured extremity, it may be difficult to find the intermuscular septum. In this setting the septum can be identified by following the perforating vessels down to it (Fig. 36.4).

Classically the fascia of the lateral lower leg is opened using an "H"-shaped incision. The crosspiece of the "H" is made using a scalpel which will expose both compartments and the septum. The legs of the "H" are made with curved scissors at least 1 cm away from the septum using just the tips which are *turned away* from the

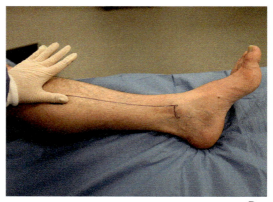

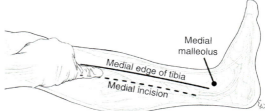

Fig. 36.3 The medial incision (*dotted line*) is marked (on the medial left lower extremity) one thumb breadth below the palpable medial edge of the tibia (*solid line*). *A thumb behind the tibia*

septum to avoid injury to the peroneal (fibular) nerves (Figs. 36.5 and 36.6). The superficial peroneal (superior fibular) nerve originates around the head of the fibula and descends to the foot within the lateral compartment becoming superficial two thirds to three fourths of the way down the leg and then crosses over to the anterior compartment (Fig. 36.6). Care must be taken to avoid injury to this nerve as the fascial incisions approach the ankle. The fascia should be opened by pushing the partially opened scissor tips in

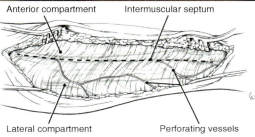

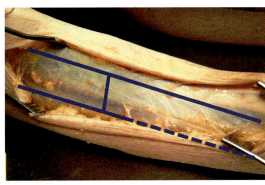

Fig. 36.4 The lateral incision on a right lower extremity demonstrates the intermuscular septum (dotted line), which separates the anterior and lateral compartments of the lower leg. Note one of the perforating vessels (arrow) which enters and helps to identify the septum

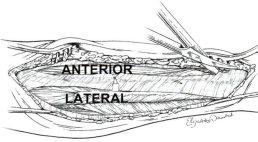

Fig. 36.5 The fascia of the right lateral lower leg (foot to the right) is opened in a classic "H"-shaped fashion for the length of the compartments with scissors turned away from the septum to avoid damage to underlying structures as seen on the right

both directions on either side of, and at least 1 cm away from, the septum, opening the fascia from the head of the fibula down to the lateral malleolus. Inspection of the septum and identification of the common peroneal (fibular) nerve and/or the anterior tibial vessels confirms entry into the anterior compartment. The skin incision should be closely inspected and extended as needed to ensure that the ends do not serve as a point of constriction.

Pitfalls of the Lower Leg Lateral Incision

The anterior compartment is the most commonly missed compartment when performing a fasciotomy of the lower extremity [34]. The most common reason the anterior compartment is missed is due to the incision being made too far posteriorly, either over or behind the fibula. If the incision is made too far posteriorly, the intermuscular septum between the lateral and superficial compartments is mistaken for the septum between the anterior and lateral compartments, and the anterior compartment is not opened (Figs. 36.7 and 36.8).

The Medial Incision of the Lower Leg

The medial incision (Fig. 36.3) is made one fingerbreadth below the palpable medial edge of the tibia (*one thumb behind the tibia*). When making this incision, it is important to identify and preserve the greater saphenous vein, as well as ligate any perforators to it. After making an incision through the skin and subcutaneous tissues, the fascia overlying the superficial posterior compartment is exposed. This compartment contains the soleus and gastrocnemius muscle. Opening this fascia from the tibial tuberosity to the medial malleolus effectively decompresses the superficial posterior compartment (Fig. 36.9).

The key to entering the deep posterior compartment is the soleus muscle. The soleus muscle attaches to the medial edge of the tibia, and dissecting these fibers (referred to by some as the

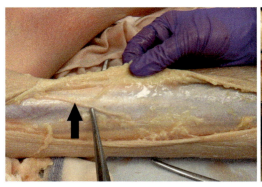

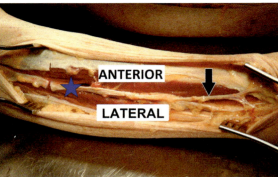

Fig. 36.6 The superficial peroneal (fibular) nerve (arrows) runs in the lateral compartment from the knee and crosses over the septum (star) into the anterior compartment 2/3–3/4 of the way down the leg toward the ankle. This must be carefully avoided by keeping the scissor tips pointed away from the septum and looking for the nerve as the fasciotomy is extended to the lateral malleolus. The left lateral lower leg is seen on the left, and the right lateral lower leg is seen on the right

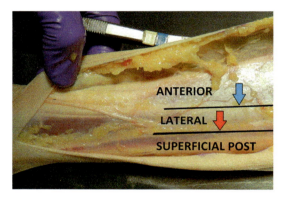

Fig. 36.7 There is an intermuscular septum (red arrow) between the lateral and superficial posterior (post) compartments which can be mistaken for the septum between the anterior and lateral compartments (blue arrow) if the incision is made too far posteriorly

soleus bridge) completely free from and exposing the underside of the tibia ensures entry into the deep posterior compartment (Fig. 36.10). Identification of the posterior tibial neurovascular bundle confirms that the compartment has been entered (Fig. 36.11). The muscle in each compartment should be assessed for viability. Viable muscle is pink, contracts when stimulated, and bleeds when cut. Dead muscle should be debrided back to healthy viable tissue. The skin incision is left open and either covered with gauze or a vacuum-assisted wound closure device which have been shown in recent studies to speed up and improve the chances definitive closure of these wounds.

Pitfalls of the Medial Incision

The deep posterior compartment (DPC) is the second most commonly missed compartment when performing a fasciotomy of the lower extremity [34]. The most common reason the DPC is missed is due to a dissection plane made between the gastrocnemius and soleus muscles and believing that opening the fascia over the soleus muscle equates to having opened the deep posterior compartment (Fig. 36.12).

In the injured extremity, a prominent plantaris tendon (also known as the "intern's nerve") may be mistaken for the posterior tibial neurovascular bundle leading one to erroneously believe that the posterior compartment has been entered and decompressed (Fig. 36.13).

Inadvertent injury to the saphenous vein can cause significant bleeding and may result in venous insufficiency if the deep venous system has also been injured.

Inadequate length of either the fascial or skin incision(s) can result in failure to reduce compartment pressures to acceptable levels.

Compartment Syndrome of the Thigh

Compartment syndrome is uncommon in the thigh because of the large volume that the thigh requires to cause an increase in interstitial

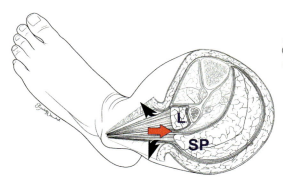
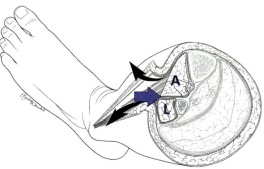

Fig. 36.8 If the lateral incision is made too posteriorly, the intermuscular septum (red arrow) between the lateral (L) and superficial posterior (SP) compartments can be mistaken for the septum (blue arrow) between the anterior (A) and lateral (L) compartments with the anterior compartment missed

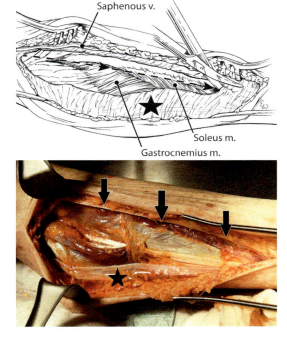

Fig. 36.9 The medial incision as seen on the left lower leg is placed such that the saphenous vein can be identified and preserved, and the fascia (star) is opened to expose the soleus and gastrocnemius muscles in the superficial posterior compartment. The superficial posterior compartment is exposed by opening the superficial fascia (star) below the edge of the tibia (arrows)

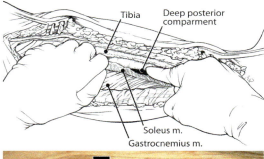
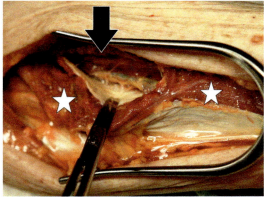

Fig. 36.10 On the left medial lower leg, the soleus muscle (stars) is dissected off of the inferior border of the tibia (arrow) allowing entry into the deep posterior compartment

pressure. In addition, the compartments of the thigh blend anatomically with the hip allowing for extravasation of blood or fluid outside the compartment. Major risk factors for thigh compartment syndrome include severe femoral fractures, vascular injury, severe blunt trauma/crush or blast injury to the thigh, iliofemoral deep vein thrombosis, and external compression of the thigh [45–49]. The thigh contains three compartments: anterior, posterior, and medial (Fig. 36.14). The anterior (not the medial) compartment contains the femoral artery and vein and is the most likely to develop a compartment syndrome.

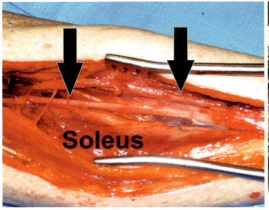 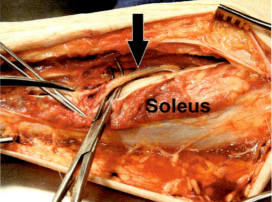

Fig. 36.11 Identification of the posterior tibial neurovascular structures (arrows) confirms entry into the deep posterior compartment after taking the soleus muscle down from the tibia as seen on the left (picture to left) and right (picture to right) medial lower leg

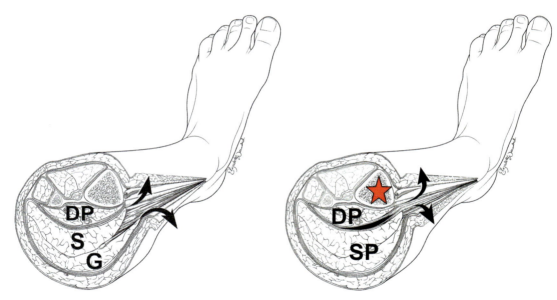

Fig. 36.12 If the dissection plane is made between the soleus (S) and gastrocnemius (G) muscles, the deep posterior (DP) compartment has not been opened, and the soleus fibers must be taken down from the underside of the tibia (star) to separate the superficial posterior (SP) from the deep posterior compartment such that it can be opened

If compartment syndrome of the thigh exists, a lateral incision is made first as this enables decompression of both the anterior and posterior compartments (Fig. 36.15). Often, the lateral incision is all that is needed, though on occasion with a severely swollen extremity a medial incision will be needed as well (Fig. 36.15). The lateral incision of the thigh extends from the intertrochanteric line to the lateral epicondyle of the femur to expose the iliotibial band or fascia latae which is opened the length of the incision. The vastus lateralis muscle is reflected superiorly and medially to expose the lateral intermuscular septum (between the anterior and posterior compartments) which incised the length of the incision. Commonly after the anterior and posterior compartments are decompressed, the pressure in the medial compartment is measured, and if elevated, this compartment is also decompressed through the medial incision.

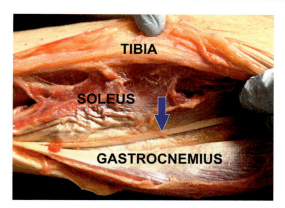

Fig. 36.13 The plantaris tendon (arrow) is found in the plane between the soleus and gastrocnemius muscles and may be mistaken for the posterior tibia neurovascular bundle. In order to enter and decompress the deep posterior compartment, the soleus muscle must be taken down from the underside of the tibia

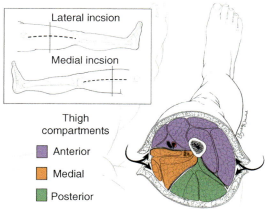

Fig. 36.15 The two incisions required to decompress the compartments of the thigh are depicted with the anterior (purple) and posterior (green) compartments opened via the lateral incision and if indicated the medial (orange) compartment opened through the medial incision

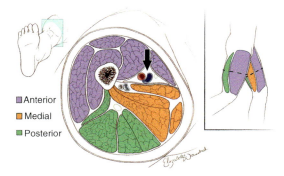

Fig. 36.14 This cross section of the mid right thigh shows the three compartments of the thigh: anterior (purple), medial (orange), and posterior (green). Note that the femoral artery and vein (arrow) are found in the anterior compartment

If needed, the medial compartment can be opened through a medial incision (Fig. 36.15) placed along the course of the saphenous vein. This is followed by rotation of the sartorius muscle and incision of the medial intermuscular septum between the medial and anterior compartments.

Compartment Syndrome of the Forearm and Hand

Compartment syndromes of the hand and forearm are much less common than in the lower extremity, but it is vital that it be recognized and

treated should it occur. Compartment syndrome of the upper arm is very unusual but may follow supracondylar fracture of the humerus. Compartment syndrome of the forearm may be associated with fractures, crush or blast injury, burns, or vascular injury [50–55]. CS of the hand can occur from trauma but is more commonly associated with infiltration of intravenous fluids [56–58]. As there are no sensory nerves in the hand compartments, physical findings do not include sensory abnormalities, and the pressure threshold for release is much less than in the legs (15–20 mmHg).

The forearm is classically described as having three compartments: volar (anterior), mobile wad, and dorsal (posterior). Some anatomy texts and practitioners subdivide the volar into superficial and deep compartments. The literature contains descriptions of multiple approaches to the volar incision [51–55]. The most commonly used and described volar fasciotomy incision of the forearm is a curvilinear incision (to release the anterior and mobile wad compartments) which is extended to the hand to release the carpal tunnel (Fig. 36.16). The incision crosses the antecubital fossa in a curvilinear fashion to the radial aspect of the upper forearm and then is carried toward the ulnar aspect down to the wrist and then across the wrist in a transverse fashion and onto the

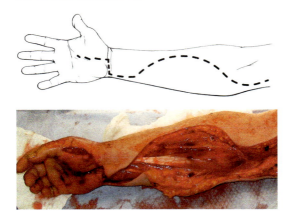

Fig. 36.16 The volar incision as seen on the right arm enabling decompression of the anterior (volar) and mobile wad compartments

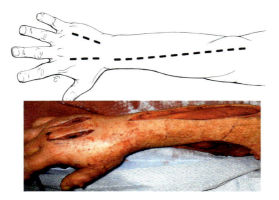

Fig. 36.17 The dorsal incision as seen on the right arm with additional incisions on the hand enabling decompression of the dorsal compartment of the forearm and the intraosseous compartments of the hand

palm to release the carpal tunnel. This volar incision allows for decompression of the volar (anterior) and mobile wad compartments as well as the carpal tunnel. This incision is preferred because of potentially better cosmetic results and maintenance of an adequate skin blood supply between it and the dorsal (Fig. 36.17) incision at the wrist.

The dorsal (posterior) compartment of the forearm is released through a linear dorsal incision, with two additional incisions on the dorsum of the hand to release the hand (Fig. 36.17). To

ensure that the compartments of the forearm are completely decompressed, it is important to do a complete episiotomy (opening the fascia overlying the muscle) of each of the muscles exposing the muscle bellies in the entire length of the forearm.

In most cases of suspected compartment syndrome of the forearm, the carpal tunnel should be opened completely at the wrist. This is accomplished by identifying the median nerve at the wrist crease and using scissors passed on either side of the transverse carpal ligament above the median nerve and divided (Fig. 36.18). The transverse carpal ligament is generally wider than one might expect (>2 cm), and there is a haptic and audible crunch that accompanies its division. If one "cuts until the crunch is gone," the carpal tunnel is fully opened. If CS of the hand is suspected, it is best to involve a hand specialist early as often additional incisions will be required to decompress the thenar and hypothenar compartments [56–58].

Aftercare and Complications

If necrotic muscle is present, it should be debrided at the time of original fasciotomy which as described above will create large wounds that must be covered. The open wounds should be covered with non-adherent dressing or moist gauze. Wound closure can be accomplished with the assistance of traction such as the "shoelace technique" or vacuum-assisted devices [59–62]. The wounds should be reevaluated 24–48 h after the initial fasciotomy with further debridement as indicated. After the acute process subsides, delayed primary closure or split-thickness skin grafting may be performed. Patients with open fasciotomy wounds are at risk for infection, and incomplete or delayed fasciotomies can lead to permanent nerve damage, loss of limb, multisystem organ failure, rhabdomyolysis, and death. Early recognition and aggressive fasciotomy will help to minimize these adverse outcomes.

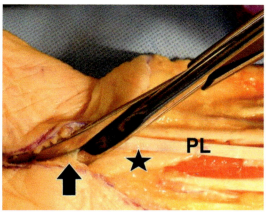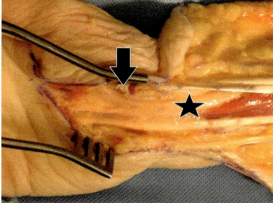

Fig. 36.18 The median nerve (star) is identified at the wrist crease running under the palmaris longus (PL) tendon. Scissors are placed above and below the transverse carpal ligament (arrow) which is divided to completely open the carpal tunnel

Conclusions

Compartment syndrome must be suspected in all polytrauma patients with extremity injury. Additionally, patients in the intensive care unit are also at risk to develop compartment syndrome from a variety of non-traumatic conditions, principally sepsis, massive resuscitation, and reperfusion. It is essential that all clinicians caring for these patients have an intimate knowledge of the pathophysiology, etiology, and evaluation of CS. Additionally, all surgeons need to have a comprehensive knowledge of the relevant anatomy and the techniques for performing a proper fasciotomy. A high index of suspicion must be maintained (especially in patients with altered levels of consciousness), and early and aggressive fasciotomy will minimize the morbidity and mortality associated with failure to adequately treat compartment syndromes.

Acknowledgment The author is grateful to Ms. Elizabeth Weissbrod, MA, CMI, for her expert illustrations contained in this manuscript.

References

1. McGee DL, Dalsey WC. Compartment syndrome and amputations. Emerg Med Clin North Am. 1992;10:783–800.
2. Matsen FA. Compartment syndrome: a unified concept. Clin Orthop. 1975;113:8–14.
3. Schreiber SN, Liebowitz MR, Berstein LH. Limb compression and renal impairment (crush syndrome) following narcotic overdose. J Bone Joint Surg. 1972;54A:1683.
4. Bowden REM, Gutman E. The fate of voluntary muscle after vascular injury in man. J Bone Joint Surg. 1949;31B:356–8.
5. Ashton H. Effect of inflatable plastic splints on blood flow. Br Med J. 1966;2:1427–30.
6. Kirby NG. Exercise ischemia in the fascial compartment of the soleus. J Bone Joint Surg. 1970;52B:738–40.
7. Cywes S, Louw JH. Phlegmasia cerulean dolens: successful treatment by relieving fasciotomy. Surgery. 1962;51:169–76.
8. Manson JW. Post-partum eclampsia complicated by the anterior tibial syndrome. Br Med J. 1964;2:1117–8.
9. Owen R, Tsimboukis B. Ischaemia complicating closed tibial and fibular shaft fractures. J Bone Joint Surg. 1967;49:268–75.

10. Sweeney HE, O'Brien GF. Bilateral anterior tibial syndrome in association with the nephrotic syndrome; report of a case. Arch Intern Med. 1965;116:487–90.

11. Weitz EM, Carson G. The anterior tibial compartment syndrome in a twenty month old infant: a complication of the use of a bow leg brace. Bull Hosp Joint Dis. 1969;30:16–20.

12. Beall S, Garner J, Oxley O. Anterolateral compartment syndrome related to drug induced bleeding. Am J Sports Med. 1983;11:454–5.

13. Aerts P, DeBoeck H, Casteleyn PP, Opdecam P. Deep volar compartment syndrome of the forearm following minor crush injury. J Pediatr Orthop. 1989;9:69–71.

14. Aprahamian C, Gessert G, Bandyk OF, Sell L, Stiehl J, Olson DW. MAST associated compartment syndrome (MACS): a review. J Trauma. 1989;29:549–55.

15. Bass RR, Allison EJ, Reines HD, Yeager JC, Pryor WH Jr. Thigh compartment syndrome without lower extremity trauma following application of pneumatic antishock trouser. Ann Emerg Med. 1983;12:382–4.

16. Black KP, Schultz TK, Cheung NL. Compartment syndromes in athletes. Clin Sports Med. 1990;9:471–87.

17. Bogaerts Y, Lameire N, Ringoir S. The compartment syndrome: a serious complication of acute rhabdomyolysis. Clin Nephrol. 1982;17:206–11.

18. DeLee JC, Stiehl JB. Open tibia fracture with compartment syndrome. Clin Orthop. 1981;160:175-184.

19. Egan TO, Joyce SM. Acute compartment syndrome following a minor athletic injury. J Emerg Med. 1989;7:353–7.

20. Garfin SR, Mubarak SJ, Evans KL, Hargens AR, Akeson WH. Quantification of intracompartmental pressure and volume under plaster casts. J Bone Joint Surg. 1981;63:449–53.

21. Halpern AA, Nagel DA. Bilateral compartment syndrome associated with androgen therapy. Clin Orthop. 1977;128:243–6.

22. Hieb LD, Alexander H. Bilateral anterior and lateral compartment syndromes in a patient with sickle cell trait. J Bone Joint Surg. 1988;228:190–3.

23. Moscati R, Moore GP. Compartment syndrome with resultant amputation following interosseous infusion. Am J Emerg Med. 1990;8:470–1.

24. Peek RD, Haynes DW. Compartment syndrome as a complication of arthroscopy. Am J Sports Med. 1984;12:464–8.

25. Reedy PK, Kaye KW. Deep posterior compartmental syndrome: a serious complication of the lithotomy position. J Urol. 1984;132:144–5.

26. Royle SG. Compartment syndrome following forearm fracture in children. Injury. 1990;21:73–6.

27. Stockley I, Harvey IA, Getty CJM. Acute volar compartment syndrome of the forearm secondary to fractures of the distal radius. Injury. 1986;19:101–4.

28. Rush RJ, Arrington E, Hsu J. Management of complex extremity injuries: touriquets, compartment syndrome detection, fasciotomy, and amputation care. Surg Clin North Am. 2012;92:987–1007.

29. Bowyer MW. Compartment syndrome. In: Gahtan V, Costanza MJ, editors. Essentials of vascular surgery

for the general surgeon. New York: Springer; 2014. p. 55–69.

30. Donaldson J, Haddad B, Khan WS. The pathophysiology, diagnosis and current management of acute compartment syndrome. Open Orthop J. 2014;8:185–93.

31. Pechar J, Lyons MM. Acute compartment syndrome of the lower leg: a review. J Nurs Pract. 2016;12:265–70.

32. Schmidt AH. Acute compartment syndrome. Orthop Clin North Am. 2016;47:517–25.

33. Branco BC, Inaba K, Barmparas G, Schnüriger B, Lustenberger T, Talving P, et al. Incidence and predictors for the need for fasciotomy after extremity trauma: a 10-year review in a mature level I trauma Centre. Injury. 2011;42:1157–63.

34. Ritenour AE, Dorlac WC, Fang R, et al. Complications after fasciotomy revision and delayed compartment release in combat patients. J Trauma. 2008;64:S153–62.

35. Blick SS, Brumback RJ, Poka A, Burgess AR, Ebraheim NA. Compartment syndrome in open tibial fractures. J Bone Joint Surg Am. 1996;68:1348–53.

36. Abouezzi Z, Nassoura Z, Ivatury RR, Porter JM, Stahl WM. A critical reappraisal of indications for fasciotomy after extremity vascular trauma. Arch Surg. 1998;133:547–51.

37. Gonzalez RP, Scott W, Wright A, Phelan HA, Rodning CB. Anatomic location of penetrating lower extremity trauma predicts compartment syndrome development. Am J Surg. 2009;197:371–5.

38. Cargile JS, Hurt JL, Perdue GF. Acute trauma of the femoral artery vein. J Trauma. 1992;32:364–71.

39. Mubarak SJ, Owen CA. Double-incision fasciotomy of the leg for decompression in compartment syndromes. J Bone Joint Surg Am. 1977;59:184–7.

40. Mubarak SJ, Owen CA, Hargens AR, Garetto LP, Akeson WH. Acute compartment syndromes: diagnosis and treatment with the aid of the wick catheter. J Bone Joint Surg Br. 1978;60:1091–5.

41. Matsen FA III, Winquist RA, Krugmire RB Jr. Diagnosis and management of compartmental syndromes. J Bone Joint Surg Am. 1980;62A:286–91.

42. Ouelette EA. Compartment syndromes in obtunded patients. Hand Clin. 1998;14:431–50.

43. Whitesides TE, Haney TC, Morimoto K, Harada H. Tissue pressure measurements as a determinant for the need for fasciotomy. Clin Orthop. 1975;113:43–51.

44. Bowyer MW. Lower extremity fasciotomy: indications and technique. Curr Trauma Rep. 2015;1:35–44.

45. Ojike N, Roberts C, Giannoudis P. Compartment syndrome of the thigh: a systematic review. Injury. 2010;41:133–6.

46. Zuchelli D, Divaris N, McCormack JE, Huang EC, Chaudry ND, Vosswinkel JA, Jawa RS. Extremity compartment syndrome following blunt trauma: a level 1 trauma center's 5-year experience. J Surg Res. 2017;217:131–6.

47. Knab LM, Abuzeid A, Rodriguez H, Issa N. Thigh compartment syndrome in urban trauma: bullets to blame, not collisions. J Surg Res. 2013;185:748–52.

48. Newnham MS, Mitchell DI. Compartment syndrome of the thigh. A case report and review of the literature. West Indian Med J. 2001;50:239–42.
49. Schwartz JT, Brumback RJ, Lakatos R, et al. Acute compartment syndrome of the thigh. A spectrum of injury. J Bone Joint Surg Am. 1989;71:392–400.
50. Dente CJ, Feliciano DV, Rozycki GS, et al. A review of upper extremity fasciotomies in a level 1 trauma center. Am Surg. 2004;70:1088–93.
51. Kalyani BS, Fisher BE, Roberts CS, Giannoudis PV. Compartment syndrome of the forearm: a systematic review. J Hand Surg [Am]. 2011;36:535–43.
52. Kistler JM, Ilyas AM, Thoder JJ. Forearm compartment syndrome: evaluation and management. Hand Clin. 2018;34:53–60.
53. Friedrich JB, Shin AY. Management of forearm compartment syndrome. Hand Clin. 2007;23:245–54.
54. Prasarn ML, Ouellette EA. Acute compartment syndrome of the upper extremity. J Am Acad Orthop Surg. 2011;19:49–58.
55. Smith J, Bowyer MW. Fasciotomy of the forearm and hand. In: Demeitriades D, Inaba K, Velmahos G, editors. Atlas of surgical techniques in trauma. Cambridge: Cambridge University Press; 2015. p. 288–93.
56. Rubinstein AJ, Ahmed IH, Vosbikian MM. Hand compartment syndrome. Hand Clin. 2018;34:41–52.
57. Oak NR, Abrams RA. Compartment syndrome of the hand. Orthop Clin North Am. 2016;47:609–16.
58. Ko JH, Hanel DP. Technique of fasciotomy: hand. Tech Orthop. 2012;27:38–42.
59. Zannis J, Angobaldo J, Marks M, et al. Comparison of fasciotomy wound closures using traditional dressing changes and vacuum-assisted closure device. Ann Plast Surg. 2009;62:407–9.
60. Jauregui JJ, Yarmis SJ, Tsai J, Onuoha KO, Illical E, Paulino CB. Fasciotomy closure techniques. J Orthop Surg (Hong Kong). 2017;25(1):2309499016684724.
61. Kakagia D. How to close a lomb fasciotomy wound: an overview of current techniques. Int J Low Extrem Wounds. 2015;14:268–76.
62. Kakagia D, Karadimas EJ, Drosos G, Ververidis A, Trypsiannis G, Verettas D. Wound closure of leg fasciotomy: comparison of vacuum-assisted closure versus shoelace technique. A randomized study. Injury. 2014;45:890–3.

Abdominal Compartment Syndrome and the Open Abdomen

37

Andrew M. Nunn and Michael C. Chang

Introduction

Compartment syndrome, first identified in the context of extremity perfusion, was described in the early 1800s. Inadequate tissue perfusion due to narrowing of the gap between perfusion pressure/flow and tissue pressure was recognized as a threat to limb perfusion and viability. This same principle can be applied to the abdomen and its visceral contents, and it was the recognition of this analogy that eventually led to the recognition of IAH and subsequent ACS as life-threatening entities. The relationship of increased abdominal pressures and its effects on the respiratory system were first described in the late 1800s. Emerson's work in the 1900s examined the true relationship of intra-abdominal pressures and the cardiovascular system in dogs [1]. The interest in IAH was reinvigorated in the 1980s with multiple publications, initially through the work of Kron et al., who described the effects of IAH and the effects of re-exploration on renal function [2, 3]. Ultimately, the World Society of the Abdominal Compartment Syndrome (WSACS), now termed the Abdominal Compartment Society, was formed in 2004 and exists to promote research and education as it relates to ACS [4, 5].

The pathophysiology of compartment syndrome is simply defined as intra-abdominal hypertension resulting in end-organ failure. The effects of intra-abdominal hypertension have vast implications including cardiac, pulmonary, renal, and even neurological function. Patients with intra-abdominal catastrophes as well as those who have undergone aggressive resuscitation in the context of dysregulated systemic inflammation are patient populations at increased risk for ACS. Once recognized, immediate attention should be directed toward relieving the IAH through consideration of both invasive and noninvasive maneuvers aimed toward decreasing abdominal pressure. These maneuvers, though beneficial in the context of decreasing abdominal pressure, often carry with them their own set of problems and issues, such as acute or chronic open abdominal wounds and challenges that come along with these wounds. Fortunately, experience has led to the creation of multiple short- and long-term options to deal with these issues.

Furthermore, as the understanding of the pathophysiology driving IAH and ACS increases, options aimed upstream of decompression are being described as being important in preventing IAH to begin with. Earlier recognition of uncompensated shock and systemic inflammation,

A. M. Nunn (✉)
Department of Surgery, Wake Forest School
of Medicine, Winston Salem, NC, USA
e-mail: amnunn@wakehealth.edu

M. C. Chang
Department of Surgery, University of South Alabama
School of Medicine, Mobile, AL, USA

© Springer International Publishing AG, part of Springer Nature 2019
C. V. R. Brown et al. (eds.), *Emergency General Surgery*, https://doi.org/10.1007/978-3-319-96286-3_37

improved fluid resuscitation strategies, and the evolution of lower tidal volume strategies for the management of respiratory failure all represent relatively recent developments in management of critically ill patients that have contributed to a decrease in the incidence and prevalence of IAH and ACS.

Definitions

Standard definitions and taxonomy have been an important focus of recent work by the WSACS. The most recent definitions, published in 2013, define IAH as intra-abdominal pressure (IAP) $\geq$ 12 mmHg. The various grades of IAP are listed in Table 37.1. ACS is defined as IAH > 20 mmHg that is associated with new organ dysfunction/failure [4]. It is important to recognize that IAH and ACS are not equivalent terms; IAH is a spectrum and ACS only occurs when there is concurrent organ dysfunction. It should be noted that the value of "normal" IAP needs to be better established in various populations including children, the obese, and pregnant women. One other important distinction made by the WSACS is primary versus secondary ACS. Primary ACS is associated with a condition, injury, or disease within the abdominopelvic region, whereas secondary ACS refers to conditions not originating in the abdominopelvic region [4].

Pathophysiology

Intra-abdominal pressure is normally atmospheric or subatmospheric. In critically ill patients, the IAP is normally 5–7 mmHg [4]. When the IAP rises to a point where organ dysfunction occurs, the diagnosis of ACS can be

Table 37.1 Intra-abdominal hypertension (IAH) grading scheme

Grade	IAP (mmHg)
I	12–15
II	16–20
III	21–25
IV	>25

made. The organ dysfunction arising from ACS can affect multiple systems including cardiovascular, pulmonary, renal, gastrointestinal, and even the central nervous system.

Traditionally, it was thought that ACS occurs when the abdominal perfusion pressure (mean arterial pressure – intra-abdominal pressure) becomes inadequate. However, recent studies suggest this may not be so straight forward. Olofsson and colleagues demonstrated that the mucosal blood flow of small bowel was less affected than other areas of microcirculation during stepwise increases in intra-abdominal pressure (IAP) in a swine model, suggesting a component of autoregulation. As cardiac output decreased, so did microcirculation; however, the small bowel mucosa was less affected relative to the seromuscular layers. This study also found that changes occur at grade 1 and 2 IAH, suggesting even mild IAH is not a benign process [6].

Primary ACS occurs when there is a direct source of increased IAP within the abdomen (trauma, pancreatitis, infection, etc.). Secondary ACS, however, occurs as a result of factors not directly related to the abdominal cavity. Examples of secondary ACS include bowel or retroperitoneal edema due to large-volume resuscitation associated with a non-abdominal source of inflammation, ACS due to massive ascites in the absence of an abdominal operation, and right heart failure associated with visceral edema. Activation of the immune system triggers cytokine release and subsequent capillary leak. This impacts the cellular function of the organ itself, along with the effects of fluid accumulation in the extravascular space. As emphasized by Malbrain, this is well recognized in the pathophysiology of acute respiratory distress syndrome, but clinicians have been slow to adopt the same physiologic blueprint to the gastrointestinal tract [7]. For these reasons, the terms acute bowel injury and acute intestinal distress syndrome were introduced by Malbrain and colleagues.

Acute bowel injury is the result of capillary leak and subsequent edema. In the so-called "two-hit" process, a first hit occurs when an insult results in neutrophil activation and cytokine release. This is followed by a second physiologic insult where capillary leak ensues resulting in persistent and worsening tissue edema and subsequent IAH. As this process continues, IAH will continue to worsen, and eventually acute intestinal distress syndrome and ACS occur. The initial insult simply opens the door to additional IAH which in and of itself will lead to decreased perfusion of the GI tract. The authors compare this to the acute lung injury progression to ARDS pathway. Inherent in this pathway is that ischemia-reperfusion likely plays a substantial role in the pathophysiology of ACS [7].

In addition to global capillary leak, ACS also has profound effects on the cardiovascular, pulmonary, genitourinary, gastrointestinal, and neurological systems. As demonstrated in multiple studies, cardiac output is negatively affected by increases in IAP [6, 8]. Decreases in global cardiovascular performance are usually a result of decreased venous return and diastolic filling (preload) combined with increases in ventricular afterload. Increases in afterload may result from both direct compression of the pulmonary artery, aorta, and their branches and sympathetic vasoconstriction secondary to metabolic stress. Continued fluid administration may be temporarily beneficial; however, ongoing fluid resuscitation without addressing the primary source and abdominal hypertension may be deleterious, as fluid cannot overcome the factors affecting low cardiac output. Fluid administration in patients with ACS has been found to increase pulmonary capillary wedge pressure (PCWP) without any concomitant increase in cardiac index (CI) [9, 10]. Fluid administration can become a viscous cycle of more fluid followed by worsening capillary leak followed by even more fluid. The lack of a systemic response to additional fluid has been appropriately termed the "futile crystalloid preloading cycle." [10] Furthermore, careful attention should be paid to how preload is being assessed in these patients, as errors in interpreting pressure-derived estimates of preload may lead to conclusions being drawn about intravascular volume status that in fact have little relationship to actual volume status. There is a positive correlation between IAH and PCWP and CVP, but this increase does not result in an increase in cardiac output as one may expect [11]. Thus, hemodynamic monitoring values should be interpreted with caution in patients with IAH.

An increase in IAP invariably leads to increased thoracic pressures and a decrease in functional residual capacity. The decrease in lung compliance is particularly noticeable in the ventilated critically ill patient. Ventilated patients on volume-limited modes will see an increase in peak inspiratory pressure, whereas those on pressure-limited modes of ventilation will have lower tidal volumes. Resultant pulmonary edema secondary to fluid administration and capillary leak results in increased PEEP requirements which then exacerbate the cardiovascular effects mentioned above. It is clear that ACS is a risk factor for the development of acute respiratory distress syndrome (ARDS), which itself is a morbid and mortal syndrome, and its development is likely multifactorial [12]. Appropriate ventilator management with lung protective strategies is crucial when managing the ACS patient.

Oliguria and subsequent renal failure were among the earliest effects of ACS noted in the surgical literature. Renal dysfunction associated with IAH is due to factors both extrinsic to the kidneys themselves and direct effects of IAH on the kidneys. Inadequate global cardiovascular function leads to relative hypotension, decreased cardiac output, and subsequent renal hypoperfusion [2]. Several investigators in the past have looked at the renal subsystem itself very carefully, focusing on both the kidneys, and the renal collecting system. Although ureteral compression was once thought to play a role, renal vein compression (outflow obstruction) along with direct compression of the renal cortex is the most plausible etiology of renal dysfunction [13].

Decompression plays a central role in the management of renal impairment associated with IAH and ACS and, if performed early in the course of the ACS, usually results in improvement in both intrinsic renal function and urine output. However, delays in recognition are often associated with either transient or no improvement in renal function at the time of decompression. Keys to early decompression center around an increased awareness of the risk of IAH in these metabolically stressed patients and definitive decision-making to move forward with decompressive maneuvers once diagnosed.

The gastrointestinal system is also vulnerable to the effects of IAH. This is likely related to the decreased perfusion secondary to the local increased pressures and the changes in the circulatory system described above. Diebel and colleagues have clearly demonstrated the profound negative effect of IAH on mesenteric perfusion using an animal model and measuring the decreases in mesenteric blood flow and mucosal pH with incremental increases in IAP [14]. Further, Chang and colleagues demonstrated a significant improvement in gut mucosal pH, indicating an improvement in intestinal perfusion, after decompression of the abdomen, which supports this concept [11].

Lastly, IAH can have a deleterious effect on the central nervous system by impairing cerebral venous outflow and thus increasing intracranial pressures (ICP). This phenomenon was first recognized with laparoscopy, and it was identified that abdominal insufflation increases ICP [15]. This can have many downstream effects including exacerbating head injury and potentially contributing to altered mental status in the critically ill patient [16]. To further demonstrate this, it has also been suggested that decompressive laparotomy can be used as an adjunctive therapy in lowering ICPs that are refractory to traditional treatments [17].

ACS affects multiple critical physiologic systems concurrently. The effect on each system can adversely potentiate the effect on another bodily system. It is the interrelation of the effects that leads to the ultimate organ failure and potential fatal consequences.

Diagnosis

IAH and ACS can result after a wide range of both anatomic and physiologic insults. The bedside clinician must be vigilant in the ICU to assess at-risk patients for IAH. It is important to always recognize that IAH is distinct from ACS. The vigilant clinician can recognize IAH

and intervene, potentially preventing ACS and its significant consequences. In a meta-analysis, large-volume crystalloid resuscitation, the respiratory status of the patient, and shock/hypotension were all risk factors for ACS; obesity, sepsis, abdominal surgery, ileus, and large-volume fluid resuscitation were notable risk factors for IAH [18]. Primary and secondary ACS vary in their presentation and course. As described by Reintam and colleagues, secondary IAH often presents late and may be characterized by a prolonged course where IAP increases over a period of days. Compared with primary IAH, secondary IAH is associated with increased mortality [19].

Early recognition of both IAH and ACS requires both a heightened suspicion of their presence in patients at risk and careful interpretation of bedside monitoring and physiologic information across all potentially affected subsystems. Changes to the respiratory status (increased peak/plateau inspiratory pressures, decreased compliance) may be among the first signs of IAH in the ventilated patient. Decreasing urine output, rising creatinine, abdominal distention, and hypotension are among other signs of IAH and impending ACS. Clinical exam alone is often not reliable in recognizing and diagnosing IAH [20].

When a concern exists for IAH or ACS, direct measurement of intra-abdominal pressure is the gold standard for diagnosis. Multiple techniques have been used to measure the pressures within the abdominal compartment. The most accepted technique involves the measurement of bladder pressure, first described by Kron et al. in 1984. Fundamentally, the bladder is filled with a specified volume of saline solution with the urinary drainage catheter clamped to maintain bladder volume. The wall of the bladder then acts as a passive diaphragm, and transduction of intravesicular pressure, done by attaching a pressure transducer to the catheter, allows a reasonable estimation of intra-abdominal pressure. Optimal volumes of bladder distention with saline have been correlated with direct measurements of intra-abdominal pressure at laparoscopy, and volumes of 25–50 cc provide the most accurate measurements [3]. The most recent recommendations of the WSACS advise to instill no more than 25 cc of saline into the bladder [4]. A schematic

Fig. 37.1 Bedside setup for measurement of bladder pressure

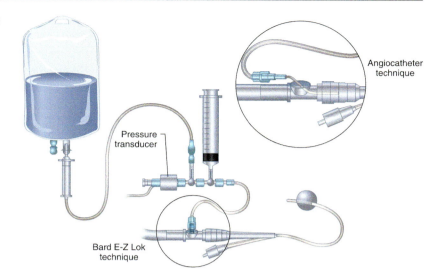

Angiocatheter technique

Pressure transducer

Bard E-Z Lok technique

of the setup to measure bladder pressures at the bedside is depicted below (Fig. 37.1). Other techniques using pressures within the vasculature, rectum, and stomach have also been described, but bladder pressure is the current standard. [2] This methodology has been validated by comparing bladder pressures to true intra-abdominal pressure during laparoscopy [21]. Optimally, bladder pressure measurements should be measured with the patient in the supine position [22]. If the patient is active or has tense abdominal muscles, the pressure may be interpreted as falsely high. In such patients, consideration should be given to sedation and potential paralysis to obtain an accurate IAP. Space-occupying materials in the pelvis, such as packs, masses, or a pelvic hematoma, may also confound bladder pressure measurements by extrinsically decreasing function bladder wall compliance, leading to elevated bladder pressures independent of increases in intra-abdominal pressure.

Ultimately, a well-defined protocol employing consistent techniques within an institution is essential to obtaining accurate and consistent bladder pressure measurements.

Management

The gold standard treatment of ACS is emergent abdominal decompression. In considering the treatment, however, one must also emphasize that

prevention is the best treatment. The WSACS has proposed a treatment algorithm which is detailed in Fig. 37.2. Once IAH is identified, steps can be taken to prevent progression to ACS, directed at both the primary physiologic insult and the secondary insult resulting from the deranged physiology due to the primary problem. Primary ACS can often not be avoided by the clinician, as the patient often has a direct insult to the abdomino-pelvic cavity. However, leaving the abdomen open after damage control surgery or in cases where the viscera cannot be reduced for abdominal closure has been a hallmark in preventing ACS and is unequivocally the reason there has been a decrease in ACS [12]. Secondary ACS may be also be preventable by intervening upon the inflammatory cascade and being judicious with fluid (particularly crystalloid) administration, with the goal being to achieve and maintain a euvolemic state.

When IAH is recognized, steps should be taken promptly to reduce IAP to prevent progression to ACS. This includes primarily medical management and close observation. Proper pain control and sedation of the patient are essential and may reduce IAP. As alluded to earlier, neuromuscular blockade may reduce IAP. At the very least, paralytics will allow for accurate IAP measurements. Although evidence is lacking, placement of enteric tubes to reduce gastric and colonic distention may be helpful [4]. As mentioned above, fluid balance plays a critical role in

Intra-abdominal hypertension (IAH) / abdominal compartment syndrome (ACS) management algorithm

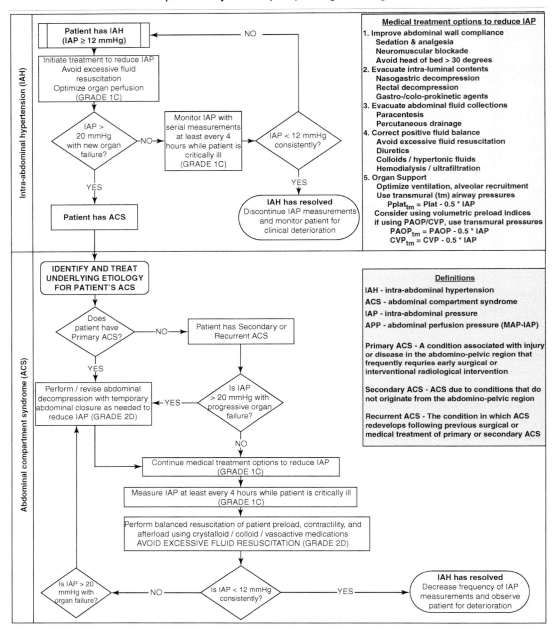

Fig. 37.2 Management algorithm for ACS. (Reprinted with permission from Kirkpatrick et al. [4])

the development of ACS (particularly secondary ACS) and should be optimized. Just as optimizing fluid balance has been shown to be favorable in ARDS, the same is likely true for ACS. Increased crystalloid volumes are associated with an increased incidence of ACS, so achieving appropriate fluid balance, which may involve strict management of fluid administration, and sometime diuresis, is critical [23]. In cases of trauma, balanced blood product resuscitation should be pursued, as this has been related to a decrease in the incidence of ACS in this population [24].

Minimally invasive strategies have been proposed to decrease IAP. This includes percutaneous drainage of fluid collections within the abdominal cavity and, in the case of severe pancreatitis, the retroperitoneum. Reports of percutaneous drainage allow for avoidance of the morbidity associated with a laparotomy and the subsequent open abdomen [25–27]. Among trauma patients with large resuscitations, percutaneous drainage was found to offer significant reduction in IAP, increase in abdominal perfusion pressure, improved pulmonary compliance, and increase in mean arterial pressure [28]. This procedure is best suited for patients with abdominal fluid after significant resuscitation with crystalloid (severe pancreatitis, sepsis) or after blunt solid organ trauma. Cheatham and colleagues demonstrated 81% treatment efficacy of this modality. These authors suggested that drainage of less than 1000 mL and a decrease in IAP of less than 9 mmHg in the first 4 h are predictive of failure [29]. Subcutaneous fasciotomy of the abdominal wall fascia has also been described in small series [30]. Leppaniemi describes a technique where the linea alba is opened through small skin incisions. This results in a hernia that must be repaired in the long term but avoids the morbidity of an open abdomen [31, 32]. Although the results are promising, this technique has only been studied in small numbers.

In light of these strategies, surgical abdominal decompression via laparotomy remains the standard. This is the most rapid and definitive method to decompress ACS. Prompt decompression results in improved preload, pulmonary function, and visceral perfusion [11]. The treatment phase of ACS not only includes this initial decompression but also includes care of the open abdomen and the subsequent closure and abdominal wall reconstruction. Appropriate management of the open abdomen and the prevention of complications are essential. Once an abdomen is opened, a negative pressure dressing should be used as a temporary closure device [4]. The open abdomen is then treated in a staged approach. This approach is very similar to the open abdomen after damage

control surgery in trauma, as described by Rotundo et al. [33] After the initial operation, a temporary closure is placed over the abdominal viscera, and the patient is taken to the intensive care unit for resuscitation and optimization. The patient is then returned to the operating room for re-exploration and definitive closure as early as possible. Potential complications of the open abdomen are inability to close, hernia, enterocutaneous fistula, infection, and even recurrent ACS. Various methods have been described for temporary abdominal closure to maximize fascial closure and minimize hernia. Bowel edema and fascial retraction often make primary abdominal wall closure difficult or impossible.

Temporary Abdominal Closure

The evolution and development of current techniques employed to manage open abdominal wounds is a relatively recent development in surgery. Before the description of the staged celiotomy [34], standard general surgical teaching was that all operations should be completed at the initial operation. In fact, failure to close the abdominal wound was considered a marker of surgical inadequacy. Advances in the understanding of IAH and ACS have driven a significant change in attitudes over the four decades, and the increased understanding of IAH and ACS has carried with it significant advances in the techniques used to safely manage temporary open abdominal wounds. Early techniques, such as skin closure with towel clips, wet dressings over open wounds, and artificial mesh sewn to the skin, are fraught with complications and have largely been abandoned. A silo-type dressing, commonly referred to as "Bogota bag," involves the placement of a sterilized IV fluid bag over the viscera and sewn to the skin edges [35, 36]. This technique is quick, simple, and inexpensive and provides a true "window" into the abdomen. The drawback to this technique is that it does not provide any tension on the fascial edges, allowing for retraction of the abdominal wall laterally.

In theory, any device or method used for temporary abdominal closure should meet certain minimum criteria. The dressing should protect the viscera, prevent spillage of ascites (with associated heat loss), allow for patient mobility, and minimize metabolic stress. Optimally, the dressing would facilitate measuring and controlling peritoneal drainage, would be flexible enough to expand should visceral edema worsen, and would not involve damage to the fascia, in anticipation of eventual delayed fascial closure.

Vacuum-assisted fascial closure (VAFC) meets most, if not all, of these criteria and has become a popular method of managing temporary open abdominal wounds. This technique involves placing a standard vacuum pack (as described by Barker et al.) to the abdomen at the index operation if the abdomen is not going to be closed [37]. If the abdomen is not able to be closed at the time of reoperation, the VAFC method is employed. Described in detail by Miller et al., this includes placement of a perforated polyethylene sheet over the viscera. A black sponge is then placed on the sheet and sutured to the skin edges with a running nylon stitch (Figs. 37.3, 37.4, and 37.5). Employing this technique allows for an abdominal closure rate of 88%. Interestingly, 48% of the patients in this study were able to be closed after 9 days, suggesting that attempts should continue to be made to close the abdomen even after 1 week or more [38]. The Denver group has described a novel vacuum technique where white sponges are placed on the viscera, followed by fascial

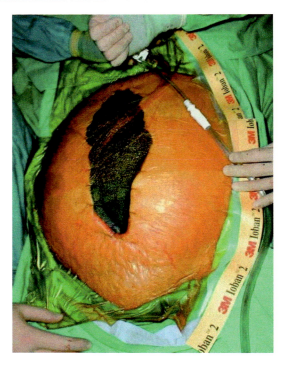

Fig. 37.4 Black sponge with nylon suture and adhesive dressing

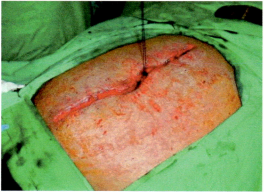

Fig. 37.5 Abdominal closure on postoperative day 21

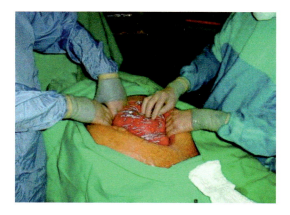

Fig. 37.3 Placement of polyethylene sheet

tension with PDS sutures, followed by a traditional sponge in the subcutaneous space. By changing this every 2 days, they claim a 100% fascial approximation rate [39]. The ABThera VAC (KCI, San Antonio, TX) is a commercially available device that accomplishes the same principles as the techniques above and has favorable abdominal closure rates. The

Wittmann Patch (Starsurgical, Burlington, WI) is a Velcro device that can be sutured to fascial edges and serially tightened until abdominal closure is adequate. Using this device has been shown to facilitate definitive abdominal closure [40, 41]. There are multiple techniques and devices that are available to maintain abdominal domain while the abdomen is open, and each individual provider must choose their preferred method. Whichever technique is employed, it is critical that the clinician recognizes that ACS can occur with a temporary abdominal dressing in place [42].

Definitive Abdominal Closure

As soon as the abdomen is initially decompressed, planning for definitive abdominal closure should begin. While the abdomen is open, appropriate fluid balance, depending on the patient's physiologic state, should be maintained. Balanced blood product resuscitation decreases the incidence of ACS and is also related to improved rates of abdominal fascial closure [43]. Enteral nutrition with adequate protein and total caloric intake should begin as soon as feasible in patients with an open abdomen, as this has been shown to improve fascial closure rates [44]. It is important to carefully monitor the protein-rich effluent from the open abdomen, as this affects both the patient's fluid balance and their nutritional status given the abdominal effluent may have 10–15 g of albumin per liter.

Management of the open abdomen can be broadly divided into three phases: phase 1 is the time after the index operation when a TAC technique is used; phase 2 is the attempted closure of the abdominal wall during the acute phase; and phase 3 is the later (6–12 months) abdominal wall reconstruction in those whom primary closures were not possible during phase 2 [45]. Primary fascial closure is by far the most desired outcome after open abdomen and can be achieved in well over half of patients, as far out as 1 month after injury [46]. In the event that primary fascial closure is unable to be attained, acute mesh repair

and component separation are techniques that may be employed to achieve abdominal closure early. Acute component separation and mesh placement, while allowing for early abdominal closure, are associated with a high complication and hernia rate, respectively [45]. When abdominal closure is not accomplished during the acute phase, planned ventral hernia with a staged approach is also an option with future definitive reconstruction.

With planned ventral hernia, the viscera must be covered in some fashion. If a visceral block has formed, the skin may be closed over the viscera with a running suture. If this skin cannot be closed, our preference is to cover the viscera with a skin graft. If a nice bed of granulation exists on the viscera, the graft may be placed directly onto it. In the more common scenario where there is not sufficient granulation or the bowel is not adhered as a block, a polyglactin mesh is sutured to the fascial edges circumferentially. This should not be placed under significant tension, as the mesh can tear; the goal of the procedure is visceral coverage, not fascial tension. Next, negative pressure wound therapy is applied until adequate granulation tissue is present, at which time a split-thickness skin graft is performed. Acellular dermal matrices are another option when closing the abdomen and can be placed to bridge the fascial defect. While this may decrease the incidence of fistula formation, it has a high rate of recurrent hernias and should be approached as a planned hernia [47]. Again, the goal of this procedure is to cover the viscera to decrease the risk of infection and fistula [48]. Many months later, often a year or more, when the skin graft heals and easily pinches away from the underlying bowel, a definitive hernia repair can be performed. Excess skin and the hernia sac are excised and primary fascial closure is attempted. There are various techniques to augment the possibility of fascial closure including external oblique release, posterior rectus release, transversus abdominis release, and Botox injections, to name just a few. Placement of mesh at the time of hernia repair significantly decreases the risk of recurrence [49]. While the techniques of abdominal hernia repair are incredibly important for long-term outcomes, they are beyond the scope of this chapter.

Conclusion

Intra-abdominal hypertension and resultant abdominal compartment syndrome are often markers of severe metabolic and physiologic stress, and patients with these conditions can be the most challenging surgical patients to manage from both a critical care and operative perspective. The decrease in incidence of abdominal compartment syndrome can be credited to the research and subsequent education that has been dedicated to this syndrome in the preceding decades, but it has been associated with a dramatic increase in the incidence of the open abdomen. The astute clinician should be familiar with the prompt recognition, diagnosis, and treatment of ACS to avoid its morbid and mortal consequences. Moreover, management of the open abdomen requires careful planning and oversight to optimize patient outcomes.

References

1. Papavramidis TS, Marinis AD, Pliakos I, Kesisoglou I, Papavramidou N. Abdominal compartment syndrome – intra-abdominal hypertension: defining, diagnosing, and managing. J Emerg Trauma Shock. 2011;4(2):279–91.
2. Bailey J, Shapiro MJ. Abdominal compartment syndrome. Crit Care. 2000;4(1):23–9.
3. Kron IL, Harman PK, Nolan SP. The measurement of intra-abdominal pressure as a criterion for abdominal re-exploration. Ann Surg. 1984;199(1):28–30.
4. Kirkpatrick AW, Roberts DJ, De Waele J, et al. Intra-abdominal hypertension and the abdominal compartment syndrome: updated consensus definitions and clinical practice guidelines from the World Society of the Abdominal Compartment Syndrome. Intensive Care Med. 2013;39(7):1190–206.
5. Kirkpatrick AW, Sugrue M, McKee JL, et al. Update from the Abdominal Compartment Society (WSACS) on intra-abdominal hypertension and abdominal compartment syndrome: past, present, and future beyond Banff 2017. Anaesthesiol Intensive Ther. 2017;49(2):83–7.
6. Olofsson PH, Berg S, Ahn HC, Brudin LH, Vikström T, Johansson KJ. Gastrointestinal microcirculation and cardiopulmonary function during experimentally increased intra-abdominal pressure. Crit Care Med. 2009;37(1):230–9.
7. Malbrain ML, De Laet I. AIDS is coming to your ICU: be prepared for acute bowel injury and acute intestinal distress syndrome. Intensive Care Med. 2008;34(9):1565–9.
8. Barnes GE, Laine GA, Giam PY, Smith EE, Granger HJ. Cardiovascular responses to elevation of intra-abdominal hydrostatic pressure. Am J Phys. 1985;248(2 Pt 2):R208–13.
9. Balogh Z, McKinley BA, Cocanour CS, Kozar RA, Cox CS, Moore FA. Patients with impending abdominal compartment syndrome do not respond to early volume loading. Am J Surg. 2003;186(6):602–7. discussion 607–8
10. Balogh Z, McKinley BA, Cocanour CS, et al. Supranormal trauma resuscitation causes more cases of abdominal compartment syndrome. Arch Surg. 2003;138(6):637–42. discussion 642–3
11. Chang MC, Miller PR, D'Agostino R, Meredith JW. Effects of abdominal decompression on cardiopulmonary function and visceral perfusion in patients with intra-abdominal hypertension. J Trauma. 1998;44(3):440–5.
12. Offner PJ, de Souza AL, Moore EE, et al. Avoidance of abdominal compartment syndrome in damage-control laparotomy after trauma. Arch Surg. 2001;136(6):676–81.
13. Harman PK, Kron IL, McLachlan HD, Freedlender AE, Nolan SP. Elevated intra-abdominal pressure and renal function. Ann Surg. 1982;196(5):594–7.
14. Diebel LN, Dulchavsky SA, Wilson RF. Effect of increased intra-abdominal pressure on mesenteric arterial and intestinal mucosal blood flow. J Trauma. 1992;33(1):45–8. discussion 48–9
15. Josephs LG, Este-McDonald JR, Birkett DH, Hirsch EF. Diagnostic laparoscopy increases intracranial pressure. J Trauma. 1994;36(6):815–8. discussion 818–9
16. Morken J, West MA. Abdominal compartment syndrome in the intensive care unit. Curr Opin Crit Care. 2001;7(4):268–74.
17. Joseph DK, Dutton RP, Aarabi B, Scalea TM. Decompressive laparotomy to treat intractable intracranial hypertension after traumatic brain injury. J Trauma. 2004;57(4):687–93. discussion 693–5
18. Holodinsky JK, Roberts DJ, Ball CG, et al. Risk factors for intra-abdominal hypertension and abdominal compartment syndrome among adult intensive care unit patients: a systematic review and meta-analysis. Crit Care. 2013;17(5):R249.
19. Reintam A, Parm P, Kitus R, Kern H, Starkopf J. Primary and secondary intra-abdominal hypertension – different impact on ICU outcome. Intensive Care Med. 2008;34(9):1624–31.
20. Kirkpatrick AW, Brenneman FD, McLean RF, Rapanos T, Boulanger BR. Is clinical examination an accurate indicator of raised intra-abdominal pressure in critically injured patients? Can J Surg. 2000;43(3):207–11.
21. Fusco MA, Martin RS, Chang MC. Estimation of intra-abdominal pressure by bladder pressure

measurement: validity and methodology. J Trauma. 2001;50(2):297–302.

22. Cheatham ML, De Waele JJ, De Laet I, et al. The impact of body position on intra-abdominal pressure measurement: a multicenter analysis. Crit Care Med. 2009;37(7):2187–90.

23. Joseph B, Zangbar B, Pandit V, et al. The conjoint effect of reduced crystalloid administration and decreased damage-control laparotomy use in the development of abdominal compartment syndrome. J Trauma Acute Care Surg. 2014;76(2):457–61.

24. Cotton BA, Au BK, Nunez TC, Gunter OL, Robertson AM, Young PP. Predefined massive transfusion protocols are associated with a reduction in organ failure and postinjury complications. J Trauma. 2009;66(1):41–8. discussion 48–9

25. Vikrama KS, Shyamkumar NK, Vinu M, Joseph P, Vyas F, Venkatramani S. Percutaneous catheter drainage in the treatment of abdominal compartment syndrome. Can J Surg. 2009;52(1):E19–20.

26. Tokue H, Tokue A, Tsushima Y. Successful interventional management of abdominal compartment syndrome caused by blunt liver injury with hemorrhagic diathesis. World J Emerg Surg. 2014;9(1):20.

27. Chen H, Li F, Sun JB, Jia JG. Abdominal compartment syndrome in patients with severe acute pancreatitis in early stage. World J Gastroenterol. 2008;14(22):3541–8.

28. Reed SF, Britt RC, Collins J, Weireter L, Cole F, Britt LD. Aggressive surveillance and early catheter-directed therapy in the management of intra-abdominal hypertension. J Trauma. 2006;61(6):1359–63. discussion 1363–5

29. Cheatham ML, Safcsak K. Percutaneous catheter decompression in the treatment of elevated intraabdominal pressure. Chest. 2011;140(6):1428–35.

30. Ouellet JF, Leppaniemi A, Ball CG, Cheatham ML, D'Amours S, Kirkpatrick AW. Alternatives to formal abdominal decompression. Am Surg. 2011;77(Suppl 1):S51–7.

31. Leppäniemi AK, Hienonen PA, Siren JE, Kuitunen AH, Lindström OK, Kemppainen EA. Treatment of abdominal compartment syndrome with subcutaneous anterior abdominal fasciotomy in severe acute pancreatitis. World J Surg. 2006;30(10):1922–4.

32. Leppäniemi A, Hienonen P, Mentula P, Kemppainen E. Subcutaneous linea alba fasciotomy, does it really work? Am Surg. 2011;77(1):99–102.

33. Rotondo MF, Schwab CW, McGonigal MD, et al. 'Damage control': an approach for improved survival in exsanguinating penetrating abdominal injury. J Trauma. 1993;35(3):375–82. discussion 382–3

34. Morris JA, Eddy VA, Blinman TA, Rutherford EJ, Sharp KW. The staged celiotomy for trauma. Issues in unpacking and reconstruction. Ann Surg. 1993;217(5):576–84. discussion 584–6

35. Fernandez L, Norwood S, Roettger R, Wilkins HE. Temporary intravenous bag silo closure in severe abdominal trauma. J Trauma. 1996;40(2):258–60.

36. Kirshtein B, Roy-Shapira A, Lantsberg L, Mizrahi S. Use of the "Bogota bag" for temporary abdominal closure in patients with secondary peritonitis. Am Surg. 2007;73(3):249–52.

37. Barker DE, Kaufman HJ, Smith LA, Ciraulo DL, Richart CL, Burns RP. Vacuum pack technique of temporary abdominal closure: a 7-year experience with 112 patients. J Trauma. 2000;48(2):201–6. discussion 206–7

38. Miller PR, Meredith JW, Johnson JC, Chang MC. Prospective evaluation of vacuum-assisted fascial closure after open abdomen: planned ventral hernia rate is substantially reduced. Ann Surg. 2004;239(5):608–14. discussion 614–6

39. Burlew CC, Moore EE, Biffl WL, Bensard DD, Johnson JL, Barnett CC. One hundred percent fascial approximation can be achieved in the postinjury open abdomen with a sequential closure protocol. J Trauma Acute Care Surg. 2012;72(1):235–41.

40. Weinberg JA, George RL, Griffin RL, et al. Closing the open abdomen: improved success with Wittmann Patch staged abdominal closure. J Trauma. 2008;65(2):345–8.

41. Tieu BH, Cho SD, Luem N, Riha G, Mayberry J, Schreiber MA. The use of the Wittmann Patch facilitates a high rate of fascial closure in severely injured trauma patients and critically ill emergency surgery patients. J Trauma. 2008;65(4):865–70.

42. Gracias VH, Braslow B, Johnson J, et al. Abdominal compartment syndrome in the open abdomen. Arch Surg. 2002;137(11):1298–300.

43. Glaser J, Vasquez M, Cardarelli C, et al. Ratio-driven resuscitation predicts early fascial closure in the combat wounded. J Trauma Acute Care Surg. 2015;79(4 Suppl 2):S188–92.

44. Collier B, Guillamondegui O, Cotton B, et al. Feeding the open abdomen. JPEN J Parenter Enteral Nutr. 2007;31(5):410–5.

45. Sharrock AE, Barker T, Yuen HM, Rickard R, Tai N. Management and closure of the open abdomen after damage control laparotomy for trauma. A systematic review and meta-analysis. Injury. 2016;47(2):296–306.

46. Miller PR, Thompson JT, Faler BJ, Meredith JW, Chang MC. Late fascial closure in lieu of ventral hernia: the next step in open abdomen management. J Trauma. 2002;53(5):843–9.

47. de Moya MA, Dunham M, Inaba K, et al. Long-term outcome of acellular dermal matrix when used for large traumatic open abdomen. J Trauma. 2008;65(2):349–53.

48. Mayberry JC, Mullins RJ, Crass RA, Trunkey DD. Prevention of abdominal compartment syndrome by absorbable mesh prosthesis closure. Arch Surg. 1997;132(9):957–61. discussion 961–2

49. Kokotovic D, Bisgaard T, Helgstrand F. Long-term recurrence and complications associated with elective incisional hernia repair. JAMA. 2016;316(15):1575–82.

Necrotizing Soft Tissue Infection

Sameer A. Hirji, Sharven Taghavi, and Reza Askari

Epidemiology

Soft tissue infections can be classified into superficial and deep infections. Superficial infections involve the skin and hypodermis, while deep infections involve the soft tissues at and below the level of the fascia [1]. Necrotizing soft tissue infections (NSTIs), in particular, are rapidly progressive infections of the deep soft tissues and are associated with high morbidity and mortality [2, 3]. In fact, these infections rank among the more difficult disease processes encountered in clinical practice and encompass a spectrum of presentations with varying severity. NSTI was first described by Hippocrates in the fifth century B.C. and later adopted by the British in the eighteenth century, where the disease was known as phagedena gangrenous, gangrenous ulcer, malignant ulcer, or hospital gangrene. The term "hospital gangrene" became the dominant term in the United States in 1871, first utilized by Confederate Army surgeon Joseph Jones who reported his initial series of over 2600 cases with a mortality rate approaching almost 50% [4].

NSTI is an uncommon clinical entity and has a reported incidence of only 1000 cases annually in the United States. In other words, it affects 0.4 to 1 person per 100,000 per year [4–6]. Furthermore, according to one study examining 9-year trends in NSTI from 1999 to 2007, the gross incidence of NSTI has more than doubled [6]. Given the varying degrees of clinical presentation, some clinicians argue that the incidence may be underestimated.

Pathophysiology: Organisms and Types

In the context of NSTI, impaired immunity is known to increase susceptibility to various infections [7]. Trauma to the skin can also precipitate these infections because of breach of integrity of underlying mucosa. The impaired immunity can either be inherent or acquired in the setting of multiple chronic conditions such as diabetes. NSTIs are also typically caused by toxin-producing bacteria and involve significant local tissue destruction as a result of toxin-mediated systematic inflammation [4].

While there is no age or gender predilection, higher rates of NSTIs are observed in diabetic, obese, alcoholic, and immunocompromised patients. Nonetheless, NSTIs can also occur in young, healthy patients without any significant comorbidities. Likewise, there are also regional and geographic differences that exist in terms of NSTI occurrence and presentation. For instance, a retrospective study involving six academic

S. A. Hirji · S. Taghavi · R. Askari (✉)
Department of Surgery, Brigham and Women's
Hospital, Harvard Medical School,
Boston, MA, USA
e-mail: raskari@bwh.harvard.edu

© Springer International Publishing AG, part of Springer Nature 2019
C. V. R. Brown et al. (eds.), *Emergency General Surgery*, https://doi.org/10.1007/978-3-319-96286-3_38

hospitals in Texas between 2004 and 2007 found that there were significant center differences in patient populations, etiology, and microbiology of NSTIs, even within a concentrated region [8].

NSTIs can be classified based on the affected anatomic part, microbial source, or infection depth [1]. For example, NSTI can affect the perineal, perianal, or genital areas, a condition also known as Fournier's gangrene (first identified in 1883 by Dr. Jean Alfred Fournier) [4]. In terms of infection depth, while NSTIs can arise primarily in the dermis and epidermis, they more commonly occur in the deeper layers of adipose tissue, fascia, or muscle causing necrotizing adiposities, fasciitis, or even myonecrosis, respectively.

Furthermore, varying amounts of early or late systemic toxicity depend on the microbial source (i.e., strain of bacteria and toxins produced). Between 55% and 80% of cases involve more than one type of bacteria [3, 9–11]. Common organisms include *Group A Streptococcus* (the most common), *Klebsiella*, *Clostridium*, *Escherichia coli*, *Staphylococcus aureus*, and *Aeromonas hydrophila*. Most of the infections involve normally residing skin flora, which coexist as commensals, and cause infections when inherent immunity is compromised. It should be noted that *Clostridium* infections typically manifest quickly and can become symptomatic within hours after initial injury or inoculation, whereas most bacterial species (except *Group A Streptococcus*) require a few days to become symptomatic [4, 7].

Thus, NSTIs can be classified into four types, depending on the infecting organism or organisms. However, no difference in clinical course, morbidity, or mortality has been demonstrated between these groups [7]:

1. Type I is the most common and caused by a mixture of bacterial types including anaerobes (*Clostridium* species). It commonly occurs at sites of surgery or sometimes blunt trauma. It can also occur in abdominal or perineal areas, both of which account for most of the cases (almost 80%) [12]. Often, these patients are typically older, with more medical comorbidities such as diabetes [4].

2. Type II is caused by *Group A Streptococcus* and usually occurs on the head, neck, arm, and legs. It often co-occurs with *Staphylococcus aureus* infection. These infections have significant potential for aggressive local spread or, in some cases, systemic toxicity including toxic shock syndrome [4]. These infections typically occur in younger, healthier patients and more commonly in patients with a history of trauma, surgery, or intravenous drug use [4].

3. Type III is caused by gram-negative marine organisms, most commonly *Vibrio vulnificus*, which often enters the skin via puncture wounds from fish or insects in sea water. Clinical presentation is similar to that of Type II infections, but there appears to be early evidence of significant systemic toxicity.

4. Type IV occurs due to fungal infection. This type of infections often coexists with the other types of NSTI.

Clinical Presentation

The hallmark presentation is intense pain and tenderness in a specific area, which clinically progresses from a prodromal phase of fever and lethargy (for 2–7 days) to fulminant, obvious gangrene formation. If the infection progresses, it can be associated with purulent drainage from the wounds and extensive subcutaneous crepitation [2–4].

In certain scenarios, obvious underlying clinical manifestations are absent, but patients may still present with pain out of proportion to physical findings. The skin overlying the affected region may be normal, erythematous, cyanotic, bronzed, indurated, or just blistered [2–4]. In some cases, the primary process may be occurring under the skin, so a high index of suspicion is warranted even if the skin appears normal. Subcutaneous emphysema, which is classic for NSTI, is rarely seen. It is for this reason that diagnosis is often hindered or delayed. Systemic symptoms, including fever, tachycardia, and hypotension, may be present once the patient becomes symptomatic and the disease has progressed significantly over time.

Diagnosis

The general approach to timely and effective diagnosis involves a thorough physical exam, labs (complete blood cell count, blood and urine culture, etc.), and imaging. A coagulation profile, including type and screen, should also be sent especially if surgical exploration is needed. Notably, immunocompromised patients pose a diagnostic challenge and may not manifest obvious systemic signs and symptoms. A recent study from our institution by Keung and colleagues found that immunocompromised patients (as defined by corticosteroid use, active malignancy, receipt of chemotherapy or radiation therapy, diagnosis of human immunodeficiency virus or AIDS, or prior solid organ or bone marrow transplantation with receipt of chronic immunosuppression) had significant delays in diagnosis and presented with lower systolic blood pressures, lower serum glucose levels, and lower WBC counts. Given the differential presentation, these patients were less likely to be transferred in, and less likely to undergo surgical debridement at the time of admission, resulting in a twofold higher mortality. In these patients, a higher index of suspicion is warranted [13].

The Role of Imaging

The role of imaging in the diagnosis of NSTI is extremely important. Imaging also helps to guide the surgical treatment approach and allows early recruitment of multiple specialties if the extent of the disease appears severe. Imaging also helps to exclude any other underlying diagnosis other than NSTI [1]. Plain radiographs should be the initial imaging study although its utility is limited in non-extremity NSTI. Gas within the soft tissues is detected more commonly than with physical exam, although absence of air on plain films does not exclude the diagnosis. Instead, computed tomography (CT) is preferred and should be considered the imaging study if choice is available, especially given its scanning speed, high spatial resolution, and multi-planar reformatting capabilities [1].

Concerning findings include soft tissue and fascial thickening, fat stranding, and soft tissue gas collections. Although magnetic resonance imaging (MRI) has better sensitivities than CT scans for soft tissues, their use in acute settings has not been validated and in fact may delay diagnosis and/or prompt treatment of NSTI. Additionally, there are logistical challenges associated with MRI. However, if time permits and when clinical suspicion of NSTI is low, MRI can be utilized to aid in the diagnosis of other soft tissue infections owing to its inherent spatial and contrast resolution [1]. MRI can also provide anatomic and pathophysiologic information about the extent and degree of soft tissue involvement, including adjacent bone.

Risk Scoring Systems

Unfortunately, true risk factors for NSTI have not been elucidated. Thus, many scoring systems have been developed to risk stratify patients. Wall et al. developed a simple risk model for discriminating NSTI from non-NSTI using their retrospective single-center cohort [14]. The study found that white blood cell count >15, 400 cells/mm^3 or a serum sodium level < 135 mmol/l was associated with NSTI, and a combination of both increased likelihood of NSTI [14]. While this tool was sensitive (90%), with a negative predictive value of 99%, it was not specific (76%) with a positive predictive value of only 26% [14].

Probably, the most widely utilized score is the Laboratory Risk Indicator for Necrotizing Fasciitis (LRINEC). This score uses six serologic measures (C-reactive protein, total white blood cell count, hemoglobin, sodium, creatinine, and glucose) to help determine the likelihood of necrotizing fasciitis being present. A score greater than or equal to 6 (maximum of 13) indicates that necrotizing fasciitis should be considered and is a reasonable cutoff to rule in the diagnosis. For intermediate- and high-risk patients (score > 6), the positive predictive value is 92% and the negative predictive value is 96%. However, a lower score doesn't rule out the diagnosis, in which case, a higher index of clinical

Table 38.1 Scoring criteria for LRINEC system

C-reactive protein (mg/L) ≥ 150: *4 points*
White blood cell count (× 10^3/mm^3): *0 points if <15, 1 point if between 15 and 25, and 2 points if >25*
Hemoglobin (g/dl): *0 point if >13.5, 1 point if between 11 and 13.5, and 2 points if <11*
Sodium (mmol/L) < 135: *2 points*
Creatinine (umol/L) > 141: *2 points*
Glucose (mmol/L) > 10: *1 point*

suspicion is warranted [15]. The scoring criteria are included in Table 38.1.

There are limited contemporary scoring systems to help predict hospital length of stay and morbidity. For instance, a retrospective review of 54 patients who were treated for Fournier's gangrene between 2010 and 2016 at one of the largest public hospitals was utilized to develop a novel scoring system, the Combined Urology and Plastics Index (CUPI) [16]. When compared to other existing scoring systems, only the newly calculated CUPI score was shown to be a significant predictor of longer hospital stay. Regardless, early emphasis on supportive care, nutrition, and prompt involvement of surgeons can, to some extent, minimize length of stay in select patients.

Management

Necrotizing soft tissue infection can progress rapidly and cause systemic toxicity. Host defense mechanisms can be rapidly overwhelmed, leading to rapid spread, hemodynamic compromise, and ultimately organ failure. Expeditious treatment must be carried out to prevent rapid decompensation. Definitive treatment is surgical debridement, and delay in operation is the major risk factor for morbidity and mortality [5].

Antibiotics

While early surgical debridement is the most important aspect of treating NSTI, timely implementation of broad-spectrum antibiotics is essential. Many NSTI patients are first seen in the ER, and implementation of antibiotics prior to going to surgery is vital. In general, antibiotic choice should include coverage against gram-positive, gram-negative, and anaerobic organisms. Consideration should be made for Group A *Streptococcus* and *Clostridium* species. Acceptable broad-spectrum regimens that should be initiated immediately include an agent from each of the following three categories:

1. A carbapenem such as imipenem, meropenem, or ertapenem or a beta-lactamase inhibitor such as piperacillin-tazobactam, ampicillin-sulbactam, or ticarcillin-clavulanate. Patients allergic to all of these agents could be treated with an aminoglycoside or a fluoroquinolone, plus metronidazole.
2. Clindamycin for its antitoxin effects against toxin-producing strains of streptococci and staphylococci [17, 18].
3. An agent with methicillin-resistant *Staphylococcus aureus* activity such as vancomycin, daptomycin, or linezolid.

Coverage of other less common organisms bears mentioning based on the patient's history and physical exam. Patients with a history of trauma in fresh or marine water may warrant coverage of *Aeromonas*. The Infectious Disease Society of America suggests that either ciprofloxacin or ceftriaxone be used in combination with doxycycline for *Aeromonas* coverage [7]. Patients with a history of trauma in sea water may need coverage of *Vibrio vulnificus*. Empiric antibiotics for *Vibrio vulnificus* include a third-generation cephalosporin plus a tetracycline. Presentation of NSTI from *Vibrio vulnificus* and *Aeromonas* can be similar, making ceftriaxone and doxycycline a good choice for empiric coverage [19].

Broad-spectrum coverage should be continued until culture results are available. Antibiotics can be tailored to gram stain, culture, and sensitivity results. For group A *streptococcal* or other beta-hemolytic *streptococcal* infection, antibiotics can be narrowed to penicillin and clindamycin. Treatment for methicillin-resistant *Staphylococcus aureus* can also be discontinued, if appropriate, when culture and sensitivity results have resulted. Optimal duration of antibiotic treatment for NSTI has not been established. At a minimum, antibiotics should be continued until no further debridement is necessary and the patient's hemodynamic status has normalized [20]. Duration of antibiotics should be individualized to each patient's clinical status.

Surgical Management

NSTIs are true surgical emergencies. Operative debridement should not be delayed by radiological studies if there are clear signs of NSTI on physical exam. Operative treatment should include aggressive debridement of all necrotic, devitalized tissue. Necrotic issue may appear swollen and fascia may have a dull-gray appearance, and tissue planes can often be easily separated. The first goal of surgery is to do a wound exploration to determine the extent of infection. The tissue necrosis usually extends well beyond the boundaries of skin infection. As a result, exposure should be wide, and excision should extend beyond the boundaries of viable tissue. It is important to extend until healthy bleeding tissue is encountered. It is imperative that some devitalized tissue be sent for gram stain and culture. However, the use of bedside or intraoperative frozen sections has limited utility likely due to lack of sensitivity and specificity and risk for delayed diagnosis and treatment [21].

After debridement is carried out, the wound should be covered with sterile dressing, and patient should be admitted to the ICU for supportive care and antibiotics. In a NSTI of the abdominal wall, a temporary abdominal closure may be necessary. A return to the operating room 24 h after the initial wound exploration is mandatory [7]. This ensures that all necrotic tissue has been debrided. In general, operative debridement should be carried out on a daily basis until the infection is well controlled. Patients that require increasing inotropes or vasopressors or whom are otherwise clinically declining should return to the operating room earlier than planned.

When the wound has been adequately debrided, a decision can be made about wound coverage. In some cases, wound healing by secondary intent is adequate, and negative pressure dressings can help the healing process. For more complex wound defects, reconstruction may be necessary. Strategies for wound coverage include skin grafts, fascio-cutaneous flaps, or myocutaneous flaps. Rarely, for NSTI of the extremities, an amputation may be necessary [22].

More recently, there is a growing interest in utilizing a skin-sparing approach for treatment of NSTI. While rapid progression of NSTI necessitates aggressive surgical debridement, this approach often leaves survivors with large surface area defects/wounds, comparable to full-thickness burns. These wounds can be challenging to manage as they often require skin grafting and extensive rehabilitation. In some instances, skin-sparing debridement may be feasible and improve reconstructive options at subsequent surgery. Using this approach, the debridement only focuses on tissues directly involved in necrosis and spares viable skin and subcutaneous tissue [23]. According to one study, this approach has decreased skin graft size and allowed some wounds to be closed by delayed primary closure alone [23], and this allows for subsequent reconstruction.

Adjunct Management

Hyperbaric oxygen therapy may improve outcomes in patients with NSTI when used as an adjunctive therapy in addition to antibiotics and surgical debridement. An animal study carried out in dogs showed a survival benefit in *Clostridium* infection [24]. Other studies have shown a benefit when using hyperbaric oxygen as an adjunct for *Clostridium* infection [25], Fournier's gangrene [20], and necrotizing fasciitis [10, 11]. Randomized controlled trials are needed to determine if there is truly an advantage to using hyperbaric oxygen for NSTI. Likewise, although IV immune globulin (IVIG) has been used as an adjunct treatment for patients with necrotizing fasciitis, multiple studies have shown that there is no benefit to administering IVIG for patients [26, 27].

Future Directions

Given the increasing prevalence of NSTI, and the challenges associated with prompt diagnosis and treatment, extensive research is ongoing to develop novel drugs for treatment of NSTI. For example, Reltecimod (previously AB103) is a peptide mimetic of the T-lymphocyte receptor, CD28, that has demonstrated safety and efficacy in modulating inflammation after NSTI in a prospective, randomized, placebo-controlled, double-blinded study across six academic medical centers in the United States [28]. This drug is currently undergoing Phase 3 trial, also known as the ACCUTE trial (Reltecimod Clinical Composite Endpoint Study in Necrotizing Soft Tissue Infections) with planned recruitment of 290 patients from approximately 60 sites in the United States. This trial will evaluate several endpoints including recovery from acute kidney injury, days in the ICU and on ventilator, 30-day hospital readmission rate, and 3-month survival [29].

Intensive Care Unity Treatment

Patients with NSTI are often intravascularly depleted, and immediate fluid resuscitation should begin as soon as the diagnosis is made. Obtaining euvolemia helps maintain adequate end-organ perfusion and tissue oxygenation. Patients that are in shock or that have concomitant cardiac or pulmonary comorbidities may benefit from adjunct methods of monitoring fluid status such as bedside ultrasound, central venous monitoring, or pulmonary artery catheterization. Vasopressors or inotropes should be used to maintain organ perfusion. Renal failure is common among patients with NSTI [30].

Furthermore, patients with NSTI should begin nutritional support as soon as possible. Enteral feeding is preferred over parenteral feeding. Patients that are ventilated for a prolonged amount of time should have enteral access for enteral feeds. Patients with NSTI often have increased total caloric demands due to a hypermetabolic state. In addition, open wounds can lead to large protein loss and increased protein requirements [30].

Outcomes

Mortality from necrotizing soft tissue is high, ranging from 14% to 59%. Several factors have been found to influence mortality. In one study, variables associated with mortality included a white blood cell count over 30,000/uL, a serum creatinine over 2.0 mg/dL, infection with *Clostridium* species, and preexisting heart disease on admission [31]. A prior study carried out in Taiwan found that liver cirrhosis, the presence of soft tissue emphysema, *Aeromonas* infection, age over 60 years, bandemia over 10%, activated partial thromboplastin time over 60 s, bacteremia, and creatinine over 2 mg/dL were significantly associated with mortality [32].

Earlier studies have also shown that delay in operative debridement for more than 24 h is strongly associated with mortality. In addition, an infection involving the head, neck, thorax, and abdomen was a risk factor for death, likely due to difficulty in debridement [33]. The mortality rate for Fournier's gangrene specifically ranges from 22% to 40% [34]. The presence of streptococcal toxic shock syndrome greatly increases the risk of mortality [35]. Survival in Fournier's gangrene is significantly associated with several laboratory parameters including urea, creatinine, bicarbonate, sodium potassium, total protein, albumin, white blood cell count, lactate dehydrogenase, and alkaline phosphatase. In addition, involvement of higher percentages of body surface area is significantly associated with mortality in Fournier's gangrene [36].

Conclusion

Necrotizing soft tissue infections are relatively infrequent but highly lethal infections, encompassing a spectrum of presentations with varying severity of soft tissue infections. Prompt diagnosis and treatment of NSTI can be challenging but are extremely crucial to survival. Given the relative rarity of this disease presentation, familiarity of epidemiology, clinical presentation, and laboratory and imaging diagnostic tools and understanding various facets of perioperative treatment, including surgical treatment, are essential. Surgical debridement remains the mainstay treatment for NSTI, combined with antimicrobial therapy and supportive adjuvant therapies in the perioperative setting. There is some role for existing risk prediction scores; however, further research is warranted to better identify high-risk patients for novel treatments and future clinical trials [7].

References

1. Hayeri MR, et al. Soft-tissue infections and their imaging mimics: from cellulitis to necrotizing fasciitis. Radiographics. 2016;36(6):1888–910.
2. Cocanour CS, et al. Management and novel adjuncts of necrotizing soft tissue infections. Surg Infect. 2017;18(3):250–72.
3. Esposito S, et al. Diagnosis and management of skin and soft-tissue infections (SSTI). A literature review and consensus statement: an update. J Chemother. 2017;29(4):197–214.
4. Hakkarainen TW, et al. Necrotizing soft tissue infections: review and current concepts in treatment, systems of care, and outcomes. Curr Probl Surg. 2014;51(8):344–62.
5. Kobayashi L, et al. Necrotizing soft tissue infections: delayed surgical treatment is associated with increased number of surgical debridements and morbidity. J Trauma. 2011;71(5):1400–5.
6. Soltani AM, et al. Trends in the incidence and treatment of necrotizing soft tissue infections: an analysis of the National Hospital Discharge Survey. J Burn Care Res. 2014;35(5):449–54.
7. Stevens DL, et al. Practice guidelines for the diagnosis and management of skin and soft tissue infections: 2014 update by the Infectious Diseases Society of America. Clin Infect Dis. 2014;59(2):e10–52.
8. Kao LS, et al. Local variations in the epidemiology, microbiology, and outcome of necrotizing soft-tissue infections: a multicenter study. Am J Surg. 2011;202(2):139–45.
9. Zhao-Fleming H, Dissanaike S, Rumbaugh K. Are anaerobes a major, underappreciated cause of necrotizing infections? Anaerobe. 2017;45:65–70.
10. Bonne SL, Kadri SS. Evaluation and management of necrotizing soft tissue infections. Infect Dis Clin N Am. 2017;31(3):497–511.
11. Chen KJ, et al. Presentation and outcomes of necrotizing soft tissue infections. Int J Gen Med. 2017;10:215–20.
12. Sarani B, et al. Necrotizing fasciitis: current concepts and review of the literature. J Am Coll Surg. 2009;208(2):279–88.
13. Keung EZ, et al. Immunocompromised status in patients with necrotizing soft-tissue infection. JAMA Surg. 2013;148(5):419–26.
14. Wall DB, et al. A simple model to help distinguish necrotizing fasciitis from nonnecrotizing soft tissue infection. J Am Coll Surg. 2000;191(3):227–31.
15. Wong CH, et al. The LRINEC (Laboratory Risk Indicator for Necrotizing Fasciitis) score: a tool for distinguishing necrotizing fasciitis from other soft tissue infections. Crit Care Med. 2004;32(7):1535–41.
16. Ghodoussipour SB, et al. Surviving Fournier's gangrene: multivariable analysis and a novel scoring system to predict length of stay. J Plast Reconstr Aesthet Surg. 2018;71(5):712–8.
17. Zimbelman J, Palmer A, Todd J. Improved outcome of clindamycin compared with beta-lactam antibiotic treatment for invasive Streptococcus pyogenes infection. Pediatr Infect Dis J. 1999;18(12):1096–100.
18. Stevens DL, Bryant AE, Hackett SP. Antibiotic effects on bacterial viability, toxin production, and host response. Clin Infect Dis. 1995;20(Suppl 2):S154–7.
19. Chen PL, et al. A comparative study of clinical Aeromonas dhakensis and Aeromonas hydrophila isolates in southern Taiwan: A. dhakensis is more predominant and virulent. Clin Microbiol Infect. 2014;20(7):O428–34.
20. Lauerman MH, et al. Less is more? Antibiotic duration and outcomes in Fournier's gangrene. J Trauma Acute Care Surg. 2017;83(3):443–8.
21. Solomon IH, et al. Frozen sections are unreliable for the diagnosis of necrotizing soft tissue infections. Mod Pathol. 2018;31(4):546–52.
22. Anaya DA, Dellinger EP. Necrotizing soft-tissue infection: diagnosis and management. Clin Infect Dis. 2007;44(5):705–10.
23. Tom LK, et al. A skin-sparing approach to the treatment of necrotizing soft-tissue infections: thinking reconstruction at initial debridement. J Am Coll Surg. 2016;222(5):e47–60.
24. Demello FJ, Haglin JJ, Hitchcock CR. Comparative study of experimental Clostridium perfringens infection in dogs treated with antibiotics, surgery, and hyperbaric oxygen. Surgery. 1973;73(6):936–41.
25. Roth RN, Weiss LD. Hyperbaric oxygen and wound healing. Clin Dermatol. 1994;12(1):141–56.
26. Madsen MB, et al. Immunoglobulin for necrotising soft tissue infections (INSTINCT): protocol for a randomised trial. Dan Med J. 2016;63(7):pii: A5250.
27. Darenberg J, et al. Intravenous immunoglobulin G therapy in streptococcal toxic shock syndrome: a European randomized, double-blind, placebo-controlled trial. Clin Infect Dis. 2003;37(3):333–40.
28. Bulger EM, et al. A novel drug for treatment of necrotizing soft-tissue infections: a randomized clinical trial. JAMA Surg. 2014;149(6):528–36.

29. Study ATB-202. http://www.atoxbio.com/pipeline/nsti/phase-3/. Accessed 26 Mar 2018.
30. Phan HH, Cocanour CS. Necrotizing soft tissue infections in the intensive care unit. Crit Care Med. 2010;38(9 Suppl):S460–8.
31. Anaya DA, et al. Predictors of mortality and limb loss in necrotizing soft tissue infections. Arch Surg. 2005;140(2):151–7. discussion 158
32. Huang KF, et al. Independent predictors of mortality for necrotizing fasciitis: a retrospective analysis in a single institution. J Trauma. 2011;71(2):467–73. discussion 473
33. Wong CH, et al. Necrotizing fasciitis: clinical presentation, microbiology, and determinants of mortality. J Bone Joint Surg Am. 2003;85-A(8):1454–60.
34. Laucks SS 2nd. Fournier's gangrene. Surg Clin North Am. 1994;74(6):1339–52.
35. Darenberg J, et al. Molecular and clinical characteristics of invasive group A streptococcal infection in Sweden. Clin Infect Dis. 2007;45(4):450–8.
36. Yeniyol CO, et al. Fournier's gangrene: experience with 25 patients and use of Fournier's gangrene severity index score. Urology. 2004;64(2):218–22.

Management of Bariatric Complications for the General Surgeon

39

Essa M. Aleassa and Stacy Brethauer

Introduction

Obesity and obesity-related comorbidities have become prevalent across the globe among all age ranges. Currently, one-third of the US population is obese [1]. The increase in the prevalence of obesity and the extensive evidence proving the safety and efficacy of bariatric surgery have led to the increased acceptance of this as a surgical discipline worldwide. More surgeons are also completing fellowship training in bariatric and metabolic surgery which has resulted in widespread application of these procedures. All of these factors have led to increased number of bariatric and metabolic procedures performed worldwide. In the United States, approximately 200,000 bariatric procedures are performed annually [2].

Managing complications in this population can present some unique challenges. Changes in the gastrointestinal anatomy, particularly the Roux-en-Y reconstruction, can present challenges when access to the excluded stomach or biliary tree is needed. Foreign bodies such as the adjustable band can obstruct or erode and occasionally present acutely. And finally, a small bowel obstruction may need to be managed differently than it would in a non-bariatric surgery

patient to avoid a catastrophic outcome. Understanding the anatomy unique to each procedure and recognizing the most serious or life-threatening complications after bariatric surgery are critical to successful management of the bariatric surgery patient. In this chapter, we aim to provide the general surgeon called to manage these patients with the information and management strategies to achieve a successful outcome.

Overview of Bariatric Procedures

Bariatric surgery is a well-established and durable treatment for obesity and its metabolic complications. The most commonly performed procedures in the United States are sleeve gastrectomy (SG) which represents about 60% of procedures currently and Roux-en-Y gastric bypass (RYGB) which represents about 35% of bariatric procedures performed. Adjustable gastric banding was widely performed a decade ago, but its utilization has decreased to about 5% of all bariatric operations due to the unpredictable outcomes and high reoperation rates seen with the band in the United States [2]. Despite the low number of bands currently being placed, there are many patients who still may present with a complication from a band place years ago.

Understanding the anatomy of different bariatric operations is essential to managing the complications after these procedures. Over 95% of

E. M. Aleassa · S. Brethauer (✉)
Department of Surgery, Cleveland Clinic,
Cleveland, OH, USA
e-mail: brethas@ccf.org

© Springer International Publishing AG, part of Springer Nature 2019
C. V. R. Brown et al. (eds.), *Emergency General Surgery*, https://doi.org/10.1007/978-3-319-96286-3_39

primary bariatric procedures are now performed laparoscopically. In RYGB, the stomach is divided to form a small proximal gastric pouch about 30 cc in volume. The distal stomach is separated from the pouch but is not resected and is referred to as the gastric remnant by bariatric surgeons. Following that, the proximal jejunum is divided 50 cm distal to the ligament of Treitz and the distal end brought up (usually antecolic, occasionally retrocolic) and anastomosed to the gastric pouch. The other (proximal) end of the divided jejunum is referred to as the biliopancreatic limb and is anastomosed 150 cm downstream from the gastrojejunostomy. The biliopancreatic juices and food then travel distally in the common channel beyond the "Roux" anastomosis (Fig. 39.1).

During sleeve gastrectomy, the gastric fundus and body are vertically resected leaving 15–20% of the stomach behind along the lesser curvature. The final product resembles a tubular banana-shaped stomach that empties normally through the pylorus. It is important to note that there are no anastomoses created in sleeve gastrectomy

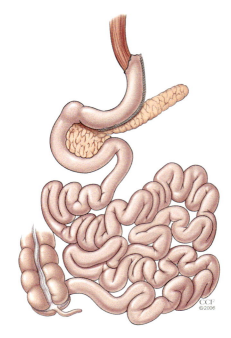

Fig. 39.2 Illustration of a sleeve gastrectomy

(Fig. 39.2). Most surgeons reinforce the long vertical staple line with synthetic buttressing material or by oversewing or inverting the staple line.

Laparoscopic adjustable gastric banding involves placement of a silicon band around the proximal stomach just below the gastroesophageal junction (Fig. 39.3). The gastric fundus is plicated over the band anteriorly with two or three interrupted sutures to help prevent prolapse of the stomach upward through the band. The inner circumference of the band is a circular balloon that is connected to tubing and a subcutaneous port. Typically, it takes several "adjustments" using saline injected into the subcutaneous port to tighten the circumference of the band enough to achieve the desired effect of decreased hunger and early satiety.

Diagnosis of Urgent Bariatric Complications

Roux-en-Y Gastric Bypass

RYGB is a safe operation in general; however a small percentage (1–2%) of patients may develop serious complications [3]. It is helpful

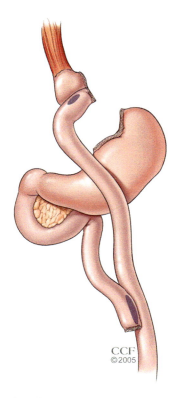

Fig. 39.1 Illustration of a Roux-en-Y gastric bypass

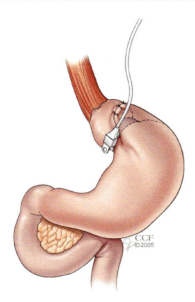

Fig. 39.3 Illustration of a laparoscopic adjustable gastric banding

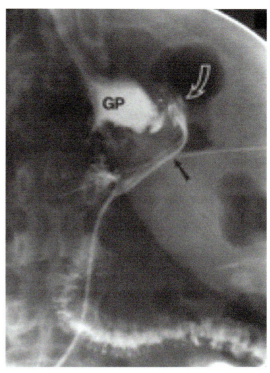

Fig. 39.4 Free extravasation of oral contrast from a leak at the gastrojejunostomy. Contrast is being picked up by the drain

to classify complications by the onset of presentation postoperatively: acute (<7 days), early (7 days–4 weeks), late (4–12 weeks), or chronic (>12 weeks). Major acute and early postoperative complications consist of anastomotic leaks, hemorrhage, and small bowel obstruction. Late and chronic complications consist of internal hernia, bowel obstruction, anastomotic ulcers and strictures, intussusception, and micronutrient deficiencies.

Anastomotic leaks after gastric bypass now occur less than 0.5% of the time but remain the second leading cause of death (after pulmonary embolism) following bariatric surgery [4]. Most early postoperative leaks occur at the gastrojejunostomy and present with early signs of sepsis. Resting tachycardia >120, tachypnea, fevers, and worsening abdominal pain, in a patient that is not progressing normally after surgery, are all concerning signs and symptoms of a leak. A high level of suspicion and early diagnosis are the keys to a favorable outcome. Any suspicion of a leak should be evaluated with imaging, either an upper GI or a CT with oral contrast (Fig. 39.4). The advantage of CT imaging is that it can also detect other complications such as an early bowel obstruction or distal leak that would not be detected with an

upper GI contrast study and may mimic the signs of a leak. If the patient is becoming ill and hypoxic but the etiology is not clear, the optimal imaging is a chest, abdomen, and pelvis CT with intravenous contrast timed for the pulmonary artery anatomy with a small amount (one or two cups) of oral contrast given before the scan to help in detecting leaks.

Small bowel obstructions can occur anytime after RYGB, and it is important to remember that these patients cannot be managed like a typical adhesive bowel obstruction in a non-bariatric patient. Because the biliopancreatic limb and gastric remnant cannot be decompressed with a nasogastric tube, a distal obstruction can result in massive dilation and perforation of this anatomy if it is not surgically decompressed.

Early postoperative bowel obstructions are typically secondary to a mechanical problem (kinking or narrowing) at the jejunojejunostomy (Fig. 39.5), an intraluminal clot at the jejunojejunostomy (Fig. 39.6) or beyond, or distal adhesive

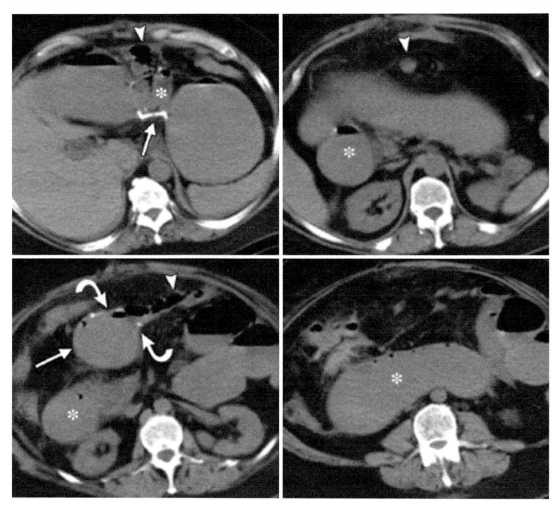

Fig. 39.5 Acute dilation of the gastric remnant and bilio-pancreatic limbs after gastric bypass due to an obstruction at the jejunojejunostomy (JJ) (curved arrows). This requires emergent surgical intervention with placement of a decompressive remnant gastrostomy tube and correction of the obstruction at the JJ anastomosis

disease from prior pelvic surgery [5]. Another cause of early postoperative bowel obstruction is a port site or abdominal wall hernia that entraps a loop of small bowel. These complications can be challenging to diagnose in patients with severe obesity, and CT imaging should be performed when concern arises. Patients with early postop bowel obstructions may look well initially but then fail to progress with their oral intake and develop worsening nausea and abdominal pain. Abdominal distension can be hard to elicit as well in this population so subjective finding of bloating, worsening nausea, pressure, and abdominal pain should prompt an evaluation. Plain film imaging can detect a distal obstruction but will often not alert the surgeon to a dilated, fluid-filled gastric remnant that needs decompression. Early postop bowel obstructions after RYGB require operative intervention and should not be managed nonoperatively. At a minimum, the gastric remnant should be decompressed with a surgical gastrostomy tube and, if possible in a stable patient, the source of the obstruction addressed.

Late bowel obstructions after RYGB most commonly result from adhesive disease or internal her-

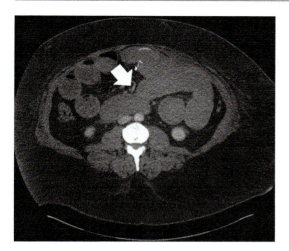

Fig. 39.6 Early postoperative small bowel obstruction secondary to intraluminal clot at the jejunojejunostomy

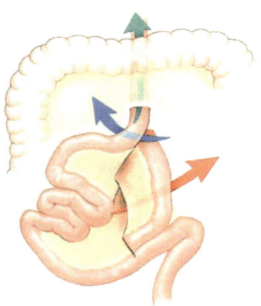

Fig. 39.7 Potential sites of internal hernia after RYGB. Most commonly, the small bowel herniates underneath the Roux limb mesentery or at the jejunojejunostomy mesenteric defect. If the Roux limb was placed retrocolic, the defect in the mesocolon is also a potential site of herniation

nias. Roux-en-Y reconstruction results in two mesenteric defects that can reopen and cause an internal hernia with mesenteric volvulus, obstruction, and bowel ischemia. These defects are located at the jejunojejunostomy behind the mesentery of the Roux limb as it passes over the colon mesentery and transverse colon. If the Roux limb is in the retrocolic position, the mesenteric defect (Peterson's defect) and the mesocolic defect are potential sites of herniation. The majority of bariatric surgeons now close these defects with nonabsorbable suture at the primary operation, but they can reopen after massive weight loss (Fig. 39.7).

Gastric bypass patients who present with sudden onset, severe mid-abdominal pain (often with an antecedent history of intermittent pain) should have CT imaging done immediately to rule out an internal hernia, volvulus, or obstruction (Fig. 39.8). Delaying the diagnosis and treatment of this problem can result in the loss of the entire midgut and a catastrophic outcome for the patient (Fig. 39.9).

If clinical concern is high and imaging is equivocal or negative, a diagnostic laparoscopy is still appropriate to rule out an internal hernia or to identify another cause of the pain [6].

Bowel intussusception is a rare cause of obstruction and most commonly occurs at the jejunojejunal anastomosis which can become dilated and patulous years after the original sur-

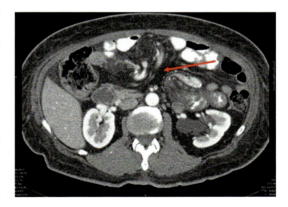

Fig. 39.8 Axial image of an internal hernia in a patient with a history of gastric bypass

gery. Small incidental intussusceptions seen on imaging in an asymptomatic patient do not require surgery, but if the intussusception is causing pain or an obstruction, operative intervention should be carried out (Fig. 39.10). In some cases, this may require resection and reconstruction of a new Roux anastomosis.

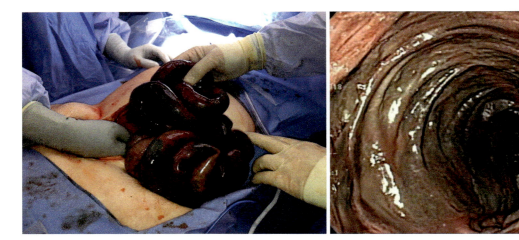

Fig. 39.9 Intraoperative findings of extensive bowel necrosis in a 56-year-old RYGB patient who presented three times to her local emergency department with severe abdominal pain prior to transfer. The entire small bowel had herniated underneath the Roux limb mesentery causing necrosis of the midgut and the Roux limb (endoscopy picture)

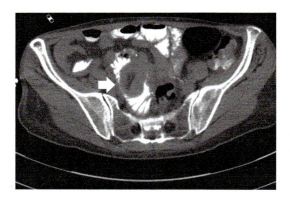

Fig. 39.10 Small bowel intussusception seen on CT imaging in a patient who presented with severe abdominal pain and obstructive symptoms

Marginal ulcers usually form chronically post-RYGB, usually on the small bowel side of the gastrojejunal anastomosis. Marginal ulcers are linked to smoking, nonsteroidal anti-inflammatory drug (NSAID) use, acid exposure from a large gastric pouch, and presence of foreign body at the anastomosis such as an eroded suture. Patients presenting with early marginal ulcers usually complain of epigastric pain after eating and nausea. The majority of ulcers after bypass can be managed medically, but patients will occasionally present with a perforation of a chronic marginal ulcer that requires emergent surgery. This problem presents as acute epigastric pain that worsens and progresses to peritonitis. Imaging will reveal free air and likely some free fluid. Management is surgical and should consist of repair if possible, omental patch, and wide drainage. There is no role for revising the anastomosis in the setting of an acute perforation. Placing a feeding gastrostomy tube in the gastric remnant should be considered depending on the condition of the patient.

Early postoperative bleeding after RYGB should be managed as with any other patient, but there are several unique circumstances in a gastric bypass patient that should be considered. Intra-abdominal bleeding most commonly occurs at one of the mesenteries that was divided during the procedure or from a staple line. Potential intraluminal bleeding sites include the pouch staple line, the gastrojejunostomy, the gastric remnant staple line, and the jejunojejunostomy staple line. While most of these events are self-limiting, they can occasionally require surgery if the intraluminal clot causes an obstruction at the jejunojejunostomy. Bleeding at the gastrojejunostomy is typically heralded by hematemesis and can be managed endoscopically.

Sleeve Gastrectomy

Sleeve gastrectomy has become the most commonly performed bariatric operation in the United States, largely because it eliminates the risk of anastomotic complications and is widely accepted by patients. The major morbidity rate is less than 2%, and adverse events mainly include staple line leaks, fistula formation, and sleeve stenosis and stricture resulting in an obstruction [7].

The most feared complication after sleeve gastrectomy is a staple line leak. Leaks after sleeve gastrectomy most often present in the first week after surgery but can occasionally present with a left upper quadrant abscess weeks later. The majority of leaks after sleeve gastrectomy occur proximally at the angle of His. Clinically, leaks will present as abdominal sepsis with fever and tachycardia. As with RYGB leaks, early detection and operative management of an early, uncontained leak are key to achieving a good outcome. In stable patients who present with a contained left upper quadrant abscess, percutaneous drainage is appropriate prior to referring the patient to a bariatric surgeon who can continue the management.

Patients with sleeve stenosis can present soon after surgery with failure to advance diet and or excessive vomiting. This can be a result of technical issues while creating the sleeve, and the most common site of narrowing is at the incisura. Twisting or kinking of the staple line can also result in a functional obstruction and severe GERD. This is not a complication that requires urgent surgical management, however, and these patients can be referred to a bariatric surgeon for further evaluation and management.

Laparoscopic Adjustable Gastric Banding

Complications after LAGB that might involve the general surgeon include acute perforation or bleeding shortly after band placement, gastric prolapse, obstruction at the band, and erosion. Mechanical problems with the tubing or port

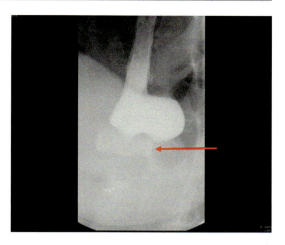

Fig. 39.11 Obstruction and pouch dilation due to an overtightened adjustable gastric band (arrow)

usually require operative repair, but these would not be emergent issues and can be referred to a bariatric surgeon.

Placing the band involves creating a small retroesophageal tunnel above the lesser sac and passing an instrument through this space to pull the band into place. This maneuver can result in a perforation or injury to the esophagus or gastric fundus that may not be immediately recognized. Since most LAGB patients are discharged the same day as surgery, they may present with abdominal sepsis secondary to a perforation several days after the injury. Upper GI contrast studies or CT imaging will confirm the diagnosis and prompt emergent operative intervention that should include removal of the band, closure of the perforation if possible, and wide drainage (Fig. 39.11). Bleeding can occur from injury to the short gastric vessels or spleen that may not be evident until the patient returns to the emergency department with hypotension or syncope at home.

Algorithmic Approach to Abdominal Pain in Patients with History of Bariatric Surgery

The American Society for Metabolic and Bariatric Surgery and the American College of Emergency Physicians have developed a practice guideline for Bariatric Examination, Assessment, and Management in the Emergency Department (BEAM-ED) to guide physicians on how to approach patients presenting to the emergency department with potential complications after bariatric surgery [8]. While this program was designed for use by ED physicians, it provides a structured, algorithmic approach to evaluating bariatric surgery patients that would be a helpful resource for the general surgeon called on to evaluate these problems.

In addition to routine history, the patient's surgical history should consist of information about the type of bariatric procedure performed, the surgeon who performed the procedure, and the center where the procedure took place. This information helps narrow down the etiology of the presenting symptom. Most complications post-bariatric procedures are unique to the procedures performed as described above. Identifying the surgeon and, if needed, contacting him/her would help provide necessary information and guide the management plan. Some surgeons work within bariatric surgery groups with associates on call round the clock. Locating the facility where the index procedure was performed can facilitate transfer of care if the patient presents with a non-emergent problem. Bariatric coverage or transfer is not always available, though, and treatment of emergent problems like perforations or internal hernias should not be delayed by transferring the patient as the additional time required may result in a worse outcome or death.

The presenting symptoms should be put into the context of the procedure performed and the timing since surgery. Gauging the duration of onset of symptoms can aid in determining the urgency of the presenting pathology; i.e., patients presenting with acute onset severe abdominal pain within the first 4 weeks postoperatively should be investigated for staple line or anastomotic leak after a sleeve gastrectomy or a gastric bypass, respectively. It is imperative to consider internal hernia and/or intestinal obstruction in patients presenting with obstructive symptoms within the same time frame. Patients with chronic abdominal pain presenting more than 4 weeks postoperatively are better managed by a bariatric surgery team as further investigation might be warranted.

Complications of bariatric surgery are not always evident. This highlights the importance of high clinical suspicion and experience dealing with bariatric surgery patients. The patient's overall status reflected in the vital signs and subjective symptomatology can help make the decision to either further investigate the patient noninvasively through imaging or invasively through a diagnostic laparoscopy or laparotomy. Signs such as fever, tachycardia, increased oxygen requirements, pain out of proportion to physcial examination or peritonitis in the setting of hemodynamic instability require prompt operative exploration after initial resuscitation.

It is important to emphasize that a general surgeon can manage all bariatric emergencies by following basic surgical principles and having some knowledge of the anatomy and potential management options. Generally speaking, damage control procedures in the deteriorating patient are appropriate, and no definitive reconstruction or repair is necessary at the initial operation. Controlling the immediate problem of contamination or bleeding, wide drainage, stabilizing the patient, and then making arrangements for transfer to a bariatric surgeon are appropriate care in this setting.

In a stable patient, there is more time to investigate the presenting symptoms. Diagnoses such as appendicitis, cholecystitis, diverticulitis, and nephrolithiasis should be considered when appropriate. In female patients, pregnancy status and other gynecological causes for abdominal symptoms should be assessed. Presence of a pulmonary embolism, deep venous thrombosis, or portomesenteric thrombus in patients presenting with concordant symptoms should be ruled out. D-dimer levels and CT angiography can be added to the work-up in these cases [9].

Management of Specific Complications

Scenario 1: Obstructing Adjustable Gastric Band

A 36-year-old female with a recent history of LAGB (8 months ago) presents with nausea, vomiting, and postprandial abdominal pain. She describes her symptoms to have started a week ago after a band adjustment in her surgeon's office. The patient otherwise looks healthy and her vital signs are within normal limits, but she continues to have dry heaves with any oral intake. She called her bariatric surgeon's office but he is out of town so she was told to report to the nearest emergency department.

Diagnostic Test Upper GI contrast study. This reveals obstruction at the level of the band with moderately dilated gastric pouch above the band and severe gastroesophageal reflux of contrast.

Management The balloon in the band needs to be deflated. A Huber™ needle can be inserted into the subcutaneous port palpated on the anterior abdominal wall. Patients typically know where their port is located. The port can be stabilized between two fingers while the patient lifts his/her head off the pillow, and the port is percutaneously accessed as any mediport would be. If a LAGB-specific Huber™ needle isn't available, any type of needle can be used in this urgent setting. Once accessed, all of the fluid should be aspirated out of the system. The patient can be given oral fluids and discharged home if symptoms are resolved and fluids are tolerated. Close follow-up with her bariatric surgeon should be arranged to further manage the band.

Scenario 2: Internal Hernia After Roux-en-Y Gastric Bypass

A 55-year-old female 3 years post laparoscopic gastric bypass presents to the emergency department with sudden, severe abdominal pain that started 6 hours ago. The abdominal pain is associated with nausea and dry heaving. When asked, she reports that her last bowel movement and flatus were on the previous morning. She has had two similar, but less severe, episodes of this pain in the last month that resolved after 2 hours. Her heart rate is 120 bpm and her blood pressure is 100/75 mmHg. On examination, she cannot get comfortable in the bed, and her abdomen is diffusely tender but soft without peritonitis.

Diagnostic Test CT of the abdomen and pelvis. Sudden onset of severe abdominal pain after gastric bypass must be considered an internal hernia or small bowel volvulus until proven otherwise. This patient may not tolerate a full dose of oral contrast for the CT, but an attempt to ingest some should be made. IV contrast should be used unless contraindicated. The pathognomonic finding on CT is the "swirl sign" of the mesenteric vasculature suggesting an internal hernia (Fig. 39.12). Other findings of bowel obstruction may or may not be present in the acute setting. Routine labs including serum lactate may further support the diagnosis of early bowel ischemia.

Management In this clinical setting, any findings on CT suggesting an internal hernia, closed loop obstruction, or bowel obstruction or ischemia require emergent operation. After resuscitation, the patient's abdomen should be explored laparoscopically or open depending on the surgeon's expertise. Internal herniation of the small bowel most commonly occurs under the mesentery of the Roux limb or through the jejunojeju-

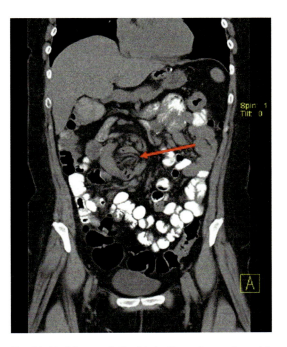

Fig. 39.12 Mesenteric "swirl sign" seen in a patient with an internal hernia after gastric bypass

nostomy mesenteric defect. The bowel should be run *distally to proximally* starting at the terminal ileum to effectively reduce the volvulus and then assessed for viability. Untwisting the bowel and identifying the site of the internal hernia can be confusing, even for an experienced bariatric surgeon, so care should be taken to slowly follow the bowel's course and reduce it to the normal position rather than performing a bowel transection to achieve this. In cases of chronic internal hernia, some adhesiolysis may be needed to restore the normal RYGB anatomy. In all cases, the original anatomy can be restored with patience and careful handling of the bowel. In a stable patient, resection (if indicated) and re-anastomosis are safe. The remaining mesenteric defects should all be re-closed with nonabsorbable suture. In an unstable patient, resection only and temporary closure of the abdomen are appropriate, and intestinal continuity can be restored when the patient stabilizes. If the Roux limb is ischemic (commonly from vascular compromise due to pressure from the bowel herniated beneath it), it should be resected up to the level of the gastric pouch. Care should be taken to divide as little of the distal gastric pouch as possible and to stay below the left gastric artery pedicle so that continuity can be restored later and the gastric bypass preserved. In cases where the majority of the midgut has become necrotic, care decisions should be presented to the patient's family and, if available, the intestinal transplant team consulted to offer their opinion regarding future reconstruction.

Scenario 3: Perforated Marginal Ulcer After RYGB

A 56-year-old male presents with severe upper abdominal pain and a rigid abdomen. His past medical history is significant for a previous myocardial infarction and a Roux-en-Y gastric bypass 7 years prior. The patient has smoked one pack of cigarettes per day for the past 5 years. He is conscious and responds to questions appropriately. His heart rate is 125 bpm and his blood pressure is 105/75 mmHg.

Diagnostic Test An upright abdominal x-ray shows free air under the diaphragm. The emergency department also obtained a CT scan of his abdomen that revealed free air, a moderate amount of free fluid, and inflammatory changes around the gastrojejunostomy in the upper abdomen.

Management This patient has a perforated marginal ulcer at the gastrojejunostomy, likely related to smoking. After adequate resuscitation, the patient should be taken to the operating room. In most cases, this problem can be managed laparoscopically. A liver retractor should be placed to expose the anterior pouch, and anastomosis and placing the patient in reverse Trendelenburg position can facilitate exposure of this area. Occasionally, omentum will have already sealed the perforation in which case it can be secured with sutures as a Graham patch. If the perforation is visible, the quality of the tissue should be assessed and primary closure attempted when possible. Omentum should then be sewn in place over the repair. If the perforation is not easily localized, intraoperative endoscopy can be used to insufflate air into the pouch while submerged in saline to identify the area of bubbling. Following repair, the abdomen should be washed out and wide drainage of the gastrojejunostomy and left upper quadrant obtained.

Whenever possible, some form of enteral access for postoperative nutritional support should be achieved. In a stable patient, time can be taken to place a remnant gastrostomy tube or a feeding jejunostomy tube. If these options aren't available, a transnasal feeding tube can be placed into the Roux limb distal to the repair to provide nutritional support.

Scenario 4: Anastomotic Leak After Gastric Bypass

A 46-year-old female presents to the emergency department feeling progressively more ill 4 days after an uneventful laparoscopic Roux-en-Y gastric bypass. She reports having progressively worse abdominal pain. Her vital signs reveal a fever of 104 F and a heart rate of 136 bpm. Her abdominal exam shows generalized tenderness with guarding.

Diagnostic Test CT of the abdomen and pelvis reveals free extravasation of oral contrast from the gastrojejunostomy with a poorly defined air and fluid collection in the left upper quadrant.

Management Patients presenting acutely within days of a Roux-en-Y gastric bypass with fever and tachycardia should be evaluated for an anastomotic leak first. The most common site for leak is the gastrojejunostomy anastomosis. Imaging may not always show extravasation of oral contrast, but other secondary findings of inflammation or fluid at one of the anastomotic sites should also prompt surgical intervention. After resuscitation and initiation of antibiotics, the patient should be taken to the operating room and explored laparoscopically or open depending on the surgeon's skill set. Reverse Trendelenburg position can facilitate exposure of the upper abdomen, and the site of the leak should be clearly identified. A gastrojejunal anastomotic leak may be severely indurated, and primary closure may not be possible. In this case, omental patch and wide drainage are appropriate. If the leak is present at the jejunojejunostomy, primary repair is usually adequate, and resection is rarely needed. Enteral access of some kind should be obtained to facilitate healing postoperatively as long as the patient is stable. Once the patient has stabilized, the patient can be transferred to a bariatric surgeon and may require additional surgical or endoscopic therapy (clips, stent).

Scenario 5: Sleeve Gastrectomy Leak

A 25-year-old male presents to the emergency department 1 week after laparoscopic sleeve gastrectomy with 2 days of persistent fever and vague abdominal pain. On examination, he is found to be febrile with a heart rate of 115 bpm

and a blood pressure of 110/75 mmHg. He is ill-appearing and his abdomen is tender in the left upper quadrant.

Diagnostic Test CT of the abdomen with IV and oral contrast will provide the diagnosis of a sleeve gastrectomy leak (Fig. 39.13). There may be free or contained extravasation of oral contrast as well as an air and fluid collection in the left upper quadrant. No other imaging is necessary, and while upper GI contrast studies may show the leak, they do not provide any information about the extent of the adjacent collections.

Management A stable patient that presents with a contained left upper quadrant abscess secondary to a sleeve leak can be managed with percutaneous drainage and transfer to a bariatric center. In this case, however, there is no defined collection and there is free extravasation that must be controlled. Primary repair is rarely possible in these cases as the leak is most commonly at the GE junction and the tissue is of very poor quality

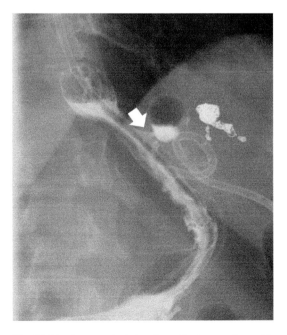

Fig. 39.13 A contrast study of a patient presenting with fever post a sleeve gastrectomy. The patient is found to have a contained leak (arrow)

by this time. The safest strategy is to wash out the left upper quadrant, sew an omental patch over the perforation, and widely drain the area. In a stable patient, a feeding jejunostomy tube should be placed as these leaks commonly evolve into chronic fistulas that require prolonged periods without oral intake to heal. Once contamination is controlled, the patient can be transferred to a bariatric center for additional endoluminal therapy to facilitate healing of the leak.

Summary

The increase in bariatric surgery procedures performed in the last decade has increased the chances that the on-call general surgeon will be faced with some of these postoperative complications. In some cases, these patients can be transferred or managed without surgical intervention, but there are some scenarios where the general surgeon should manage the acute complication to avoid progression of the problem, delays in treatment, and increased risk for patient mortality. These emergent problems in the bariatric surgery patient can be managed by the general surgeon by following basic surgical principles: stabilize the patient, identify the anatomy, identify the problem, stop contamination or bleeding, wide drainage, and enteral access if indicated. General surgeons are familiar with Roux-en-Y reconstructions, staple line leaks, internal hernias, and bowel obstructions after many other types of general surgery procedures, and it is critical that they manage these problems in bariatric patients the same way they would in patients who have had surgery for gastric cancer, biliary malignancies, and small bowel disease.

Gaining familiarity of bariatric surgery anatomy and the initial diagnosis and management of bariatric surgery complications is an important skill for the general surgeon given the increasing number of bariatric surgery patients in our soci-

ety. While bariatric surgery consultation or transfer is often appropriate and necessary, it should never delay treatment for a life-threatening complication that can be initially managed by the general surgeon on call.

References

1. Ogden CL, Carroll MD, Fryar CD, Flegal KM. Prevalence of obesity among adults and youth: United States, 2011-2014. NCHS Data Brief. 2015:1–8.
2. English WJ, DeMaria EJ, Brethauer SA, Mattar SG, Rosenthal RJ, Morton JM. American Society for Metabolic and Bariatric Surgery estimation of metabolic and bariatric procedures performed in the United States in 2016. Surg Obes Relat Dis. 2018;14:259–63.
3. Hutter MM, Schirmer BD, Jones DB, Ko CY, Cohen ME, Merkow RP, et al. First report from the American College of Surgeons Bariatric Surgery Center Network: laparoscopic sleeve gastrectomy has morbidity and effectiveness positioned between the band and the bypass. Ann Surg. 2011;254:410–20. discussion 20–2
4. Carrasquilla C, English WJ, Esposito P, Gianos J. Total stapled, total intra-abdominal (TSTI) laparoscopic Roux-en-Y gastric bypass: one leak in 1000 cases. Obes Surg. 2004;14:613–7.
5. Shimizu H, Maia M, Kroh M, Schauer PR, Brethauer SA. Surgical management of early small bowel obstruction after laparoscopic Roux-en-Y gastric bypass. Surg Obes Relat Dis. 2013;9:718–24.
6. Pitt T, Brethauer S, Sherman V, Udomsawaengsup S, Metz M, Chikunguwo S, et al. Diagnostic laparoscopy for chronic abdominal pain after gastric bypass. Surg Obes Relat Dis. 2008;4:394–8. discussion 8
7. Brethauer SA, Hammel JP, Schauer PR. Systematic review of sleeve gastrectomy as staging and primary bariatric procedure. Surg Obes Relat Dis. 2009;5:469–75.
8. American College of Emergency Physicians, American Society for Metabolic and Bariatric Surgery. BEAM-ED: Bariatric Examination, Assessment, and Management in the Emergency Department. https://www.acep.org/beam/#sm.00001uj1yvg2ccdrqtrzezeif 0xkd. 26 March 2018.
9. Shaheen O, Siejka J, Thatigotla B, Pham DT. A systematic review of portomesenteric vein thrombosis after sleeve gastrectomy. Surg Obes Relat Dis. 2017;13:1422–31.

Emergency General Surgery in the Elderly

40

Bellal Joseph and Mohammad Hamidi

Introduction

The Growing Elderly Population

It is estimated that between 2014 and 2060, the United States (USA) population will increase from 319 million to 417 million, reaching 400 million by 2051 [1]. The elderly group is the fastest-growing segment as by 2030, those 65 and older are projected to make up 20% of the American population; in other words one in every five people will be 65 and older [1].

Burden of Emergency General Surgery Conditions in the Elderly

Emergency general surgery (EGS) is referred to surgery performed when a patient has a condition that requires an emergency surgical intervention (e.g., acute appendicitis, acute cholecystitis, or acute mesenteric ischemia) [2]. Such interventions require special attention in the geriatric population (age $\geq$ 65 years) because, for instance, as an individual grows older, the number of ailing systems in the body increases. In general, emer-

gency surgery carries an abundant global health burden and is associated with high rates of mortality [3]. It's worth elaborating more on emergency surgery burden in elderly, as a Danish study by Svenningsen et al. found that emergency laparotomy carried a 48% mortality rate in patients aged >75 years [4]. A further study found that mortality rate is doubled in patients who aged 90 years and above undergoing emergency surgery as compared to younger patients. And, of notice, 1-year mortality was high after both elective (29%) and emergency surgery (49%) [5]. Another study has found that surgeries that involve bowel resection are associated with higher rates of mortality (43%) [6].

Aging and the Impact of Multiple Comorbidities

Aging is a process characterized by progressive and unavoidable physiological and biological changes. Gradually, the accumulation of such changes decreases performance and increases physiological function impairment, which results in a decreased ability to tolerate the pathological process and stress. Multiple comorbidities defined as the presence of two or more chronic conditions. The prevalence of multiple chronic conditions increases with age and is more robust in the elderly. In addition, multiple comorbidities interact synergistically instead of producing

B. Joseph (✉) · M. Hamidi
Division of Trauma, Critical Care, Burns & Emergency Surgery, Department of Surgery, Banner – University Medical Center Tucson, Tucson, AZ, USA
e-mail: bjoseph@surgery.arizona.edu

© Springer International Publishing AG, part of Springer Nature 2019
C. V. R. Brown et al. (eds.), *Emergency General Surgery*, https://doi.org/10.1007/978-3-319-96286-3_40

isolated effects. They compromise a patient's overall medical condition and usually coexist with other problems, such as addiction disorders (e.g., opioid use), mental illnesses (e.g., depression), dementia, and other cognitive impairment disorders [7–9]. The impact of aging and comorbidities in patients requiring EGS is further intensified by the risk of surgery itself as well as a lack of appropriate preoperative assessment, preparation, or optimization of the patient's general condition [10].

Common Emergency General Surgery Procedures in the Elderly

Acute Appendicitis

Acute appendicitis is the most common EGS procedure. Approximately 7–14% of the general population will develop acute appendicitis at some point in their lifetime. In the elderly, the risk of the disease is only 1:35 for women and 1:50 for men [11]. However, the manifestations of appendicitis in the elderly are associated with increased mortality and morbidity that are mainly due to a delay in the diagnosis [12]. Such a delay can be attributable to many factors, including a failure on the part of the physician to consider the diagnosis early on because of its low incidence in this population, a reluctance to operate on elderly patients, and excessive laboratory and radiographic studies prior to reaching the final diagnosis. Likewise, the blunted inflammatory response in the elderly prevents the development of significant clinical features of acute appendicitis and delays the presentation [13–15]. While the pathophysiology of appendicitis is similar in the elderly and the young, there are several differences that make the elderly more vulnerable to increased progression and early perforation. In the elderly, the lumen of the appendix is narrowed due to fibrosis, lipid accumulation, and mucosal atrophy. Moreover, the atherosclerosis of vessels compromises the blood flow to the appendix. As a result, blockage of the appendix lumen due to any cause with a mild increase in intraluminal pressure can lead to ischemia, gangrene, and perforation. Perforation rates are higher in the elderly; the reported incidence of perforation in elderly patients with acute appendicitis is as high as 70% [14]. In terms of prognosis, elderly and young patients have a similar prognosis, but when perforation occurs, the elderly have a worse prognosis and higher mortality rates compared to younger patients [16, 17].

Currently, the most commonly used scores for diagnosing appendicitis are the Alvarado score and the comparatively more accurate appendicitis inflammatory response score. While each clinical sign associated with each score has a low predictive value by itself, the predictive value becomes stronger when they are combined [18]. There is a controversy regarding the operative and non-operative management of appendicitis in elderly patients. It has been reported that the use of an antibiotic alone produces favorable outcomes, but no one has yet demonstrated the superiority of antibiotic therapy compared to operative management [19]. In the elderly patients, laparoscopic appendectomy remains the gold standard for the early treatment of appendicitis. In comparison to an open appendectomy, laparoscopic approach is associated with lower morbidity, lower mortality rates, lower hospital stays, and reduced hospital charges [20–25].

Acute Cholecystitis

Acute cholecystitis is a common cause of emergency general surgery in elderly patients especially in female and may have an atypical course with serious complications and high mortality [26]. Abdominal pain remains a common presenting symptom, but nausea, vomiting, fever, or leukocytosis is often absent. In the elderly, a positive Murphy's sign is useful. However, a negative sign should be further investigated in combination with other diagnostic tests because it has a lower negative predictive value [27, 28]. For patients with suspected gallbladder disease, liver function tests remain the most important type of laboratory investigation. An ultrasound is the diagnostic gold standard for the diagnosis of acute cholecystitis.

The management of gallstone disease in the elderly is quite challenging because of their frailty status and associated comorbidities. In addition, their course of management is associated with higher rates of complications, such as choledocholithiasis and gallstone pancreatitis. The first line of treatment of acute cholecystitis is a laparoscopic cholecystectomy. However, in elderly or critically ill patients with underlying comorbidities, an emergency cholecystectomy is associated with higher rates of mortality and morbidity. Decompression by tube cholecystostomy allows the inflammation to subside and gives the patient extra time to recover from the acute illness [29, 30]. In the literature, percutaneous cholecystostomy in selected patients especially critically ill patients at time of presentation followed by interval laparoscopic cholecystectomy has been described as a safe option of management of acute cholecystitis [29–32].

Acute Diverticulitis

The acquired form of diverticulitis is highly common in the western society. It affects about 5–10% of the population over 45 years old and approximately 80% of those over age 85 [33]. Symptomatic diverticulitis develops in around 20% of patients. The pathophysiology of acute diverticulitis mainly attributed to two mechanisms: increased intraluminal pressure and weakening of the bowel wall. The latter usually happens near the sites of vasa recta penetration and occurs primarily in the sigmoid colon [34]. The majority of patients present with abdominal pain that usually starts at the hypogastrium and then migrates to localize in the left lower quadrant. Some patients present with a change in their bowel habits (i.e., diarrhea and/or constipation). Physical examination reveals tenderness to palpation in the left lower quadrant, and lower abdominal or rectal mass may present.

The gold standard imaging test for the diagnosis of acute diverticulitis is a computed tomographic (CT) scan, which has a high sensitivity and specificity. The use of colonoscopy and sigmoidoscopy should be avoided in the acute stage of the disease because of a high risk of colonic perforation and concomitant peritonitis due to the fragility of the inflamed colonic wall. Usually, a colonoscopy is recommended 4–6 weeks after the acute phase of the inflammation in order to rule out other coexisting diseases such as malignancy, especially in people older than 50 years of age.

Conservative management of acute uncomplicated diverticulitis is successful in 70–100% of cases [35]. Geriatric patients with acute diverticulitis can be managed safely with outpatient therapy. For these patients, the treatment of choice is 7–10 days of oral broad-spectrum antibiotics [36]. Hospitalization is indicated only for those who require analgesia, who cannot tolerate any diet, or who have complicated diverticulitis. Such patients should be made NPO (nil per os), and broad-spectrum antibiotics should be administered intravenously [37]. These patients are followed serially with white cell counts, abdominal examinations, and repeat CT scans. Many organizations, however, recommended bowel resection after two attacks of diverticulitis. Nonetheless, a review paper concluded that there is no evidence to support elective surgery after two such attacks because the surgical intervention in the elderly is usually associated with higher rates of morbidity and mortality [38]. Moreover, surgery of diverticular disease has a high complication rate and a 25% chance of ongoing symptoms after the diverticular resection [38].

Acute Mesenteric Ischemia

Acute mesenteric ischemia is a serious, relatively rare disorder of the elderly with an overall mortality rate of 60–80% [39, 40]. It refers to a wide spectrum of bowel injury ranging from partial reversible ischemic changes to full-thickness bowel wall infarction [41]. It occurs within the distribution of the celiac artery, the superior mesenteric artery (the most common artery involved), and/or the inferior mesenteric artery. It is categorized into four types based on its cause: (1)

arterial embolism, (2) arterial thrombosis, (3) nonocclusive mesenteric ischemia, and (4) mesenteric venous thrombosis [40].

Patients with acute mesenteric ischemia typically present with sudden, severe, periumbilical abdominal pain, often accompanied by nausea and vomiting. Elderly patients frequently have antecedent symptoms of chronic mesenteric ischemia, including postprandial abdominal pain, avoidance of meals, and unintentional weight loss. The most common laboratory abnormalities seen in patients with acute mesenteric ischemia are hemoconcentration, leukocytosis, a high anion gap, and possibly lactic acidosis in more advanced cases. High amylase, aspartate aminotransferase, and lactate dehydrogenase can also be observed.

The first-line imaging modality for diagnosing acute intestinal ischemia is contrast-enhanced CT, which has a high sensitivity and specificity [42, 43]. Findings on the CT scan include bowel wall thickening (which is seen more frequently with venous occlusion compared to arterial occlusion), pneumatosis intestinale, dilation of the bowel lumen, and, in most of the cases, emboli or thrombi in the mesenteric arteries and veins [44].

Acute mesenteric ischemia management should include a high index of clinical suspicion, rapid preoperative evaluation, revascularization with open surgical techniques, resection of infarcted bowel, liberal use of second-look procedures, sophisticated postoperative care for the prevention of multi-organ failure, and recognition of recurrent mesenteric ischemia. The overall clinical outcome in these patients is still poor, yet the aforementioned management approach will result in the early survival of two-thirds of the patients with embolism and thrombosis [45].

A Perforated Peptic Ulcer

A perforated peptic ulcer in the elderly is associated with high rates of morbidity (up to 50%) and mortality (up to 30%) and is more common in females than males [46, 47]. The prevalence of *Helicobacter pylori* increases with age, and it has a well-established role in the development of ulcers. In the elderly, nonsteroidal anti-inflammatory medications also contribute to the increased incidence of ulcers and the development of complications [48, 49]. In addition, the presence of other concomitant diseases (e.g., diabetes mellitus, chronic obstructive pulmonary disease, hypertension, and congestive heart failure) is a significant risk factor for peptic ulcer disease.

Clinical presentation in the elderly is less specific than in younger patients. It presents with vague abdominal pain rather than intense epigastric pain [50]. During the clinical assessment of elderly patients, other differential diagnoses (i.e., ruptured abdominal aortic aneurysm or acute pancreatitis) should be considered and excluded. Laboratory markers are not diagnostic in a perforated peptic ulcer. However, they are helpful in estimating the degree of inflammatory response and assessing organ functions.

On an erect abdominal X-ray, the most classical sign of a perforated peptic ulcer and other viscus perforations is air under the diaphragm. This sign has a sensitivity of only 75% and cannot specify the origin of the pneumoperitoneum which limits its use in making definitive diagnosis [51]. Recent surgical research concerns whether a definitive surgical approach should be sought at the time of presentation. A study by Trevor et al. indicates that a period of observation before operating on a suspected perforation of a peptic ulcer is unlikely to be harmful in patients over 70 years old [52]. Indeed, many patients may avoid an operation altogether. Period of observation allows to restore circulating intravascular volume and to administer antibiotics. Although non-operative treatment may seem the most logical in elderly patients who face higher risks under surgery, there is evidence that they do not fare well with this approach. Another issue has to be taken into consideration that perforation is less likely to seal spontaneously in elderly patients. Therefore, early surgical management (i.e., laparotomy) for these patients is recommended, unless they experience a rapid improvement in their symptoms.

Perioperative Care

In recent years, there has been an increased interest in the impact of surgery on the elderly patients. As the baby boomers age, the number of geriatric patients undergoing surgery in general is increasing. It is therefore crucial that surgeons gain substantial knowledge and understanding of the care and optimization of elderly patients. It is also important for surgeons and healthcare providers to understand the differences between elderly patients and their younger counterparts and how management needs to be modified to improve outcomes. Pre- and postoperative care is critical in the elderly as they have higher rates of morbidity, which can alter the potential benefits of surgery in this population.

Preoperative Assessment

Preoperative assessment highlights risk factors that can lead to adverse events. The identification of these risk factors allows for their optimization prior to surgery and improves surgical outcomes in these patients [53–55]. The pathophysiology of the disease as well as the surgical procedure itself is important prognostic factors. However, the most important factors in the determination of postoperative morbidity and mortality are related to the general health and physiological capacity of the patient [56]. Diminished physiologic capacities have a direct impact on the patient's ability to tolerate the additional stress of surgery and possible postoperative complications.

There are many available tools that can be used preoperatively which can objectively assess the elderly patients in the setting of emergency general surgery; in this review we are going to discuss frailty assessment, the role of geriatric consultation, and goals of care.

Elderly Assessment Tools

Assessing and optimizing elderly patient's medical conditions in the context of emergency surgery is not an easy task. It can be very subjective and limited, especially with the narrow time frame available in the preoperative period. This review discusses some of the widely used, objective assessment tools that can predict postoperative outcomes among the elderly, optimize the degree of preparedness and the decision-making capacity of surgeons, and enhance the prognostic discussion with the patient's family members [57, 58]. There is, for instance, a general consensus about the value of the assessment of frailty, and it has been thoroughly described in the literature as a one such tool [59].

Frailty Assessment

Frailty is a decrease in physiological function or reserve that increases vulnerability to stressors. Among the many ways to assess frailty, the two most common tools define it phenotypically or as an accumulation of deficits [60–63]. Frailty phenotypes include the following five measures: weight wastage, low endurance, grip strength, sluggishness, and low energy expenditure [64] (Table. 40.1). A patient is frail if three or more of these factors are present. Patients with one or two factors are pre-frail, and those with none of the factors are non-frail. Nonetheless, it is not always clear what the appropriate clinical steps should be based on such phenotypic factors. Unlike the phenotype model, the cumulative deficit model of frailty developed by the Canadian study of health and aging (CHSA), which is also known as the frailty index [66], is a quantitative measure based on 92 variables of

Table 40.1 Phenotypic model of frailty

Weight wastage
Self-reported, unintentional weight loss ≥10 pounds (4.5 kg) or weight loss of ≥5% per year
Low endurance
Indicated by self-report of exhaustion. Self-reported exhaustion, identified by two questions from the CES–D scale [65]
Grip strength
Decreased grip strength by 20% compared to baseline, along with adjustment for sex and body mass index
Sluggishness
Decreased time to walk 15 feet (4.57 m), along with adjustment for sex and height
Lower energy expenditure
Energy expenditure <383 kcal/week (men) or <270 kcal/week (women)

symptoms, signs, abnormal lab values, disease status, and disabilities. Calculating frailty based on this index is done by simply dividing the total positive signs and symptoms over 92 (e.g., 30/92 = 0.32).

Emergency General Surgery Frailty Index (EGSFI)

Frailty can be assessed using the 50-variable Rockwood frailty index [66] which is an extensive and difficult to apply in the setting of emergency surgery. Based on that we developed and validated the emergency general surgery frailty index which has a 15-variable questionnaire that is simple, quick, and reliable bedside tool for EGS patients [67]. It comprises of patient's comorbidities, daily activity, health attitude, and one lab-based result, which is the albumin level (Table. 40.2). Univariate analysis identified 15 variables significantly associated with complications that were used to develop the EGSFI. A cutoff frailty score of 0.325 was identified using receiver operating characteristic curve analysis for frail status. Frailty status determined by this EGSFI is an independent predictor of postoperative complications and mortality in geriatric EGS patients.

Geriatrician Consultation

Hospitals and healthcare providers will need to invest in quality improvement initiatives in optimizing the care among elderly patients [68]. This entails quality measures directed at the care of elderly patients and/or inpatient geriatric consultation. Relatively speaking, geriatric consultation is an easily implemented, generalizable intervention for the frail elderly who are hospitalized. Previous studies have reported various results with geriatric consultation. One study has shown that inpatient geriatric consultation had a beneficial role in the acute care of older patients comprising a variety of surgical populations (e.g., emergency general surgery, orthopedic surgery), including decreasing patient's mortality, hospital length of stay, and cost of care. Another study also demonstrated that geriatric consultation is associated with a significant reduction in postoperative delirium [69, 70].

Postoperative Complications

Delirium

Delirium is defined as a multifactorial neuropsychiatric disorder with well-defined predisposing and precipitating factors, and it is the

Table 40.2 Emergency general surgery frailty index

Comorbidities				
Cancer history	Yes (1)	No (0)		
Hypertension	Yes (1)	No (0)		
Coronary artery disease	MI (1)	CABG (0.75)	PCI (0.5)	Medication (0.25)	None (0)
Dementia	Severe (1)	Moderate (0.5)		Mild (0.25)	No (0)
Daily activities				
Help with grooming	Yes (1)		No (0)	
Help managing money	Yes (1)		No (0)	
Help doing house work	Yes (1)		No (0)	
Help toileting	Yes (1)		No (0)	
Help walking	Wheel chair (1)	Walker (0.75)	Cane (0.5)	No (0)
Health attitude				
Feel less useful	Most times (1)	Sometimes (0.5)	Never (0)	
Feel sad	Most times (1)	Sometimes (0.5)	Never (0)	
Feel effort to do everything	Most times (1)	Sometimes (0.5)	Never (0)	
Feel lonely	Most times (1)	Sometimes (0.5)	Never (0)	
Feel sexually active	Yes (1)		No (0)	
Nutrition				
Albumin	<3 (1)		>3 (0)	

most common complication in hospitalized older patients [71]. Two types of delirium usually present in the postoperative period: emergence delirium (ED) and postoperative delirium (POD) [72]. ED is a benign cognitive disorientation that can occur during the transition period from anesthesia to wakefulness and resolves within minutes or hours, while POD is an acute organic brain disorder that usually develops within the first few postoperative days. POD has been associated with a wide range of negative long-term outcomes in the elderly patients, even though patients may initially recover completely. Almost 15% of all elderly patients experience POD after elective procedures, with a higher rates (30–70%) among elderly who undergo emergency operations [73]. Several risk factors and precipitating factors can lead to postoperative delirium (Table. 40.3) [74]. Delirium can be managed and prevented by the prompt identification and treatment of precipitant factors, early mobilization, hydration, nutrition, and withdrawal of drugs [75].

Postoperative Hospital Acquired Infections
Postoperative infection accounts for about 28% of hospital acquired infections [76]. Nowadays, although there is an improvement of aseptic and surgical techniques, postoperative infectious complication rates range from 0.5% to 23% [77]. The most frequent postoperative infections include wound infection, pulmonary infections, and urinary tract infections [77].

Table 40.3 Delirium risk factors and precipitating factors

Risk factors	Precipitating factors
Elderly (age > 65)	Pain
Frailty	Surgery
Dementia	Sleep deprivation
Infection	Respiratory and urinary infections
Dehydration	Electrolytes disturbance
Polypharmacy	Drugs with anticholinergic activity
Malnutrition	Hypoxia
Deafness/visual impairment	Neurological disorder

• *Urinary tract infection*

Urinary tract infection (UTI) in surgical patients is typically due to prolonged bladder catheterization [78]. Around 80% of patients with hospital acquired UTIs underwent urinary bladder catheterization [79]. In addition to increase the risk of UTI, Wald et al. have found that urinary catheterization for longer periods than normal postoperatively is associated with increased mortality and a decreased chance of the patient being discharged to home [56]. There is an increase in the need for urinary bladder catheterization in elderly patients for several reasons, including medication side effects, neurogenic bladder or obstruction secondary to spinal cord injury/disease, multiple sclerosis, enlarged prostate, or cerebrovascular accident. Elderly patients usually present with the classic symptoms of dysuria, fever, and frequency, which are commonly present in younger people; however, they may present with vague presentation, such as an acute confusion state or delirium, decreased mobility, or newly developed urinary incontinence [80]. Thus, it is important to recognize a diagnosis of a UTI in the absence of the classical symptoms. It is, therefore, necessary to examine the patient completely for other possible diagnoses and obtain objective laboratory data. The most important preventive strategies for UTI in elderly patients are minimization of the use of urinary catheters and the early removal of catheters.

• *Surgical site infection*

A surgical site infection (SSI) is an infection related to an operative procedure that occurs at or near the surgical incision within 30 days of the procedure or within 1 year if a prosthetic material is implanted at the time of surgery [81, 82]. SSI has a huge impact on morbidity and creates a substantial economic burden for patients and the healthcare system-multidisciplinary teams who are involved in managing them. Most significant, elderly patients with an SSI have a two-time higher mortality compared to elderly patients without infections [83]. Advanced age independently is considered as a host-derived risk factor for developing surgical site infections. SSI is caused by organisms that contaminate the surgical wound at the time of operation. Most of these organisms originate from the patient's own microflora; however, bacteria from other sources (e.g., aseptic techniques) can also lead to infection [82]. SSI can be prevented by the use of prophylactic measures, such as antibiotic administration, intraoperative maintenance of body temperature (i.e., normothermia), the avoidance of shaving the surgical site for long period prior to the skin incision, and ensuring perioperative blood sugar control (i.e., euglycemia) [53, 84]. Preoperative antibiotic prophylaxis is an effective method of prevention [82]. Because resistant pathogens are common among elderly patients, physicians should consider switching the antibiotic agent to cover the resistant pathogen. Careful observation of surgical wounds postoperatively is necessary to ensure early identification and treatment of SSI. Upon the development of SSI, treatment approaches include opening the incision and allowing adequate drainage along with antibiotic coverage.

Cardiac Complications

Cardiac complications such as myocardial infarction and heart failure are among the common causes of postoperative morbidity and mortality that occur in 1–5% of patients undergoing non-cardiac surgery [85, 86]. Multiple comorbidities such as hypertension, diabetes mellitus, and history of cardiac or renal failure are risk factors for higher incidence of perioperative myocardial infarction (5.1%), cardiac death (5.7%), or ischemia (12–17.7%) in elderly patients [87].

Most perioperative MIs that occur early after surgery are asymptomatic, of the non-Q-wave type, and are most commonly preceded by ST-segment depression rather than ST-segment elevation [88]. Most ischemic episodes often happen at the end of surgery and during emergence from general anesthesia. This period is characterized by tachycardia, increased arterial pressure, sympathetic system overdrive, and pro-coagulation processes [89].

Eighty percent of elderly patients don't experience infarction pain [90] and may present in a nonclassical symptoms of myocardial ischemia or infarction, which makes the diagnosis obscure and challenging. Additional factors that could mislead the diagnosis of ischemic attacks postoperatively include inability to discriminate between the incisional pain and the ischemic pain, residual anesthesia, and postoperative analgesia.

Two major strategies should be sought to reduce the incidence of perioperative MI, as well as other cardiac events and complications: preoperative assessment and revascularization of the stenotic lesions as well as pharmacological treatment [91]. The latter specifically refers to the use of beta-blockers. Perioperative B-blockade improves cardiac outcome in patients with, or at risk of, coronary artery disease, as well as in patients with documented inducible MI undergoing non-cardiac surgery [92].

Pulmonary Complications

Postoperative pulmonary complications (PPCs) are not exclusive to thoracic surgeries as 5–10% of patients undergoing non-thoracic surgery develop PPCs [93]. They are considered as the second most common serious morbid condition after the cardiovascular events [93]. PPCs include atelectasis, pneumonia, bronchitis, bronchospasm, pulmonary collapse due to mucus plugging pulmonary embolism, and respiratory failure that requires ventilation [94]. Development of these complications can extend the intensive care unit stay and increase mortality. As compared to younger patients, elderly patients especially those 70 years of age and above have a higher risk of developing respiratory complications, including pneumonia, pulmonary edema of the non-cardiogenic type, and respiratory failure requiring intubation [95]. Elderly patients are more prone to develop respiratory complications due to age-related alterations in pulmonary function combined with postoperative pulmonary pathophysiologic changes.

Risk factors for PPCs are preoperative and procedure-related (Table. 40.4) [93]. In order to prevent or minimize PPCs, risk reduction strategies can be planned from the preoperative period itself. Optimization of surgical and anesthetic techniques, as well as meticulous postopera-

Table. 40.4   Postoperative pulmonary complications risk factors

Patient-related risk factors		Procedure-related risk factors	
Risk factor	Relevance to complication	Risk factor	Relevance to complication
Age > 65 years	Independent, unmodifiable	Duration of the surgery	Independent risk factor
Smoking	Higher incidence of complications, only if associated with COPD	Type of anesthesia	RA decreases the risk of complications. Long-acting NBMs during GA increase the risk
Chronic obstructive pulmonary disease	Most important risk factor. Preoperative preparation decreases significantly	Site of surgery	Neck, thorax, upper abdominal surgeries, neurological surgery and lonely aortic aneurysm surgery
Obstructive sleep apnea	Higher risk of developing postoperative hypoxemia, hypercarbia, aspiration pneumonia, and ARDS	Type of surgery	Laparoscopic vs. open. Emergency vs. elective surgery

tive care, can prevent the progression to severe pulmonary complications [96].

Goals of Care

As our population is aging, older patients are living longer with chronic illness. Discussion on the goals of care should be initiated with the admission of geriatric patients. A multidisciplinary approach involving the patient and family with the discussion on the risk and benefits will allow the patients to make informed decision toward the end of life. Advance care planning can decrease the suffering, increase the quality of life, and improve the experience of family members and decrease healthcare costs [97, 98]. Establishing goals of care that correspond with the patient's values and preferences; and communication between the patient and all those involved in their care should be part of the assessment of any geriatric patient for emergency general surgery. It is important for surgeons to identify high-risk patients and initiate the discussion of a definitive curative surgery vs. a temporizing procedure based on the goals of care. A study by Olson et al. found that about 40% of surgeons who frequently perform high-risk procedures reported a conflict with critical care physicians and nurses regarding the goals of care for their patients with poor postoperative outcomes. This can be only improved with effective communication with all the team members involved in the care of elderly patients [99].

Failure to Rescue

Failure to rescue (FTR), mortality after developing a major complication following surgery, is an important marker of patient safety and healthcare quality [100]. Several previous studies have shown that in-hospital mortality rates are significantly affected by the variation in the management of complications that develop after surgery. Recent evidence suggests that minimizing the rates of FTR events might be the most appropriate target for quality improvement in the elderly population.

A study performed Sheetz et al. demonstrated a significant difference in FTR rates between elderly and younger patients, especially when pulmonary and infectious complications are the first complication to develop. However, the study found no significant difference between the two groups regarding cardiovascular complications. They had almost the same FTR rates [101]. Another study by Joseph, et al. shows an association between frailty status and FTR. It concluded that frail elderly trauma patients are more likely to die after developing a major complication following surgery. Thus, they have a higher FTR rate than non-frail patients [102]. Predicting FTR in elderly undergoing EGS has been described in the literature, a study described the use of geriatric rescue after surgery (GRAS) score, which can accurately predict the probability of dying from complications in elderly patients undergoing EGS [103, 104].

Discharge Disposition and Readmission

Discharge disposition is the person's anticipated location or status following the hospital encounter (e.g., death, transfer to home/hospice/skilled nursing facility). One third of the patients undergoing EGS are discharged to skilled nursing facility [105]. More than half of these patients stay greater than a year, with only less than 12% returning to home eventually [105]. In elderly who undergo emergency general surgery, the risk factors that decrease the chances of the patients to discharge home are the advancing age, lower American Society of Anesthesiologists (ASA) physical status classification, and the development of in-hospital complications [106]. Frailty plays a major role in predicting the discharge disposition. A study by Makary et al. has shown in their adjusted model that frailty independently predicts the odds of being discharged to skilled or assisted living facility and intermediately frail patients had 3.16-fold higher odds of being discharged to a skilled or assisted living facility [107].

Among elderly EGS patients, the most common reason for readmission is gastrointestinal illnesses followed by surgical infections [108]. In addition, older patients are more likely to return to hospital due to malnutrition, genitourinary, vascular, pulmonary, and cardiac reasons, compared to younger patients who get readmitted mainly due to surgical infections [108]. Predictors of readmission include higher score on an index of coexisting illnesses, being discharged against medical advice, and insurance status.

Withdrawal of Care

An elderly patient's decision to undergo an emergent surgical procedure is time sensitive and usually made while experiencing severe physical discomfort. One study found that that many elderly patients will consent to emergency surgery, but they are more likely to decline aggressive medical intervention postoperatively, especially if they had a prior DNR (do not resuscitate) order before the operation [109]. According to the study by Scarborough et al., patients consent to emergency surgery for various reasons, including the use of general anesthesia during surgery and the chance that emergency surgery will reduce their pain and treat the underlying cause. However, the procedure might make them more debilitated, or the postoperative discomfort might be worse than expected, leading to a decreased willingness to undergo continued aggressive management [110]. The same study found that mortality rates are higher in the elderly who have a preoperative DNR order and who underwent emergency surgery. This is mainly due to their unwillingness to pursue rescue when major postoperative complications occur.

Conclusion

Managing risks and predicting postoperative outcomes in elderly patients who undergo emergency general surgery is a complex process due to their acute presentation, which renders many preoperative preparations difficult to apply. However, there are certain preoperative and most often postoperative opportunities to improve outcomes. Therefore, focusing on preoperative and postoperative outcomes in such patients should be the target for both the surgeon and the hospital. In comparison to age alone, frailty is used as an objective tool to predict the postoperative outcomes in elderly and helps surgeons to formulate their decisions in managing this group of patients. Geriatric consultation is recommended in the hospital setting as it is associated with reduction in mortality rates, hospital length of stay, as well as lower costs of care.

Conflict of Interest There are no identifiable conflicts of interests to report.

Financial Statement The authors have no financial or proprietary interest in the subject matter or materials discussed in the manuscript.

References

1. Colby SL, Ortman JM. Projections of the size and composition of the US population: 2014 to 2060. US Census Bureau. 2015. 9.
2. Shafi S, et al. Emergency general surgery: definition and estimated burden of disease. J Trauma Acute Care Surg. 2013;74(4):1092–7.
3. Stewart B, et al. Global disease burden of conditions requiring emergency surgery. Br J Surg. 2014;101(1):e9.
4. Svenningsen P, et al. Increased mortality in the elderly after emergency abdominal surgery. Dan Med J. 2014;61(7):A4876.
5. Racz J, et al. Elective and emergency abdominal surgery in patients 90 years of age or older. Can J Surg. 2012;55(5):322.
6. Green G, et al. Emergency laparotomy in octogenarians: a 5-year study of morbidity and mortality. World J Gastrointest Surg. 2013;5(7):216.
7. Vogeli C, et al. Multiple chronic conditions: prevalence, health consequences, and implications for quality, care management, and costs. J Gen Intern Med. 2007;22(3):391–5.
8. Lee TA, et al. Mortality rate in veterans with multiple chronic conditions. J Gen Intern Med. 2007;22(3):403.
9. Wolff JL, Starfield B, Anderson G. Prevalence, expenditures, and complications of multiple chronic conditions in the elderly. Arch Intern Med. 2002;162(20):2269–76.
10. Yancik R, et al. Report of the national institute on aging task force on comorbidity. J Gerontol Ser A Biol Med Sci. 2007;62(3):275–80.
11. Peltokallio P, Jauhiainen K. Acute appendicitis in the aged patient: study of 300 cases after the age of 60. Arch Surg. 1970;100(2):140–3.
12. Horattas MC, Guyton DP, Wu D. A reappraisal of appendicitis in the elderly. Am J Surg. 1990;160(3):291–3.
13. Omari AH, et al. Acute appendicitis in the elderly: risk factors for perforation. World J Emerg Surg. 2014;9(1):6.
14. Freund H, Rubinstein E. Appendicitis in the aged. Is it really different? Am Surg. 1984;50(10):573–6.
15. Paajanen H, Kettunen J, Kostiainen S. Emergency appendectomies in patients over 80 years. Am Surg. 1994;60(12):950–3.
16. Eldar S, et al. Delay of surgery in acute appendicitis. Am J Surg. 1997;173(3):194–8.
17. Peltokallio P, Tykkä H. Evolution of the age distribution and mortality of acute appendicitis. Arch Surg. 1981;116(2):153–6.
18. Kollár D, et al. Predicting acute appendicitis? A comparison of the Alvarado score, the Appendicitis Inflammatory Response Score and clinical assessment. World J Surg. 2015;39(1):104–9.
19. Khalil M, et al. Antibiotics for appendicitis! Not so fast. J Trauma Acute Care Surg. 2016;80(6):923–32.
20. Masoomi H, et al. Does laparoscopic appendectomy impart an advantage over open appendectomy in elderly patients? World J Surg. 2012;36(7):1534–9.
21. Harrell AG, et al. Advantages of laparoscopic appendectomy in the elderly. Am Surg. 2006;72(6):474–80.
22. Guller U, et al. Laparoscopic appendectomy in the elderly. Surgery. 2004;135(5):479–88.
23. Wu S-C, et al. Laparoscopic appendectomy provides better outcomes than open appendectomy in elderly patients. Am Surg. 2011;77(4):466–70.
24. Salminen P, et al. Antibiotic therapy vs appendectomy for treatment of uncomplicated acute appendicitis: the APPAC randomized clinical trial. JAMA. 2015;313(23):2340–8.
25. Hui TT, et al. Outcome of elderly patients with appendicitis: effect of computed tomography and laparoscopy. Arch Surg. 2002;137(9):995–1000.
26. Hafif A, et al. The management of acute cholecystitis in elderly patients. Am Surg. 1991;57(10):648–52.
27. Kahng KU, Wargo JA. Gallstone disease in the elderly. In: Principles and practice of geriatric surgery. New York: Springer; 2001. p. 690–710.
28. Adedeji O, McAdam W. Murphy's sign, acute cholecystitis and elderly people. J R Coll Surg Edinb. 1996;41(2):88–9.
29. Winbladh A, et al. Systematic review of cholecystostomy as a treatment option in acute cholecystitis. HPB. 2009;11(3):183–93.
30. Borzellino G, et al. Emergency cholecystostomy and subsequent cholecystectomy for acute gallstone cholecystitis in the elderly. Br J Surg. 1999;86(12):1521–5.
31. McGillicuddy E, et al. Non-operative management of acute cholecystitis in the elderly. Br J Surg. 2012;99(9):1254–61.
32. Sugiyama M, Tokuhara M, Atomi Y. Is percutaneous cholecystostomy the optimal treatment for acute cholecystitis in the very elderly? World J Surg. 1998;22(5):459–63.
33. Ferzoco L, Raptopoulos V, Silen W. Acute diverticulitis. N Engl J Med. 1998;338(21):1521–6.
34. Fischer MG, Farkas AM. Diverticulitis of the cecum and ascending colon. Dis Colon Rectum. 1984;27(7):454–8.
35. Kellum JM, et al. Randomized, prospective comparison of cefoxitin and gentamicin-clindamycin in the treatment of acute colonic diverticulitis. Clin Ther. 1992;14(3):376–84.
36. Jacobs DO. Diverticulitis. N Engl J Med. 2007;357(20):2057–66.
37. Chabok A, et al. Randomized clinical trial of antibiotics in acute uncomplicated diverticulitis. Br J Surg. 2012;99(4):532–9.
38. Janes S, Meagher A, Frizelle F. Elective surgery after acute diverticulitis. Br J Surg. 2005;92(2):133–42.
39. Lock G. Acute intestinal ischaemia. Best Pract Res Clin Gastroenterol. 2001;15(1):83–98.
40. Oldenburg WA, et al. Acute mesenteric ischemia: a clinical review. Arch Intern Med. 2004;164(10):1054–62.

41. Kaleya RN, Boley SJ. Acute mesenteric ischemia. Crit Care Clin. 1995;11(2):479–512.
42. Taourel PG, et al. Acute mesenteric ischemia: diagnosis with contrast-enhanced CT. Radiology. 1996;199(3):632–6.
43. Menke J. Diagnostic accuracy of multidetector CT in acute mesenteric ischemia: systematic review and meta-analysis. Radiology. 2010;256(1):93–101.
44. Furukawa A, et al. CT diagnosis of acute mesenteric ischemia from various causes. Am J Roentgenol. 2009;192(2):408–16.
45. Park WM, et al. Contemporary management of acute mesenteric ischemia: factors associated with survival. J Vasc Surg. 2002;35(3):445–52.
46. Møller M, et al. Multicentre trial of a perioperative protocol to reduce mortality in patients with peptic ulcer perforation. Br J Surg. 2011;98(6):802–10.
47. Søreide K, et al. Perforated peptic ulcer. Lancet. 2015;386(10000):1288–98.
48. Borum ML. Peptic-ulcer disease in the elderly. Clin Geriatr Med. 1999;15(3):457–71.
49. Pilotto A, et al. Optimal management of peptic ulcer disease in the elderly. Drugs Aging. 2010;27(7):545–58.
50. Chang C-C, Wang S-S. Acute abdominal pain in the elderly. Int J Gerontol. 2007;1(2):77–82.
51. Furukawa A, et al. Gastrointestinal tract perforation: CT diagnosis of presence, site, and cause. Abdom Imaging. 2005;30(5):524–34.
52. Crofts TJ, et al. A randomized trial of nonoperative treatment for perforated peptic ulcer. N Engl J Med. 1989;320(15):970–3.
53. Jehan F, et al. Perioperative glycemic control and postoperative complications in patients undergoing emergency general surgery: what is the role of HbA1c? J Trauma Acute Care Surg. 2018;84(1):112–7.
54. Jehan F, et al. CT-measured waist-to-hip ratio: a reliable predictor of outcomes after emergency general surgery. J Am Coll Surg. 2017;225(4):S81.
55. Ho C, et al. Can sarcopenia quantified by CT predict adverse outcomes in emergency general surgery? J Am Coll Surg. 2017;225(4):S80.
56. Wald HL, et al. Indwelling urinary catheter use in the postoperative period: analysis of the national surgical infection prevention project data. Arch Surg. 2008;143(6):551–7.
57. Rosenthal RA, Kavic SM. Assessment and management of the geriatric patient. Crit Care Med. 2004;32(4):S92–S105.
58. McGory ML, et al. Developing quality indicators for elderly surgical patients. Ann Surg. 2009;250(2):338–47.
59. Joseph B, et al. Superiority of frailty over age in predicting outcomes among geriatric trauma patients: a prospective analysis. JAMA Surg. 2014;149(8):766–72.
60. Bortz WM. A conceptual framework of frailty: a review. J Gerontol Ser A Biol Med Sci. 2002;57(5):M283–8.
61. Robinson TN, et al. Frailty for surgeons: review of a National Institute on Aging Conference on Frailty for Specialists. J Am Coll Surg. 2015;221(6):1083.
62. Rockwood K, et al. Prevalence, attributes, and outcomes of fitness and frailty in community-dwelling older adults: report from the Canadian study of health and aging. J Gerontol Ser A Biol Med Sci. 2004;59(12):1310–7.
63. Fried LP, et al. Frailty in older adults: evidence for a phenotype. J Gerontol Ser A Biol Med Sci. 2001;56(3):M146–57.
64. Clegg A, et al. Frailty in elderly people. Lancet. 2013;381(9868):752–62.
65. Orme JG, Reis J, Herz EJ. Factorial and discriminant validity of the center for epidemiological studies depression (CES? D) scale. J Clin Psychol. 1986;42(1):28–33.
66. Rockwood K, et al. A global clinical measure of fitness and frailty in elderly people. Can Med Assoc J. 2005;173(5):489–95.
67. Jokar TO, et al. Emergency general surgery specific frailty index: a validation study. J Trauma Acute Care Surg. 2016;81(2):254–60.
68. Ingraham AM, et al. Variation in quality of care after emergency general surgery procedures in the elderly. J Am Coll Surg. 2011;212(6):1039–48.
69. Marcantonio ER, et al. Reducing delirium after hip fracture: a randomized trial. J Am Geriatr Soc. 2001;49(5):516–22.
70. Ansaloni L, et al. Risk factors and incidence of postoperative delirium in elderly patients after elective and emergency surgery. Br J Surg. 2010;97(2):273–80.
71. McCusker J, et al. The course of delirium in older medical inpatients. J Gen Intern Med. 2003;18(9):696–704.
72. Radtke F, et al. Risk factors for inadequate emergence after anesthesia: emergence delirium and hypoactive emergence. Minerva Anestesiol. 2010;76(6):394–403.
73. Strøm C, Rasmussen L. Challenges in anaesthesia for elderly. Singap Dent J. 2014;35:23–9.
74. Young J, Inouye SK. Delirium in older people. BMJ. 2007;334(7598):842.
75. Dyer CB, Ashton CM, Teasdale TA. Postoperative delirium: a review of 80 primary data-collection studies. Arch Intern Med. 1995;155(5):461–5.
76. Eriksen H, Iversen B, Aavitsland P. Prevalence of nosocomial infections in hospitals in Norway, 2002 and 2003. J Hosp Infect. 2005;60(1):40–5.
77. Datuashvili G, Tabutsadze T. Postoperative hospital acquired infections. Tbilisi State Medical University; Tbilisi, Georgia, XLV: p. 55.
78. Beliveau MM, Multach M. Perioperative care for the elderly patient. Med Clin N Am. 2003;87(1):273–89.
79. Cunha BA, Tamminga C, Blair B. Urinary tract infections in males. In: Conns current therapy. WB Saunders Company; Philadelphia, PA, 2003. p. 733–5.
80. Burton JR, Lee AG, Potter JF. Geriatrics for specialists. Cham: Springer; 2017.
81. Kaye KS, et al. The effect of surgical site infection on older operative patients. J Am Geriatr Soc. 2009;57(1):46–54.

82. Kirby JP, Mazuski JE. Prevention of surgical site infection. Surg Clin N Am. 2009;89(2):365–89.
83. Kirkland KB, et al. The impact of surgical-site infections in the 1990s: attributable mortality, excess length of hospitalization, and extra costs. Infect Control Hosp Epidemiol. 1999;20(11):725–30.
84. Dellinger EP, et al. Hospitals collaborate to decrease surgical site infections. Am J Surg. 2005;190(1):9–15.
85. McGory ML, Maggard MA, Ko CY. A meta-analysis of perioperative beta blockade: what is the actual risk reduction? Surgery. 2005;138(2):171–9.
86. Auerbach AD, Goldman L. β-Blockers and reduction of cardiac events in noncardiac surgery: scientific review. JAMA. 2002;287(11):1435–44.
87. Mehta RH, et al. Acute myocardial infarction in the elderly: differences by age. J Am Coll Cardiol. 2001;38(3):736–41.
88. Landesberg G, et al. Myocardial infarction after vascular surgery: the role of prolonged, stress-induced, ST depression-type ischemia. J Am Coll Cardiol. 2001;37(7):1839–45.
89. Hemmings HC, Hopkins PM. Foundations of anesthesia: basic sciences for clinical practice. Philadelphia: Elsevier Health Sciences; 2006.
90. Badner NH, et al. Myocardial infarction after noncardiac surgery. Anesthesiology. 1998;88(3):572–8.
91. Priebe H-J. Perioperative myocardial infarction—aetiology and prevention. BJA. 2005;95(1):3–19.
92. Eagle KA, et al. ACC/AHA guideline update for perioperative cardiovascular evaluation for noncardiac surgery. J Am Coll Cardiol. 2002;39(3):542–53.
93. Kelkar KV. Post-operative pulmonary complications after non-cardiothoracic surgery. Indian J Anaesth. 2015;59(9):599.
94. Ergina PL, Gold SL, Meakins JL. Perioperative care of the elderly patient. World J Surg. 1993;17(2):192–8.
95. Polanczyk CA, et al. Impact of age on perioperative complications and length of stay in patients undergoing noncardiac surgery. Ann Intern Med. 2001;134(8):637–43.
96. Miller RD, et al. Miller's anesthesia e-book. Elsevier Health Sciences; Philadelphia, PA, 2014.
97. Wright AA, et al. Associations between end-of-life discussions, patient mental health, medical care near death, and caregiver bereavement adjustment. JAMA. 2008;300(14):1665–73.
98. Detering KM, et al. The impact of advance care planning on end of life care in elderly patients: randomised controlled trial. BMJ. 2010;340:c1345.
99. Olson TJP, et al. Surgeon-reported conflict with intensivists about postoperative goals of care. JAMA Surg. 2013;148(1):29–35.
100. Silber JH, et al. Hospital and patient characteristics associated with death after surgery: a study of adverse occurrence and failure to rescue. Med Care. 1992;30:615–29.
101. Sheetz KH, et al. The importance of the first complication: understanding failure to rescue after emergent surgery in the elderly. J Am Coll Surg. 2014;219(3):365–70.
102. Joseph B, et al. The impact of frailty on failure-to-rescue in geriatric trauma patients: a prospective study. J Trauma Acute Care Surg. 2016;81(6):1150–5.
103. Khan M, et al. Geriatric rescue after surgery (GRAS) score to predict failure-to-rescue in geriatric emergency general surgery patients. Am J Surg. 2018;215(1):53–7.
104. Khan M, et al. Impact of frailty on failure-to-rescue in geriatric emergency general surgery patients: a prospective study. J Am Coll Surg. 2017;225(4):S96–7.
105. Beck JC. Geriatrics review syllabus: a core curriculum in geriatric medicine. New York: Wiley; 2002.
106. Lees MC, et al. Perioperative factors predicting poor outcome in elderly patients following emergency general surgery: a multivariate regression analysis. Can J Surg. 2015;58(5):312.
107. Makary MA, et al. Frailty as a predictor of surgical outcomes in older patients. J Am Coll Surg. 2010;210(6):901–8.
108. Havens JM, et al. Defining rates and risk factors for readmissions following emergency general surgery. JAMA Surg. 2016;151(4):330–6.
109. Kaldjian LC, Broderick A. Developing a policy for do not resuscitate orders within a framework of goals of care. Jt Comm J Qual Patient Saf. 2011;37(1):11–AP1.
110. Scarborough JE, et al. Failure-to-pursue rescue: explaining excess mortality in elderly emergency general surgical patients with preexisting "do-not-resuscitate" orders. Ann Surg. 2012;256(3):453–61.

Non-obstetric Emergency Surgery in the Pregnant Patient

41

Ram Nirula, Ronald Buczek, and Milos Buhavac

Introduction

Pregnant patients are often a fear-inducing population for the general surgeon. These patients present a unique and sometimes difficult challenge, representing one of the few situations in surgery where decisions have the potential to directly affect two lives. Despite this, little emphasis seems to be placed on teaching general surgeons specific considerations about this population. Though there are actually "two patients," the well-being of the mother always takes precedence over that of the fetus, since in emergent situations especially, the optimal management of the condition of the fetus is appropriate resuscitation, diagnosis, and management of the mother. There are many important anatomic and physiologic changes to consider in the pregnant patient, and these changes effect practically every organ system. These changes must be considered whether pregnant mothers present with emergency general surgical conditions or injuries, as

R. Nirula (✉) · M. Buhavac
Department of Surgery, University of Utah School of Medicine, University of Utah,
Salt Lake City, UT, USA
e-mail: r.nirula@hsc.utah.edu; milos.buhavac@hsc.utah.edu

R. Buczek
Department of Surgery, University of Utah,
Salt Lake City, UT, USA
e-mail: ronald.buczek@hsc.utah.edu

they carry the need for specific considerations in both the evaluation and treatment of these patients.

Evaluation of the Pregnant Surgical Patient

A full history and physical exam should be obtained, and this should include all past and current obstetric history, gestational age, prenatal care, and issues with any pregnancy, including the current one. While general surgical conditions affect pregnant patients, one should still consider and rule out other obstetric-related causes, such as ectopic pregnancy, placental abruption, preeclampsia, or rupture of visceral aneurysms. It is prudent to also consider changes in anatomic relationships and landmarks that occur during pregnancy.

Evaluation should include a sterile speculum exam and fetal heart tone monitoring if indicated, as adjuncts to a thorough physical exam. Fetal monitoring is generally recommended to begin at 24 weeks gestation, when patients present with significant medical conditions. If performing a laparoscopic procedure, it is not possible to obtain transabdominal signal with pneumoperitoneum, therefore transvaginal monitoring should be employed. A transabdominal tocodynamometer can be placed immediately following operation to monitor for uterine contractions. Prolonged, regular contractions (eight per hour for greater than 4 h) are associated with placental abruption, which carries a high fetal mortality rate [1]. If fetal monitoring remains normal for more than 4 h, in the absence of concerning findings on physical exam (vaginal bleeding, uterine tenderness, membrane rupture), it is generally considered safe to discontinue [2] (Fig. 41.1). Though this figure is from trauma literature, it is likely applicable to emergency general surgery conditions as well, as these patients may also present in various forms of shock with heightened physiologic stress. If continuous fetal monitoring is not available, calculation of fetal heart rate can be done with bedside ultrasound as a temporary substitute [3].

Imaging

The amount of radiation the mother is exposed to is not necessarily the same amount presented to the fetus, and this varies based on fetal positioning as well as maternal tissue thickness. The detrimental effects of radiation exposure include lethality early in gestation, teratogenicity during organogenesis, and finally growth retardation in later stages; each of these effects occurs above a certain threshold level. For lethality, it is difficult to determine a threshold level due to the high number of fertilized embryos that naturally abort, often without knowledge of the production of a conceptus. Regarding teratogenicity, exposure of 10 rad or higher is proven to create substantial risk to the fetus [4]. Risk of growth restriction is

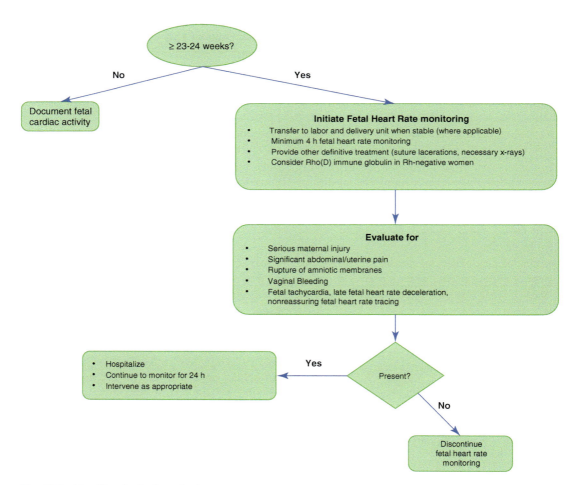

Fig. 41.1 Algorithm for fetal monitoring

increased at any dose above 5 rad [5]. Due to these risks, the radiation dose should be limited to no more than 5–10 rad during the first 25 weeks of pregnancy, with no single dose exceeding 5 rad [6]. A list of radiation exposure from common procedures is available in Table 41.1.

The first imaging modality of choice is often ultrasound. It utilizes no ionizing radiation, and is an excellent first imaging choice for many obstetric and gynecologic causes of abdominal pain. However, one should not delay imaging studies that do use radiation if they are indeed

Table 41.1 Average radiation exposure for common imaging techniques

Procedure	Mean exposure (rad)	Maximum exposure (rad)
Conventional radiographic examination		
Chest	<0.001	<0.001
Abdomen	0.14	0.42
Intravenous urogram	0.17	1
Pelvis	0.11	0.4
Lumbar spine	0.17	1
Skull	<0.001	<0.001
Thoracic spine	<0.001	<0.001
Fluoroscopic examination		
Barium meal (upper GI)	0.11	0.58
Barium enema	0.68	2.4
Computed tomography		
Abdomen	0.8	4.9
Head	0.006	0.096
Chest	<0.0005	<0.0005
Lumbar spine	0.24	0.86
Pelvis	2.5	7.9
Procedure	**Estimate (rad)**	**Range (rad)**
Cardiac catheter ablation	0.015–0.06[a]	
ERCP	0.31	0.001–5.59
TIPS creation	0.55	
Pulmonary angiography	0.002–0.046	
Uterine fibroid embolization	4.2	
Cerebral angiography	0.006	

[a]Depending on procedure duration

truly warranted. There is no evidence that properly performed diagnostic ultrasonography presents any harm to the fetus [7].

Each abdomen and pelvis CT scan results in an exposure of 5–10 rad, but if the exam is deemed clinically necessary, it must be done. Clinical necessity should be based on a risk versus benefit analysis. MRI without contrast is considered safe in pregnancy, but as there may be a considerable delay in performance and interpretation of MRI versus alternate imaging modalities, it may delay further workup or resuscitation. Gadolinium contrast is a teratogen and should be avoided.

Physiology

There are significant differences in the physiology of pregnant patients, which affect almost every organ system. Changes are apparent in baseline physiology, as well as anatomy and laboratory values.

Hematologic System

A large increase in circulating volume occurs in pregnancy until about 32–34 weeks, where it then plateaus in order to maintain perfusion and prepare for anticipated blood loss during delivery [8, 9]. The average blood loss during vaginal delivery is approximately 500 cc, while it is closer to 1000 cc for cesarean delivery. Twin pregnancies may increase blood volume by as much as 70%. Total body water increases by 4–5 L and is regulated by changes in the renin-angiotensin-aldosterone system. This leads to increased sodium reabsorption and water retention. Estrogens and progesterone both act to increase aldosterone levels. Most of this increase in total body water is within the fetus, placenta, and amniotic fluid. Blood volume is augmented by 1.2–1.3 L of plasma and 300–400 cc of erythrocytes. There is a disproportionate increase in plasma volume; therefore a normal hematocrit during pregnancy is 31–35% [10]. The pregnant patient can bleed 1.2–1.5 L before exhibiting hypovolemia-related symptoms [11]. In this situation, the only presenting evidence of fetal distress may be fetal tachycardia.

Leukocytosis also may be present during pregnancy and can be normal. Levels of around 15,000/mm^3 are not unusual during pregnancy, with levels of 25,000/mm^3 often present during labor. Fibrinogen and other serum clotting factors are elevated mildly. Albumin drops somewhat to around 2.2–2.8 g/dL, which also decreases serum protein, though osmolarity remains roughly normal. The hypervolemia of pregnancy leads to a mild reduction in serum sodium (125–138 mEq/L).

Cardiovascular System

Cardiac output increases by 1.0–1.5 L/min in order to increase perfusion, due to increased plasma volume and decreased uterine and placental vascular resistance. These structures receive as much as 20% of the maternal cardiac output. As stroke volume increases, cardiac output concomitantly increases as well to 6 L/min in the first two trimesters – an increase of 50%. This is augmented by an increase in heart rate, up to 10–20 bpm faster, by the third trimester. Stroke volume eventually decreases as the pregnancy advances due to compression of the aorta and vena cava by the uterus. Uterine blood flow is ~25% of cardiac output at term. Fetal perfusion is reliant on the maternal mean arterial pressure, as uteroplacental circulation lacks autoregulatory mechanisms. Therefore, maternal MAP must be maintained to sufficiently perfuse the fetus, and anything that decreases maternal MAP (or cardiac output) may impair fetal perfusion.

In terms of positional effects on cardiovascular status, second or third trimester patients in the supine position will have compression on the vena cava, resulting in reduction of the cardiac output of up to 30% [11]. This compressive effect on venous return can be exaggerated in women with poorly developed venous collaterals. Systemic vascular resistance can be expected to decrease by around 15% due to progesterone-mediated blood vessel dilation, as well as low vascular resistance in the uteroplacental circula-

tion. Venodilation causes higher venous pressures and greater distensibility, which is more pronounced in dependent areas such as the lower extremities.

Systolic blood pressure can decrease by 5–15 mmHg by the second trimester but trends toward or returns to normal by term. Some studies suggest blood pressure may increase, particularly in obese women [12]. Additional cardiovascular changes can include JVD, mild hypotension and/or tachycardia, and increased peripheral edema. There may be a leftward axis shift by as much as 15 degrees, which can result in flattened or inverted T waves in leads III, AVF, and precordial, which would be considered normal. Most of these pregnancy-related changes return to normal within the few days following delivery. On the other hand, cardiac output can take up to 3 months to return to normal.

Several remodeling changes occur in the heart through the first month of pregnancy. All of the heart's chambers increase in size, as do the valvular annular diameters and left ventricular wall. It is not unusual to have systolic flow murmurs or a third heart sound during pregnancy, and over 90% of pregnant women will have tricuspid and pulmonic regurgitation [13, 14]. On the other hand, sounds that may indicate underlying heart disease are diastolic, pansystolic, or late systolic murmurs. Hematologic and cardiovascular changes are listed in Table 41.2.

Pulmonary System

As the fetus grows and the uterus expands, upward forces from the abdomen compress the thorax and result in multiple changes to pulmonary mechanics, as well as the prominence of pulmonary vasculature on chest radiography. Lung volume can be expected to decrease by around 5%. Inspiratory capacity will increase, and residual volume can be expected to decrease. Tidal volume, however, will increase, which results in an increase in minute ventilation by 30–50%, as respiratory rate remains relatively constant. As minute ventilation increases, $PaCO_2$ can be expected to decrease, and hypocapnia is

Table 41.2 Mean values of hemodynamic changes during pregnancy

Parameter	Nonpregnant	Trimester 1	Trimester 2	Trimester 3
Heart rate (beats/min)	70	78	82	85
Systolic blood pressure (mm Hg)	115	112	112	114
Diastolic blood pressure (mm Hg)	70	60	63	70
Central venous pressure (mm/Hg)	9	7.5	4	3.8
Cardiac output (L/min)	4.5	4.5	4	3.8
Blood volume (mL)	4000	4200	5000	5600
White blood cells (cells/mm^3)	7200	9100	9700	9800
Hematocrit with iron (%)	40	36	34	36

Data from Refs. [57–60]

common late in pregnancy. Conversely, a $PaCO_2$ of 35–40 may indicate impending respiratory failure in the pregnant patient, though this is obviously normal otherwise. These changes are thought to be mediated by progesterone, which stimulates the respiratory system. As $PaCO_2$ decreases, this establishes a gradient to facilitate transfer of carbon dioxide from fetal to maternal circulation across the placenta. As mentioned previously, maternal oxygen reserve is decreased, due to increased maternal oxygen consumption as well as by the placenta and fetus. Difficult intubation leading to hypoxia is therefore a significant cause of morbidity and mortality during pregnancy, and the risk of failed intubation is up to 11 times higher in pregnant patients [15, 16]. Additionally, there may be generalized airway edema, which also makes intubation more difficult. In the trauma setting, if a pregnant patient requires tube thoracostomy, it may need to be placed more cephalad to account for upward displacement of the diaphragm by the gravid uterus.

Renal System

Due to increased cardiac output and decreased systemic vascular resistance, there will be a rise in GFR, as well as an increase in renal blood flow. Alterations in sodium reabsorption result in water retention and plasma expansion. With an increased GFR, there will also be a decrease in serum creatinine. Importantly, one must make necessary adjustments to medications that are cleared by the renal system. Progesterone also works in the renal system, causing smooth mus-

cle relaxation and thus dilation of the collecting system. This may be a dilation of the renal system, including the calices, pelvis, and ureters. Collecting system dilation can also be exacerbated by physical compression of the ureters due to the enlarging uterus, which can result in increased dilation of the right renal collecting system in comparison to the left. The dilated collecting system lends itself to urinary stasis, which predisposes pregnant women to urinary system infections and stones [17]. Glycosuria may be present, because of impaired tubular resorption of glucose as well as increased GFR.

Gastrointestinal System

Gastrointestinal changes are mostly anatomic, due to physical compression or displacement of intra-abdominal structures due to the gravid uterus (Fig. 41.2). The uterus remains a pelvic organ until approximately the 12th week of gestation, gradually rising to the level of the umbilicus around 20 weeks and to the costal margin around 34 weeks. Taking this into account, operative intervention for common gastrointestinal procedures may require a modified or alternate incision location. Pregnancy alters the relationship of the esophagus and stomach, resulting in decreased function of the lower esophageal sphincter [18–21]. Physiologically, gastric motility and emptying decrease during pregnancy, though some studies dispute any effect on emptying [22]. Due to larger stomach volume and decreased motility, pregnant women have a larger risk of aspiration when sedated. There is also

Fig. 41.2 Changes in
fundal height during
pregnancy, which can be
used as an estimate of
gestational age

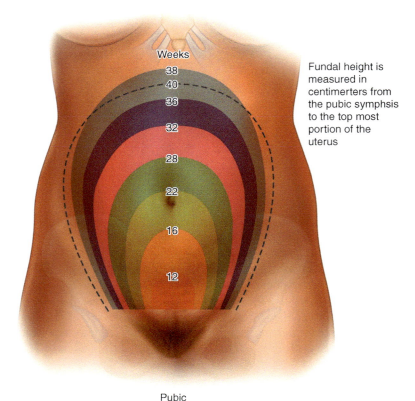

generalized relaxation of smooth muscle, and gastric emptying time is lengthened during pregnancy.

Hematologic System

Contributing factors to physiologic anemia include the transfer of iron stores to the fetus as well as a disproportionate increase in plasma volume versus red cell volume. Leukocytosis can be found during pregnancy, especially peripartum, and should not be mistaken as a marker for infection. Pregnant patients do undergo hematologic changes that result in hypercoagulability. These changes include an increase in all procoagulant factors as well as decrease in fibrinolysis. Thus, pregnant patients are at an up to fivefold higher risk for thrombotic events, including DVT and PE [23]. The baseline increase in hypercoagulability is important to consider, as it is increased further by trauma or emergency surgery, as well

as the immobility and elaboration of inflammatory factors that subsequently follows. The frequency of deep venous thrombosis is the same across the trimesters and is reported as 0.7 in 1000 women [24], though it is more common in the left leg [25]. Diagnosis can be difficult in the pregnant patient, as leg pain and swelling tend to be quite common in those without DVT as well. However, unilateral swelling or pain should prompt evaluation with venous compression ultrasonography. In contrast to DVT, pulmonary embolism tends to be more common in the post-partum period. Treatment is with low molecular weight heparin, with warfarin being reserved for use postpartum, due to its teratogenic effects. Low molecular weight heparin is preferred over unfractionated heparin by the American College of Chest Physicians [26]. Following a thrombotic event, treatment should be for 3–6 months, to include 6 weeks postpartum. Twelve months of treatment is indicated for those with recurrent thrombosis or history of a hypercoagulable state.

Endocrine System

Pituitary gland hypertrophy can be up to three-fold, which may result in pituitary insufficiency, especially when the mother may have experienced hypotensive episodes. Synthesis of TSH, prolactin, and ACTH increases, while gonadotropin and growth hormone production decrease during pregnancy. Cortisol levels, both free and bound, are increased [27]. Patients may have a relative adrenal insufficiency that results in rapid decompensation during the stress of labor. This should be immediately treated with hydrocortisone if suspected.

Levels of T3 and T4 increase, but free levels of both are unchanged. Thyroid size may increase in 15% of women [28, 29]. If the patient has pre-existing hypothyroidism, levothyroxine dose should be increased by 30% [30].

Pre- and Perioperative Considerations

As previously mentioned, this patient population has a high aspiration risk and a low oxygen reserve. When performing emergent procedures, early and rapid intubation is essential to attempt to mitigate morbidity and mortality both to mother and fetus from airway complications. In a study performed by Olson et al., women undergoing cesarean delivery were at roughly a three-fold higher risk for aspiration than the general population undergoing anesthesia [31]. However, there are other studies that do not show increased risk with cesarean delivery, but rather with emergency surgery [32, 33]. Though pregnant women are at significantly increased risk in terms of aspiration, this risk has decreased within the last few decades, likely due to significant increases in the utilization of neuraxial anesthesia. It is important to note that in this population, the reported risk of aspiration upon emergence from anesthesia is just as high as the risk upon induction, and thus clinicians should remain especially vigilant and utilize protective strategies during the entire course of intervention [33].

The American Society of Anesthesiologists obstetric anesthesia practice guidelines recommend administration of H2 blockers, non-particulate antacids, and/or reglan prior to surgical procedures in this population [34].

Fluid management should be judicious but aggressive, in an attempt to limit use of vasopressors as much as possible. If necessary, the preferred agent is phenylephrine, due to its limited effects on uterine and placental perfusion. The two most studied vasopressor agents in obstetrics seem to be ephedrine and phenylephrine. In contrast to ephedrine, phenylephrine can be administered in doses that maintain maternal blood pressure while preventing nausea and vomiting and without causing fetal acidosis. Phenylephrine, however, is associated with decreases in maternal heart rate and cardiac output [35].

If possible, the patient should be placed in a left lateral decubitus position to augment venous return by relieving compression from the vena cava. If this is not possible, one may utilize a bolster placed under the right hip or tilt the table toward the patient's left. There is some concern as to whether chest compressions are as effective when the patient is placed in positions other than supine. An alternative to positioning changes is to place the patient supine and utilize manual retraction of the uterus to the patient's left side. Pregnant patients may require significant modifications to the way in which cardiopulmonary resuscitation is performed (Table 41.3).

Table 41.3 Modifications to CPR performed on the pregnant patient

Chest compressions: place the hands slightly higher on the sternum
Obtain intravenous access above the diaphragm
Anticipate difficult airway management
Discontinue magnesium sulfate (if applicable) and administer calcium chloride or calcium gluconate
Perform manual left uterine displacement, or place a firm wedge under the resuscitation board to tilt patient approximately 30°
Defibrillation: remove both internal and external fetal monitors
If spontaneous circulation does not return within 4 min of cardiac arrest, immediate hysterotomy or cesarean delivery should be performed if gestational age is 20 weeks or greater, aiming for delivery within 5 min of cardiac arrest

In this population, a consult should be placed to an obstetrician as soon as is possible for their assistance in determining need for and performance of emergent cesarean section.

General and Emergency Surgical Considerations

General surgery procedures are required in about 1 in 500 pregnant patients [36]. The incidence of surgical disease in the pregnant population is similar to the nonpregnant population [36] for the most part, though some conditions, such as cholelithiasis, may have an increased incidence.

Appendicitis

The most common general surgical condition affecting pregnant patients is acute appendicitis, which accounts for approximately 25% of all non-obstetric surgical interventions in pregnant patients. Acute appendicitis seems to have an equal frequency across all three trimesters [37]. However,

this population does have a higher rate of perforated appendicitis, which correlates with an increased maternal and fetal morbidity and mortality. The presence of peritonitis from a perforated viscus can lead to preterm labor and delivery in up to 50% of cases during the third trimester [38]. Increased vascularity and lymphatic drainage within the abdomen during pregnancy lead to more rapid dissemination of infection and potential complications for both mother and fetus. During gestation, the position of the appendix within the abdomen changes, as it becomes progressively displaced into the right mid- to upper quadrant (Fig. 41.3). Therefore, location of pain in the right lower quadrant is common only earlier on in the gestational period. As the abdominal wall musculature also demonstrates increased laxity and the uterus may be interposed between the appendix and the abdominal wall, guarding and rebound tenderness can be diminished or absent. The position and size of the uterus may also contribute to decreased ability of the omentum to reach and wall off a ruptured appendix [38]. Nausea, vomiting, and anorexia are common in pregnant patients with appendicitis, appearing in 58–72% of cases [37].

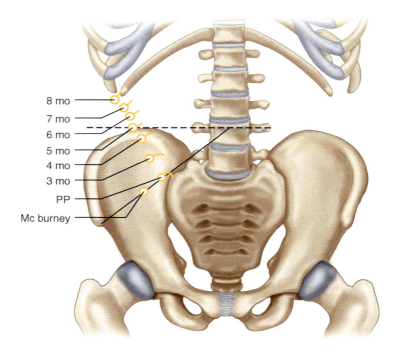

Fig. 41.3 Changes in the position of the appendix throughout pregnancy

This may cloud the clinical picture early in the pregnancy, since nausea and emesis are common during the first trimester. In later stages of gestation, these signs should arouse suspicion and result in investigation, especially when coupled with abdominal pain. Though CT scan is highly sensitive and specific for appendicitis, its concomitant radiation exposure usually leads to ultrasound being the most common initial imaging modality, unless the diagnosis is in question. An appendiceal wall thickness over 3 mm and a diameter of greater than 6 mm are findings that suggest appendicitis. Of course, ultrasound is an operator-dependent modality, and it can be difficult to obtain a high-quality exam during pregnancy. Abdominal wall thickness, alteration of usual landmarks, and displacement of intra-abdominal structures may complicate the exam. If necessary, CT scan can and should be performed. Performing a CT with rectal contrast decreases the radiation exposure to roughly one-third of that of a regular CT scan [39]. It is important to remember that while the amount of radiation to perform a CT scan is unlikely to result in fetal loss or teratogenicity (though possible), low levels of radiation can and do increase the risk

and incidence of childhood malignancies. This increased lifetime risk of cancer is estimated to increase from 20% to 21% for those exposed to at least 10 rad [40]. It is important to use discretion in performing CT scan and other radiologic studies in pregnant patients and should be reserved for those cases in which the diagnosis is not clear after performing a thorough history and physical, as well as ultrasound examination.

MRI is another potential imaging modality for diagnosis of appendicitis. One study reports sensitivity and specificity of MRI for acute appendicitis in pregnancy to be 100% and 93.6%, respectively [41].

Appendectomy tends to be well-tolerated both by mother and fetus. Laparoscopy becomes increasingly challenging with increasing uterine size, particularly after the second trimester. Regardless of trimester, it is recommended that an open technique of initial trocar placement be utilized, in order to attempt to avoid injury to the uterus or fetus. A proposed alternate port placement for laparoscopic appendectomy is shown in Fig. 41.4. Indications for laparoscopy in the pregnant patient, as presented by the Society of

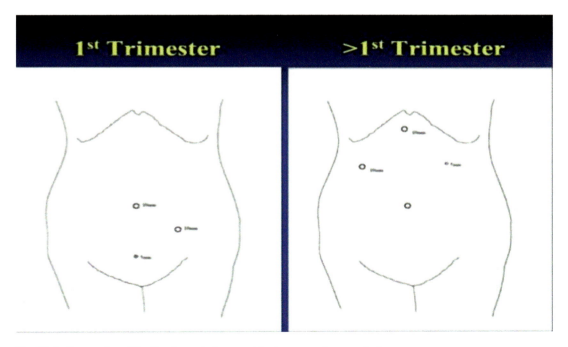

Fig. 41.4 Proposed modification for port placement for laparoscopic appendectomy

American Gastrointestinal and Endoscopic Surgeons, are shown in Table 41.4. If an open operative technique is utilized, the safest approach is generally a right-sided transverse incision overlying the point of maximal tenderness [37, 42]. The second trimester seems to be the optimal time for operation, as fetal organogenesis is complete and maternal anatomic changes will not be as marked as in the third trimester. Operative intervention, of course, can be performed during any trimester for urgent or emergent indications and should only be delayed for active labor, in which case appendectomy may be performed immediately afterward. Cesarean delivery should be performed if there is evidence of sepsis or septic shock. Pregnant patients have a higher incidence of false-negative appendiceal pathology, though this is acceptable due to the significant fetal and maternal risks that come with a delay in diagnosis or management. If the appendix is found to appear grossly normal, an appendectomy should still be performed, as it only mildly impacts morbidity and eliminates the organ as a source of potential confusion if there is recurrence of symptoms in the future [37].

Table 41.4 SAGES guidelines for laparoscopy in the pregnant patient

Indications for laparoscopic treatment of acute abdominal processes are the same as for nonpregnant patients
Laparoscopy can be safely performed during any trimester of pregnancy
Preoperative obstetric consultation should be obtained
Intermittent lower extremity pneumatic compression devices should be used intraoperatively and postoperatively to prevent venous stasis (i.e., as prophylaxis for deep vein thrombosis)
The fetal heart rate and uterine tone should be monitored both preoperatively and postoperatively
End-tidal CO_2 should be monitored during surgery
Left uterine displacement should be maintained to avoid aortocaval compression
An open (Hassan) technique, a Veress needle, or an optical trocar technique may be used to enter the abdomen
Low pneumoperitoneum pressures (between 10 and 15 mm Hg) should be used
Tocolytic agents should not be used prophylactically but should be considered when evidence of preterm labor is present

Biliary Disease

The second most common non-obstetric surgical condition is biliary tract disease. Again, the signs and symptoms closely follow those of nonpregnant patients, though Murphy's sign may not be present. The gallbladder empties more slowly during pregnancy, and there is also an increase in residual volume. Bile is supersaturated by cholesterol, which is mediated by estrogen, and progesterone mediates relaxation of the gallbladder [43]. These changes increase the likelihood of lithogenesis during pregnancy [44]. In fact, the risk of developing gallstones increases with increasing pregnancies [43, 45, 46]. Gallbladder physiology returns to normal as early as 2 weeks postpartum, but if stones have formed, they may persist. Ultrasound is the imaging modality of choice in pregnant women with complaints of right upper quadrant pain. Symptomatic cholelithiasis is likely to be managed conservatively in the pregnant patient, with planned cholecystectomy postpartum. However, with conservative management, there is an increased risk of progression of biliary disease or continuation of symptoms. Between 57% and 70% of patients treated medically for gallstone disease during the gestational period will have a recurrence at some point during their pregnancy [47, 48], and the risk of recurrence is proportional to the amount of remaining gestational time. Additionally, if these patients progress to acute cholecystitis or choledocholithiasis, they are at higher risk compared to nonpregnant patients for complications such as cholangitis and gallstone pancreatitis. Patients who develop these complications are at a much higher risk for fetal loss and maternal mortality, as high as 15% for the mother and 60% for the fetus [49]. For these reasons, some advocate for early operative management in those presenting early in their pregnancy, with the second trimester being the optimal time for operation. Despite the increased prevalence of gallstones, fortunately acute cholecystitis is not frequent and occurs in 0.01–0.08% of pregnancies [50, 51]. As in appendectomy, laparoscopy is acceptable and seems to be well-tolerated by mother and fetus. A proposed alternate port placement for the pregnant patient is shown in Fig. 41.5. If necessary, ERCP can be performed in this population. With judicious

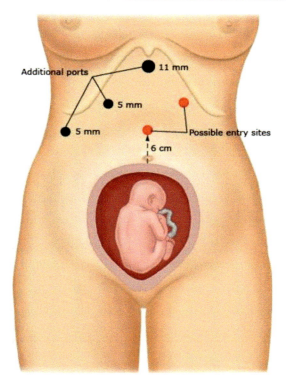

Fig. 41.5 Proposed alternate port placement for laparoscopic cholecystectomy during pregnancy

management including bowel rest, nasogastric tube decompression, and IV fluids being an acceptable starting point. However, the diagnosis of ischemia can be difficult in this patient population, as pain can sometimes be attributed to the pregnancy, and since the WBC count is mildly elevated in pregnancy, it can erroneously be dismissed. Delayed diagnosis of ischemic bowel can be detrimental to both mother and fetus creating a difficult dilemma. A discussion regarding the risks of radiation exposure for CT scan versus diagnostic laparoscopy or exploration must be undertaken when uncertainty arises. The surgeon must be prepared to take the patient to the operating room if there is suspicion for bowel compromise, even in the absence of definitive diagnostics, prior to perforation as fetal and maternal outcomes will be compromised if this diagnosis is missed. The overall rate of fetal loss during bowel obstruction is 17%, with a maternal mortality rate of 2% [54].

Umbilical Hernia

Umbilical hernias are common in pregnancy, though most do not incarcerate or strangulate. For patients that present with hernia, an attempt should be made at reduction and observation, assuming there are no signs pointing to bowel ischemia or necrosis, such as overlying cellulitis or peritoneal signs. Operative repair should be urgently undertaken if the hernia is irreducible or if there are signs of peritonitis or fetal distress. At our institution, umbilical hernias in this population are generally repaired primarily if possible. Contrary to the general surgery population, mesh repair is not associated with a lower recurrence rate compared to suture repair for patients with subsequent pregnancy [55]. It may also be advisable to avoid implantation of foreign material during pregnancy, and the growing uterus and forces exerted on the abdominal wall during labor may lend the hernia to recurrence if repair is undertaken during pregnancy, regardless of employed technique. Suture or mesh repair is therefore best avoided until at least the postpartum period. The risk of recurrence and reoperation

use of fluoroscopy and adequate shielding, fetal radiation exposure can be kept to a minimum. If the uterus is shielded, one series reported no radiation exposure of the uterus as measured by dosimeter [52].

Bowel Obstruction

The third most common non-obstetric surgical condition affecting pregnant women is bowel obstruction. Most of these obstructions are caused by adhesions from previous surgeries. Due to rapid changes in shape and size of the uterus and the shifting of intra-abdominal organs, volvulus is more common in pregnant patients [53]. The affected segment of the bowel is usually the sigmoid, as the gravid uterus causes a redundant sigmoid to rise out of the pelvis and twist around its mesentery. Treatment for bowel obstruction follows the same principles as for nonpregnant patients, with a trial of nonsurgical versus strangulation or incarceration during pregnancy should be weighed against each other. Some studies suggest any subsequent pregnancy following hernia repair is associated with a higher risk of recurrence. It may be beneficial to wait until no future pregnancies are desired to repair umbilical hernias if symptoms are minimal [55, 56].

References

1. Shah S, Miller PR, Meredith JW, Chang MC. Elevated admission white blood cell count in pregnant trauma patients: an indicator of ongoing placental abruption. Am Surg. 2002;68:644–7.
2. Pearlman MD, Tintinallli JE, Lorenz RP. A prospective controlled study of outcome after trauma during pregnancy. Am J Obstet Gynecol. 1990;162:1502–7.
3. Raja AS, Zabbo C. Trauma in pregnancy. Emerg Med Clin North Am. 2012;30(4):937–48.
4. Schwartz HM, Reichling BA. Hazards of radiation exposure for pregnant women. JAMA. 1978;239:1908.
5. Brent RL. The effects of embryonic and fetal exposure to x-ray, microwaves, and ultrasound: counseling the pregnant and non-pregnant patient about these risks. Semin Oncol. 1989;16:347–68.
6. Karam PA. Determining and reporting fetal radiation exposure from diagnostic radiation. Health Phys. 2000;79(5 Suppl):S85–90.
7. Reece AE, Goldstein I, Hobbins JC. Fundamentals of obstetric and gynecologic ultrasound. Norwalk: Appleton & Lange; 1994.
8. Carbillon L, Uzan M, Uzan S. Pregnancy, vascular tone, and maternal hemodynamics. Obstet Gynecol Surv. 2000;55:574–81.
9. Pacheco L, Constantine MM, Hankins GDV. Physiological changes during pregnancy. In: Clinical pharmacology during pregnancy. San Diego: Academic; 2013. p. 5–14.
10. Allen LH. Anemia and iron deficiency: effects on pregnancy outcome. Am J Clin Nutr. 2000;71:1280S–4s.
11. Hill CC, Pickinpaugh J. Physiologic changes in pregnancy. Surg Clin North Am. 2008;88:391–401.
12. Gaillard R, Bakker R, Willemsen SP, et al. Blood pressure tracking during pregnancy and the risk of gestational hypertensive disorders: the Generation R study. Eur Heart J. 2011;32:3088–97.
13. Scirica BM, O'Gara PT. Valvular heart disease in pregnancy. Curr Cardiol Rep. 2006;8:83–9.
14. Campos O, Andrade JL, Bocanegra J, et al. Physiologic multivalvular regurgitation during pregnancy: a longitudinal Doppler echocardiographic study. Int J Cardiol. 1993;40:265.
15. Lyons G. Failed intubation. Six years' experience in a teaching maternity unit. Anaesthesia. 1985;40:759–62.

16. Rocke DA, Murray WB, Rout CC, Gouws E. Relative risk analysis of factors associated with difficult intubation in obstetric anesthesia. Anesthesiology. 1992;77:67–73.
17. Rasmussen PE, Nielse FR. Hydronephrosis during pregnancy: a literature survey. Eur J Obstet Gynaecol Reprod Biol. 1988;27:249–59.
18. Hey VM, Cowley DJ, Ganguli PC, et al. Gastro-oesophageal reflux in late pregnancy. Anaesthesia. 1977;32:372–7.
19. Lind JF, Smith AM, McIver DK, et al. Heartburn in pregnancy—a manometric study. Can Med Assoc J. 1968; 98:571–4.
20. Van Thiel DH, Gavaler JS, Joshi SN, et al. Heartburn of pregnancy. Gastroenterology. 1977;72:666–8.
21. Vanner RG, Goodman NW. Gastro-oesophageal reflux in pregnancy at term and after delivery. Anaesthesia. 1989;44:808–11.
22. Davison JS, Davison MC, Hay DM. Gastric emptying time in late pregnancy and labour. J Obstet Gynaecol Br Commonw. 1970;77:37–41.
23. Toglia MR, Weg JG. Venous thromboembolism during pregnancy. N Engl J Med. 1996;335:108–14.
24. Snow V, Qaseem A, Barry P, et al. Management of venous thromboembolism: a clinical practice guideline from the American College of Physicians and the American Academy of Family Physicians. Ann Intern Med. 2007;146:204–10.
25. Dresang LT, Fontaine P, Leeman L, et al. Venous thromboembolism during pregnancy. Am Fam Physician. 2008;77:1709–16.
26. Bates SM, Greer IA, Pabinger I, et al. Venous thromboembolism, thrombophilia, antithrombotic therapy, and pregnancy: American College of Chest Physicians evidence-based clinical practice guidelines 8th edition. Chest. 2008;133.(suppl:8445–65.
27. Mastorakos G, Ilias I. Maternal hypothalamic-pituitary-adrenal axis in pregnancy and the postpartum period: postpartum-related disorders. Ann N Y Acad Sci. 2000;900:95.
28. Casey BM, Levenek K. Thyroid disease in pregnancy. Obstet Gynecol. 2006;108:1283–92.
29. Neale D, Cootauco A, Burrow G. Thyroid disease in pregnancy. Clin Perinatol. 2007;34:543–57.
30. Alexander EK, Marqusee E, Lawrence J, et al. Timing and magnitude of increases in levothyroxine requirements during pregnancy in women with hypothyroidism. N Engl J Med. 2004;351:241–9.
31. Olsson GL, Hallen B, Hambraeus-Jonzon K. Aspiration during anaesthesia: a computer-aided study of 185,358 anaesthetics. Acta Anaesthesiol Scand. 1986;30:84–92.
32. Kluger MT, Short TG. Aspiration during anaesthesia: a review of 133 cases from the Australian Anaesthetic Incident Monitoring Study (AIMS). Anaesthesia. 1999;54:19–26.
33. Warner MA, Warner ME, Weber JG. Clinical significance of pulmonary aspiration during the perioperative period. Anesthesiology. 1993;78:56–62.

34. American Society of Anesthesiologists Committee on Standards and Practice Parameters. Practice guidelines for obstetric anesthesia. Anesthesiology. 2015;124(2):1–31.
35. Ngan Kee WD, Khaw K. Vasopressors in obstetrics: what should we be using? Curr Opin Anaesthesiol. 2006;19(3):238–43.
36. Kammerer WS. Nonobstetric surgery during pregnancy. Med Clin North Am. 1979;63(6):1157–64.
37. Babaknia A, Parsa H, Woodruff JD. Appendicitis during pregnancy. Obstet Gynecol. 1977;50:40–4.
38. Dietrich CS III, Hill CC, Hueman M. Surgical diseases presenting in pregnancy. Surg Clin North Am. 2008;88:403–19.
39. Rao PM, Rhea JT, Novelline RA, et al. Helical CT combined with contrast material administered only through the colon for imaging of suspected appendicitis. AJR Am J Roentgenol. 1997;169:1275–80.
40. NCRP Commentary No. 9. Considerations regarding the unintended radiation exposure of the embryo, fetus or nursing child. National Council on Radiation Protection: Bethesda; 1994.
41. Pedrosa I, Levine D, Eyvazzadeh AD, Siewert B, Ngo L, Rofsky NM. MR imaging evaluation of acute appendicitis in pregnancy. Radiology. 2006;238:891–9.
42. Weingold AB. Appendicitis in pregnancy. Clin Obstet Gynecol. 1983;26:801–9.
43. Everson GT. Gastrointestinal motility in pregnancy. Gastroenterol Clin N Am. 1992;21:751–76.
44. Everson GT, McKinley C, Lawson M, et al. Gallbladder function in the human female: effect of the ovulatory cycle, pregnancy, and contraceptive steroids. Gastroenterology. 1982;82:711–9.
45. Valdivieso V, Covarrubias C, Siegel F, et al. Pregnancy and cholelithiasis: pathogenesis and natural course of gallstones diagnosed in early puerperium. Hepatology. 1993;17:1–4.
46. Barbara L, Sama C, Morselli Labate AM, et al. A population study on the prevalence of gallstone disease: the Sirmione Study. Hepatology. 1987;7:913–7.
47. Curet MJ, Allen D, Josloff RK, et al. Laparoscopy during pregnancy. Arch Surg. 1996;131:546–51.
48. Dixon NP, Faddis DM, Silberman H. Aggressive management of cholecystitis during pregnancy. Am J Surg. 1987;154:292–4.
49. Simon JA. Biliary tract disease and related surgical disorders during pregnancy. Clin Obstet Gynecol. 1983;26:810–21. Eichenberg BJ, Vanderlinden J, Miguel C, et al. Laparoscopic cholecystectomy in the third trimester of pregnancy. Am Surg. 1996;62:874–7
50. Basso L, McCollum PT, Darling MN, et al. A study of cholelithiasis during pregnancy and its relationship with age, parity, menarche, breast-feeding, dysmenorrhea, oral contraception, and a maternal history of cholelithiasis. Surgery. 1992;175:41–6.
51. Mayer IE, Hussain H. Abdominal pain during pregnancy. Gastroenterol Clin N Am. 1998;27:1–36.
52. Howden JK, Robuck-Mangum G, Jowell PS, et al. Endoscopic management of choledocholithiasis during pregnancy: safety and efficacy of endoscopic retrograde cholangiopancreatography and endoscopic sphincterotomy. Gastrointest Endosc. 2001;53(5):AB96.
53. Alshawi JS. Recurrent sigmoid volvulus in pregnancy: report of a case and review of the literature. Dis Colon Rectum. 2005;48(9):1811–3.
54. Webster PJ, Bailey MA, Wilson J, et al. Small bowel obstruction in pregnancy is a complex surgical problem with a high risk of fetal loss. Ann R Coll Surg Engl. 2015;97(5):339–44.
55. Oma E, Jensen KK, Jorgensen LN. Recurrent umbilical or epigastric hernia during and after pregnancy: a nationwide cohort study. Surgery. 2016;159(6):1677–83.
56. Lappen JR, Sheyn D, Hackney DN. Does pregnancy increase the risk of abdominal hernia recurrence after prepregnancy surgical repair? Am J Obstet Gynecol. 2016;215(3):390.e1–5.
57. de Swiet M. The cardiovascular system. In: Hytten F, Chamberlain G, editors. Clinical physiology in obstetrics. Oxford: Blackwell Scientific Publications; 1980. p. 3–42.
58. Colditz RB, Josey WE. Central venous pressure in supine position during normal pregnancy. Comparative determinations during first, second and third trimesters. Obstet Gynecol. 1970;36:769.
59. Letsky E. The hematological system. In: Hytten RF, Chamberlin G, editors. Clinical physiology in obstetrics. Oxford: Blackwell Scientific Publications; 1980. p. 43–78.
60. Cruikshank DP. Anatomic and physiologic alterations of pregnancy that modify the response to trauma. In: Buchsbaum HJ, editor. Trauma in pregnancy. Philadelphia: WB Saunders; 1979. p. 21–39.

Emergency General Surgery in the Immunocompromised Surgical Patient

42

Shawn Tejiram and Jack A. Sava

Introduction

The immunocompromised patient presents unique challenges to the general surgeon. These patients usually present in a delayed fashion with atypical symptoms and an unreliable physical exam. Even common diagnoses can be difficult. Immune compromise can come from many sources (Table 42.1) [1]. While the general management of immunosuppression may not traditionally fall under the purview of the general surgeon, it is critical to understand the basic pathophysiology and effects of immune suppression in the emergent setting when considering operative intervention. This chapter will review common causes of immune compromise and their impact on decision for surgery, operative care, and perioperative management.

Evaluating the Immunocompromised Patient

Immune compromise is usually readily apparent when taking the history and performing physical examination. Once identified, it is critical to note details related to the cause and management of a patient's immune compromise. The indication, timing, and current dose of any immunosuppression medication, for example, will be even more crucially important than details of other medica-

Table 42.1 Causes of immune compromise

HIV
Transplant
Recent transplant
Long-term transplant on immunosuppressive therapy
Cancer/malignancy/neutropenic patients
Rheumatologic diseases
Systemic lupus erythema
Rheumatoid arthritis
Sarcoidosis
Inflammatory bowel disease
Iatrogenic
Steroids
Chemotherapeutics (tacrolimus, cyclosporin, methotrexate, etc.)
Anti-inflammatory medications (anti-TNF-alpha, NSAIDs)
Diabetes
Liver failure
Renal failure
Elderly

S. Tejiram
General Surgery, Medstar Washington Hospital,
Washington, DC, USA

J. A. Sava (✉)
Department of General Surgery, Trauma Service,
Washington Hospital Center, Washington, DC, USA
e-mail: Jack.A.Sava@medstar.net

© Springer International Publishing AG, part of Springer Nature 2019
C. V. R. Brown et al. (eds.), *Emergency General Surgery*, https://doi.org/10.1007/978-3-319-96286-3_42

tions. Furthermore, the general surgeon will need to come to an understanding of the patient's prognosis in the condition causing immune compromise. In an era of increasingly specialized care, this will often require multidisciplinary help from many fields of expertise.

The physical exam is notoriously blunted by immune suppression. Signs such as peritonitis are absent, and commonly used decision rubrics or scoring systems may be difficult to apply safely. Even general indicators of disease such as fever and leukocytosis may not be present, leaving the surgeon with precious little to base a clinical diagnosis. Suspicion, however, should remain elevated for any diagnosis under consideration, and final decision-making should not be made until all information is made available [2, 3].

Laboratory testing may be more comprehensive than in immunocompetent patients with typical presentations. A complete blood count, comprehensive metabolic panel, electrolytes, arterial blood gas, lactate, and lipase form the basis of a general laboratory evaluation. In patients with solid organ transplantation, organ-specific biomarkers should be evaluated for any risk or presence of transplant rejection. A renal transplant patient, for example, may need evaluation of urine, creatinine, or other renal-related studies, while liver function testing is necessary when evaluating a liver transplant recipient. Specialized stains and cultures may also be necessary in neutropenic or immunocompromised patients such as those with human immunodeficiency virus (HIV) or acquired immunodeficiency syndrome (AIDS) to determine the presence of opportunistic infection [2, 4].

Imaging may also have a heightened importance in the workup of immunocompromised patients. With paradoxical presentations and exam findings, imaging sometimes may be the only diagnostic finding in a presenting immunocompromised patient. Imaging can often identify disease pathology that may not have been apparent or considered based on clinical examination or blood tests alone. Computed tomography (CT) is commonly used in the search for septic sources,

but other tools such as Doppler ultrasound or magnetic resonance imaging (MRI) may be needed after transplantation. Protocols which serve to limit overuse of imaging (e.g., clinical diagnosis pathways for acute appendicitis) may not apply to patients with altered immune function and should not be used until validated in those populations.

Decision for Surgery

When managing immunocompromised patients, the decision to operate is often particularly challenging for the surgeon [5]. Compared to other patient encounters, there is likely to be more diagnostic uncertainty. Assessment of severity and host response is similarly difficult. Two overarching and contrary concerns accompany the decision for possible operation. First, it may be clear that the patient will tolerate surgery poorly. Wound and respiratory complications will be more likely than usual, and a complicated postoperative course may be anticipated. These factors lead the surgeon away from the operating room and toward less invasive strategies, which may include percutaneous drainage or observation.

In contrast, the surgeon will likely appreciate that these patients have little reserve for fighting infection. Their ability to heal perforations or resorb small abscesses may be significantly diminished. Worse, they may not show early signs of unresolved infection, but instead may collapse suddenly from septic shock. Clearly, patients with immune compromise cannot afford delayed or incomplete source control and may have only one chance at success.

These concerns – often summarized into the question, "too sick to operate or too sick not to operate?" – can be confounding. Many experienced surgeons have concluded that in operations involving source control (cholecystitis, perforated diverticulitis, appendicitis, etc.), the surgeon should lean toward aggressive surgical source control in immunocompromised patients. Many exciting, less invasive treatment plans for abdominal infections have arisen in recent years, including laparoscopic lavage for perforated diverticulitis, non-operative treatment of acute appendicitis, and ileostomy with colonic lavage for fulminant *Clostridium difficile* colitis. Until these strategies are validated in immunocompromised patients, it may be more prudent to ask the question, "Can my patient afford to fail" a new noninvasive strategy? If the answer is no, it is reasonable to select early, definitive surgical source control while acknowledging the potential consequences.

When surgery is contemplated for other reasons – e.g., symptom control or lifestyle improvement – the surgeon may reasonably be more cautious in choosing an operative approach. This does not mean that immune compromise is an absolute contraindication to non-lifesaving surgery but rather that the risks and benefits need to be carefully weighed and explained to the patient as part of a shared decision. Immune compromise is not a binary "yes or no" phenomenon, and while some such patients may be too ill to tolerate any surgery, others with well-controlled immune modulation may achieve surgical outcomes nearly identical to their non-compromised counterparts.

Disease-Specific Considerations

Familiarity with the care of immunocompromised patients allows the general surgeon to become more proficient in preparing patients for surgery and better optimize their chances for success [2, 3]. Following the decision to proceed with surgery, the patient must be optimized with focus on any active immunosuppressive disease process. Maintenance of fluid balance, restoration of hemodynamics, circulatory function optimization, electrolyte replacement, and correction of acidosis should all be emphasized [6]. Basic considerations such as minimizing exposure to invasive lines, ensuring early extubation after surgery, or selecting appropriate anesthetic management in patients with organ failure have led to an overall improvement in care.

Human Immunodeficiency Virus and Acquired Immunodeficiency Syndrome

Patients with human immunodeficiency virus (HIV) and the more advanced acquired immunodeficiency virus (AIDS) can be a diagnostic challenge for the emergency general surgeon. Not only do they have the atypical presentations inherent to the immunocompromised population, but the possibility of opportunistic infection can further complicate their course. Important elements to note while obtaining a history in patients with HIV/AIDS include the use of antiretroviral therapy, compliance with management, and last known CD4 count and viral load. Evaluation of CD4 count is critical – worse outcomes are associated with those patients who have CD4 counts less than 200 [7–9]. Common complications in this patient population include poor wound healing, surgical site infections, postoperative pneumonias, or the development of opportunistic infections following operative intervention [10–12].

The introduction of highly active antiretroviral therapy (HAART) in the 1990s has improved patient survival and made this deadly virus increasingly manageable. Despite this, however, compliance with this regimen is incomplete, and patients still oftentimes present in the emergent setting whether they are well-managed or not [9]. Patients with HIV and AIDS can present for a variety of emergent reasons such as appendicitis, hernias, cholecystitis, opportunistic infections, and malignancies such as Kaposi sarcoma and lymphoma [13–15].

Emergent procedures in this patient population are notably associated with increasing complications, and some literature report mortality rates as high as 50% [16, 17]. Immune status as identified by viral load and CD4 count must be considered in the evaluation of the patient. Susceptible opportunistic organisms include *Candida*, *Helicobacter pylori*, *Cryptosporidium*, *Mycobacterium avium complex (MAC)*, *spirochete*, and *Cytomegalovirus (CMV)* and have been implicated in gastrointestinal perforations, cholecystitis, and cholangitis [18–21]. Anorectal disease is also a common among these patients and presents as simple and deep, complex perianal abscesses, HPV-associated anorectal warts, and anal intraepithelial neoplasia (AIN).

A 10-year retrospective review of HIV-positive patients examined whether CD4 count was predictive of outcomes following emergent abdominal operations. They noted patients who underwent urgent operations were more likely to have lower CD4 counts preoperatively and were more likely to suffer a major or fatal complication [9]. Some studies have also suggested a correlation between lower CD4 counts and increased complications in both aortic and gynecologic surgeries [22–24]. Other studies have suggested a relationship with lower CD4 count and increased risk of death [25, 26]. Viral load (HIV-1 RNA) has also been considered as a marker for immune status, but results comparing outcomes appear to be more discordant [9]. Compared to the uninfected population, there is decreased morbidity with the laparoscopic approach in HIV-infected patients [20, 27].

Some simple steps may mitigate the increased morbidity seen in these patients. Current evidence supports early infectious disease consultation in the surgical management of patients with HIV disease. They can help manage and advise in the use of antiretroviral therapy, manage postoperative infections, and optimize CD4 counts and viral loads in preparation for operative intervention. Their inclusion has been shown to reduce the rate of postoperative complications, mortality, and hospital costs and shorten length of stay [28–30].

Opportunistic organisms can be a source of surgical pathology [31]. In one series, more than 80% of patients undergoing operative intervention were found to be due to HIV-related pathology such as opportunistic infections. Preoperative antibiotic selection may be different than in other patients due to the potential for opportunistic infections such as *Pneumocystis jirovecii*, MAC, *Candida*, and CMV. Related antibiotic prophylactic regimens typically include bactrim, azithromycin, fluconazole, and valganciclovir [32–34]. Patients already on antiretroviral medications

with suppressed viral loads and a CD4 count >200, however, may not need a specialized prophylactic regimen [35].

AIDS patients requiring emergency abdominal surgery have increased morbidity and mortality [20, 22, 36]. Patients presenting emergently typically have CD4 counts significantly lower than those undergoing elective procedures [9]. Antiretroviral therapy can have a protective effect on a patient's immune system by decreasing viral load while increasing CD4 count in an attempt to reestablish the immune system. This may prevent opportunistic infections and potentially improve survival [37].

Solid Organ Transplantation

Patients who have undergone solid organ transplantation are unique even among the immunocompromised population, due to their medication-induced immunosuppression and prior history of major surgery. As the field of organ transplantation has matured, graft survival and life expectancy have improved. This longevity has increased the likelihood of these patients needing emergency surgery [38–40]. These patients are typically managed by transplant teams, are chronically on immunosuppressive medications, and present atypically. It is crucial that the consulting general surgeon performs a thorough examination of these patients even in the presence of mild abdominal pain, to avoid missing atypical presentations of significant pathology [1].

Emergency surgery in the transplant patient is not a rare event. All surgeons should be familiar with the factors that influence surgical outcomes in these patients. A recent meta-analysis showed that, among transplanted patients who underwent emergency surgery, 2.5% of these patients were due to graft-unrelated acute abdominal disease. The most common presentations for emergency abdominal surgery included gallbladder disease followed by gastrointestinal perforations, complicated diverticulitis, small bowel obstruction, and appendicitis. Overall mortality was reported at 5.5% [5].

Timing can factor into the differential diagnosis of posttransplant complications. Typically within the first month, nosocomial infections should be considered first. These can present as cellulitis, catheter-associated urinary tract infection (CAUTI), central line-associated blood stream infection (CLABSI), hospital- or community-associated pneumonia, *Clostridium difficile*, intra-abdominal abscesses, or fungal infections. However, up to 6 months afterward, higher risks for opportunistic infections should be considered including CMV, MAC, tuberculosis, amebiasis, *Salmonella*, and *Campylobacter*. After the first year, patients with no graft issues or signs of rejection present with abdominal surgical emergencies similar to those in immunocompetent patients. Those with immunosuppressive issues or more intense rejection signs are more likely to have opportunistic infection [1]. Current evidence does not support the use of any specific preoperative antibiotic in transplant patients. However, standard perioperative antibiotic guidelines and practices should be followed [41, 42].

Preoperative evaluation should note the type, location, and timing of transplantation as well as current immunosuppressive medications. The immunosuppressive regimen may be influenced by a patient's history of adverse reactions, previous rejections, or tolerance to the medications themselves [43, 44]. Immunosuppressive medications can have an important impact on surgical outcomes. The use of calcineurin inhibitors, antiproliferative agents, and corticosteroids can predispose patients to gastrointestinal diseases, lymphoproliferative disorders, and infectious complications. They have additionally been implicated as a cause of the atypical and masked symptoms of presentation [44, 45]. A complete understanding on the reasoning behind a patient's current regimen can help identify what available alternative immunosuppressive options are available.

Immunosuppressive agents can have important cross-reaction with perioperative medications, including anesthetic agents. Calcineurin inhibitors work to suppress the immune system by preventing IL-2 production and include medications like cyclosporine or tacrolimus. Their combined use with other medications can alter bloodstream concentrations and affect metabolism of the inhibitors itself. For example, combination use of paralytics such as vecuronium or pancuronium with calcineurin inhibitors may increase neuromuscular blockade. Its concomitant use with fluconazole, erythromycin, or phenytoin may alter calcineurin inhibitor levels [2, 46, 47]. This can potentially put the transplanted organ at risk. Medication levels must therefore be measured postoperatively and daily thereafter. Antiproliferatives work to prevent DNA replication through a purine pathway and include such medications as mycophenolate mofetil and azathioprine. One of the most important side effects of antiproliferative use is chronic and extensive myelosuppression. Preoperative evaluation should thus also focus on preoperative and daily medication levels as well as daily evaluation of blood counts in anticipation of any signs or symptoms of toxic dosing and to evaluate the need for transfusion [48, 49].

Meta-analyses of gallbladder disease in solid organ transplantation identified acute cholecystitis as the most common presenting problem requiring emergent abdominal surgery in transplanted patients [5]. The prevalence of biliary tract disease may be due to cyclosporine-induced perturbation of the enterohepatic circulation, resulting in increased biliary stone formation. Other factors that may potentially affect the enterohepatic system include vagotomy associated with transplantation, hemolysis, or rapid posttransplant weight loss [50–52]. In transplanted patients undergoing cholecystectomy, a morbidity rate of 13.6% was reported. Common postoperative complications included surgical site infection, deep venous thrombosis, pulmonary embolus, respiratory failure, pneumonia, and bleeding. The mortality rate was 3.4% with a median hospital length of stay of 9.3 days [5, 40, 53–55]. Consequently, some authors have advocated prophylactic cholecystectomy in asymptomatic patients awaiting transplantation [56, 57]. Comparing open versus laparoscopic approach for gallbladder disease in transplanted patients, there is some evidence to suggest that the laparoscopy has fewer postoperative complications than open approach – as seen in nontransplant patients – and can be performed safely after lung and kidney transplant [53].

Gastrointestinal perforations are serious and multifactorial, with causes ranging from perioperative hypoperfusion to high-dose immunosuppressant or invasive infectious colonic disease [58–61]. Gastrointestinal perforations are the second most frequent cause of emergent abdominal surgery subsequent to organ transplantation [5, 62, 63]. Meta-analyses of transplanted patients identified diverticulitis, peptic disease, ischemia, chronic inflammatory bowel disease, posttransplantation lymphoproliferative disorders, *Clostridium difficile* colitis, and CMV as the most frequent causes of perforation. Signs and symptoms may be absent, nonspecific, or obvious with acute peritonitis [64–66]. The interval from clinical onset to surgery ranges as high as 8 days. Diagnosis is often confirmed by CT. Perforations are mostly located in the colon and, to a lesser extent, small bowel and stomach. Meta-analysis of transplanted patients with gastrointestinal perforation noted that a colostomy was required in 2.5% of patients, median hospital length of stay was 22.2 days, and the overall mortality rate was 17.5% [5].

Complicated diverticulitis in transplant patients carries a complication rate as high as 32.7% and typically manifests as respiratory disease or wound infection. A mortality rate of 13.6% has been reported, with most deaths due to sepsis. Diagnosing diverticular disease in transplanted patients is known to be challenging due to the masked signs and symptoms that hinder diagnosis [67]. These patients typically present with fever, abdominal pain, peritonitis, anorexia, diarrhea, and leukocytosis. In this setting, abdominal CT is reliable in identifying the location and severity of disease. Significantly higher morbidity and mortality have been reported after emergency colectomy for diverticulitis in a solid organ transplant patient compared to those performed on immunocompetent individuals [68, 69].

The most frequent cause of small bowel mechanical obstruction following organ transplantation is adhesive disease [5]. Diagnosis is made based on a combination of abdominal radiographs and CT and usually occurs within the first 2 years following transplantation. Small bowel obstruction is strongly associated with high levels of immunosuppression, and up to a third of patients may have both small and large bowel involvement [70, 71]. A course of nonoperative management can be attempted initially with bowel rest, intravenous fluid administration, and serial abdominal exams, but adhesiolysis must be considered in patients who fail to progress. Mortality rates may be up to 14%, which has been attributed mainly to sepsis and surgical-related complications [5].

Appendicitis presenting with nonspecific gastrointestinal symptoms may be confused with other transplant complications. While atypical symptoms may occasionally occur in the transplanted patient, evidence suggests that the clinical presentation overall still resembles that of a nonimmunosuppressed patients – right lower quadrant pain is typical, often with nausea, emesis, fevers, and diarrhea. Laboratory findings may be unreliable. In one study of liver-transplanted patients who presented with appendicitis, most patients showed no leukocytosis (>10 K) which may have contributed to delayed diagnosis and treatment [72]. Imaging can be used to take advantage of its noninvasiveness and accessibility, but computed tomography still remains the diagnostic gold standard, with the highest sensitivity and specificity [73, 74]. Delay in diagnosis is associated with a higher incidence of appendiceal rupture, gangrene, increased likelihood of laparotomy, and other related complications making early surgical intervention the treatment of choice [5, 72]. Length of stay may be high in these patients [73], but overall mortality rates associated with appendectomy are lower compared to other gastrointestinal complications [75].

Opportunistic infections can similarly affect the gastrointestinal system. Tuberculosis (TB) of the colon, for example, represents a clinical, diagnostic, and therapeutic challenge for a variety of reasons. *Mycobacterium tuberculosis* is difficult to identify on samples taken from lower GI endoscopy and has been reported to be definitively identified in less than 18% of cases. Even its gross appearance on endoscopic evaluation more closely resembles Crohn's disease and further compounds its misdiagnosis. Due to these factor, as well as a paucity of guidelines or evidence compared to pulmonary TB, colonic TB is more often a diagnosis of exclusion [76]. Up to 12% of gastrointestinal tuberculosis occurs in the colon with the most common site of colitis or enteritis occurring in the distal ileus and ileocecal region, making differentiation clinically from Crohn's disease more difficult. Up to 50% of patients with TB colitis will have no pulmonary etiology. One way to distinguish from Crohn's disease is the presence of diarrhea, which is encountered in Crohn's disease or overgrowth of the enteric flora but absent in colonic TB. Endoscopic evaluation will reveal inflamed or ulcerated mucosa and possible pseudopolyps near the ileocecal region. Histopathologic analysis will similarly exhibit chronic inflammation with ulceration of the mucosa, granulomatous changes with central necrosis, and lymph node invasion. Large granulomatous pseudopolyps are diagnostic and can cause obstruction. With concomitant thinning of the colonic wall and lymphadenopathy, vascular ischemia can result in perforation and become a surgical emergency [76]. Without perforation, treatment usually focuses on the avoidance of corticosteroids during microbiological and serologic testing, as well as a 9–12 month antituberculous treatment regimen with follow-up endoscopy to evaluate progression [76].

Other posttransplant complications may present to the general surgeon. Patients undergoing pancreatic transplantation, for example, may experience an early, posttransplant pancreatitis known as physiologic acute graft pancreatitis. This entity may occur up to 72 h post procedure. However, graft pancreatitis may present with abdominal pain up to 3 months after transplantation. Other considerations should include vascular thrombosis, infection, or rejection response. Evaluation at this point should include pancreas function studies such as amylase, lipase, and glucose as well as CT and Doppler imaging to examine the transplanted organ [1]. Graft-versus-host disease is a rare disease with high mortality rates in liver transplant patients. The disease develops due to the presence of lymphoid tissue in the donor organ. The presence of skin rash, diarrhea symptoms, and abdominal pain should raise suspicion [1]. Posttransplant bowel edema, ascites, and donor/recipient mismatch can also lead to increased intra-abdominal pressures. This is usually seen in the postoperative inpatient setting with worsening ascites or increasing abdominal pressure. Treatment should follow standard compartment syndrome protocols with measurements of bladder pressures to fully assess the degree of this condition with considerations given for decompressive laparotomy [1].

Neutropenic Patients

Cancer is a leading cause of death worldwide, and therapeutic advances have allowed extended survival in many malignancies. As with other immunocompromised patients, an increasing population of neutropenic patients are presenting to the general surgeon with potential life-threatening complications related to malignancy and its treatment [77]. The patients that present with neutropenia are usually undergoing extensive chemotherapy. A review of gastrointestinal emergencies in critically ill cancer patients revealed a variety of presentations that included neutropenic enterocolitis, mucosal toxicity, bowel infiltration by malignancy, and infectious colitis. A hospital mortality rate up to 35% was reported. Higher Simplified Acute Physiology Score (SAPS) II and Logistic Organ Dysfunction System (LODS) and neutropenia were independently associated with hospital mortality [77]. Evaluation of the neutropenic patient should begin with a thorough history noting the current disease process, location, and treatment regimen. Laboratory testing should identify preoperative anemia, thrombocytopenia, coagulopathy, or other hematologic dyscrasias that should be addressed prior to surgery. Bone marrow suppression and, as a result, coagulation function may similarly be affected either due to the disease process or treatment regimen and should also be considered in preoperative evaluation [78, 79].

Chemotherapeutic agents can potentially alter the metabolism of anesthetic agents, and a complete medication list should be obtained. For example, agents like anthracyclines can cause cardiotoxicity-associated dysrhythmias [80], bleomycin can cause pulmonary toxicity [81], and cisplatinum can cause neurotoxicity [82]. Due to the anesthetic needs required for operative intervention, a thorough understanding of drug-related reactions should be reviewed with the anesthesia team to determine an appropriate anesthetic regimen.

Like HIV and AIDS patients, neutropenic patients are at considerably increased risk for both common and opportunistic infections. Appropriate contact precautions should be set up limiting the number of staff interacting with the patient and providing appropriate personal protective equipment. Antibiotic prophylaxis should be considered particularly in patients with a low neutrophil count. No established consensus guidelines have been reached to suggest a standardized preoperative antibiotic regimen, but broad-spectrum antibiotics considered include piperacillin-tazobactam for its antipseudomonal properties, ciprofloxacin, or levofloxacin in high-risk patients. Fluconazole is an effective antifungal therapy to consider against *Candida* and *Aspergillus* pathogens while acyclovir can be used to manage patients with herpes simplex virus [83].

In the emergent setting, the risk of postoperative complications that include anastomotic leak can increase considerably. A retrospective analysis of patients who underwent segmental colectomy with anastomosis in the 2012 American College of Surgeons National Surgical Quality Improvement Program (NSQIP) identified several risk factors associated with anastomotic leak. Upon multivariate analysis, preoperative chemotherapy was significantly associated with increased rates of anastomotic leak. Radiation therapy has similarly been implicated in the association of anastomotic complications as well [84]. It is prudent for the general surgeon to consider all possible outcomes in this setting and consider diversion options, which can include diverting ileostomy, colostomy, or end ostomy.

Diverting ileostomy has been associated with a decreased incidence of leak compared to those with primary anastomosis [85].

Neutropenic enterocolitis (NEC), otherwise known as typhlitis, has become an increasingly recognized intestinal pathologic entity in the neutropenic patient. Presentation typically includes the triad of neutropenia, fever, nausea, emesis, abdominal pain, and distention following antineoplastic chemotherapy. It may encompass the entire bowel from small intestines to colon and may be identified with signs of colitis on CT imaging [1]. Affected patients can deteriorate quickly with rapidly progressing sepsis and multisystem organ failure. Improved outcomes critically depend on rapid diagnosis and intervention [86].

Several chemotherapeutic agents have been implicated in the pathogenesis of NEC and include paclitaxel, vincristine, doxorubicin, 5-fluorouracil, and leucovorin, among others. Associated malignancies were originally exclusively identified among pediatric leukemia, but adult leukemia, lymphoma, and solid tumors of breast, lung, colorectal, and ovarian origin have since been implicated. Symptoms appear as white blood cell counts reach their lowest point. Terminal ileum and cecum are commonly affected, due the distensibility and limited blood supply [86].

The pathophysiology of NEC is related to numerous factors including neutropenia, chemotherapeutic damage to the intestinal mucosa, and alteration of the gut lining that allows pathogenic bacterial invasion. The ensuing endotoxin produced allows the cascade of bacteremia, septic shock, and enteric necrosis. Initial care is supportive, with broad-spectrum antibiotic coverage and resuscitation. Diagnosis can be still be difficult at this point and relies on a high index of suspicion. CT imaging can be helpful, revealing bowel wall thickening, distention, and pneumatosis [86].

Treatment for NEC has traditionally involved bowel resection. Recent evidence suggests that some cases may be nonsurgical via careful hemodynamic support, bowel rest, and broad-spectrum antibiotics. Still, surgical intervention remains an important tool in refractory cases [86].

Corticosteroid Use

Corticosteroids are potent anti-inflammatory and immunosuppressive medications used broadly in the medical management of various disease processes. An estimated 0.9% of the population are said to use oral corticosteroids with approximately 22% having long-term use in excess of 6 months. The most common diseases causing corticosteroid use are respiratory disease, disease of the musculoskeletal system, and disease of the skin [87]. A review of the 2012 NSQIP data identified the association of corticosteroid use with increased risk of anastomotic leak. Patients in this population with anastomotic leak were noted to have longer hospital length of stay, higher rates of mortality, and a higher likelihood of multiple returns to the OR [85].

The general surgeon should expect higher rates of complications with steroid use, including wound complications, and should counsel their patients appropriately [88]. The association of corticosteroid use with gastrointestinal perforation is clear. In a large study examining diverticular perforations over a 15-year period, a threefold increase in diverticular perforation risk was associated with corticosteroid use [89]. The diagnosis of peritonitis from the onset of symptoms has been suggested to take as long as 2 weeks [90].

The underlying mechanisms of bowel perforation in chronic corticosteroid use are likely multifactorial. Corticosteroid use disturbs the cyclooxygenase enzyme responsible for prostaglandin synthesis necessary for intestinal mucosal defense [91]. The absence of such defensive mechanisms predisposes the gut to noxious agents like bacterial pathogens and related toxins [87]. As in other immunocompromised patients, the chronic corticosteroid use has been reported to mask peritoneal signs during evaluation for emergency abdominal surgery [92–94].

Historically, perioperative stress dosing was widely used to avoid adrenal insufficiency in patients with chronic corticosteroid use. These strategies included preoperative or intraoperative cortisol levels, with supplemental steroid administration if levels are inadequate [95, 96]. Current evidence, however, suggests a lack of benefit to this use [97]. Newer recommendations involve maintaining the patient's baseline dose with additional intraoperative dosing only in the case of unexplained clinical deterioration [98, 99].

Immune Compromise Following Burn Injury

Burn injury can cause pronounced changes in intestinal physiology that may result in gastrointestinal ischemia or infarction, often associated with pneumatosis intestinalis. Due to marked fluid shifts, changes in cardiac output, and decreased regional organ perfusion, gas may be identified within the bowel wall on diagnostic imaging. Several theories exist to explain the accumulation of gas in the bowel wall. Mucosal injury and loss of structural integrity may allow the passage of intraluminal gas into the bowel wall. Alternatively, the translocation of bacteria into the abdominal wall may produce gas. A 6-year review at an Army burn ICU noted that pneumatosis intestinalis was associated with intestinal ischemia in 91% of patients and an overall survival rate of 27% [100].

Most patients in this setting will require a laparotomy with potential resection and diversion. When definitive abdominal closure is not performed, abdominal negative pressure wound dressings can be a challenge due to difficulty in achieving adequate seals to burned skin. Bowel infarction usually – though not always – occurs in patients with large burns [100].

Diabetes

Diabetes has been identified as a significant risk factor for postoperative complications in emergency surgery patients, which may lead to prolonged hospital stay and additional healthcare costs. The pathophysiology underlying the detrimental effects of hyperglycemia is complex. Changes in glucose homeostasis are compounded by acute illness, anesthesia administration, and the surgical intervention itself. Stress responses involving glucagon, epinephrine, cortisol, growth hormone, epinephrine, and cortisol impair glucose utilization and increase insulin resistance. This in turn reduces T cell response, neutrophil function, and immunoglobulin behavior to increase a patient's susceptibility to infection.

Diabetes in recent decades has been a national public health issue after initiatives such as the Diabetes Control and Complications Trial showed that glycemic control could decrease microvascular-associated complications [101]. Poor glycemic control has been linked to worse outcomes in cardiac surgery and other critically ill patients. In contrast, reductions in multi-organ failure, systemic infections, and mortality have been demonstrated with appropriate glycemic control [102]. In a large retrospective review of patients undergoing non-cardiac surgery, 1-year mortality was significantly related to preoperative blood glucose [102, 103]. Additional risks identified in the literature include a higher risk for surgical site infection, complicated appendicitis, perforation, and development of intra-abdominal abscess [104]. These patients may have atypical or absent clinical signs and symptoms due to their blunted inflammatory response. They are less likely to have expected findings such as elevated temperature, white blood cell count, or pain-related findings on physical exam. As such, clinical suspicion should remain high for any abdominal pathology [105, 106].

A retrospective study of appendicitis in diabetic patients noted that patients were more likely to present with comorbid disease such as obesity, chronic kidney disease, hypertension, coronary artery disease, peripheral vascular disease, and chronic obstructive pulmonary disease. These patients had a lower white blood cell count compared to nondiabetics and a higher rate of appendiceal perforation. Complications were also notably higher in the diabetic population, and, on multivariate analysis, a longer length of stay was noted [107]. The general surgeon should remain wary of poor glycemic control when diabetic patients present in this setting.

Gallstone disease is more prevalent in diabetic patients than in the general population [108]. Diabetic patients with biliary disease also have poorer surgical outcomes, higher rates of complications, and higher rates of conversion from laparoscopy to open cholecystectomy [109–111]. A recent study examining the effect of diabetes on outcomes in patients undergoing emergent cholecystectomy for acute cholecystitis noted just above 14% of the total population had concomitant diabetes and that diabetes was an independent risk factor for renal failure, infectious complications, cardiovascular events, and death [112]. A retrospective review of the NSQIP data noted that delay of cholecystectomy more than 24 h following admission in diabetic patients was associated with higher odds of surgical site infection and longer hospital length of stay compared to nondiabetics [113].

Fournier's gangrene is a progressive necrotizing fasciitis involving the perineum, perianal, and genital area. The gangrene results from polymicrobial aerobic and anaerobic infection arising from the colorectal, genitourinary, or skin systems. Early diagnosis and treatment is critical to achieving successful outcomes. Despite this, mortality rates remain high. Recent studies have evaluated predisposing factors for this disease and have identified diabetes mellitus as a significant factor. Aggressive early surgical debridement, hemodynamic stabilization, and broad-spectrum antibiotic therapy remain the mainstay of treatment. However, good glycemic control is equally important in maximizing optimal outcomes in this patient group [114].

Evaluation of these patients should focus on the level of glycemic control, history of related complications, cardiovascular issues, and previous hospitalizations. A thorough review of all diabetic medications, oral glycemics, and insulin use should be performed with a focus on adequacy of glycemic control [105, 106]. Possible mitigation strategies include delaying procedures when possible and normalizing the glycemic levels of any diabetic patient [115]. Several algorithms exist to assist in the glycemic management of the surgery patient, such as the Emory University Perioperative Algorithm for the Management of Hyperglycemia and Diabetes in Non-Cardiac Surgery Patients. According to this tool, in the critically ill patient, IV insulin infusion should be considered at a threshold of 180 mg/dL or higher with a goal glucose level of 140–180 mg/dL. In the non-critically ill patient, rapid-acting insulin can be used to obtain glycemic control in both the operating room and on the surgical floor with a focus on converting to a basal-bolus or oral glycemic control with oral intake that has been reestablished. Glycemic control is often directed by the surgeon or surgical intensivist but may include anesthesiology, critical care medicine, internal medicine, endocrinology, and a primary care provider in an outpatient setting [102].

End-Stage Renal Disease

Breakthroughs in hemodialysis and peritoneal dialysis have resulted in the prolongation of life and a steady increase in the number of dialysis patients presenting with acute surgical problems. End-stage renal disease itself is associated with complex and multifactorial perturbations of the immune system. The buildup of uremic toxins can impair function of the cells involved in innate immunity. Decreased cytokine production, endocytosis, and impaired maturation have all been described. The decrease in renal elimination can additionally introduce the issue of volume overload, oxidative stress, and accumulation of pro-inflammatory cytokines that can each have their own downstream effect on the immune system, explaining the high infection rates seen in this patient population. These effects are compounded by the fact that these patients present with significant comorbidity including cardiovascular disease, diabetes, or pulmonary issues [116].

Common indications for emergency abdominal surgery include biliary tract disease, gastrointestinal perforation, and bleeding. Those undergoing emergency surgery have high reported morbidity and mortality rates – up to 50% and 70%, respectively [117, 118]. When planning

urgent or emergent operation, the general surgeon should document the renal function of the patient and determine current dialysis methods, timing of last dialysis, adequacy, and whether dialysis access is currently available. The surgical team should anticipate possible high volume fluid resuscitation and possible consequent volume overload. Critically ill and hemodynamically unstable patients who require filtration may benefit from continuous venous hemofiltration for more hemodynamic-sensitive filtration.

Conclusion

General surgeons are often called upon to manage immunocompromised patients, and these consultations will grow increasingly frequent as more Americans undergo organ transplantation. While immunocompromised patients will most often suffer from common and familiar conditions, their presentation may be subtle or paradoxical and their outcomes worse. Infection prevention and management require extra consideration and may trigger additional consultation. Details of medication management may be even more important than in other patients. The decision for surgery will be particularly challenging, recognizing the increased burden of operative complications as well as the dire consequences of delayed source control in infected patients.

Conflict of Interest The authors report no proprietary or commercial interest in any product mentioned or concept discussed in this chapter.

References

1. McKean J, Ronan-Bentle S. Abdominal pain in the immunocompromised patient-human immunodeficiency virus, transplant, cancer. Emerg Med Clin North Am. 2016;34(2):377–86.
2. Hammel L, Sebranek J, Hevesi Z. The anesthetic management of adult patients with organ transplants undergoing nontransplant surgery. Adv Anesth. 2010;28(1):211–44.
3. Hannaman MJ, Ertl MJ. Patients with immunodeficiency. Med Clin North Am. 2013;97(6):1139–59.
4. Gohh RY, Warren G. The preoperative evaluation of the transplanted patient for nontransplant surgery. Surg Clin North Am. 2006;86(5):1147–66. vi

5. de'Angelis N, et al. Emergency abdominal surgery after solid organ transplantation: a systematic review. World J Emerg Surg. 2016;11(1):43.

6. Yang XL, et al. Anesthesia management of surgery for sigmoid perforation and acute peritonitis patient following heart transplantation: case report. Int J Clin Exp Med. 2015;8(7):11632–5.

7. Carter JT, et al. Thymoglobulin-associated Cd4+ T-cell depletion and infection risk in HIV-infected renal transplant recipients. Am J Transplant. 2006;6(4):753–60.

8. Bahebeck J, et al. Implant orthopaedic surgery in HIV asymptomatic carriers: management and early outcome. Injury. 2009;40(11):1147–50.

9. Deneve JL, et al. CD4 count is predictive of outcome in HIV-positive patients undergoing abdominal operations. Am J Surg. 2010;200(6):694.

10. Günthard HF, et al. Antiretroviral treatment of adult HIV infection: 2014 recommendations of the International Antiviral Society-USA Panel. JAMA. 2014;312(4):23–30.

11. Ng TB, et al. Pharmacotherapy approaches to antifungal prophylaxis. Expert Opin Pharmacother. 2012;13(12):1695–705.

12. Dworkin MS, et al. HIV/AIDS – prophylaxis with trimethoprim-sulfamethoxazole for human immunodeficiency virus-infected patients: impact on risk for infectious diseases. Clin Infect Dis. 2001;33(3):393.

13. Safai B, Diaz B, Schwartz J. Malignant neoplasms associated with human immunodeficiency virus infection. CA Cancer J Clin. 1992;42(2):74–95.

14. Friedman SL, Wright TL, Altman DF. Gastrointestinal Kaposi's sarcoma in patients with acquired immunodeficiency syndrome. Endoscopic and autopsy findings. Gastroenterology. 1985;89(1):102–8.

15. Ziegler JL, et al. Non-Hodgkin's lymphoma in 90 homosexual men. N Engl J Med. 1984;311(9):565–70.

16. Robinson G, Wilson SE, Williams RA. Surgery in patients with acquired immunodeficiency syndrome. Arch Surg. 1987;122(2):170–5.

17. Wexner SD, et al. The surgical management of anorectal diseases in AIDS and pre-AIDS patients. Dis Colon Rectum. 1986;29(11):719–23.

18. Huppmann AR, Orenstein JM. Opportunistic disorders of the gastrointestinal tract in the age of highly active antiretroviral therapy. Hum Pathol. 2010;41(12):1777–87.

19. Michalopoulos N, Triantafillopoulou K, Beretouli E, Laskou S, Papavramidis TS, Pliakos I, Hytiroglou P, Papavramidis ST. Small bowel perforation due to CMV enteritis infection in an HIV-positive patient. BMC Res Notes. 2013;6:45.

20. Foschi D, et al. Impact of highly active antiretroviral therapy on outcome of cholecystectomy in patients with human immunodeficiency virus infection. Br J Surg. 2006;93(11):1383–9.

21. Aronson NE, et al. Biliary giardiasis in a patient with human immunodeficiency virus. J Clin Gastroenterol. 2001;33(2):167–70.

22. Emparan C, et al. Infective complications after abdominal surgery in patients infected with human immunodeficiency virus: role of CD4+ lymphocytes in prognosis. World J Surg. 1998;22(8):778–82.

23. Savioz D, et al. Preoperative counts of CD4 T-lymphocytes and early postoperative infective complications in HIV-positive patients. Eur J Surg. 1998;164(7):483–7.

24. Yii MK, Saunder A, Scott DF. Abdominal surgery in HIV/AIDS patients: indications, operative management, pathology and outcome. Aust N Z J Surg. 1995;65(5):320–6.

25. Albaran RG. CD4 cell counts as a prognostic factor of major abdominal surgery in patients infected with the human immunodeficiency virus. Arch Surg. 1998;133(6):626.

26. Tran HS, et al. Predictors of operative outcome in patients with human immunodeficiency virus infection and acquired immunodeficiency syndrome. Am J Surg. 2000;180(3):228–33.

27. Csikesz N, et al. Current status of surgical management of acute cholecystitis in the United States. World J Surg. 2008;32(10):2230–6.

28. Horberg MA, et al. Surgical outcomes in human immunodeficiency virus-infected patients in the era of highly active antiretroviral therapy. Arch Surg. 2006;141(12):1238–45.

29. Hamandi B, et al. Impact of infectious disease consultation on the clinical and economic outcomes of solid organ transplant recipients admitted for infectious complications. Clin Infect Dis. 2014;59(8):1074–82.

30. Schmitt S, et al. Infectious diseases specialty intervention is associated with decreased mortality and lower healthcare costs. Clin Infect Dis. 2014;58(1):22–8.

31. Yoshida D, Caruso JM. Abdominal pain in the HIV infected patient. J Emerg Med. 2002;23(2):111–6.

32. Zhang L, et al. Prevention and treatment of surgical site infection in HIV-infected patients. BMC Infect Dis. 2012;12:115.

33. Freeman AF, Holland SM. Antimicrobial prophylaxis for primary immunodeficiencies. Curr Opin Allergy Clin Immunol. 2009;9(6):525–30.

34. Stewart MW. Optimal management of cytomegalovirus retinitis in patients with AIDS. Clin Ophthalmol. 2010;4:285–99.

35. Kirk O, et al. Safe interruption of maintenance therapy against previous infection with four common HIV-associated opportunistic pathogens during potent antiretroviral therapy. Ann Intern Med. 2002;137(4):239–50.

36. Ferguson CM. Surgical complications of human immunodeficiency virus infection. Am Surg. 1988;54(1):4–9.

37. Gulick RM, et al. Treatment with indinavir, zidovudine, and lamivudine in adults with human immunodeficiency virus infection and prior antiretroviral therapy. N Engl J Med. 1997;337(11):734–9.

38. Goldberg HJ, et al. Colon and rectal complications after heart and lung transplantation. J Am Coll Surg. 2006;202(1):55–61.

39. Bravo C, et al. Prevalence and management of gastrointestinal complications in lung transplant patients: MITOS study group. Transplant Proc. 2007;39(7):2409–12.
40. Paul S, et al. Gastrointestinal complications after lung transplantation. J Heart Lung Transplant. 2009;28(5):475–9.
41. Whiting J. Perioperative concerns for transplant recipients undergoing nontransplant surgery. Surg Clin North Am. 2006;86(5):1185–94. vi–vii
42. Bratzler DW, Houck PM, Surgical Infection Prevention Guideline Writers. Antimicrobial prophylaxis for surgery: an advisory statement from the National Surgical Infection Prevention Project. Am J Surg. 2005;189(4):395–404.
43. Littlewood KE. The immunocompromised adult patient and surgery. Best Pract Res Clin Anaesthesiol. 2008;22(3):585–609.
44. Lin S, Cosgrove CJ. Perioperative management of immunosuppression. Surg Clin North Am. 2006;86(5):1167–83. vi
45. Popov Z, et al. Postoperative complications following kidney transplantation. Ann Urol (Paris). 2000;34(5):323–9.
46. Kostopanagiotou G, et al. Anesthetic and perioperative management of adult transplant recipients in nontransplant surgery. Anesth Analg. 1999;89(3):613–22.
47. Miller LW. Cyclosporine-associated neurotoxicity. The need for a better guide for immunosuppressive therapy. Circulation. 1996;94(6):1209–11.
48. Sakhuja V, et al. Azathioprine induced myelosuppression in renal transplant recipients: a study of 30 patients. Nephrology. 1995;1(4):285–9.
49. Connell WR, et al. Bone marrow toxicity caused by azathioprine in inflammatory bowel disease: 27 years of experience. Gut. 1993;34(8):1081–5.
50. Hulzebos CV, et al. Cyclosporine A-induced reduction of bile salt synthesis associated with increased plasma lipids in children after liver transplantation. Liver Transpl. 2004;10(7):872–80.
51. Moran D, et al. Inhibition of biliary glutathione secretion by cyclosporine A in the rat: possible mechanisms and role in the cholestasis induced by the drug. J Hepatol. 1998;29(1):68–77.
52. Steck TB, Costanzo-Nordin MR, Keshavarzian A. Prevalence and management of cholelithiasis in heart transplant patients. J Heart Lung Transplant. 1991;10(6):1029–32.
53. Taghavi S, et al. Postoperative outcomes with cholecystectomy in lung transplant recipients. Surgery. 2015;158(2):373–8.
54. Kilic A, et al. Outcomes of cholecystectomy in US heart transplant recipients. Ann Surg. 2013;258(2):312–7.
55. Englesbe MJ, et al. Gallbladder disease in cardiac transplant patients: a survey study. Arch Surg. 2005;140(4):399–403. discussion 404
56. Graham SM, et al. The utility of prophylactic laparoscopic cholecystectomy in transplant candidates. Am J Surg. 1995;169(1):44–8. discussion 48–9
57. Kao LS, Kuhr CS, Flum DR. Should cholecystectomy be performed for asymptomatic cholelithiasis in transplant patients? J Am Coll Surg. 2003;197(2):302.
58. Osawa H, et al. Surgical management of perforated gastrointestinal posttransplantation lymphoproliferative disorder after heart transplantation. Int Surg. 2015;100(2):358–64.
59. Maurer JR. The spectrum of colonic complications in a lung transplant population. Ann Transplant. 2000;5(3):54–7.
60. Watson CJ, et al. Early abdominal complications following heart and heart-lung transplantation. Br J Surg. 1991;78(6):699–704.
61. Rodriguez-Larrain JM, et al. Incidence of adenomatous colorectal polyps in cardiac transplant recipients. Transplantation. 1997;64(3):528–30.
62. Andreoni KA, et al. Increased incidence of gastrointestinal surgical complications in renal transplant recipients with polycystic kidney disease. Transplantation. 1999;67(2):262–6.
63. Fleming TW, Barry JM. Bilateral open transperitoneal cyst reduction surgery for autosomal dominant polycystic kidney disease. J Urol. 1998;159(1):44–7.
64. Merrell SW, et al. Major abdominal complications following cardiac transplantation. Utah Transplantation Affiliated Hospitals Cardiac Transplant Program. Arch Surg. 1989;124(8):889–94.
65. Beaver TM, et al. Colon perforation after lung transplantation. Ann Thorac Surg. 1996;62(3):839–43.
66. Stelzner M, et al. Colonic perforations after renal transplantation. J Am Coll Surg. 1997;184(1):63–9.
67. Detry O, et al. Acute diverticulitis in heart transplant recipients. Transpl Int. 1996;9(4):376–9.
68. Catena F, et al. Gastrointestinal perforations following kidney transplantation. Transplant Proc. 2008;40(6):1895–6.
69. Reshef A, et al. Case-matched comparison of perioperative outcomes after surgical treatment of sigmoid diverticulitis in solid organ transplant recipients versus immunocompetent patients. Color Dis. 2012;14(12):1546–52.
70. Patel H, et al. Posttransplant lymphoproliferative disorder in adult liver transplant recipients: a report of seventeen cases. Leuk Lymphoma. 2007;48(5):885–91.
71. Younes BS, et al. The involvement of the gastrointestinal tract in posttransplant lymphoproliferative disease in pediatric liver transplantation. J Pediatr Gastroenterol Nutr. 1999;28(4):380–5.
72. Fonseca-Neto OC, et al. Acute appendicitis in liver transplant recipients. Arq Bras Cir Dig. 2016;29(1):30–2.
73. Andrade RdO, et al. Acute appendicitis after liver transplant: a case report and review of the literature. OJOTS. 2014;04(04):29–32.
74. Wei CK, et al. Acute appendicitis in organ transplantation patients: a report of two cases and a literature review. Ann Transplant. 2014;19:248–52.
75. Hoekstra HJ, et al. Gastrointestinal complications in lung transplant survivors that require surgical intervention. Br J Surg. 2001;88(3):433–8.

76. Sikalias N, et al. Acute abdomen in a transplant patient with tuberculous colitis: a case report. Cases J. 2009;2:9305.
77. Lebon D, et al. Gastrointestinal emergencies in critically ill cancer patients. J Crit Care. 2017;40:69–75.
78. Arain MR, Buggy DJ. Anaesthesia for cancer patients. Curr Opin Anaesthesiol. 2007;20(3):247–53.
79. Lefor AT. Surgical problems affecting the patient with cancer : interdisciplinary management. Philadelphia: Lippincott-Raven; 1996.
80. Ganz WI, et al. Review of tests for monitoring doxorubicin-induced cardiomyopathy. Oncology. 1996;53(6):461–70.
81. Donat SM, Levy DA. Bleomycin associated pulmonary toxicity: is perioperative oxygen restriction necessary? JURO. 1998;160(4):1347–52.
82. Huettemann E, Sakka SG. Anaesthesia and anti-cancer chemotherapeutic drugs. Curr Opin Anaesthesiol. 2005;18(3):307–14.
83. Freifeld AG, et al. Clinical practice guideline for the use of antimicrobial agents in neutropenic patients with cancer: 2010 Update by the Infectious Diseases Society of America. Clin Infect Dis. 2011;52(4):427–31.
84. Hayden DM, et al. Patient factors may predict anastomotic complications after rectal cancer surgery. Anastomotic complications in rectal cancer. Ann Med Surg. 2015;4(1):11–6.
85. Midura EF, et al. Risk factors and consequences of anastomotic leak after colectomy: a national analysis. Dis Colon Rectum. 2015;58(3):333–8.
86. Cloutier RL. Neutropenic enterocolitis. Hematol Oncol Clin North Am. 2010;24(3):577–84.
87. Gravante G, Yahia S. Medical influences, surgical outcomes: role of common medications on the risk of perforation from untreated diverticular disease. World J Gastroenterol. 2013;19(36):5947–52.
88. Wang AS, Armstrong EJ, Armstrong AW. Corticosteroids and wound healing: clinical considerations in the perioperative period. Am J Surg. 2013;206(3):410–7.
89. Humes DJ, et al. Concurrent drug use and the risk of perforated colonic diverticular disease: a population-based case-control study. Gut. 2011;60(2):219–24.
90. Fadul CE, et al. Perforation of the gastrointestinal tract in patients receiving steroids for neurologic disease. Neurology. 1988;38(3):348–52.
91. Kaya B, et al. Steroid-induced sigmoid diverticular perforation in a patient with temporal arteritis: a rare clinical pathology. Clin Med Insights Pathol. 2012;5:11–4.
92. Behrman SW. Management of complicated peptic ulcer disease. Arch Surg. 2005;140(2):201–8.
93. Piekarek K, Israelsson LA. Perforated colonic diverticular disease: the importance of NSAIDs, opioids, corticosteroids, and calcium channel blockers. Int J Color Dis. 2008;23(12):1193–7.
94. Kouyialis A, et al. Delayed diagnosis of steroid-induced colon diverticulum perforation. N Z Med J. 2003;116(1183):U631.
95. Merry WH, et al. Postoperative acute adrenal failure caused by transient corticotropin deficiency. Surgery. 1994;116(6):1095–100.
96. Salem M, et al. Perioperative glucocorticoid coverage. A reassessment 42 years after emergence of a problem. Ann Surg. 1994;219(4):416–25.
97. Mathis AS, Shah NK, Mulgaonkar S. Stress dose steroids in renal transplant patients undergoing lymphocele surgery. Transplant Proc. 2004;36(10):3042–5.
98. Kelly KN, Domajnko B. Perioperative stress-dose steroids. Clin Colon Rectal Surg. 2013;26(3):163–7.
99. MacKenzie CR, Goodman SM. Stress dose steroids: myths and perioperative medicine. Curr Rheumatol Rep. 2016;18(7):47.
100. Huzar TF, et al. Pneumatosis intestinalis in patients with severe thermal injury. J Burn Care Res. 2011;32(3):e37–44.
101. Diabetes C, et al. The effect of intensive treatment of diabetes on the development and progression of long-term complications in insulin-dependent diabetes mellitus. N Engl J Med. 1993;329(14):977–86.
102. Duggan EW, et al. The Emory University Perioperative Algorithm for the management of hyperglycemia and diabetes in non-cardiac surgery patients. Curr Diab Rep. 2016;16(3)
103. Abdelmalak BB, et al. Preoperative blood glucose concentrations and postoperative outcomes after elective non-cardiac surgery: an observational study. Br J Anaesth. 2014;112(1):79–88.
104. Sivrikoz E, et al. The effect of diabetes on outcomes following emergency appendectomy in patients without comorbidities: a propensity score-matched analysis of National Surgical Quality Improvement Program database. Am J Surg. 2015;209(1):206–11.
105. Gusberg RJ, Moley J. Diabetes and abdominal surgery: the mutual risks. Yale J Biol Med. 1983;56(4):285–91.
106. Stewart CL, Wood CL, Bealer JF. Characterization of acute appendicitis in diabetic children. J Pediatr Surg. 2014;49(12):1719–22.
107. Bach L, et al. Appendicitis in diabetics: predictors of complications and their incidence. Am Surg. 2016;82(8):753–8.
108. Noel RA, et al. Increased risk of acute pancreatitis and biliary disease observed in patients with type 2 diabetes: a retrospective cohort study. Diabetes Care. 2009;32(5):834–8.
109. Paajanen H, et al. Laparoscopic versus open cholecystectomy in diabetic patients and postoperative outcome. Surg Endosc. 2011;25(3):764–70.
110. Landau O, et al. The risk of cholecystectomy for acute cholecystitis in diabetic patients. Hepato-Gastroenterology. 1992;39(5):437–8.
111. Shpitz B, et al. Acute cholecystitis in diabetic patients. Am Surg. 1995;61(11):964–7.
112. Karamanos E, et al. Effect of diabetes on outcomes in patients undergoing emergent cholecystectomy for acute cholecystitis. World J Surg. 2013;37(10):2257–64.

113. Gelbard R, et al. Effect of delaying same-admission cholecystectomy on outcomes in patients with diabetes. Br J Surg. 2014;101(2):74–8.

114. Tarchouli M, et al. Analysis of prognostic factors affecting mortality in Fournier's gangrene: a study of 72 cases. Can Urol Assoc J. 2015;9(11–12):E800–4.

115. Silvestri M, et al. Modifiable and non-modifiable risk factors for surgical site infection after colorectal surgery: a single-center experience. Surg Today. 2018;48(3):338–45.

116. Kato S, et al. Aspects of immune dysfunction in end-stage renal disease. Clin J Am Soc Nephrol. 2008;3(5):1526–33.

117. Toh Y, et al. Abdominal surgery for patients on maintenance hemodialysis. Surg Today. 1998;28(3):268–72.

118. Ozel L, et al. Elective and emergency surgery in chronic hemodialysis patients. Ren Fail. 2011;33(7):672–6.

Cirrhosis

43

Jessica K. Reynolds and Andrew C. Bernard

Introduction

Cirrhosis increases morbidity and mortality in patients requiring emergency surgery [1]. In these patients, every phase of care is challenging, from preoperative risk stratification and optimization to operative intervention and management. Efforts have been made to predict survival in patients with cirrhosis under various clinical circumstances, yet a single predictive model that encompasses the patients' clinical condition and the specific emergency procedure has yet to be established. Emergency surgery in cirrhotic patients confers an additional four to five times higher mortality risk compared to elective surgery [1]. However, increased awareness of risk has to date not translated into substantial improvement in outcomes [2]. Preoperative planning relies upon the stage of cirrhosis, timing of surgery, comorbid conditions, and the type of operation [3]. In all situations, surgeons will benefit from understanding the pathophysiology of cirrhosis as it relates to the treatment of the acute disease process. In urgent situations, the opportunity for optimization is minimal. To achieve optimal outcomes, surgeons must recognize the disease, defer surgery when appropriate, optimize physiology, and perform a technically excellent operation.

Epidemiology

Liver cirrhosis is the 8th most common cause of death in the United States with a prevalence of 0.27% [4, 5]. However, cirrhosis is underdiagnosed, with as many as 70% of patients being unaware of their clinical condition [5]. For that reason, patients with risk factors for liver disease such as obesity, chronic alcohol abuse, previous transfusions, substance abuse, tattooing, known hepatitis exposure, high-risk sexual behavior, and family history should be evaluated for chronic liver disease prior to surgical intervention [1]. Due to the endemic nature of obesity in the United States, nonalcoholic steatohepatitis (NASH) accounts for a large proportion of undiagnosed patients with cirrhosis.

Pathophysiology

Advanced liver disease affects every organ system and is frequently associated with life-threatening complications [1]. Hemodynamic changes associated with liver dysfunction include increased cardiac output, diastolic dysfunction, and decreased systemic vascular resistance (SVR). Patients will

J. K. Reynolds · A. C. Bernard (✉)
Section of Trauma and Acute Care Surgery,
Department of Surgery, University of Kentucky
College of Medicine, UK Healthcare,
Lexington, KY, USA
e-mail: andrew.bernard@uky.edu

© Springer International Publishing AG, part of Springer Nature 2019
C. V. R. Brown et al. (eds.), *Emergency General Surgery*, https://doi.org/10.1007/978-3-319-96286-3_43

frequently demonstrate inappropriate response to surgical stress. For the cirrhotic patient requiring operative intervention, the surgeon and anesthesia provider should make every effort to avoid arterial hypotension in order to preserve hepatic arterial blood flow and hepatic function. General anesthesia alone causes reduced hepatic arterial blood flow. When combined with sepsis, acute blood loss, and the intraoperative effects of reflex sympathetic hypotension from traction of abdominal viscera, normotension can be difficult to achieve. Patients may also experience rising intra-abdominal pressures from laparoscopic surgery or positive pressure ventilation. The compounded effects of vasodilation and resultant ischemic injury to the remaining functioning hepatocytes in a cirrhotic liver will increase the risk of acute decompensation [1].

Initial Evaluation

Performing a thorough physical exam is critical in the preoperative evaluation of the cirrhotic patient. Suspicion for chronic liver disease should arise in any patient who is obese or displays clinical features of chronic liver disease or portal hypertension [1]. Patients with cirrhosis may exhibit obesity, ascites, jaundice, asterixis, peripheral edema, and hepatosplenomegaly. Subtle exam findings such as palmar erythema, spider nevi, temporal wasting, parotid gland enlargement, testicular atrophy, and gynecomastia should not be overlooked. If planning a laparoscopic operation, a careful examination for periumbilical varices should be performed. A history of esophageal varices on prior endoscopy, or upper gastrointestinal hemorrhage, should raise suspicion of cirrhosis.

The etiology of cirrhosis is frequently multifactorial as a single patient may have multiple risk factors. Obtaining a detailed history may assist the surgeon in identifying patients with risk factors for cirrhosis, prompting further work-up and optimization. The provider should give special attention to social history including alcohol and intravenous drug abuse, tattooing, high-risk sexual behavior, and known hepatitis exposure. A

history of previous blood transfusion, travel history to areas where liver infections are endemic, or family history of liver disease should also be noted. Obesity is frequently overlooked as a significant risk factor, and its potential impact should not be underestimated. A detailed review of prescription and over-the-counter medications should be performed to exclude possible drug-induced liver disease [1].

The cirrhotic will present in one of two distinct clinical phases: compensated or decompensated cirrhosis [1]. Decompensated cirrhosis is defined by the presence of complications such as ascites, spontaneous bacterial peritonitis (SBP), variceal hemorrhage, encephalopathy, hepatocellular carcinoma (HCC), hepatorenal syndrome (HRS), or hepatopulmonary syndrome (HPS) [1]. Patients with compensated cirrhosis have a median survival of more than 12 years, compared to the patient with decompensated cirrhosis, who demonstrate a markedly diminished median survival rate of less than 2 years [6]. Patients who present with compensated cirrhosis in the emergency surgery setting can quickly transition to a decompensated state with development of acute liver failure, severe coagulopathy, portal vein thrombosis, electrolyte imbalance, acute renal failure, and sepsis [1]. Clinicians must be vigilant in monitoring for early signs of decompensation and be proactive in preventing decompensation.

Risk Assessment and Scoring Systems

Once the presence of cirrhosis has been identified, the next step is to perform risk stratification in order to guide decision making and determine overall prognosis. Laboratory tests should include a complete blood count, INR, and comprehensive metabolic panel including liver function tests, electrolytes, and renal function. Incidental findings of low platelets, coagulopathy, hyponatremia, elevated bilirubin, low albumin, or elevated liver enzymes warrant a thorough assessment to evaluate the severity of liver disease [7]. Available imaging studies including ultrasonography or computed tomography (CT) should be reviewed to assess the size and contour of the liver as well as the presence of ascites or signs of portal hypertension (splenomegaly and varices).

The degree of decompensation is the most important factor in determining perioperative outcomes [8–13]. The two most commonly used scoring systems to help predict morbidity and mortality are the Child-Turcotte-Pugh (CTP) and Model for End-Stage Liver Disease (MELD) score. Although neither model is perfect, both are reasonable predictors of short-term complications [12].

The CTP score has been used to assess the severity of cirrhosis, prognosis, and management of surgical patients. The CTP score has five measures, each given a score of 1–3, with 3 representing the most severe derangement (Table 43.1) [14, 15]. Although frequently used in clinical practice, the CTP score has not been validated [1]. Inherent problems to the reproducibility of this score include its subjective assessment of ascites and encephalopathy. Additionally, arbitrary thresholds were chosen for the objective components – albumin, bilirubin, and INR. Table 43.1 highlights the components used to calculate the CTP score.

The MELD score was historically used in transplantation to predict mortality after transjugular intrahepatic portosystemic shunt (TIPS) procedure. This model was later found useful in assessing prognosis of liver cirrhosis and prioritizing patients as candidates for transplantation [16, 17]. Today, the score is often used to assess the severity of cirrhosis and perioperative risk in emergency general surgery. MELD is a calculated formula using objective data including serum bilirubin, INR, and serum creatinine.

MELD = $3.78 \times \ln[\text{serum bilirubin (mg/dL)}] + 11.2 \times \ln[\text{INR}] + 9.57 \times \ln[\text{serum creatinine (mg/dL)}] + 6.43$ [17]. Lack of reliance on subjective measures makes MELD a more consistent predictive tool. In practice, mortality increases 1% for each point up to 20 and then 2% for each point thereafter when using the MELD score [18]. MELD may be a better predictive model for the decompensated cirrhotic given the importance of creatinine in the determination [6]. The MELD score has been validated in many studies and is used extensively [1].

When comparing CTP to MELD, scores of <10, 10–14, and >14 are comparable to CTP classes A, B, and C [1]. Thus, advanced stages of cirrhosis are defined as MELD >14 and CTP class C. Patients with this severity of cirrhosis have consistently demonstrated higher morbidity and mortality in emergent cases. Historically, studies by Garrison and Mansour showed similar mortality rates of 10%, 31%, and 76% when comparing CTP classes A, B, and C to corresponding MELD scores [8, 9]. In contrast, a recent study by Telem et al. showed significantly lower mortality rates of 2%, 12%, and 12% in CTP classes A, B, and C [10].

Perioperative Optimization

Patients with cirrhosis can achieve better outcomes by undergoing perioperative optimization directed at addressing factors that increase morbidity and mortality in the cirrhotic population. Emergency surgery frequently does not afford such an opportunity for true preoperative optimization; however there are still opportunities to minimize risk. The first steps are to identify the

Table 43.1 CTP score calculation

Parameter	1 point	2 points	3 points
Albumin, g/dL	>3.5	2.8–3.5	<2.8
Bilirubin, mg/dL	<2	2–3	>3
INR	<1.7	1.7–2.3	>2.3
Hepatic encephalopathy	None	Grades 1–2	Grades 3–4
Ascites	None	Mild and moderate	Severe

Abbreviations: *CTP* Child-Turcotte-Pugh, *INR* international normalized ratio
CTP score = addition of each parameter score. CTP class: A = 5–6 points, B = 7–9 points, C = 10–15 points

cause of cirrhosis and determine the level of compensation. Efforts should then be focused on optimizing liver function, with particular attention to nutrition, correction of coagulopathy and electrolytes, and management of ascites.

Nutrition

Malnutrition affects more than 80% of patients with cirrhosis. Hypoalbuminemia is a hallmark of malnutrition and liver disease, resulting in decreased oncotic pressure and intravascular hypovolemia [1]. Malnutrition is an independent predictor of mortality in the cirrhotic surgical patient [19]. A serum albumin of 2.1 g/dL compared to a level of 4.6 g/dL is associated with morbidity rates of 65% versus 10% and mortality rates of 29% versus 1% [20]. Despite this association, albumin replacement is not recommended as it has not been shown to improve mortality.

Accurate assessment of malnutrition in the cirrhotic remains a challenge. Factors such as malabsorption with fat-soluble vitamin deficiency and reduced food intake due to ascites and anorexia can contribute to malnutrition. Perioperative nutrition support improves outcomes [21, 22]. Use of immune-enhancing formulas should be considered after trauma and before and after surgery. If hepatic encephalopathy is present, a diet high in carbohydrates and lipids with milk-based and branched chain amino acids is preferred [23].

Coagulopathy and Thrombocytopenia

Liver disease results in complex alterations of all three phases of hemostasis: primary hemostasis, coagulation, and fibrinolysis [24]. Both platelet number and function may be reduced in the cirrhotic, with the majority of patients demonstrating mild to moderate thrombocytopenia [24]. Bone marrow suppression by antiviral therapy, alcohol, or folate deficiency can impair platelet production. Platelet sequestration also occurs as a result of portal hypertension and congested splenomegaly. Despite the quantitative effects of cirrhosis on platelets, the procoagulant activity of thrombin generation is typically preserved [24]. In chronic liver disease, synthesis of procoagulant proteins is reduced (factors II, V, VII, IX, and XI). Natural anticoagulant proteins such as proteins C and S are also reduced and found to be similar to the range of values seen in patients with inherited deficiencies [24]. Fibrinolytic activity varies among individuals. Reabsorption of large-volume ascites may contribute to enhanced fibrinolysis [24]. Due to the relative deficiency of both procoagulant and anticoagulant factors, patients may develop hemorrhage or thrombosis depending on the clinical circumstances [24].

Conventional coagulation tests such as prothrombin time (PT) and activated partial thromboplastin time (aPTT) do not fully reflect the derangement in hemostasis and do not accurately predict the risk of bleeding [24]. Prevention of bleeding should not be sought by correction of these conventional tests as a high INR does not equate with hypocoagulability. Prophylactic infusion of plasma prior to invasive procedures is unlikely to have clinical benefit [24]. Large-volume plasma may paradoxically increase the bleeding risk by exacerbating portal hypertension from volume overload. Waiting for plasma may also delay procedures, thus exposing the patient to unnecessary risks [24]. For the patient who is actively bleeding, plasma (10–20 cc/kg) should be given, noting that the effect of plasma transfusion on INR is negligible if INR is <1.7 [25]. Thrombocytopenia may be a better predictor of bleeding than INR. Platelet counts <50–60 K have been associated with an increased rate of post-procedure bleeding. However, a threshold platelet count for prophylactic transfusion in patients with liver disease has not been established [24]. For the actively bleeding patient, the platelet count should be maintained >50 K to ensure adequate thrombin generation [24]. Transfusion of cryoprecipitate to maintain a fibrinogen level > 100 has been recommended in cirrhotic patients, although an evidence base is lacking [24]. There is insufficient data to support the use of prothrombin complex concentrates (PCCs), recombinant factor VII, or tranexamic acid in acute hemorrhage. Use of these products may increase thrombotic risk while providing minimal if any benefit [24]. Vitamin K administration will not reverse the liver synthetic impairment; however it may contribute to correction of coagulopathy if malabsorption and fat-soluble vitamin deficiency are contributing [1]. Currently, no evidence-based guidelines exist for acute hemorrhage in patients with cirrhosis.

The clinical utility of whole blood assays of hemostasis is evolving [24]. Although use of thromboelastography (TEG) and thromboelastometry (ROTEM) has not been validated for predicting bleeding risk in patients with liver disease, these diagnostic tests can provide insight into the dynamics of clot formation, clot strength, and clot stability [24]. In a recent randomized trial, TEG-guided transfusion strategy resulted in transfusion of only 17% of patients compared to 100% of patients in whom transfusion was based upon INR and platelets, without an increase in bleeding complications [26]. These tests show promise but are not universally available and require expertise in interpretation.

Ascites

Ascites is a common presentation of decompensated cirrhosis. The development of ascites is an important landmark in the natural history of cirrhosis, and its presence is associated with a 50% mortality rate over 2 years [27]. Presence of ascites is a risk factor for development of dilutional hyponatremia, spontaneous bacterial peritonitis, and acute kidney injury (AKI), all of which contribute to increased morbidity and mortality [28]. First-line treatment for uncomplicated ascites is sodium restriction combined with diuretic therapy [28]. Sodium is typically restricted to a no-added salt diet with <5 g of salt per day [27]. Water restriction is only employed in uncomplicated ascites if serum sodium level is <125 mmol/L. [27] Spironolactone is the initial drug of choice in treatment of ascites, starting with a dose of 100 mg/day that may be progressively increased to 400 mg/

day. If spironolactone fails to resolve ascites, furosemide can be added at an initial dose of 40 mg/day which may be gradually increased to a dose of 160 mg/day [27]. With diuretic therapy, electrolytes, renal function, and volume status should be closely monitored. In the emergency surgical setting, ascites control will be impossible preoperatively, and postoperative diuretic use may be precluded by physiology. Restriction of I.V. fluid use, when appropriate, may reduce ascites [29].

For refractory ascites, paracentesis with albumin replacement is feasible. Large-volume paracentesis with colloid replacement has been shown to be rapid, safe, and effective [27]. However, failure to give volume expansion after paracentesis can result in electrolyte disturbances and impairment of renal function [27]. If a therapeutic tap is performed, or large-volume ascites are removed during an emergency operation, published guidelines suggest that albumin should be replaced with albumin 25% solution at a dose of 6–8 g/L of fluid removed in excess of 5 L [29]. TIPS is a rescue measure for refractory ascites and a good alternative for some patients.

Fluids and Electrolytes

Fluid and electrolyte balance should be meticulously monitored [1]. In cases of volume depletion such as diarrhea, emesis, or excessive diuresis, fluid replacement should consist of isotonic crystalloids (0.9% NaCl) [30]. Balanced salt solutions such as Plasmalyte® may be preferred in the patient with hyperchloremic acidosis [30]. With presence of elevated lactate, non-lactate-containing solutions should be used [1]. The patient with hemorrhagic shock should be resuscitated with blood products. For a patient with suspected bacterial infection, a combination of crystalloids and 5% albumin is preferred [1]. Three particular situations exist where albumin should be favored: SBP, large-volume paracentesis, and type 1 hepatorenal syndrome [31]. Hydroxyethyl starch (HES) has potential nephrotoxic effects and should be avoided [31].

Hyponatremia occurs in up to 50% of patients with cirrhosis and ascites, with 10–20% of patients presenting with severe hyponatremia (serum sodium ≤125 mEq/L) [32]. Hyponatremia is not only a predictor of complications but also a predictor of mortality [33]. For each mEq drop in sodium below 135 mEq/L, the mortality risk has been shown to increase by 10% in patients considered for transplantation [32]. Hyponatremia develops from systemic vasodilation with subsequent activation of compensatory neurohormonal mechanisms that function to restore effective circulatory volume [33, 34]. First, vasodilation results in activation of the sympathetic nervous system, renin-angiotensinogen system, and non-osmotic release of antidiuretic hormone (ADH) [33]. Resulting hyponatremia can occur with hypovolemia or hypervolemia. Hypovolemic hyponatremia occurs due to fluid loss from the kidneys or gastrointestinal tract. Treatment should be focused on volume replacement and correction of the underlying cause of volume loss [34]. Hypervolemic hyponatremia occurs with volume overload and is attributed to the inability of the kidneys to excrete solute-free water proportionate to the amount of free water ingested [34]. This form of hyponatremia is an ominous sign and is difficult to manage. The mainstay of treatment is to increase renal excretion of free water through diuresis [32]. The decision to treat should be based on the patient's clinical status and symptoms rather than absolute serum sodium level [33]. The rate of sodium correction should be closely monitored to avoid neurologic complications such as seizures and central pontine myelinolysis [34].

Serum potassium levels should also be monitored and replaced accordingly. Correction appears to be important for two reasons: (1) correction tends to raise serum sodium and osmolality and (2) hypokalemia promotes development of hepatic encephalopathy by increasing synthesis of ammonia in the proximal tubules [34, 35].

Esophageal Varices

Despite advances in endoscopic therapy, the mortality rate of acute variceal hemorrhage remains around 15% [36]. Standard treatment for acute variceal hemorrhage includes the combination of endoscopic band ligation, vasoactive drugs, and prophylactic antibiotics [24, 36]. Effective hemostasis and volume management are essential in preventing complications [36]. If bleeding cannot be controlled with endoscopic ligation, or bleeding recurs, TIPS should be performed to reduce portal hypertension. In cases of massive life-threatening hemorrhage, balloon tamponade (Sengstaken-Blakemore or Minnesota tube) or a covered esophageal stent may be used as a salvage therapy or a bridge to definitive banding or TIPS.

Anesthetic Considerations

Emergency general surgeons should have a basic knowledge of anesthetic agent use in the cirrhotic. Given the physiologic derangements of this patient population, there are multiple factors to take into consideration. As previously stated, avoidance of hypotension is of utmost importance.

In general, benzodiazepines should be avoided. Propofol has been shown to be a safer alternative due to its faster elimination. Etomidate can be safely used. In regard to opiate analgesics, remifentanil is the safest, as it is metabolized by red cell esterase as opposed to hepatocytes [1]. Other opiates such as morphine and fentanyl have decreased clearance and should be monitored accordingly. Among inhalation anesthetics, desflurane is considered the safest for patients with cirrhosis due to preservation of hepatic blood flow and cardiac output [1]. Additionally, desflurane undergoes minimal hepatic metabolism [37]. Atracurium and cisatracurium undergo Hoffman degradation and are considered safe neuromuscular blocking agents. Caution should be taken with spinal or epidural anesthesia to avoid hypotension and prevent local bleeding complications related to coagulopathy or thrombocytopenia [1].

Pain Management

Pain management in the cirrhotic can be challenging. Contrary to popular belief, acetaminophen is not contraindicated and may be used with caution at a recommended dose of 2–3 g/day. Nonsteroidal anti-inflammatories should be avoided due to potential for nephrotoxicity, platelet dysfunction, and gastrointestinal bleeding [38]. In patients with compensated liver disease, I.V. patient-controlled anesthesia is well tolerated [37]. Opiate dose and frequency should be reduced to avoid over-sedation and encephalopathy. For abdominal operations, use of regional anesthesia in the form of local infiltration or transversus abdominis plane block may be beneficial to decrease need for narcotics.

Considerations for Specific Procedures

Abdominal Wall Hernias

Increased intra-abdominal pressure, weakening of the abdominal wall fascia, and recanalization of the umbilical vein increase the risk of development of abdominal wall hernias in patients with cirrhosis and ascites [39]. Patients may present with complications including incarceration or strangulation of bowel, hernia rupture with ascites leak, and evisceration [39]. Despite evidence that elective repair is safe, many hernias in cirrhotic patients with ascites are observed until becoming a surgical emergency.

Marsam et al. found that conservative management of umbilical hernia (UH) in cirrhosis was successful in only 23% of patients, with nearly 50% requiring an emergent hernia repair [40]. Acute rupture of UH in patients with cirrhosis carries a high mortality rate, and emergency repair can require prolonged length of stay with significant consumption of hospital resources [41, 42]. Early elective repair of UHs should be considered, as repair has proven to be safe, even in advanced cirrhosis [40, 43–46]. Although no clear method exists to determine when cirrhosis is severe enough to preclude elective repair, a recent retrospective study comparing outcomes of UH repair in patients with cirrhosis suggested to avoid elective repair of UHs in patients older than 65 years, with MELD score ≥ 15 and serum albumin <3.0 g/dL [47].

The same study found the mortality rate for emergency repair of UH to be 11% in patients with MELD ≥15 compared to 1.3% in patients with MELD <15 [47].

Hernia repair must include meticulous surgical technique and adequate control of ascites. Ascites can usually be controlled with a combination of diuretic therapy, surgical drainage, and intermittent paracentesis. Some patients may benefit from TIPS, although this is usually reserved for optimization in elective hernia repair [39]. Use of mesh and the optimal surgical technique is controversial. Options for repair include open primary tissue repair, open mesh repair, and laparoscopic mesh repair. Primary tissue repair with permanent suture is the most frequently performed procedure. However, UH recurrence in cirrhotic patients has been shown to be decreased at 6 months with mesh repair compared to primary repair (14% vs. 2.7%) without substantial increase in morbidity [48]. The presence of ruptured UH, infected ascites, or bowel obstruction will increase risk of mesh infection.

Cirrhotic patients are sevenfold more likely to die with emergent ventral hernia repair (VHR) compared to elective VHR [49]. Although there is little data regarding the repair of ventral, incisional, and parastomal hernias with ascites in the emergency setting, early elective repair should be considered when feasible in order to prevent an acute surgical emergency [39]. In the elective setting, laparoscopic VHR compared to open VHR has lower wound-related complications and shorter hospital length of stay [49]. However, with the presence of ascites, laparoscopic VHR has been associated with significantly higher mortality, systemic complications, and unplanned return to the operating room [49].

Elective inguinal hernia (IH) repair is generally well-tolerated and should be considered if the patients' nutritional status can be optimized and ascites can be controlled [39]. Although superficial wound complications are common, there is no evidence to suggest against use of mesh in emergency inguinal hernia (IH) repair in a non-contaminated field [39].

Cholecystectomy

The incidence of gallstones in cirrhotic patients is 29%, compared to 12% in the non-cirrhotic population [50]. Prior to the advent of laparoscopic surgery, the mortality rate of open cholecystectomy was reported to be as high as 87% [51]. Laparoscopic cholecystectomy has since proven to be safe and led to decreased mortality, overall complications, and length of hospital stay compared to open cholecystectomy in cirrhotic patients [52–55]. For CTP class C, conservative management with antibiotics and percutaneous cholecystostomy tube placement should be considered as an alternative to surgery [56]. In patients with symptomatic cholelithiasis at risk of developing biliary pancreatitis or acute cholecystitis, elective laparoscopic cholecystectomy should be considered.

Gastrointestinal Tract and the Open Abdomen

In the cirrhotic patient, complications of gastroduodenal ulcer disease, including perforation and bleeding, carry mortality rates of 42% and 49% [57]. In the emergency setting, surgical intervention should not be aimed at treatment of peptic ulcer disease but rather focused on control of perforation or bleeding [57]. Resectional treatment should be avoided when possible [57]. If the surgeon is technically facile with complex laparoscopy, a laparoscopic approach for repair of gastric perforation should be used [1]. Percutaneous endoscopic gastrostomy (PEG) is advised against in patients with cirrhosis and ascites [29].

Colorectal surgery in a patient with cirrhosis is associated with a morbidity of 50% and mortality of 25% [58]. In a recent study examining risk of anastomotic leak after colorectal surgery in cirrhosis, the leak rate was found to be 12.5% compared to 2.5% in patients without cirrhosis [58]. Despite the increased risk of anastomotic failure, stoma creation is also not without risk when bowel resection is needed [59]. Although a temporary loop ileostomy may decrease the sequelae of anastomotic leak, the risks of parastomal hernia, bleeding peristomal varices, and complications related to stoma closure should be taken into consideration [58].

Damage control laparotomy with temporary abdominal closure (TAC) is frequently used in patients with hemodynamic instability or with massive intra-abdominal contamination. A recent study showed that cirrhotic patients managed with TAC are susceptible to early acidosis, persistent coagulopathy, large negative pressure wound therapy (NPWT) fluid losses, prolonged vasopressor requirements, multiple organ failure, and early mortality [60]. Use of TAC should be avoided when possible.

Key Points

- Cirrhosis increases morbidity and mortality in patients requiring emergency surgery.
- Preoperative planning relies upon the stage of cirrhosis, timing of surgery, comorbid conditions, and the type of operation.
- To achieve optimal outcomes, surgeons must recognize the disease, defer surgery when appropriate, optimize physiology, and perform a technically excellent operation.
- MELD and CTP scores can be useful in predicting perioperative morbidity and mortality.
- TEG has shown promise in reducing unnecessary empiric blood product transfusion.
- Management of ascites and albumin replacement help prevent surgical complications and hemodynamic side effects of large-volume paracentesis.
- Avoid factors that exacerbate worsening liver failure (hypotension, general anesthesia, hepatotoxins, AKI).
- Early repair of hernias in patients with cirrhosis and ascites is a safe option for select patients and may help prevent increased morbidity and mortality associated with need for emergent repair.
- Consider referral to a high-volume tertiary care facility when appropriate.

References

1. Abba N, Makker J, Abbas H, Balar B. Perioperative care of patients with liver cirrhosis: a review. Health Serv Insights. 2017;10:1178632917691270. https://doi.org/10.1177/1178632917691270. eCollection 2017.

2. Neff HP, Streule GC, Drognitz O, et al. Early mortality and long-term survival after abdominal surgery in patients with liver cirrhosis. Surgery. 2014;155:623–32.

3. Bhangui P, Laurent A, Amathieu R, Azoulay D. Assessment of risk for non-hepatic surgery in cirrhotic patients. J Hepatol. 2012;57:874–84.

4. GBD 2013 Mortality and Causes of Death Collaborators. Global, regional, and national age-sex specific all-cause and cause-specific mortality for 240 causes of death, 1990–2013: a systematic analysis for the Global Burden of Disease Study 2013. Lancet. 2015;385:117–71.

5. Scaglione S, Kliethermes S, Cao G, et al. The epidemiology of cirrhosis in the United States: a population-based study. J Clin Gastroenterol. 2015;49:690–6.

6. D'Amico G, Garcia-Tsao G, Pagliaro L. Natural history and prognostic indicators of survival in cirrhosis: a systematic review of 118 studies. J Hepatol. 2006;44:217–31.

7. Millwala F, Nguyen GC, Thuluvath PJ. Outcomes of patients with cirrhosis undergoing non-hepatic surgery: risk assessment and management. World J Gastroenterol. 2007;13:4056–63.

8. Garrison RN, Cryer HM, Howard DA, Polk HC Jr. Clarification of risk factors for abdominal operations in patients with hepatic cirrhosis. Ann Surg. 1984;199:648–55.

9. Mansour A, Watson W, Shayani V, Pickleman J. Abdominal operations in patients with cirrhosis: still a major surgical challenge. Surgery. 1997;122:730–5. discussion 735–6.

10. Telem DA, Schiano T, Goldstone R, et al. Factors that predict outcome of abdominal operations in patients with advanced cirrhosis. Clin Gastroenterol Hepatol. 2010;8:451–7. quiz e458.

11. Befeler AS, Palmer DE, Homan M, Longo W, Solomon H, Di Bisceglie AM. The safety of intra-abdominal surgery in patients with cirrhosis: model for end-stage liver disease score is superior to Child-Turcotte-Pugh classification in predicting outcome. Arch Surg. 2005;140:650–4. discussion 655.

12. Farnsworth N, Fagan SP, Berger DH, Awad SS. Child-Turcotte-Pugh versus MELD score as a predictor of outcome after elective and emergent surgery in cirrhotic patients. Am J Surg. 2004;188(5):580–3.

13. Nee H, Mariaskin D, Spangenberg HC, Hopt UT, Makowiec F. Perioperative mortality after non-hepatic general surgery in patients with liver cirrhosis: an analysis of 138 operations in the 2000s using Child and MELD scores. J Gastrointest Surg. 2011;15:1–11.

14. Child CG, Turcotte JG. The liver and portal hypertension. In: Child CG, editor. Surgery and portal hypertension. Philadelphia: Saunders; 1964.

15. Pugh RN, Murray-Lyon IM, Dawson JL, Pietroni MC, Williams R. Transection of the oesophagus for bleeding oesophageal varices. Br J Surg. 1973;60:646–9.

16. Malinchoc M, Kamath PS, Gordon FD, et al. A model to predict poor survival in patients undergoing transjugular intrahepatic portosystemic shunts. Hepatology. 2000;31:864–71.

17. Kamath PS, Kim WR. Advanced liver disease study G. The model for end-stage liver disease (MELD). Hepatology. 2007;45:797–805.

18. Northup PG, Wanamaker RC, Lee VD, Adams RB, Berg CL. Model for End-Stage Liver Disease (MELD) predicts nontransplant surgical mortality in patients with cirrhosis. Ann Surg. 2005;242(2):244–51.

19. Alberino F, Gatta A, Amodio P, et al. Nutrition and survival in patients with liver cirrhosis. Nutrition. 2001;17:445–50.

20. Gibbs J, Cull W, Henderson W, Daley J, Hur K, Khuri SF. Preoperative serum albumin level as a predictor of operative mortality and morbidity: results from the National VA Surgical Risk Study. Arch Surg. 1999;134:36–42.

21. Jie B, Jiang ZM, Nolan MT, Zhu SN, Yu K, Kondrup J. Impact of preoperative nutritional support on clinical outcome in abdominal surgical patients at nutritional risk. Nutrition. 2012;28:1022–7.

22. Tsiaousi ET, Hatzitolios AI, Trygonis SK, Savopoulos CG. Malnutrition in end stage liver disease: recommendations and nutritional support. J Gastroenterol Hepatol. 2008;23:527–33.

23. Wiklund RA. Preoperative preparation of patients with advanced liver disease. Crit Care Med. 2004;32:S106–15.

24. Kujovich JL. Coagulopathy in liver disease: a balancing act. Hematology Am Soc Hematol Educ Program. 2015;2015:243–9.

25. Holland LL, Brooks JP. Toward rational fresh frozen plasma transfusion: the effect of plasma transfusion on coagulation test results. Am J Clin Pathol. 2006;126:133–9.

26. De Pietri L, Bianchini M, Montalti R, et al. Thromboelastography-guided blood product use before invasive procedures in cirrhosis with severe coagulopathy: a randomized, controlled trial. Hepatology. 2016;63:566–73.

27. Moore KP, Aithal GP. Guidelines on the management of ascites in cirrhosis. Gut. 2006;55(Suppl VI):vi1–vi12.

28. Piano S, Tonon M, Angeli P. Management of ascites and hepatorenal syndrome. Hepatol Int. 2018;12(Suppl 1):122–34.

29. Runyon BA, AASLD. Introduction to the revised American Association for the Study of Liver Diseases Practice Guideline management of adult patients with ascites due to cirrhosis 2012. Hepatology. 2013;57:1651–3.

30. Finfer S, Bellomo R, Boyce N, French J, Myburgh J, Norton R. A comparison of albumin and saline for fluid resuscitation in the intensive care unit. N Engl J Med. 2004;350:2247–56.

31. Nadim MK, Durand F, Kellum JA. Management of the critically ill patient with cirrhosis: a multidisciplinary perspective. J Hepatol. 2016;64:717–35.

32. Fortube B, Cardenas A. Ascites, refractory ascites and hyponatremia in cirrhosis. Gastroenterol Rep. 2017;5(2):104–12.

33. Sinha VK, Ko B. Hyponatremia in cirrhosis-pathogenesis, treatment, and prognostic significance. Adv Chronic Kidney Dis. 2015;22(5):361–7.

34. Savio J, Thiluvath PJ. Hyponatremia in cirrhosis: pathophysiology and management. World J Gastroenterol. 2015;21(11):3197–205.

35. Abu Hossain S, Chaudhry FA, Zahedi K, Siddiqui F, Amlal H. Cellular and molecular basis of increased ammoniagenesis in potassium deprivation. Am J Physiol Renal Physiol. 2011;301:F969–78.

36. Cabrera L, Tandon P, Abraldes JG. An update on the management of acute esophageal variceal bleeding. Gastroenterol Hepatol. 2017;40(1):34–40.

37. Vaja R, McNicol L, Sisley I. Anaesthesia for patients with liver disease. Contin Educ Anaesth Crit Care Pain. 2010;10:15–9.

38. Imani F, Motavaf M, Safari S, Alavian SM. The therapeutic use of analgesics in patients with liver cirrhosis: a literature review and evidence-based recommendations. Hepat Mon. 2014;14:e23539.

39. Odom SR, Gupta A, Talmor D, et al. Emergency hernia repair in cirrhotic patients with ascites. J Trauma Acute Care Surg. 2013;75:404–9.

40. Marsman HA, Heisterkamp J, Halm JA, Tilanus HW, Metselaar HJ, Kazemier G. Management in patients with liver cirrhosis and an umbilical hernia. Surgery. 2007;142:372–5.

41. Chatzizacharias NA, Bradley JA, Harper S, et al. Successful surgical management of ruptured umbilical hernias in cirrhotic patients. World J Gastroenterol. 2015;21:3109–13.

42. Violi F, Basili S, Raparelli V, Chowdary P, Gatt A, Burroughs AK. Patients with liver cirrhosis suffer from primary haemostatic defects? Fact or fiction? J Hepatol. 2011;55:1415–27.

43. Carbonell AM, Wolfe LG, DeMaria EJ. Poor outcomes in cirrhosis-associated hernia repair: a nationwide cohort study of 32,033 patients. Hernia. 2005;9:353–7.

44. Choi SB, Hong KD, Lee JS, Han HJ, Kim WB, Song TJ, Suh SO, Kim YC, Choi SY. Management of umbilical hernia complicated with liver cirrhosis: an advocate of early and elective herniorrhaphy. Dig Liver Dis. 2011;43:991–5.

45. Hansen JB, Thulstrup AM, Vilstup H, Sorensen HT. Danish nationwide cohort study of postoperative death in patients with liver cirrhosis undergoing hernia repair. Br J Surg. 2002;89:805–6.

46. Gray SH, Vick CC, Graham LA, Finan KR, Neumayer LA, Hawn MT. Umbilical herniorrhaphy in cirrhosis: improved outcomes with elective repair. J Gastrointest Surg. 2008;12:675–81.

47. Cho SW, Bhayani N, Newell P, et al. Umbilical hernia repair in patients with signs of portal hypertension: surgical outcome and predictors of mortality. Arch Surg. 2012;147:864–9.

48. Ammar SA. Management of complicated umbilical hernias in cirrhotic patients using permanent mesh: randomized clinical trial. Hernia. 2010;14:35–8.

49. Juo YY, Skancke M, Holzmacher J, et al. Laparoscopic versus open ventral hernia repair in patients with chronic liver disease. Surg Endosc. 2017;31:769–77.

50. Zhang J, Ye L, Zhang J, et al. MELD scores and Child-Pugh classifications predict outcomes of ERCP in cirrhotic patients with choledocholithiasis: a retrospective cohort study. Medicine. 2015;94(3):e433.

51. Aranha GV, Sontag SJ, Greenlee HB. Cholecystectomy in cirrhotic patients: a formidable operation. Am J Surg. 1982;143:55–60.

52. Cheng Y, Xiong XZ, Wu SJ, Lin YX, Cheng NS. Laparoscopic vs. open cholecystectomy for cirrhotic patients: a systematic review and meta-analysis. Hepato-Gastroenterology. 2012;59:1727–34.

53. de Goede B, Klitsie PJ, Hagen SM, et al. Meta-analysis of laparoscopic versus open cholecystectomy for patients with liver cirrhosis and symptomatic cholecystolithiasis. Br J Surg. 2013;100:209–16.

54. Laurence JM, Tran PD, Richardson AJ, Pleass HC, Lam VW. Laparoscopic or open cholecystectomy in cirrhosis: a systematic review of outcomes and meta-analysis of randomized trials. HPB (Oxford). 2012;14:153–61.

55. Puggioni A, Wong LL. A metaanalysis of laparoscopic cholecystectomy in patients with cirrhosis. J Am Coll Surg. 2003;197:921–6.

56. Curro G, Iapichino G, Melita G, et al. Laparoscopic cholecystectomy in Child-Pugh class C cirrhotic patients. JSLS. 2005;9:311–5.

57. Lehnert T, Herfarth C. Peptic ulcer surgery in patients with liver cirrhosis. Ann Surg. 1993;217(4):338–46.

58. Kaser SA, Hofmann I, Willi N, et al. Liver cirrhosis/severe fibrosis is a risk factor for anastomotic leakage after colorectal surgery. Gastroenterol Res Pract. 2016;2016:1563037. 5 pages.

59. Belghiti J, Desgrandchamps F, Farges O, Fekete F. Herniorrhaphy and concomitant peritoneovenous shunting in cirrhotic patients with umbilical hernia. World J Surg. 1990;14:242–6.

60. Loftus TJ, Jordan JR, Croft CA, et al. Emergent laparotomy and temporary abdominal closure for the cirrhotic patient. J Surg Res. 2017;210:108–14.

Surgical Palliative Care, "Heroic Surgery," and End-of-Life Care

Franchesca Hwang and Anastasia Kunac

Case Vignette

Urgent surgical consultation is requested in the emergency department (ED) at 2:30 a.m. The patient is an 87-year-old female with the following comorbidities: congestive heart failure with ejection fraction of 30% and a recently diagnosed stage IV ovarian cancer. According to the patient's son, she is not undergoing treatment for her ovarian cancer because the patient expressed to her oncologist that she did not want to pursue any intervention that would "make her sick." She resides at home with her son, daughter-in-law, and grandchildren and a 24-hour health aide. She uses a walker for ambulation and rarely leaves her residence. According to her son, in the last week, her oral intake has decreased, and her chronic constipation has worsened. Her only complaint is abdominal pain for the last few days. This evening, she began vomiting profusely at which time the son brought her into the ED. On initial assessment in the ED, she is lying in bed confused and lethargic with her heart rate in 110's and systolic BP in the 90's—her heart rate and blood pressure improve with initiation of intravenous fluids. Her exam reveals a distended abdomen, tender to palpation in all four quadrants. A CT scan has already been performed and shows diffuse peritoneal metastasis with complete obstruction in the proximal jejunum. Now you are going to talk to the son—what treatment will you offer?

The vignette represents a variation of a case that nearly all surgeons have encountered—a very ill patient, possibly even moribund, with a diagnosis that "could" be treated with surgery. The diagnoses may differ: bowel perforation, intestinal ischemia, cholangitis, or gastrointestinal bleeding. Comorbidities that make this high-risk surgery also vary and include heart failure, cancer, advanced cirrhosis, or frailty. No matter what the exact clinical picture, it is cases such as this that leave the surgeon wondering what is best for the patient. There are many potential treatment options for the patient presented above: (1) operate for obstruction despite the high risk for morbidity and mortality, (2) offer only comfort care with adequate pain control, (3) conservative management of obstruction with nasogastric decompression and IV hydration, or (4) recommend a palliative gastrostomy to relieve vomiting. How does one decide among these options? If one of the above options does not achieve the desired outcome, when should the clinician revisit alternate options?

The management decision must consider the patient's preferences. The surgeon first needs to elicit if the patient has had an advance directive and ask if the patient has discussed her wishes with her family previously. Depending on the answers to these inquiries, the surgeon will

F. Hwang · A. Kunac (✉)
Department of Surgery, Rutgers New Jersey Medical School, Newark, NJ, USA
e-mail: kunacan@njms.rutgers.edu

© Springer International Publishing AG, part of Springer Nature 2019
C. V. R. Brown et al. (eds.), *Emergency General Surgery*, https://doi.org/10.1007/978-3-319-96286-3_44

choose among the different care pathways. This chapter will offer tools to help guide these complicated and difficult discussions and subsequent management decisions.

Surgical Palliative Care

The World Health Organization (WHO) defines palliative care as an approach that improves the quality of life of patients and their families facing problems associated with life-threatening illness, through the prevention and relief of suffering by means of early assessment and treatment of physical, psychological, and spiritual pain [1]. Palliative care has been shown to improve symptom management and satisfaction in patients, with overall improvement in the quality of life for patients with serious illness and their caregivers [2, 3]. Its positive effects on patient-centered outcomes also translate into reduction in the intensity of care and overall healthcare costs at the end of life in regions with more palliative care services [4]. The same approach has been shown to be beneficial when caring for patients with surgical diagnoses.

In a systematic review of palliative care in surgical patients, palliative care has been linked to improved quality of communication and symptom management and decreased healthcare resources and cost [5]. In the trauma intensive care unit (ICU) setting, early integration of palliative care approach with goals-of-care (GOC) communications within 72 h of admission led to improved patient and family satisfaction, quality of care, and length of ICU stay without changing the overall mortality [6]. Another study in geriatric trauma patients demonstrated decreased ICU and hospital days in patients who had palliative medicine consultation within 2 days of admission [7]. The earlier the goals of care are established, the less conflict will occur later regarding futile life-prolonging procedures, end-of-life decisions, do-not-resuscitate (DNR) orders, or withholding life-sustaining treatments. These conflicts frequently prolong patients' suffering.

Recognizing the significance of palliative care in surgery, the American College of Surgeons

(ACS) has been advocating it since the late 1990s. The ACS collaborated with the Robert Wood Johnson Foundation to form a surgical palliative care workgroup in 2001, and in 2005, the College issued the Statement of Principles of Palliative Care.

The Palliative Care Task Force later became part of the Division of Education and then evolved into the Committee on Surgical Palliative Care (CSPC). The College continued to endorse the efforts of the CSPC by publishing the "Surgical Palliative Care: A Resident's Guide" in 2009, again demonstrating the value of training surgical residents on palliative care [8].

Optimal surgical palliative care meets the following objectives: (1) to address the surgical issues, (2) to improve quality of life, and most importantly, (3) to meet patients' goals. To meet these objectives, the key step is to consider patients' values and preferences in the context of prognosis. The values important to patients may be different from what surgeons believe to be important. Mortality is undoubtedly a patient-centered outcome as no one wishes for it. Nonetheless, not everyone may consider death the worst outcome. In fact, more than half of older hospitalized patients with serious illnesses reported bowel and bladder incontinence, relying on a breathing tube or feeding tube to live or needing care all the time as health states that would be worse than death [9]. This finding emphasizes the magnitude of finding out patients' values prior to any operative procedures.

Palliative Care in Emergency General Surgery

Palliative care does not necessarily equate to end-of-life care. If we revisit the first two core principles of surgical palliative care as defined by the American College of Surgeons, outlined in Table 44.1, we are reminded that patient autonomy and shared decision-making are core principles in surgical palliative care. Decision-making in emergency general surgery (EGS) poses challenges for both surgeons and the patients and their families. EGS alone is an independent risk factor

Table 44.1 Statement of Principles of Palliative Care developed by the American College of Surgeons Task Force on Surgical Palliative Care and the Committee on Ethics [10]

1. Respect the dignity and autonomy of patients, patients' surrogates, and caregivers
2. Honor the right of the competent patient or surrogate to choose among treatments, including those that may or may not prolong life
3. Communicate effectively and empathically with patients, their families, and caregivers
4. Identify the primary goals of care from the patient's perspective, and address how the surgeon's care can achieve the patient's objectives
5. Strive to alleviate pain and other burdensome physical and nonphysical symptoms
6. Recognize, assess, discuss, and offer access to services for psychological, social, and spiritual issues
7. Provide access to therapeutic support, encompassing the spectrum from life-prolonging treatments through hospice care, when they can realistically be expected to improve the quality of life as perceived by the patient
8. Recognize the physician's responsibility to discourage treatments that are unlikely to achieve the patient's goals, and encourage patients and families to consider hospice care when the prognosis for survival is likely to be less than a half year
9. Arrange for continuity of care by the patient's primary and/or specialist physician, alleviating the sense of abandonment patients may feel when "curative" therapies are no longer useful
10. Maintain a collegial and supportive attitude toward others entrusted with care of the patient

for mortality and major postoperative complications compared to non-emergency general surgery, adjusting for preoperative characteristics and procedure types [11]. This mandates in-depth conversations regarding the risks and potential benefits of surgery. For patients who have pre-existing life-limiting comorbidities, the outcomes are even worse. Over one third of patients with advanced cancer, who underwent emergency abdominal surgery, died in 30 days, and two thirds experienced complications [12]. These findings underline the need for palliative care in this at-risk patient population undergoing emergency general surgery to encourage shared decision-making and goals-of-care discussion perioperatively.

The nature of surgical emergency, however, makes extensive discussion challenging. Yet, the decision to undergo an operation, or not to, is not simply a unidirectional decision from the surgeon that affects the patient. It is rather a shared decision-making process where all parties *together* make decisions about patient care. These decisions should be made after considering the likelihood of many factors such as surviving the operation, developing complications, returning home to a functionally independent lifestyle, or needing assistance to varying degrees with the activities of daily living. In cases such as the case vignette presented, where consideration is given to operating for obstruction in the setting of metastatic cancer, the patient and family must understand that the purpose of the operation is symptom relief and will not cure the malignancy; if the cancer is not being treated, the malignancy will progress whether or not the patient has an operation. Through this process, goals of care are established that are consistent with the patients' wishes. Therefore, having goals-of-care discussion is of the utmost importance when caring for patients with emergency general surgical diagnoses.

Shared Decision-Making

The key to surgical palliative care is grounded in the shared decision-making between the surgeons and the patients and their families. It is different from the informed consent process in which the physician "provides" the patient with the purpose, benefits, and potential risks of an intervention, and the patient "receives" the information and signs the document after understanding it. Shared decision-making is, rather, a process to which both parties are contributing. The physician shares the information about treatment options, prognosis, and expected outcomes, and the patient shares his or her expectations, preferences, and wishes. Both parties *together* then make decisions that best meet the patient's goals.

Determination of Decision-Making Capacity

Shared decision-making implies that both the surgeon and the patient understand the nature of the patient's disease and can engage in a two-way discussion. At times, patients are too ill to participate in these discussions. The principle of autonomy is built on the assumption that the patient can make decisions regarding his or her own care and understands the risks and benefits of the treatment, or no treatment. This capacity is often compromised in the setting of emergency general surgery when the patient may have impaired cognition due to shock or other metabolic derangements.

Alternately, the patient at baseline may have cognitive deficits, such as dementia secondary to advanced age, that would preclude their ability to make appropriate decisions. As the US population is growing older, and people over the age of 65 are projected to represent more than 20% by 2030, the issues of geriatric surgery are relevant to any general surgeon in practice now. Many older adults have surgery, and as many as one third of Medicare beneficiaries undergo inpatient surgery during the last year of life [13]. As surgery in older patients is increasingly prevalent, it has become more critical for surgeons to understand decision-making capacity. All surgeons in practice who operate on adult patients can expect to be faced with geriatric patients with acute surgical emergency.

The following criteria may be useful as a guide to establish a person's decision-making capacity [14] (Table 44.2):

If the patient does not meet all the criteria or has already been deemed incompetent, a surrogate decision-maker must be involved in the discussion about treatment plan. If the patient is competent to make decisions, it is important to remember that the concept of autonomy justifies the patient's right to refuse treatments. This refusal should be honored regardless of the potential benefits of the plan discussed and even if the proposed treatment is lifesaving. A patient may weigh the risks and benefits of a surgical intervention and refuse an operation.

Discussions Regarding Goals of Care

People have different values and naturally have different goals of care. Goals also change depending on the stage of life at which patients face

Table 44.2 Guide to ascertain patient's decision-making capacity

1. Acknowledgment of relevant information	The patient should understand his/her diagnosis and the treatment options.
2. Appreciating one's circumstances	The patient should acknowledge the disease he/she has and understand how it will impact his/her life. He/she should be able to answer what the outcome may be with or without treatment.
3. Logical use of information	The patient should be able to give evidence for his/her decision. Even if the patient comes to a decision against the physician's recommendation, this is acceptable if it was made in a logical fashion.
4. Communication of choices	This is a paramount condition of judging competence. The patient must be able to communicate his/her preference of one choice over another. If he/she says "yes" to every treatment option choice, he/she is not appropriately integrating information. The patient can change his/her mind over time but should be able to provide a meaningful reason for the change.

medical decisions. Goals of care in a young, healthy person will most likely be different from those of an older person with many comorbidities. Nevertheless, a previously healthy, relatively young man who acutely developed bowel perforation and spent numerous days in the ICU with prolonged respiratory failure will now have different sense of what brings him the greatest meaning and value in life. Some potential goals of care are presented in Table 44.3. Although not comprehensive, the table lists relevant goal-concordant treatment option examples encountered in surgery [15].

As listed above, goals of care are not based on a simple dichotomous approach: curative versus comfort care. The perception among many surgeons, regardless of the number of years they have been practicing, is that symptom management and surgery are in opposition to each

Table 44.3 Potential goals of care and examples of goal-concordant treatment options

Cure of disease	Pain relief
Complete resection of cancer	*Hip or knee replacement to relieve chronic arthritic pain*
Avoidance of premature death	Prolongation of life
Evacuation of intracranial hematoma in the setting of severe traumatic brain injury	*Feeding tube placement in patients with severe dysphagia after stroke*
Maintenance/improvement of function	Maintenance of control
Femoral-tibial arterial bypass for claudication symptoms	*Reversal of colostomy months after developing perforated diverticulitis*
Death with dignity	Support for family or loved ones
Symptom management without surgery for malignant perforation in a patient with stage IV colon cancer that has not responded to chemotherapy	*Offering in-home hospice care for a dying patient when the patient's needs exceed family capacity for offering care*

The goals-of-care discussion, as outlined in Table 44.4, is comprehensive and lengthy—it takes 30–60 min to have this serious discussion, and it may have to take place in stages. Even in emergency general surgery, it is important to consider that this decision about whether to operate or not does not always have to be made within moments—often, the patient can be managed non-operatively with close monitoring until a thoughtful decision is reached regarding the next appropriate treatment option.

Following these steps not only helps uncover concerns or questions that patients may have prior to surgery but also ensures that both patients and surgeons are on the same page about expectations. Some patients have misconceptions of surgery as a "cure-all." This may be due in part to commercial advertising or other misleading portrayals in media. For instance, many people believe that bariatric surgery is a cure for obesity or coronary artery bypass surgery for heart disease. If patients' expectations are not realistic, their goals of care are often not feasible. Thus, it is critical to set the common ground for expectations. If operating on a patient with peritonitis

another. Instead, goals of care are usually more fluid and can change over the course of patients' illness. Patients' conditions may improve or worsen. No matter how their condition changes, the ultimate objective remains the same: to maximize their quality of life and preserve their autonomy.

It is, therefore, extremely important to assess patient preferences in goals-of-care (GOC) discussions prior to procedures and postoperatively throughout the recovery process. Any surgical procedure has inherent risks, however common the procedure is. Perioperative morbidity is higher in emergency surgery as compared to elective surgery, and yet most surgeons do not discuss goals of care at all in an emergent setting even if they routinely do so while obtaining consent for elective cases in the office. The following table shows a step-by-step structured template for preoperative GOC discussion applicable to any major surgery whether elective or emergent.

Table 44.4 Template for goals-of-care discussion

Sequence	Rationale
1. Introduction	Identity/role of participants
2. Ask patient to explain his/her disease condition and/or planned surgery in his/her own words	Establish foundation of discussion
	Establish whether patient has decision-making capacity
3. Ask patient if any questions/fears	Provide opportunities to address concerns
4. Describe perioperative care including in the ICU, if expected	Establish range of outcomes
5. Establish healthcare proxy	Begin advance directive, if possible
6. Discuss goals of care	Establish patient's expectations/hopes
7. Discuss/document advance directive	Preferences regarding life support
8. New questions/concerns	Provide emotional support
	Bring session to a close

secondary to a perforated malignancy, surgeons must clearly explain that the surgery may help to control sepsis but will not cure the cancer.

Once the surgeon has clearly laid out the disease condition and potential option of surgical treatment, asking the patient to explain the planned surgery in his or her own words helps to confirm understanding. If the patient cannot explain the surgery just described, he or she may not have decision-making capacity and perhaps should not be the person to give consent. If he or she can understand risks and benefits of the proposed procedure, this is a great opportunity to address questions and speak about fears. As outlined above, in emergency general surgery, there are frequently undesirable outcomes—stroke, myocardial infarction, profound sepsis, multiorgan failure, prolonged ICU stays, and the need for long-term mechanical support are all possibilities and are difficult to discuss.

A useful transition into the next part of the discussion is to talk about the "what ifs," as in "what if things don't go well?" The first "what if" to establish is who to contact if the patient is unable to speak for him- or herself—name a healthcare proxy. This person is frequently not the next of kin. Sometimes patients fear that their spouse would be too emotional to "make the right decision" and instead ask that an adult child or a sibling be named proxy. Sometimes a patient has several adult children and believes that one is more suited than the others in assisting with these decisions. Many of us as healthcare professionals might be named proxy for our parents, siblings, and adult children by virtue of our training. Asking patients to assign their own healthcare proxy allows them to disclose who they think is best suited to honor their wishes regarding medical treatment decisions.

It is important to ensure that this identification of healthcare proxy is documented in the medical record to prevent any medicolegal issues. If possible, this person should be notified that he or she has been named to this role and should be invited to participate in the remainder of the preoperative discussion, even in the emergency setting. Family conflicts, in the setting of no assigned healthcare proxy, prolong decision-making processes related

to end-of-life care, leading to prolonged suffering or suboptimal care for patients. Surrogates who have not participated in preoperative discussions with the patient are often influenced by their own needs and preferences which may be at odds with patient-centered preferences [16]. If the patient is too ill to name a proxy, the preoperative discussion is with the next of kin. Under these circumstances, it is important to remind the surrogate decision-makers that they are to consider what the patient would have wanted for him- or herself.

Once a healthcare proxy has been identified and invited to join the conversation, surgeons need to then paint the picture of what the recovery process is like. This should include in-hospital postoperative care and expectations beyond the hospital after the patients are discharged. When the prognosis is not clear, the most helpful approach to establish a range of outcomes is by describing the "best-case/worst-case" scenarios. This range of outcomes should be personalized to individual patients, rather than simply reporting numbers such as the expected in-hospital or 30-day mortality [17]. For example, if we revisit the case vignette above, and if the patient's son is favoring an operative intervention for her malignant obstruction, the best-case scenario may be a relatively straightforward operation to relieve obstruction secondary to a simple adhesive band, and she returns home to her previous quality of life within a few days postoperatively. The worst-case scenario may be that the operation could not be carried out successfully due to diffuse peritoneal metastases and a "frozen abdomen," and the patient has prolonged ventilator-dependent respiratory failure postoperatively and a large painful laparotomy wound that is chronically draining malignant ascites. By presenting these potential outcomes, the surgeons help patients and their families understand the implications of the proposed treatment plans.

Additionally, using objective prognostic tools may be valuable in certain situations. The ACS National Surgical Quality Improvement Program (NSQIP) Surgical Risk Calculator, which is readily available online, offers estimated risks of postoperative complications based on specific patient characteristics along with the type of planned procedure and whether it is an emergency case. For geriatric patients specifically, age or comorbidities alone do not predict outcomes; frailty has been shown to independently predict postoperative complications, length of stay, and discharge to facilities in older surgical patients [18]. Utilizing these adjunctive tools for prognostication may provide surgeons and patients a common ground to establish expected outcomes for shared decision-making.

Once both parties agree regarding expectations, the goals-of-care conversation continues with gathering more information regarding their preferences for life support and advance directives. Some patients may opt out of surgery once they find out about the expected outcomes. Others may elect to have surgery but will ask to enact a do-not-resuscitate order and will indicate that if they do not recover well, they would not want to be kept alive on mechanical support. Hence, it is essential to have a GOC discussion preoperatively, even in the emergency setting, to ensure that patients receive the treatments that are aligned with their preferences postoperatively. The discussion about advance directives is difficult—patients have a hard time considering their own mortality, and it is especially difficult when faced with a surgical emergency. Patients may simply state that they are comfortable with a named proxy making end-of-life decisions on their behalf. No matter what decisions are made, this is a good time to provide assurances that the patient will be well cared for throughout their hospitalization and that these concepts can be revisited at any time. Closing the GOC discussion by determining if the patient or surrogate has any new questions, concerns, or worries may shed additional light on the patient's wishes, goals, and even advance directives; practically speaking, addressing new concerns helps ease the patient into the next step of his or her care.

"Heroic Surgery": To Intervene, or Not to Intervene?

The term "heroic" refers to a behavior that is excessively bold. There is no better example of "heroic surgery" than the controversial repair of

aortic dissection in Dr. Michael Ellis DeBakey. Dr. DeBakey was the pioneer in cardiac surgery after whom the standard classification system of aortic dissection was named. At the age of 97, on December 31, 2005, he self-diagnosed acute aortic dissection after a sudden chest pain. It took him 3 days to undergo CT scan which showed type II aortic dissection, and yet he refused to be admitted to the hospital until almost a month after his first symptoms. His dissection had worsened by this time, and he still refused surgery repeatedly saying, "I prefer to die." By the time his clinical condition deteriorated, he lost consciousness in early February. The hospital ethics committee was convened late at night as Dr. DeBakey had previously signed an advance directive indicating that a do-not-resuscitate order should be in effect, and the anesthesiologist refused to put him to sleep. This meeting lasted about an hour until Mrs. DeBakey charged in and demanded surgery to be done immediately. Subsequently, Dr. DeBakey was taken to the operating room for a 7-hour-long surgery. He became the oldest patient to survive this surgery, but not without its consequences. He endured a long, painful, and difficult recovery with numerous complications: ventilator-dependent respiratory failure for 6 weeks, tracheostomy, dialysis, parenteral feedings, and multiple episodes of infection. He was later readmitted for another 4 months. The hospital bill for his care was estimated to be well over a million dollars. A year after the surgery, he could walk but was mostly limited to a motorized wheelchair. He ultimately died of an unspecified cause in 2008, 2 months before his 100th birthday.

This story of Dr. DeBakey generates many questions about the decision-making process—surgery was carried out with a lack of respect for his wishes and rights. He survived the surgery and eventually recovered, albeit painfully. Nonetheless, his wish not to undergo surgery was not honored, and the stakeholders, his wife and his surgeons, chose to operate based on their own preferences. The principle of patient autonomy was completely disregarded in his case. This brings back the question: "To intervene, or not to intervene?" The answer always lies in the patient's wishes. This anecdote highlights why the preoperative discussion is so very important.

Futility

The concept of futility, like the concepts of beneficence and non-maleficence, was recognized as early as the time of Hippocrates when he himself suggested to "refuse to treat those who are overmastered by their disease, realizing that in such cases medicine is powerless." Physicians should serve in a role to preserve the processes of life but should not look to prolong death. There are many cases in which death is inevitable, and a surgical incision could inflict more pain and more suffering without saving the patient's life.

In the modern time when medical care advances are continuously made, the natural response to a critically ill patient with surgical diagnoses is to "do something." Pursuing heroic measures when they are most likely futile is ill-advised. The term *medical futility* carries both technical and ethical weights. It is defined as "a clinical action serving no useful purpose in attaining a specified goal for a given patient." [19] Hence, futility is defined by the patients' goal whether it is survival, neurological recovery, or returning to independent lifestyle.

The "Grey Zone"

Many surgeons are comfortable with a complex consent process in emergency general surgery and with respecting patient autonomy. Still others pride themselves on not offering or rendering futile care. There are clinical situations where it is very difficult to determine if an operative intervention is futile or not—we will call this the "grey zone." Surgeons should consider a time-limited trial in complicated cases such as this. In the "grey zone," some patients unexpectedly do extraordinarily well, while others linger in the intensive care unit for months before dying. It is important to remember that goals of care can be revisited at any time. A surgeon may decide to pursue "heroic measures" at the direction of a

patient, or by the persuasion of a surrogate decision-maker, or because the surgeon really did not understand the breadth of disease. When this happens, the outcome may be undesirable and not consistent with a quality of life that would have been acceptable to the patient. Under these circumstances, it is crucial that the physician revisits GOC and considers altering the course of treatment accordingly.

End-of-Life Care

Even after we as surgeons determine that further aggressive interventions, such as surgery, would not promote patients' quality of life, our role does not simply end there. Patients who are nearing the end of life with surgical diagnoses still benefit from hospice care, and surgeons need to take the initiative to help patients and their families during this process. For instance, the woman in the case vignette is most likely eligible for hospice services either at her home or in a facility. Generally, to be eligible for hospice services, she must be certified by a physician as terminally ill with a prognosis of 6 months or less. It is still very important to be reminded that palliative care can be offered to patients at any stage of illness, whether terminal or not.

For surgical patients who are in their last days of life, it is essential for surgeons to first recognize that death is imminent and reassess the patients' goals of care to ensure they are met. Most experienced surgeons are familiar with the signs and symptoms of dying patients, as well as symptom management, such as pain. Yet, the more difficult and time-consuming aspect of end-of-life care is providing the psychological support to the family during this process; this can be achieved by being available for multiple goals-of-care discussions and ensuring that both patients and families understand the treatment plans. When the time comes to discuss withdrawal of life-sustaining treatments in the intensive care unit, it is critical to have GOC discussions as families often become frustrated if they feel that suffering is prolonged. It is often helpful to involve the patient's primary nurse, social worker, and counselors for family support/bereavement, if available, during these meetings to facilitate the discussion. Issues that need to be addressed during these meetings are withdrawal or withholding of ventilator support, artificial hydration and feeding, blood products, and vasopressive/inotropic agents. Detailed documentation of the decisions and a do-not-resuscitate (DNR) order must be written in the medical record, and thorough discussion with the staff caring for the patient regarding the plan must be carried out. If available, bereavement support from religious leaders, counselors, or social workers should be offered to the family.

New Paradigm

It is difficult for surgeons to recommend *no surgery* to patients and their families. Frequently, having a conversation about operative or non-operative options with patients and families is more time-consuming and painstaking than simply obtaining the signed surgical consent. Furthermore, surgeons rarely are reimbursed, or almost always underpaid, for the time spent on GOC discussions, while their time will certainly be compensated much more for operating. Consequently, surgeons often turn to the traditional paradigm of "patriarchal" approach to make decisions on what they believe to be the best on behalf of the patients, instead of asking for patients' values and preferences.

Times are changing. Recently, at the 76th Annual Meeting of American Association for the Surgery of Trauma (AAST) and Clinical Congress of Acute Care Surgery, Dr. Ronald Maier presented the Fitts Lecture named "Patients are First," calling to incorporate palliative care in trauma, emergency general surgery, and surgical critical care (Fig. 44.1). He emphasized that the surgeons' traditional practice using the Golden Rule "Do unto others as you would have them do unto you" reflects only surgeons' perspective and as such does not necessarily lead to decision-making that is aligned with the patients' wishes. He then pro-

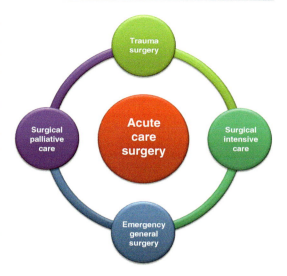

Fig. 44.1 Service components provided by acute care surgeons [20]

posed a new paradigm of the Platinum Rule: "Treat the patients the way *they* want to be treated." This paradigm brings the focus onto the patients and their *autonomy* as this is one of the central principles in medical ethics and acute care surgery.

Conclusion

Caring for patients in emergency general surgical setting is challenging and requires not only operative skills but excellent communication skills. Honoring patient autonomy is of the foremost importance in surgical palliative care and is now also considered preeminent in acute care surgery. As such, surgeons caring for ill patients and considering emergency surgical procedures must assess patients' goals and preferences through structured goals-of-care discussions with patients and/or surrogate decision-makers. Together, via a process of shared decision-making, clinicians along with patients and families will develop treatment plans that are concordant with patient goals. Time spent in developing these treatment plans leads to improved patient and family satisfaction, decreased healthcare costs, and less patient suffering.

References

1. World Health Organization (WHO). WHO definition of palliative care. [Cited 11 Nov 2017]. 2015. Available at: http://www.who.int/cancer/palliative/definition/en/
2. Cauley CE, Panizales MT, Reznor G, Haynes AB, Havens JM, Kelley E, Mosenthal AC, Cooper Z. Outcomes after emergency surgery in patients with advanced cancer: opportunities to reduce complications and improve palliative care. J Trauma Acute Care Surg. 2015;79(3):399–406.
3. Gade G, Venohr I, Conner D, McGrady K, Beane J, Richardson RH, et al. Impact of an inpatient palliative care team: a randomized control trial. J Palliat Med. 2008;11:180–90.
4. Teno JM, Mor V, Ward N, Roy J, Clarridge B, Wennberg JE, Fisher ES. Bereaved family member perceptions of quality of end-of-life care in U.S. regions with high and low usage of intensive care unit care. J Am Geriatr Soc. 2005;53:1905–11.
5. Lilley EJ, Khan KT, Johnston FM, Berlin A, Bader AM, Mosenthal AC, Cooper Z. Palliative care interventions for surgical patients: a systematic review. JAMA Surg. 2016;151:172–83.
6. Mosenthal AC, Murphy PA, Barker LK, Lavery R, Retano A, Livingston DH. Changing the culture around end-of-life care in the trauma intensive care unit. J Trauma. 2008;64:1587–93.
7. Kupensky D, Hileman BM, Emerick ES, Chance EA. Palliative medicine consultation reduces length of stay, improves symptom management, and clarifies advance directives in the geriatric trauma population. J Trauma Nurs. 2015;22(5):261–5.
8. Dunn GP, Martensen R, Weissman D, editors. Surgical palliative care: a resident's guide. Chicago: American College of Surgeons, Cunniff-Dixon Foundation; 2009.
9. Rubin EB, Buehler AE, Halpern SD. States worse than death among hospitalized patients with serious illnesses. JAMA Intern Med. 2016;176:1557–9.
10. Task Force on Surgical Palliative Care: Committee on Ethics. Statement of principles of palliative care. Bull Am Coll Surg. 2005;90:34–5.
11. Havens JM, Peetz AB, Do WS, Cooper Z, Kelly E, Askari R, Reznor G, Salim A. The excess morbidity and mortality of emergency general surgery. J Trauma Acute Care Surg. 2015;78(2):306–11.
12. Cauley CE, Panizales MT, Reznor G, Haynes AB, Havens JM, Kelley E, Mosenthal AC, Cooper Z. Outcomes after emergency abdominal surgery in patients with advanced cancer: opportunities to reduce complications and improve palliative care. J Trauma Acute Care Surg. 2015;79(3):399–406.
13. Kwok AC, Semel ME, Lipsitz SR, Bader AM, Barnato AE, Gawande AA. The intensity and variation of surgical care at the end of life: a retrospective cohort study. Lancet. 2011;378:1408–13.
14. University of Illinois at Chicago College of Medicine. Ethics in clerkships; surrogate decision making. [cited 20 Nov 2017]. Available at: http://www.uic.edu/depts/mcam/ethics/surrogate.htm.
15. Stone MJ. Goals of care at end of life. BUMC Proc. 2001;14:134–7.
16. Fritsch J, Petronio S, Helft PR, Torke AM. Making decisions for hospitalized older patients: ethical factors considered family surrogates. J Clin Ethics. 2013;24(2):125–34.
17. Kruser JM, Nabozny MJ, Steffens NM, Brasel KJ, Campbell TC, Gaines ME, Schwarze ML. "Best case/worst case": qualitative evaluation of a novel communication tool for difficult in-the-moment surgical decisions. J Am Geriatr Soc. 2015;63:1805–11.
18. Makary MA, Segev DL, Pronovost PJ, Syin D, Bandeen-Roche K, Patel P, et al. Frailty as a predictor for surgical outcomes in older patients. J Am Coll Surg. 2010;210:901–8.
19. Kasman DL. When is medical treatment futile? J Gen Intern Med. 2004;19:1053–6.
20. O'Connell K, Maier R. Palliative care in the trauma ICU. Curr Opin Crit Care. 2016;22(6):584–90.

Index

Printed by Printforce, the Netherlands

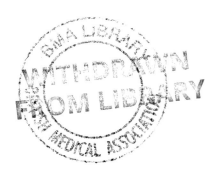